A Quick Guide to Pediatric Retina

Wei-Chi Wu • Wai-Ching Lam
Editors

A Quick Guide to Pediatric Retina

Springer

Editors
Wei-Chi Wu
Department of Ophthalmology
Chang Gung Memorial Hospital
Linkou, Taoyuan
Taiwan

Wai-Ching Lam
Department of Ophthalmology
University of Hong Kong
Hong Kong
China

Department of Ophthalmology and
Vision Science
Hospital for Sick Children
Toronto
Canada

ISBN 978-981-15-6551-9 ISBN 978-981-15-6552-6 (eBook)
https://doi.org/10.1007/978-981-15-6552-6

This Springer imprint is published by the registered company Springer Nature Singapore Pte Ltd.
The registered company address is: 152 Beach Road, #21-01/04 Gateway East, Singapore 189721, Singapore

Preface

This textbook on pediatric retina is our effort to provide an overview of the state-of the-art management for pediatric retina patients. We hope that it is both practical and easy to understand. In this 33 chapters, grouped into two major sections, we tried to cover the essence in the understanding, diagnosis, and management of pediatric retina diseases. We hope this book will be a handy guide for the ophthalmic surgeons at all levels, from the novice, the occasional caregiver for the pediatric retina patients, to the expert leaders in this field.

Our aim is not only to cover the medical aspects but also to explore the surgical advances of these diseases, as well as not only just the clinical presentations but also the basic theory and hypotheses of the diseases, such as understanding of the foveal development.

Pediatric retina is a not only a challenging field but also a lonely one. It is a specialty that has received little attention in the past, but has been gaining traction recently. However, we all know how important this field is, because it affects the vision of newborns and growing children. As physicians, we also know how time-consuming and difficult it can be to deal with a child patient.

Recognizing the cliché "kids are not small adults," the anatomy, pathophysiology, and management philosophy in kids are very different from those in adults. In addition, their visual system is still developing. Therefore, while handling these cases especially during surgery, the surgical settings, the instruments used, and the surgical goals are very dissimilar from those of adults. Without such knowledge, a doctor can actually do far more harm than good for this unique population of pediatric patients.

In the past, there were very few people focusing on work related to this topic. Most of us work "part-time" in this field, thinking of it as a burden and praying that each case is the last. There were very few surgical instruments available for these small children. There are barely any dedicated textbooks available. Relevant topics at conferences were also scant. As a result, the surgical outcomes have been unsatisfactory, due to a lack of dedicated doctors, proper instruments, proper training, and information. But gradually, with the efforts of pioneers such as Dr. Mary Elizabeth Hartnett on the pathophysiology of ROP using animal models [1–3], Dr. Michael Trese in the vitrectomy for Stage 4 and 5 ROP [4–6], Dr. William V Good in the work of early treatment of ROP [7, 8], and Dr. HA Mintz-Hittner on "Bevacizumab Eliminates the Angiogenic Threat" (BEAT ROP) [9], we have seen much improved understanding and outcomes in the recent management of ROP patients. Young doctors may feel encouraged by the improved outcomes of the patients. Access to knowledge and information about pediatric retina has made significant strides; there are an increasing number of panels and symposia related to pediatric retina at the major international conferences. The industry has also started to pay more attention to this field. For instance, the launching of vitrectomies for the pediatric population (e.g., 25 + Short, Alcon), specifically designed for tiny eyes with thick vitreous and a thin sclera, is making ROP surgery safer.

We would like to express our sincere appreciation for the huge efforts from these world-renowned experts in contributing to this special issue. We are extremely lucky to know these scholars, great teachers, and close friends. We feel like standing on the shoulder of many giants so we could see much further and learn so much faster with their help. Dr. Lam and I also owe a great debt of gratitude to the professional team from Springer, especially the project coordinator, Miss Kripa Guruprasad. Without their professional assistance, it would be impossible to achieve this remarkable outcome.

There are not many reference textbooks on pediatric retina. We hope this will be the one that people love to read and reference. For the young ophthalmologists or those new in this field, we hope they could get a good picture of this special subspecialty with the help of these contributing authors. If our readers could pick up some useful points for their practice in pediatric retina, it will be our joy and honor to see the changes this book has brought about. Finally, we hope to see more and more devoted young doctors get inspired to "fall in love" with this field and act as an invigorating force to propel this specialty into a better future in the care of the children.

Linkou, Taoyuan, Taiwan — Wei-Chi Wu
Hong Kong, China — Wai-Ching Lam
Toronto, Canada

References

1. Hartnett ME. The effects of oxygen stresses on the development of features of severe retinopathy of prematurity: knowledge from the 50/10 OIR model. Doc Ophthalmol. 2010;120(1):25–39.
2. Hartnett ME, et al. Neutralizing VEGF decreases tortuosity and alters endothelial cell division orientation in arterioles and veins in a rat model of ROP: relevance to plus disease. Invest Ophthalmol Vis Sci. 2008;49(7):3107–14.
3. Hartnett ME, Penn JS. Mechanisms and management of retinopathy of prematurity. N Engl J Med. 2012;367(26):2515–26.
4. Capone A Jr, Trese MT. Take good care of my baby: evolving standards of care for retinopathy of prematurity. Ophthalmology. 2002;109(5):831–3.
5. Trese MT. Visual results and prognostic factors for vision following surgery for stage V retinopathy of prematurity. Ophthalmology. 1986;93(5):574–9.
6. Trese MT. Two-hand dissection technique during closed vitrectomy for retinopathy of prematurity. Am J Ophthalmol. 1986;101(2):251–2.
7. Good WV, G. Early Treatment for Retinopathy of Prematurity Cooperative. Final results of the Early Treatment for Retinopathy of Prematurity (ETROP) randomized trial. Trans Am Ophthalmol Soc. 2004;102:233–48; discussion 248–50.
8. Good WV, Hardy RJ. The multicenter study of Early Treatment for Retinopathy of Prematurity (ETROP). Ophthalmology. 2001;108(6):1013–4.
9. Mintz-Hittner HA, et al. Efficacy of intravitreal bevacizumab for stage 3+ retinopathy of prematurity. N Engl J Med. 2011;364(7):603–15.

Acknowledgments

When I was a resident in ophthalmology, I could never dream of the career path I had for the next two decades: to focus on the research in pediatric retina. More often, I pictured myself to be a wealthy local medical doctor practicing an easy ophthalmic clinic. At that time, when I had to see the ROP patients in the NICU, I always felt this was a job that is not very pleasant, even painful because nobody could give me good guidance. I was like being thrown to the sea before learning how to swim. I was panicking because of the lack of support and proper guidance. Later, I was lucky to perform a couple of cases of laser photocoagulation in the NICU with a senior doctor. I felt happy to see the very positive effect after laser treatment for the patients. Then I was "assigned" to become a doctor specialized in this field by my retina section chief, Prof. Chi-Chun Lai, at that time. That have dramatically changed my life. That was a turning point for me because I have never seen any surgery for ROP associated with retinal detachment, including vitrectomy or scleral buckling. How could I start from ground zero?

I know I could not learn this knowledge by myself. I had to find a great teacher to guide me. I have heard of Dr. Michael Trese, who started vitrectomy for these premature babies with severe ROP, a giant in this field. But I did not have any connection nor my colleagues. How could I approach him?

I handed in my CV to Dr. Trese at an ARVO meeting after a pediatric retina session. I tried to chat with him about my admiration for him and expressed my hope to learn from him. But then I did not hear back from him for a couple of months. During those time, I was thinking, perhaps they did not like me and I might have to find somewhere else. One day, I got an email from Dr. Kimberly Drenser, saying they had a research fellow spot for me and asked if I could take it? I was exuberant in saying yes! Thank God! Later, I realized that it was Prof. Lai who contacted Prof. Stanley Chang, the teacher of Prof. Lai, who had helped to reach out to Dr. Trese to land the position. I owed Prof. Lai and Chang for their generous support.

At Associated Retinal Consultants (ARC), I was extremely lucky to learn from Dr. Michael Trese, Dr. Antonio Capone, and Dr. Kimberly Drenser. Please forgive my subjectivity, I think they are the best teachers in pediatric retina you could think of on this planet. Besides, you could also learn the best adult retina management from Dr. George Williams, MD. I really felt I could reach the sky because I was standing on the shoulder of these giants! Thanks so much for my teachers' teaching.

So, with their help and introduction, I was able to meet these world-class experts in this field. Most of them are the contributing authors of this book. I am extremely lucky to work with them and learn from their knowledge. From my close observation, the doctors who are interested in pediatric retina are all special people with a kind heart and mind.

Finally, I would like to thank my families for their unwavering support. My parents, my wife, and my son are my pillars. It is a bit selfish to say: with their support, I have the luxury to do a lot of projects, including this one, without needing to worry about the things at home. I am deeply indebted to them.

—Wei-Chi Wu

It was a couple of years ago, during one of the international meetings, I met up with Dr Wei-Chi Wu. I believe we were presenting at one of the pediatric retina sessions. He was all excited to share the news that Springer has approached him to prepare a book on pediatric retina. He asked me to join him to do that together. I agreed on the spot without any hesitation. We then embarked on this wonderful journey together. This has been a journey of learning and excitements. His tireless effort to follow up with each and every author and his unwavering determination have made this project from a dream to reality. I am so thankful to have this opportunity to work with Wei-Chi.

I also want to thank Springer Nature and especially the projector coordinator Ms. Kripa Guruprasad for their support and guidance.

Of course, we are not only grateful but very much in debt to all the contributing authors for sharing their passion of knowledge, insights, expertise, and their personal collection of great illustrative pictures....

My children, Dawn and Alexander, are my inspiration for working on this book. I am so fortunate to have two healthy children, who constantly remind me the importance of what we do toward the well-being of our pediatric patients and their parents.

Finally, I want to thank my wife who is my soulmate and support. She is always there by my side supporting my every decision whether sensible or not. She has made everything possible and worthwhile.

—Wai-Ching Lam

Contents

Part I

ROP

The Pathophysiology of Retinopathy of Prematurity

1

M. Elizabeth Hartnett

Abstract

The pathophysiology of retinopathy of prematurity (ROP) is evolving as advances in prenatal care allow extremely premature infants to survive. In addition, throughout the world, there is variability in the presentations of ROP. In regions that lack resources to support prenatal and perinatal care, ROP develops in infants of older gestational ages and larger birth weights and has potentially different pathophysiologic factors. This chapter will review the pathophysiology of ROP and factors involved in the presentation of ROP based on what is known through clinical studies and from experimental studies using animal models of oxygen-induced retinopathy (OIR), which are critical to study molecular mechanisms and cell–cell interactions. Although the main areas involve clinical study, it is impossible to discuss pathophysiology without including evidence from the most representative animal models of oxygen-induced retinopathy (OIR) and other models adapted to study maternal–fetal interactions. Understanding the role of vascular endothelial growth factor (VEGF) in the physiology of retinal and vascular development and survival and the pathology in stage 3 and plus disease of ROP is important in discussing pathophysiology. Thoughts regarding areas of future study will be briefly described.

The work in the chapter was supported by the National Institutes of Health/National Eye Institute as grant support to MEH (PI): R01 EY015130, R01 EY017011, T35EY026511, and R13EY029900, by an Unrestricted Grant from Research to Prevent Blindness (to the Department of Ophthalmology & Visual Sciences) and by the National Eye Institute Vision Core Grant EY014800.

M. E. Hartnett (✉)
Calvin S. and JeNeal N. Hatch Presidential Endowed Chair and Distinguished Professor in Ophthalmology and Visual Sciences, John A. Moran Eye Center, Department of Ophthalmology and Visual Sciences, University of Utah, Salt Lake City, UT, USA
e-mail: me.hartnett@hsc.utah.edu

Keywords

Retinal angiogenesis · Pathophysiology of ROP Vascular endothelial growth factor (VEGF) · Reactive oxygen · Oxidative stress · Erythropoietin · ROP phases Angiogenesis · Oxygen fluctuations · IGF-1

1.1 Introduction

ROP occurs because of a delay in physiologic retinal vascular development (PRVD) and damage to newly developed retinal vasculature often from high supplemental oxygen or other oxygen stresses. The initial two-phased hypothesis proposed by Ashton described oxygen-induced damage to newly developed retinal capillaries, called vaso-obliteration in Phase I [1]. Infants who survived premature birth during Ashton's time were only about 2 months premature so their retinas and retinal vasculature were more developed than premature infants at risk of treatment-warranted ROP today, who are born 3 or more months premature. In addition, at the time of Ashton, little was known about the effects of oxygen. Later clinical trials by Patz and Kinsey provided evidence of the damage to newly formed capillaries from high oxygen at birth [2, 3]. Today, however, the original Phase I "vaso-obliteration" no longer is accurate. Rather Phase I is better described as compromised physiologic vascularity and delayed physiologic retinal vascular development (PRVD), and both increase avascular retina. Although only the peripheral avascular retina is appreciated clinically on retinal examinations with indirect ophthalmoscopy or with retinal imaging using contact fundus cameras (see also Chap. 8). The peripheral avascular retina is described by the International Classification of ROP by zones [4]. Avascular areas within already vascularized retina are noted as reduced capillary density in experimental models but likely to be undetected on most clinical evaluations unless fluorescein angiography is performed [5, 6]. Once an infant is removed from high supplemental oxygen, then avascular retinal areas

W.-C. Wu, W.-C. Lam (eds.), *A Quick Guide to Pediatric Retina*, https://doi.org/10.1007/978-981-15-6552-6_1

become hypoxic and cells within the retina are stimulated to express angiogenic growth factors. However, instead of causing angiogenesis to grow into the retina, it grows into the vitreous. This Phase II, vasoproliferation, leads to common causes of vision loss from ensuing retinal detachment or dragging of the retina.

The original two-phased hypothesis is based on animal models of oxygen-induced retinopathy (OIR). However, the current clinical stages of ROP (Fig. 1.1) have necessitated that the original hypothesis be refined (Fig. 1.2) [7, 8]. No longer is high oxygen at birth the main cause of ROP, but rather it is recognized that other stresses, including fluctuations in oxygenation are important [9]. Animal models will be covered extensively in Chap. 2. It must be emphasized that the most representative models of ROP are OIR models in the rat and beagle, but these species require newer techniques to study molecular mechanisms. The mouse OIR model may not be as representative of the oxygen stresses or of common presentations of ROP but it provides greater ease in testing molecular mechanisms through the use of knockout or transgenic mice. Nonetheless, all animal models share the limitation of using full-term newborn animals that develop retinal vasculature after birth. Therefore, as with any translational study of human pathophysiology, it is necessary to integrate evidence from multiple sources when developing a hypothesis.

In humans, there is a third phase of fibrovascular retinal detachment (Fig. 1.1) that is not well modeled in most animals (Fig. 1.2). Most treatment strategies have been to treat treatment-warranted, vascularly active ROP with stage 3 and plus disease [10, 11] to prevent retinal detachment, clinically known as stages 4 and 5 ROP. However, there are other causes of vision loss in premature infants beside retinal detachment. As premature infants survive at younger gestational ages, the vascular beds of the choroid or retina and retinal neurons and glia are incompletely developed [12]. Neural connections within the retina are also incomplete, and the interactions among neural, glial, and vascular cells and signaling cascades can affect physiologic function. Infants born at gestational ages below 28 weeks who never developed ROP have been shown to have reduced ERG functions at age 6 [13, 14], suggesting that extremely preterm birth itself affects the retina and visual function. Finally, prematurity can also cause cortical visual impairment, which broadly includes connections through the brain to the occipital cortex and can affect visual acuity and function.

Genetic studies have not found any variant associated with severe ROP, but many studies have been regional and studies have had small sample sizes [15, 16]. Infant characteristics also vary across studies and this can affect outcomes. If infants enrolled have already survived extreme premature birth, genetic variants associated with severe ROP in less

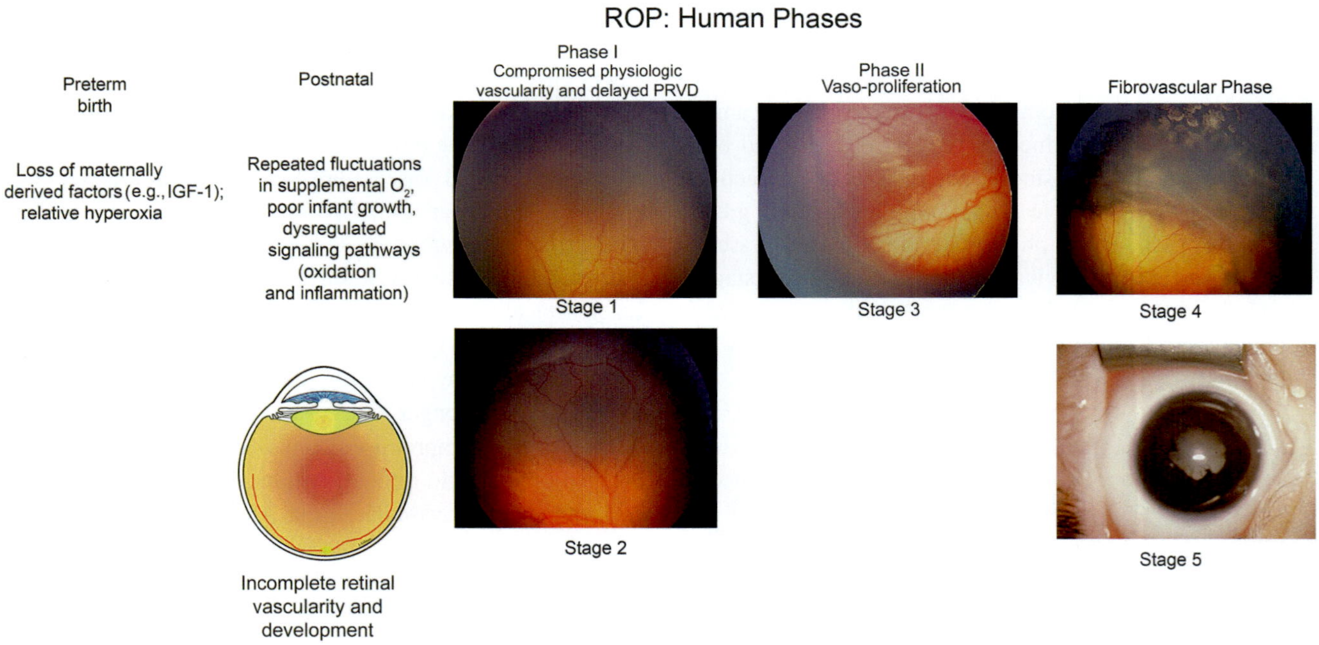

Fig. 1.1 ROP is characterized by zone of vascular development and the stage of disease. There are five stages. The stages relate to phases of OIR. Stages 1 and 2 ROP relate to Phase I OIR with compromised physiologic vascularity and delayed physiologic retinal vascular development (delayed PRVD). Stage 3 ROP relates to Phase II OIR with vasoproliferation in the form of intravitreal neovascularization, clinically known as Stage 3 ROP. Stage 1 has a line between the vascularized and avascular retina. Stage 2 has a thickened ridge. Stage 3 has intravitreal neovascularization and Stage 4 has a partial retinal detachment. Stage 5 is a total retinal detachment and may appear like a white pupil in an infant eye (not shown). Drawing by James Gilman CRA, FOPS. *Adapted from Hartnett ME. Pathophysiology and mechanisms of severe retinopathy of prematurity. Ophthalmology 2015;122:200–210, Figure 1*

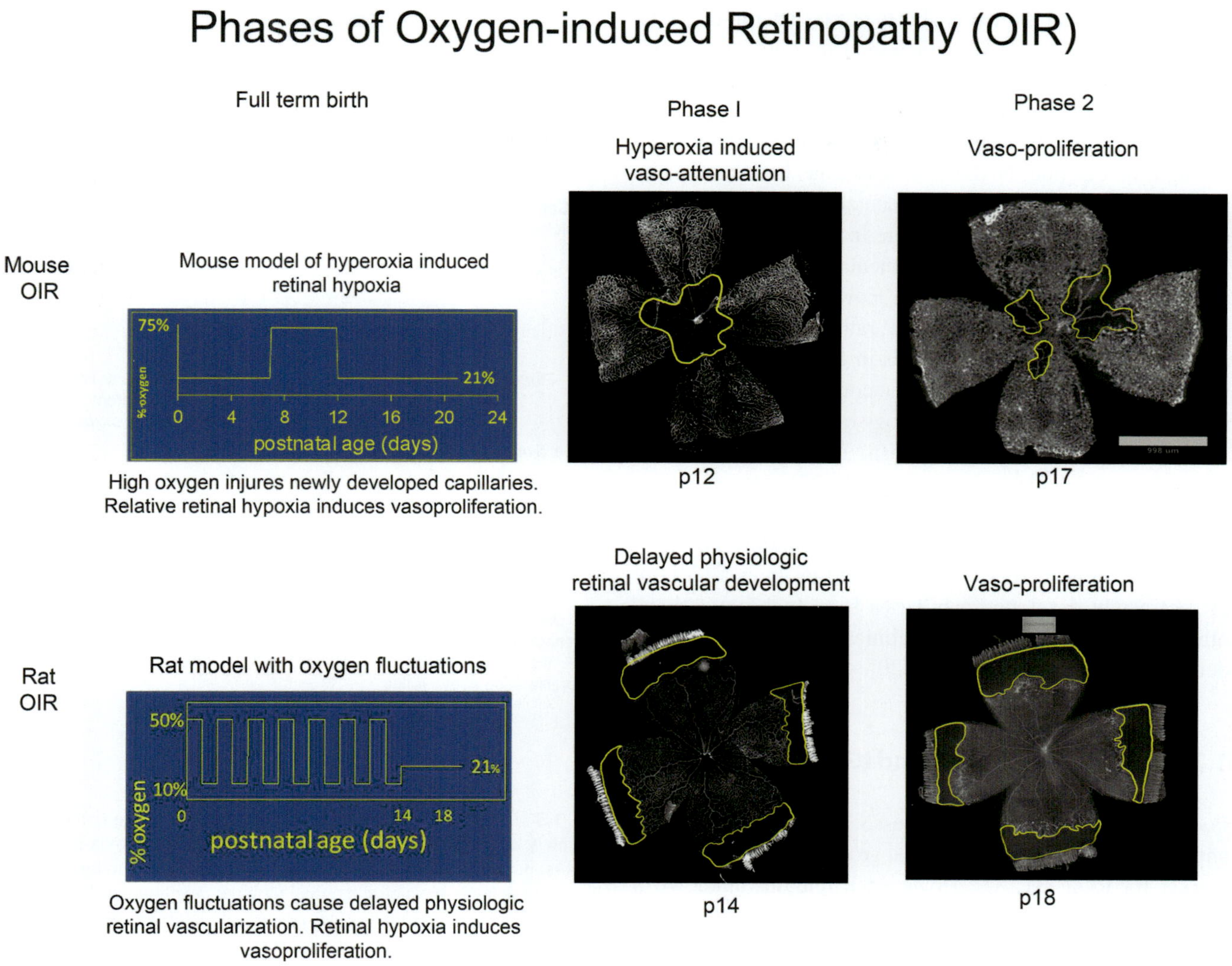

Fig. 1.2 The original two-phase hypothesis of ROP was based on animal models of oxygen-induced retinopathy OIR in kittens. The most often used models today are in mouse and rat. The rat OIR model is more representative of the pathophysiology of human. The mouse OIR model is easier to test genetic mechanisms involved in high oxygen-induced injury to newly formed capillaries. Phase I and Phase II are shown for both OIR models. Yellow lines depict avascular nonperfused retina in Phases I and II OIR. Drawing by James Gilman CRA, FOPS. *Adapted from Hartnett ME. Pathophysiology and mechanisms of severe retinopathy of prematurity. Ophthalmology 2015;122:200–210, Figure 2*

hardy infants may not be present and, therefore, not be detected. One example from the Neonatal Research Network in the US tested blood spots from infants born <1000 g and discovered variants in brain-derived neurotrophic factor (BDNF) associated with severe ROP. Other studies in larger and older premature infants did not find *BDNF* variants involved. On the other hand, several factors have been reported associated with ROP in the Wnt signaling pathway [17, 18]. Such variants can also cause the variably expressed condition, familial exudative vitreoretinopathy (FEVR). FEVR is classically described as occurring in full-term infants but there can be overlap with ROP if infants with FEVR are born prematurely [19]. Evidence suggests that premature infants with known Wnt variants should be monitored for severe forms of ROP [18].

1.2 Pathophysiology Associated with Reduced Vascularity in Phase I and Events Leading into Phase II

Early clinical trials provided evidence that high oxygen at birth was associated with the loss of newly developed capillaries. Since then, efforts are made to avoid high oxygen at birth. However, in regions with insufficient resources to regulate or monitor oxygen, high oxygen-induced retinopathy has been reported [20].

There are maternal–fetal interactions that are believed to affect ROP. Infants at risk of developing ROP are usually born before the third trimester of gestation when maternal factors are transferred through the placenta to the fetus. Therefore, the premature infant has no benefit of maternally derived factors and is often unable to produce them (Fig. 1.1). In addition, the process of premature birth is associated with the generation of oxidative compounds, but the premature infant has insufficient ability to quench reactive oxygen species. Generation of reactive oxygen species, particularly through the enzyme, NADPH oxidase, has been associated with vascular cell death in experimental models and in larger areas of peripheral avascular retina in Phase I [21]. Antioxidant treatment in experimental OIR models have reduced avascular retina [22, 23]. However, clinical studies have not shown a reduction in ROP, rather it has been associated with increased risks of sepsis in the use of exogenous vitamin E [24]. Deficiency of some compounds are believed to be involved in the pathophysiology of Phase I by not being available to promote angiogenesis or tissue protection, including insulin-like growth factor 1 [25], omega-3 fatty acids [26], erythropoietin (EPO) [27], lutein [28], and hypoxia-inducible factors [29] (Fig. 1.3). Studies are ongoing to determine if these factors would promote PRVD or protect newly developed capillaries from high oxygen and other stresses. However, current clinical trials have not led to definitive recommendations [28, 30].

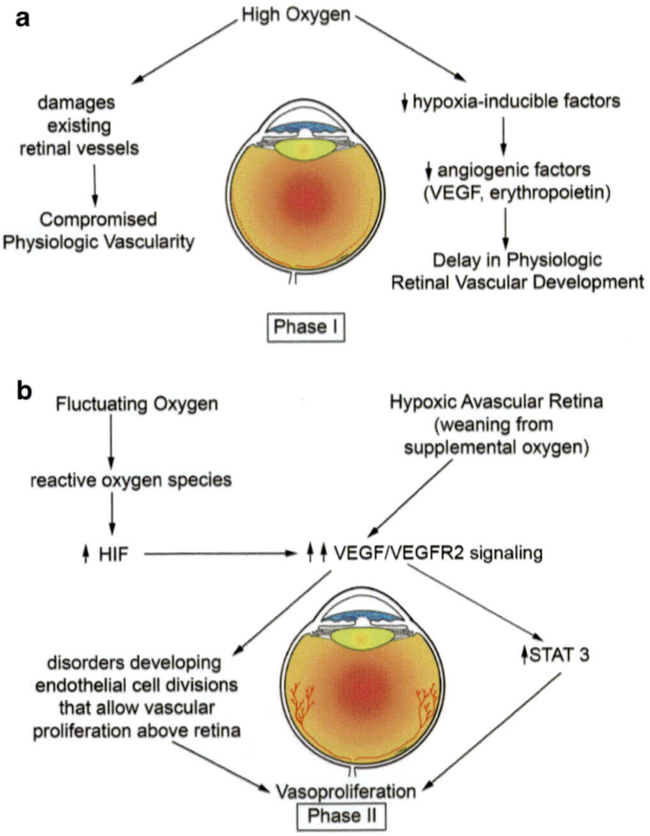

Fig. 1.3 Diagrams showing (**a**) the effects of high oxygen on damage of newly developed blood vessels and on reducing hypoxia-inducible factors, both of which lead to Phase I compromised physiologic vascularity and delay in physiologic retinal vascular development. Activation of VEGF/VEGFR2 disorders angiogenesis and interferes with PRVD in Phase I. (**b**) Fluctuations in oxygen that increase the generation of reactive oxygen species and lead to hypoxia-inducible factors while hypoxic avascular retina from Phase I can trigger VEGF expression when the infant is weaned from supplemental high oxygen. These events lead to vasoproliferation in Phase II. Activation of the transcription factor, STAT3, specifically in retinal endothelial cells by VEGF/VEGFR2 signaling contributes to vasoproliferation, but does not interfere with PRVD. Drawing by James Gilman CRA, FOPS

1.2.1 Postnatal Growth and IGF-1

Poor postnatal growth has been associated with lower zone and worse ROP, and poor postnatal growth has become a biomarker for ROP [31, 32]. However, it remains unknown if interventions to improve growth will affect the development of ROP. Infant growth has been linked to IGF-1 levels and ROP [33, 34]. A hypothesis was developed based on the findings that premature infant IGF-1 levels fall rapidly after birth and remain low compared to in utero levels (Fig. 1.1). IGF-1 has been experimentally shown to permit VEGF to be angiogenic and have protective mechanisms against oxygen-induced retinopathy [25, 35, 36]. A recent multicenter phase 2 clinical trial tested the effect from an infusion of IGF-1/IGF-BP3 versus standard care to reduce ROP but did not find a reduction in ROP or an increase in infant growth parameters [37]. However, only 28 of 61 infants achieved target goals of serum IGF-1 levels. Nonetheless, there was a reduction in severe levels of bronchopulmonary dysplasia in treated infants compared to those with standard care, and more studies may provide greater sample size, optimized drug delivery, and additional information.

1.2.2 Oxygen

Besides early oxygen studies [2, 3, 38], a number of studies have been done regionally testing varying oxygen levels. The Supplemental Therapeutic Oxygen for Prethreshold ROP found no benefit or harm on the progression of prethreshold ROP in 96–99% oxygen saturations compared to 89–94% [39]. Several recent multicenter clinical trials have tested low oxygen saturation targets on the risk of ROP. The Surfactant, Positive Pressure, and Oxygenation Randomized Trial (SUPPORT) and the Benefits of Oxygen Saturation Targeting II (BOOSTII) trials found a lower oxygenation target of 85–89% are associated with decreased ROP but also increased mortality compared to infants with a higher target of 91–95% [40, 41]. The Canadian Oxygen Trial did not find these associations [42].

Fluctuations in oxygenation have been associated with ROP clinically and in experimental models, most notably the rat OIR model [9]. Experimentally, there are several pathophysiologic events that occur in the retina in association with oxygen fluctuations (Fig. 1.3). There is differential expression of VEGF splice variants, specifically greater expression of the prevalent VEGF164/165 variant that is most commonly found in pathologic angiogenesis in retinal diseases, compared to hypoxia alone [43]. There is also activation of the enzyme NADPH oxidase that generates ROS and triggers signaling events that lead to the death of vascular cells in Phase I [21] and to intravitreal neovascularization in Phase II [44]. In addition, intermittent hypoxemic episodes have been associated with treatment-warranted ROP [45, 46]. Some neonatologists recommend testing the effects of low oxygen saturation targets early followed by higher SaO2 targets when ROP develops or at an older post-gestational age [47–49].

1.2.3 Light

The initial Light ROP study tested the effect of goggles to reduce ambient light to preterm infants upon birth on the risk of ROP, but there was no difference compared to control [50]. Experimental studies in mice reported that more light even through the abdomens of pregnant dams was important for physiologic intraretinal vascular development through a melanopsin dependent signaling pathway in the fetus [51]. Subsequent clinical studies have also suggested that higher average day length was associated with lower risk of severe ROP [52]. There is current interest in circadian studies on cycled light and the idea that infants might have better retinal vascular development and less severe ROP if kept on a circadian rhythm within neonatal nurseries, rather than be sheltered from light during daytime.

1.2.4 Erythropoietin and Role of Stress-Induced Factors in Infant

Erythropoietin has additional properties besides its role as a hematopoietic hormone, including in neuronal and tissue protection and angiogenesis [53]. The effect is believed to depend on the dimerization between the erythropoietin receptor (EPOR) and other receptors including the beta-common receptor (CD131) subunit for tissue-protective effects or the VEGFR2 receptor for angiogenesis [54]. EPO has been associated with the stabilization of vessels in Phase I but also with vascular activity in Phase II [27, 55]. Difficulty in experimental studies has been due to the inconsistency of EPO receptor (EPOR) antibodies that identify the location of the receptor in various tissues. Experimental studies are ongoing, but clinical studies have not identified the EPO promoter variant related to diabetic retinopathy to be present in infants with ROP [56]. Clinical trials testing supplemented EPO or derivatives for protection have not resulted in clear recommendations regarding ROP [57]. The Preterm Erythropoietin Neuroprotection Trial (PENUT) did not increased risk of ROP. Experimental data has also led to the interesting premise that stress due to conditions surrounding prematurity may induce protective mechanisms that support vascularization of the retina during Phase I in certain animals [58]. Additional studies to identify such protective pathways are warranted.

1.3 Pathophysiology Related to Phase II

1.3.1 Vascular Endothelial Growth Factor Signaling

Aberrant angiogenesis manifesting as growth of blood vessels into the vitreous rather than into the retina is a hallmark of treatment-warranted ROP. Although a number of angiogenic factors are associated with aberrant angiogenesis, the one that has been studied the most and is likely a causative factor in treatment-warranted ROP is vascular endothelial growth factor (VEGF). VEGF is expressed as a result of hypoxia or reactive oxygen species, both stresses are associated with ROP, and there are feed-forward loops that can drive pathologic angiogenic signaling. VEGF-induced activation of receptor 2 (VEGFR2) causes disordered developmental growth of dividing endothelial cells allowing them to grow on top of one another into the vitreous rather than into the retina to extend vasculature to the ora serrata (Fig. 1.3). Experimental and clinical evidence has supported the hypothesis that overactive VEGF/VEGFR2 signaling causes intravitreal stage 3 and interferes with PRVD in ROP. (VEGF/VEGFR2 activation of the transcription factor, signal transducer, and activator of transcription 3 (STAT3) contributes to intravitreal neovascularization, but does not interfere with PRVD.) (Fig. 1.3) Neutralizing antibodies delivered into the vitreous that bind VEGF inhibited stage 3 ROP and extended physiologic retinal vascularization [59–61]. Additional experimental evidence using similar antibodies that bind rat VEGF in the rat OIR model has reduced the dilation of retinal veins and tortuosity of retinal arterioles, reducing plus disease [62]. Knockdown of VEGFR2 specifically in retinal endothelial cells using a novel gene therapy approach has reduced intravitreal neovascularization and extended physiologic retinal vascularization in the rat OIR model [63].

However, the molecular mechanisms and roles of other receptors are still being discerned as is the understanding of inhibition of VEGF ligand and its potential adverse effect to the developing stressed retina that has been found using experimental models [64]. In addition, neural guidance molecules and the role of glial, neural, and vascular interactions have been and are being studied [65].

1.3.2 Reactive Oxygen Species

Reactive oxygen species generated through the enzyme, NADPH oxidase, may affect Phase II through several signaling pathways [44, 63]. However, to date, the only interventions that have reduced vasoproliferation in Phase II are strategies to inhibit VEGF signaling.

References

1. Ashton N, Ward B, Serpell G. Effect of oxygen on developing retinal vessels with particular reference to the problem of retrolental fibroplasia. Br J Ophthalmol. 1954;38:397–430.
2. Patz A. Oxygen studies in retrolental fibroplasia. Am J Ophthalmol. 1954;38(3):291–308.
3. Kinsey VE. Cooperative study of retrolental fibroplasia and the use of oxygen. Arch Ophthalmol. 1956;56:481–543.
4. No Authors. An international classification of retinopathy of prematurity. The Committee for the Classification of Retinopathy of Prematurity. Arch Ophthalmol. 1984;102(8):1130–4.
5. Klufas MA, Patel SN, Ryan MC, Patel Gupta M, Jonas KE, Ostmo S, et al. Influence of fluorescein angiography on the diagnosis and management of retinopathy of prematurity. Ophthalmology. 2015;122(8):1601–8.
6. Lepore D, Quinn GE, Molle F, Baldascino A, Orazi L, Sammartino M, et al. Intravitreal bevacizumab versus laser treatment in type 1 retinopathy of prematurity: report on fluorescein angiographic findings. Ophthalmology. 2014;121(11):2212–9.
7. Hartnett ME, Penn JS. Mechanisms and management of retinopathy of prematurity. N Engl J Med. 2012;367(26):2515–26.
8. Hartnett ME. Pathophysiology and mechanisms of severe retinopathy of prematurity. Ophthalmology. 2015;122(1):200–10.
9. York JR, Landers S, Kirby RS, Arbogast PG, Penn JS. Arterial oxygen fluctuation and retinopathy of prematurity in very-low-birth-weight infants. J Perinatol. 2004;24(2):82–7.
10. Early Treatment for Retinopathy of Prematurity Cooperative Group. Revised indications for the treatment of retinopathy of prematurity: results of the early treatment for retinopathy of prematurity randomized trial. Arch Ophthalmol. 2003;121(12):1684–94.
11. CfRoPC Group. Multicenter trial of cryotherapy for retinopathy of prematurity: snellen visual acuity and structural outcome at 51/2 years after randomization. Arch Ophthalmol. 1996;114:417–24.
12. Hartnett ME. Electroretinographic responses in the smallest eyes. JAMA Ophthalmol. 2017;135(8):862–3.
13. Molnar AEC, Andreasson SO, Larsson EKB, Akerblom HM, Holmstrom GE. Reduction of rod and cone function in 6.5-year-old children born extremely preterm. JAMA Ophthalmol. 2017;135(8):854–61.
14. Austeng D, Kallen KB, Ewald UW, Jakobsson PG, Holmstrom GE. Incidence of retinopathy of prematurity in infants born before 27 weeks' gestation in Sweden. Arch Ophthalmol. 2009;127(10):1315–9.
15. Swan R, Kim SJ, Campbell JP, Paul Chan RV, Sonmez K, Taylor KD, et al. The genetics of retinopathy of prematurity: a model for neovascular retinal disease. Ophthalmol Retina. 2018;2(9):949–62.
16. Hartnett ME, Cotten CM. Genomics in the neonatal nursery: focus on ROP. Semin Perinatol. 2015;39(8):604–10.
17. Kondo H, Kusaka S, Yoshinaga A, Uchio E, Tawara A, Tahira T. Genetic variants of FZD4 and LRP5 genes in patients with advanced retinopathy of prematurity. Mol Vis. 2013;19:476–85.
18. Dailey WA, Gryc W, Garg PG, Drenser KA. Frizzled-4 variations associated with retinopathy and intrauterine growth retardation: a potential marker for prematurity and retinopathy. Ophthalmology. 2015;122(9):1917–23.
19. John VJ, McClintic JI, Hess DJ, Berrocal AM. Retinopathy of prematurity versus familial exudative vitreoretinopathy: report on clinical and angiographic findings. Ophthalmic Surg Lasers Imaging Retina. 2016;47(1):14–9.
20. Martinez-Castellanos MA, Velez-Montoya R, Price K, Henaine-Berra A, Garcia-Aguirre G, Morales-Canton V, et al. Vascular changes on fluorescein angiography of premature infants with low risk of retinopathy of prematurity after high oxygen exposure. Int J Retina Vitreous. 2017;3:2.
21. Saito Y, Geisen P, Uppal A, Hartnett ME. Inhibition of NAD(P)H oxidase reduces apoptosis and avascular retina in an animal model of retinopathy of prematurity. Mol Vis. 2007;13:840–53.
22. Hartnett ME, DeAngelis MM. Studies on retinal and choroidal disorders. In: Armstrong D, editor. Studies on retinal and choroidal disorders. 1st ed. New York: Humana Press; 2012. p. 559–84.
23. Soghier LM, Brion LP. Cysteine, cystine or N-acetylcysteine supplementation in parenterally fed neonates. Cochrane Database Syst Rev. 2006;4:Cd004869.
24. Brion LP, Bell EF, Raghuveer TS. Vitamin E supplementation for prevention of morbidity and mortality in preterm infants. Cochrane Database Syst Rev. 2003;4:Cd003665.
25. Smith LEH, Kopchick JJ, Chen W, Knapp J, Kinose F, Daley D, et al. Essential role of growth hormone in ischemia-induced retinal neovascularization. Science. 1997;276:1706–9.
26. Connor KM, SanGiovanni JP, Lofqvist C, Aderman CM, Chen J, Higuchi A, et al. Increased dietary intake of [omega]-3-polyunsaturated fatty acids reduces pathological retinal angiogenesis. Nat Med. 2007;13(7):868–73.
27. Chen J, Connor KM, Aderman CM, Smith LE. Erythropoietin deficiency decreases vascular stability in mice. J Clin Invest. 2008;118(2):526–33.
28. Manzoni P, Guardione R, Bonetti P, Priolo C, Maestri A, Mansoldo C, et al. Lutein and zeaxanthin supplementation in preterm very low-birth-weight neonates in neonatal intensive care units: a multicenter randomized controlled trial. Am J Perinatol. 2013;30(1):25–32.
29. Sears JE, Hoppe G, Ebrahem Q, Anand-Apte B. Prolyl hydroxylase inhibition during hyperoxia prevents oxygen-induced retinopathy. Proc Natl Acad Sci. 2008;105(50):19898–903.
30. Najm S, Lofqvist C, Hellgren G, Engstrom E, Lundgren P, Hard AL, et al. Effects of a lipid emulsion containing fish oil on polyunsaturated fatty acid profiles, growth and morbidities in extremely premature infants: a randomized controlled trial. Clin Nutr ESPEN. 2017;20:17–23.
31. Wu C, Vanderveen DK, Hellstrom A, Lofqvist C, Smith LE. Longitudinal postnatal weight measurements for the prediction of retinopathy of prematurity. Arch Ophthalmol. 2010;128(4):443–7.
32. Binenbaum G, Bell EF, Donohue P, Quinn G, Shaffer J, Tomlinson LA, et al. Development of modified screening criteria for retinopathy of prematurity: primary results from the postnatal growth and retinopathy of prematurity study. JAMA Ophthalmol. 2018;136(9):1034–40.
33. Hellstrom A, Hard AL, Engstrom E, Niklasson A, Andersson E, Smith L, et al. Early weight gain predicts retinopathy in preterm infants: new, simple, efficient approach to screening. Pediatrics. 2009;123(4):e638–e45.
34. Hellstrom A, Engstrom E, Hard A-L, Albertsson-Wickland K, Carlsson B, Niklasson A, et al. Postnatal serum insulin-like growth factor I deficiency is associated with retinopathy of prematurity and other complications of premature birth. Pediatrics. 2003;112(5):1016–20.
35. Smith LEH, Shen W, Peruzzu C, Soker S, Kinose F, Xu X, et al. Regulation of vascular endothelial growth factor-dependent retinal

neovascularization by insulin-like growth factor-1 receptor. Nat Med. 1999;5:1390–5.
36. Chang KH, Chan-Ling T, McFarland EL, Afzal A, Pan H, Baxter LC, et al. IGF binding protein-3 regulates hematopoietic stem cell and endothelial precursor cell function during vascular development. Proc Natl Acad Sci. 2007;104(25):10595–600.
37. Ley D, Hallberg B, Hansen-Pupp I, Dani C, Ramenghi LA, Marlow N, et al. rhIGF-1/rhIGFBP-3 in preterm infants: a phase 2 randomized controlled trial. J Pediatr. 2018;206:56–65.e8.
38. Flynn JT, Bancalari E, Snyder ES, Goldberg RN, Feuer W, Cassady J, et al. A cohort study of transcutaneous oxygen tension and the incidence and severity of retinopathy of prematurity. N Engl J Med. 1992;326(16):1050–4.
39. Group TS-RMS. Supplemental therapeutic oxygen for prethreshold retinopathy of prematurity (STOP-ROP), a randomized, controlled trial. I: primary outcomes. Pediatrics. 2000;105(2):295–310.
40. Carlo WA, Finer NN, Walsh MC, Rich W, Gantz MG, Laptook AR, et al. Target ranges of oxygen saturation in extremely preterm infants. N Engl J Med. 2010;362(21):1959–69.
41. Stenson BJ, Tarnow-Mordi WO, Darlow BA, Simes J, Juszczak E, Askie L, et al. Oxygen saturation and outcomes in preterm infants. N Engl J Med. 2013;368(22):2094–104.
42. Schmidt B, Whyte RK, Asztalos EV, Moddemann D, Poets C, Rabi Y, et al. Effects of targeting higher vs lower arterial oxygen saturations on death or disability in extremely preterm infants: a randomized clinical trial. JAMA. 2013;309(20):2111–20.
43. McColm JR, Geisen P, Hartnett ME. VEGF isoforms and their expression after a single episode of hypoxia or repeated fluctuations between hyperoxia and hypoxia: relevance to clinical ROP. Mol Vis. 2004;10:512–20.
44. Saito Y, Uppal A, Byfield G, Budd S, Hartnett ME. Activated NAD(P)H oxidase from supplemental oxygen induces neovascularization independent of VEGF in retinopathy of prematurity model. Investig Ophthalmol Vis Sci. 2008;49(4):1591–8.
45. Di Fiore JM, Bloom JN, Orge F, Schutt A, Schluchter M, Cheruvu VK, et al. A higher incidence of intermittent hypoxemic episodes is associated with severe retinopathy of prematurity. J Pediatr. 2010;157(1):69–73.
46. Di Fiore JM, Kaffashi F, Loparo K, Sattar A, Schluchter M, Foglyano R, et al. The relationship between patterns of intermittent hypoxia and retinopathy of prematurity in preterm infants. Pediatr Res. 2012;72(6):606–12.
47. Gaynon MW, Wong RJ, Stevenson DK, Sunshine P. Prethreshold retinopathy of prematurity: VEGF inhibition without VEGF inhibitors. J Perinatol. 2018;38(10):1295–300.
48. Colaizy TT, Longmuir S, Gertsch K, Abramoff MD, Klein JM. Use of a supplemental oxygen protocol to suppress progression of retinopathy of prematurity. Invest Ophthalmol Vis Sci. 2017;58(2):887–91.
49. Sears JE, Pietz J, Sonnie C, Dolcini D, Hoppe G. A change in oxygen supplementation can decrease the incidence of retinopathy of prematurity. Ophthalmology. 2009;116(3):513–8.
50. Reynolds JD, Hardy RJ, Kennedy KA, Spencer R, van Heuven WAJ, Fielder AR. Lack of efficacy of light reduction in preventing retinopathy of prematurity. N Engl J Med. 1998;338:1572–6.
51. Rao S, Chun C, Fan J, Kofron JM, Yang MB, Hegde RS, et al. A direct and melanopsin-dependent fetal light response regulates mouse eye development. Nature. 2013;494(7436):243–6.
52. Yang MB, Rao S, Copenhagen DR, Lang RA. Length of day during early gestation as a predictor of risk for severe retinopathy of prematurity. Ophthalmology. 2013;120(12):2706–13.
53. Juul SE et al, A Randomized Trial of Erythropoietin for Neuroprotection in Preterm Infants. N. Engl J Med 2020 Jan 16;382(3):233–43.
54. Brines M, Cerami A. Discovering erythropoietin's extra-hematopoietic functions: biology and clinical promise. Kidney Int. 2006;70(2):246–50.
55. Chen J, Connor KM, Aderman CM, Willett KL, Aspegren OP, Smith LEH. Suppression of retinal neovascularization by erythropoietin siRNA in a mouse model of proliferative retinopathy. Invest Ophthalmol Vis Sci. 2009;50(3):1329–35.
56. Dame C, Sciesielski LK, Rau C, Badur CA, Buhrer C. The erythropoietin promoter variant rs1617640 is not associated with severe retinopathy of prematurity, independent of treatment with erythropoietin. J Pediatr. 2018;199:256–9.
57. Ohlsson A, Aher SM. Early erythropoiesis-stimulating agents in preterm or low birth weight infants. Cochrane Database Syst Rev. 2017;11:Cd004863.
58. Becker S, Wang H, Yu B, Brown R, Han X, Lane RH, et al. Protective effect of maternal uteroplacental insufficiency on oxygen-induced retinopathy in offspring: removing bias of premature birth. Sci Rep. 2017;7:42301.
59. Mintz-Hittner HA, Kennedy KA, Chuang AZ. Efficacy of intravitreal bevacizumab for stage 3+ retinopathy of prematurity. N Engl J Med. 2011;364(7):603–15.
60. Stahl A, Krohne TU, Eter N, Oberacher-Velten I, Guthoff R, Meltendorf S, et al. Comparing alternative ranibizumab dosages for safety and efficacy in retinopathy of prematurity: a randomized clinical trial. JAMA Pediatr. 2018;172(3):278–86.
61. Wallace DK, Kraker RT, Freedman SF, Crouch ER, Hutchinson AK, Bhatt AR, et al. Assessment of lower doses of intravitreous bevacizumab for retinopathy of prematurity: a phase 1 dosing study. JAMA Ophthalmol. 2017;135(6):654–6.
62. Hartnett ME, Martiniuk D, Byfield G, Geisen P, Zeng G, Bautch VL. Neutralizing VEGF decreases tortuosity and alters endothelial cell division orientation in arterioles and veins in rat model of ROP: relevance to plus disease. Invest Ophthalmol Vis Sci. 2008;49:7–3107. Mar 31 epub
63. Simmons AB, Bretz CA, Wang H, Kunz E, Hajj K, Kennedy C, et al. Gene therapy knockdown of VEGFR2 in retinal endothelial cells to treat retinopathy. Angiogenesis. 2018;21(4):751–64.
64. Becker S, Wang H, Simmons AB, Suwanmanee T, Stoddard GJ, Kafri T, et al. Targeted knockdown of overexpressed VEGFA or VEGF164 in Muller cells maintains retinal function by triggering different signaling mechanisms. Sci Rep. 2018;8(1):2003.
65. Sapieha P. Eyeing central neurons in vascular growth and reparative angiogenesis. Blood. 2012;120(11):2182–94.

Animal Models of Retinopathy of Prematurity

2

Chi-Hsiu Liu and Jing Chen

Abstract

Retinopathy of prematurity (ROP) is a leading cause of blindness in preterm infants. It is a biphasic disease characterized by an initial phase of arrested vascular growth caused by hyperoxia exposure and loss of maternal–fetal interaction, followed by a second phase of hypoxia-induced neovascularization, which may lead to retinal detachment and vision loss. Animal models of ROP are crucial for studying the cellular and molecular mechanisms underlying ROP pathogenesis and for the development of potential therapeutics. Early animal models of oxygen-induced ROP were developed in the 1950s in multiple species including feline, canine, and murine, after the recognition of supplemental oxygen use as a risk factor. Refined mouse and rat models of oxygen-induced retinopathy were modernized in the 1990s with standardized oxygen protocols and improved methods for assessing retinopathy severity. More recently, murine models of hyperglycemia-associated neonatal retinopathy were developed to mimic neonatal hyperglycemia, a newly identified ROP risk factor. This chapter summarizes the basic concepts, advantages, and limitations of animal models of ROP, with a focus on the most widely used mouse model of oxygen-induced retinopathy.

Keywords

Retinopathy of prematurity · Animal models
Oxygen-induced retinopathy · Vaso-obliteration
Neovascularization

C.-H. Liu · J. Chen (✉)
Department of Ophthalmology, Boston Children's Hospital and Harvard Medical School, Boston, MA, USA
e-mail: Chi-Hsiu.Liu@childrens.harvard.edu; Jing.Chen@childrens.harvard.edu

2.1 Introduction

Retinopathy of prematurity (ROP), a potentially blinding disorder caused by abnormal retinal blood vessel growth affecting premature infants, was first reported as "retrolental fibroplasia" by Theodore L. Terry during its epidemic in the 1940s [1]. In the 1930s and 1940s, oxygen administration became a common practice in neonatal care to improve the health of preterm infants with underdeveloped pulmonary function [2, 3]. The epidemic of ROP and ROP-associated blindness soon followed in the 1940s and early 1950s [4], which led to the recognition that unrestricted supplemental oxygen therapy was associated with ROP risk, as initially suggested by Kate Campbell [5] and confirmed by subsequent studies [6, 7]. This discovery of oxygen use as a key risk factor for ROP enabled early development of animal models of ROP in the 1950s. These models recapitulated the detrimental vascular effects of excess oxygen on retinal vascular growth in feline, canine, and murine pups, although inconsistencies remained. Modernization of murine ROP models in the 1990s [8, 9] standardized the protocols of oxygen exposure and methods for evaluation of ROP severity. Combined with the availability of genetically manipulated mice, these newer models greatly advanced research investigating the molecular basis of ROP pathogenesis and the development of potential therapeutics.

Decades of clinical and experimental ROP research have led to the consensus that ROP is a biphasic disease consisting of an initial phase of incomplete retinal vessel growth followed by a second phase of hypoxia-driven pathologic vessel proliferation [10–12]. Unlike full-term infants whose retinal vessels are almost completely developed, infants born prematurely have incompletely developed retinal vasculature with a peripheral avascular zone. After premature birth, the development of retinal vessels is delayed by the relatively hyperoxic postnatal room air environment (compared with in utero) and further worsened by the supplemental oxygen therapy. The first phase of ROP occurs between birth and approximately 30–32 weeks postmenstrual age. As the infant

W.-C. Wu, W.-C. Lam (eds.), *A Quick Guide to Pediatric Retina*, https://doi.org/10.1007/978-981-15-6552-6_2

matures, the peripheral avascular retina becomes increasingly metabolically active, leading to tissue ischemia and hypoxia, which is often exacerbated by the termination of oxygen therapy [13–16]. Hypoxia stimulates upregulation of pro-angiogenic growth factors, such as vascular endothelial growth factor (VEGF) and erythropoietin (EPO), leading to uncontrolled vascular growth into the vitreous, occurring at the junction of avascularized and vascularized retina, and, in severe cases, tractional retinal detachment and blindness [10–12]. The second phase of ROP begins around 32–34 weeks postmenstrual age. Both ROP phases can be closely mimicked in the animal models of oxygen-induced retinopathy (OIR) to allow investigation on the mechanisms of vaso-obliteration, vascular regeneration, and pathological neovascularization processes.

Unlike humans, in whom retinal vessels develop fully before birth, in animal models of feline, canine, and rodent, retinal vessels develop and mature postnatally [16, 17]. Therefore, although these oxygen-induced ROP models reproduce the essential vascular features of ROP, they model only the oxygen influence without taking into account the prematurity itself, which is challenging to model in utero. Factors related to prematurity, such as essential fatty acids and insulin-like growth factors (provided in the third trimester in utero and often decreased or missing after premature birth), are commonly investigated experimentally using supplemental treatments in the OIR model [18, 19]. As additional risk factors (such as neonatal hyperglycemia, a common problem in extremely preterm infants) have been associated with severe ROP [20–23], new murine models of neonatal hyperglycemia-associated retinopathy [24, 25] have also been generated recently. This chapter mainly reviews the historical development of ROP models and focuses primarily on the most commonly used mouse and rat models [8, 9], with a brief discussion of hyperglycemia-associated neonatal retinopathy models [24, 25].

2.2 Experimental Models of ROP

The OIR models have been valuable tools with which to explore the role of oxygen and oxygen-related factors in the pathogenesis of ROP. These models were developed by exposing newborn experimental animals, including feline [26], murine [8, 9], canine [27–29], and piscine (fish) [30], to constantly high or cycling high and low oxygen environments. These animal models of OIR reproduce both the initial vaso-obliteration phase and subsequent ischemia- and hypoxia-induced neovascularization phase, resembling ROP in humans. Due to their simplicity in the induction of pathological neovessels and the ease of monitoring and quantification, the animal models of OIR are widely used for studying the mechanisms and evaluating new therapeutics for treating the sight-threatening neovascularization in ROP and other ischemic proliferative retinopathies, albeit the consistency and reproducibility of neovascularization vary across different species.

2.2.1 Early Animal Models of OIR: The Feline and Canine Models

In light of the clinical observations linking oxygen with ROP, in the early 1950s Ashton et al. exposed kittens to 70–80% of oxygen for at least 4 days, causing retinal vascular closure and obliteration, then returned them to ambient air (21% oxygen), resulting in hypoxia-induced vaso-proliferation [26, 31]. This feline model of OIR is one of the earliest experimental models establishing the effects of altering oxygen concentration on retinal vascular development [16, 26]. The model successfully mimics the early stages of ROP closely and characterizes both the vaso-obliterative and the vaso-proliferative phases.

Attempts at using the canine OIR model for studying ROP were made at about the same time, in which the first model was developed by Patz's group, to determine the effects of oxygen on the immature retinal vasculature in puppies [29, 32], and modified in subsequent studies [27, 28, 33]. Beagle puppies were exposed to 95–100% of oxygen for 4 days to induce retinopathy. Similar to the kitten model, exposure to hyperoxia arrests the retinal vascular development, causing vaso-obliteration. After moving the puppies from hyperoxia back to room air, the resultant relative hypoxia leads to the vaso-proliferative stage [27, 34]. In addition, retinal detachment, which can be observed in the late, severe stage of human ROP, occurs in the canine but not feline or murine OIR model. Whereas feline and canine models are still occasionally used, achieving a statistically significant number of animals can be challenging. Usage of OIR models in mice and rats has been much more common, largely due to the standardization of the murine models and genetic manipulation in mice since the 1990s.

2.2.2 The Mouse Model of OIR

2.2.2.1 Postnatal Development of Mouse Retinal Vasculature

Mouse retinal vascular development follows similar morphological patterns as in humans [17, 35]. A major difference is the temporally delayed nature of retinal angiogenesis and neuron maturation in mice. In a human fetus, the retinal vasculature develops relatively early during the second trimester, whereas in mice it does not begin to develop until after birth [17, 36, 37]. Therefore, human full-term infants are born with mostly mature retinal vasculature while neonatal mice possess underdeveloped vasculature in the eyes in the first few postnatal weeks, allowing studies of physiological and pathological retinal angiogenesis. The development of the mouse retinal vasculature starts with sprouting from the optic nerve head, parallel to the regression of hyaloid vasculature. The hyaloid vasculature is a transient circulatory system providing oxygen and nutrient to the developing lens and inner retina as well as the primary vitreous in embryonic eyes [38–40]. During the first postnatal week, the retinal vessels expand radially, forming the superficial vascular plexus; the hyaloid vasculature starts to degenerate at the same time (Fig. 2.1a) [40]. From the second week onward,

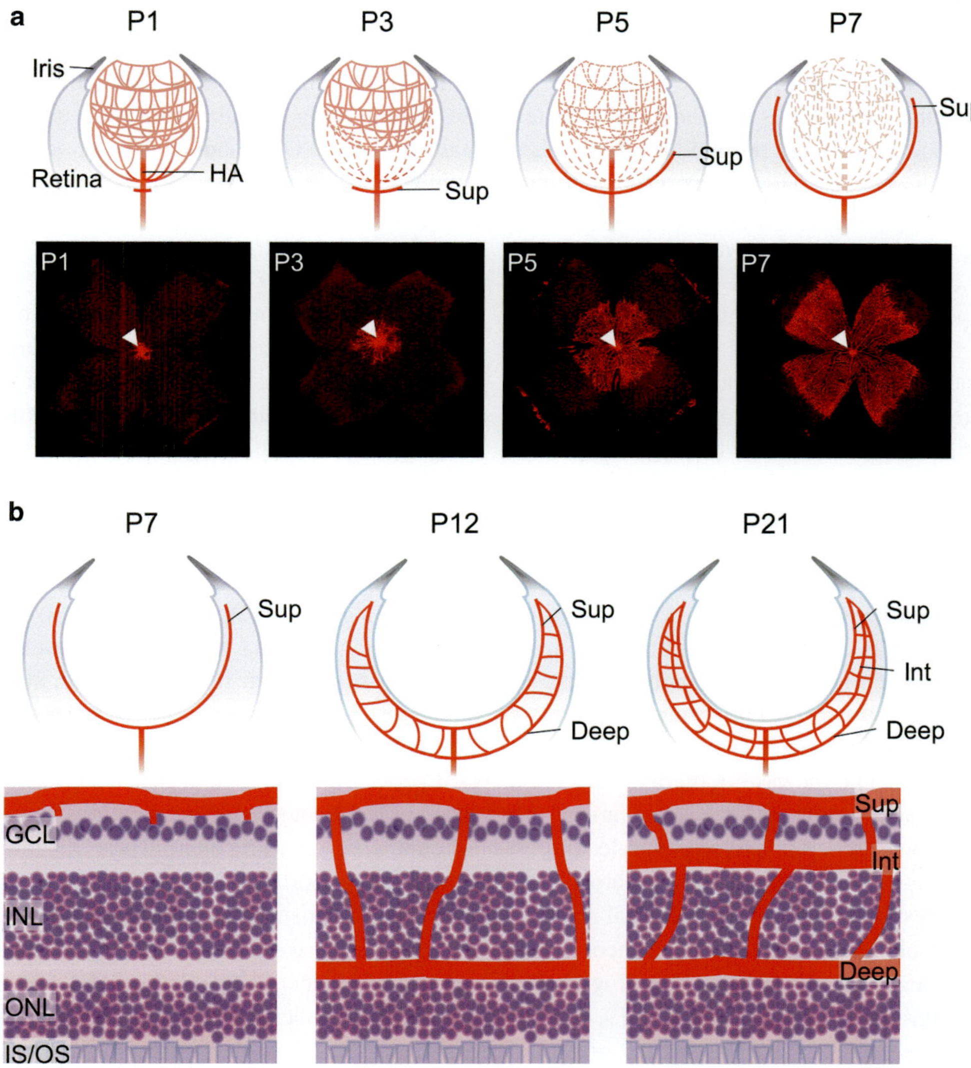

Fig. 2.1 Postnatal development of mouse retina vasculature. (**a**) Development of mouse retinal vessels occurs postnatally. The upper panels illustrate cross-section diagrams of mouse eyes with developing superficial retinal vascular plexus (Sup; indicated in red) from postnatal day (P) 1 to 7, parallel to regression of hyaloid vasculature (indicated in light red), which is a transient embryonic vascular bed providing blood supply to the developing eye. The lower panels are representative images of the retinal flat mounts from C57BL/6J mice. The vasculature was stained with isolectin (red). At P1, the mouse retina is nearly devoid of blood vessels. Originating from the optic nerve head (white arrowheads), the superficial vascular plexus extends radially from the central retina and reaches the peripheral retina by the end of the first week of postnatal development. (**b**) Development of the deep and intermediate vascular plexus in mouse retina occurs from the second week postnatally onward. The upper panels are cartoons of eye cross-sections overviewing the organization of three retinal layers (at P7, P12, and P21) during the development of superficial, intermediate, and deep vascular layers. The lower panels are schematic images of retinal cross-sections showing the maturation process of the three retinal vascular plexuses (in red). During the first postnatal week, the superficial plexus reaches out to the edge of the peripheral retina. From the second week onward, the superficial vascular plexus starts to grow perpendicularly into the retina to form the deep vascular plexus between the INL and ONL, which is fully developed at P12. Further growth and maturation of the intermediate plexus continue between the GCL and INL and are mostly complete by P21. Deep, deep retinal vessels; GCL, ganglion cell layer; INL, inner nuclear layer; Int, intermediate retinal vessel; IS/OS, inner segment/outer segment of photoreceptors; ONL, outer nuclear layer; Sup, superficial retinal vessels. The retinal flat mount images in panel a were adapted and reprinted with permission from Stahl et al. [17]

the superficial capillaries grow perpendicularly into the inner retina, forming the deep and then the intermediate vascular plexuses (Fig. 2.1b). By the end of the third postnatal week, a complete retinal vasculature is developed, and hyaloid vessels are mostly regressed [37]. During this period, especially in the first week, the immature retinal vasculature and remnant hyaloid vessels in neonatal mouse pups resemble those of preterm human infants, having a largely avascular retina and highly susceptible to oxygen-induced retinopathy [17].

2.2.2.2 The Mouse OIR Model

In the 1950s, around the same time as the studies in the kitten OIR model, pathologic features resembling ROP were reported in mouse retinas exposed to high oxygen conditions [29, 41]. Subsequent studies in mice further examined the effects of varying oxygen conditions on reproducing ROP-like pathological ocular characteristics [42, 43], providing insights that helped shape the current standardized OIR models.

Coupled with advanced technology in the visualization of retinal vasculature, uniform and thorough assessment of retinopathy severity, as well as the advantage of genetic manipulation in mice, the current mouse model of OIR described by Smith et al. in the 1990s is one of the most commonly used OIR models [9, 44]. In this model, neonatal mice are exposed to 75% ± 2% of oxygen for 5 days starting at postnatal day (P) 7, followed by 5 days in room air starting from P12 to P17 (Fig. 2.2a). Hyperoxia conditions from P7 to P12 result in central retinal vessel regression, leading to vaso-obliteration and mimicking the initial stage of ROP. The maximal amount of vessel loss is observed at P9, followed by slow revascularization into the vaso-obliterated areas [45, 46]. After returning to room air at P12, the retinal areas with vaso-obliteration become ischemic and hypoxic, leading to stimulation of hypoxia-induced pro-angiogenic factors, such as VEGF and EPO, resulting in both physiological revascularization of the vaso-obliteration area and also uncontrolled compensatory pathological neovascularization (Fig. 2.2b), resembling the proliferative stage of human ROP [9, 47–50]. These pathological neovessels, also known as preretinal tufts, are disorganized, small-caliber clumps of neovascularization growing at the border between vascular and avascular areas and protruding intravitreally (Fig. 2.2c, d). At P17, the typical endpoint of this mouse model, the extent of pathological neovessels reaches the maximal severity and is also accompanied by increased vascular leakage and breakdown of the blood–retinal barrier. After P17, abnormal preretinal neovascularization starts gradual regression spontaneously and completely disappears by about P25 [44].

The mouse retinal vasculature can be visualized by fluorescent angiography, which highlights the lumen of blood vessels, or (more efficiently) by staining with blood vessel markers such as isolectin in retinal flat mounts. Both methods allow for easy quantification of pathological vascular features with computer-aided imaging software. Both vaso-obliteration and neovascularization levels can be quantified as a percentage of total retinal areas in flat mounts [44, 51]. Moreover, preretinal neovascular tufts protruding into the vitreous cavity can also be visualized and quantified in cross-sections of eyes [9] (Fig. 2.2d). Vascular permeability can be visualized using fluorescent angiography and quantified by Miles assay [51–55]. Delayed retinal neuronal development or retinal thinning also occurs in OIR, mostly in the inner retina. Overall, the accessibility of genetic manipulation and the consistent and reliable induction of neovascularization make the mouse OIR model a popular one for studying ROP pathogenesis. In addition, OIR is a reliable model for the proliferative aspect of diabetic retinopathy and useful for investigating other diseases related to abnormal neovascularization.

The mouse OIR model reproduces vaso-obliteration and neovascularization consistently, contributing to its broad use in ROP research. Yet one limitation is that the area of vaso-obliteration locates in the central part of the retinas, unlike the peripheral avascular regions in humans. This geographic localization of the peripheral avascular region is recapitulated better in the rat OIR model with cycling oxygen exposure. In addition, there are strain-dependent differences in mouse angiogenic response and hence OIR susceptibility [56, 57]. In general, 129S strains with mixed background are more angiogenic and show higher levels of neovascular response in OIR than inbred C57BL/6 strains do, and the albino BALB/cByJ strain is even less angiogenic than C57BL/6. Moreover, vender-related substrain differences in OIR neovascularization may also exist, even within the same strain [17]. These strain considerations need to be taken into account when choosing appropriate OIR mouse strains.

Another important consideration for interpreting the OIR phenotype is postnatal weight gain of mouse pups during OIR. Postnatal weight gain is a reliable predictor for the severity of clinical ROP in infants [58–60]. Similarly, in the mouse OIR model, pups with poor postnatal weight gain (<5 g at P17) reveal dampened vascular response and prolonged phase of retinopathy compared with medium postnatal weight gain (5 g-7.5 g at P17) and extensive postnatal weight gain (>7.5 g at P17) pups [61]. Monitoring mouse weight gain and keeping them in the normal range is necessary for proper interpretation of OIR data. Runty pups (<5 g) with poor OIR responses should be excluded from data analysis. Other factors, such as the hypoxic effect on lactating mothers [42, 62], may affect maternal care of pups and the susceptibility and severity of the OIR phenotype, hence surrogate mouse mothers may be used when needed.

The mouse OIR model greatly facilitated the investigation of various molecular pathways in developmental and pathological retinal angiogenesis, particularly the discovery of

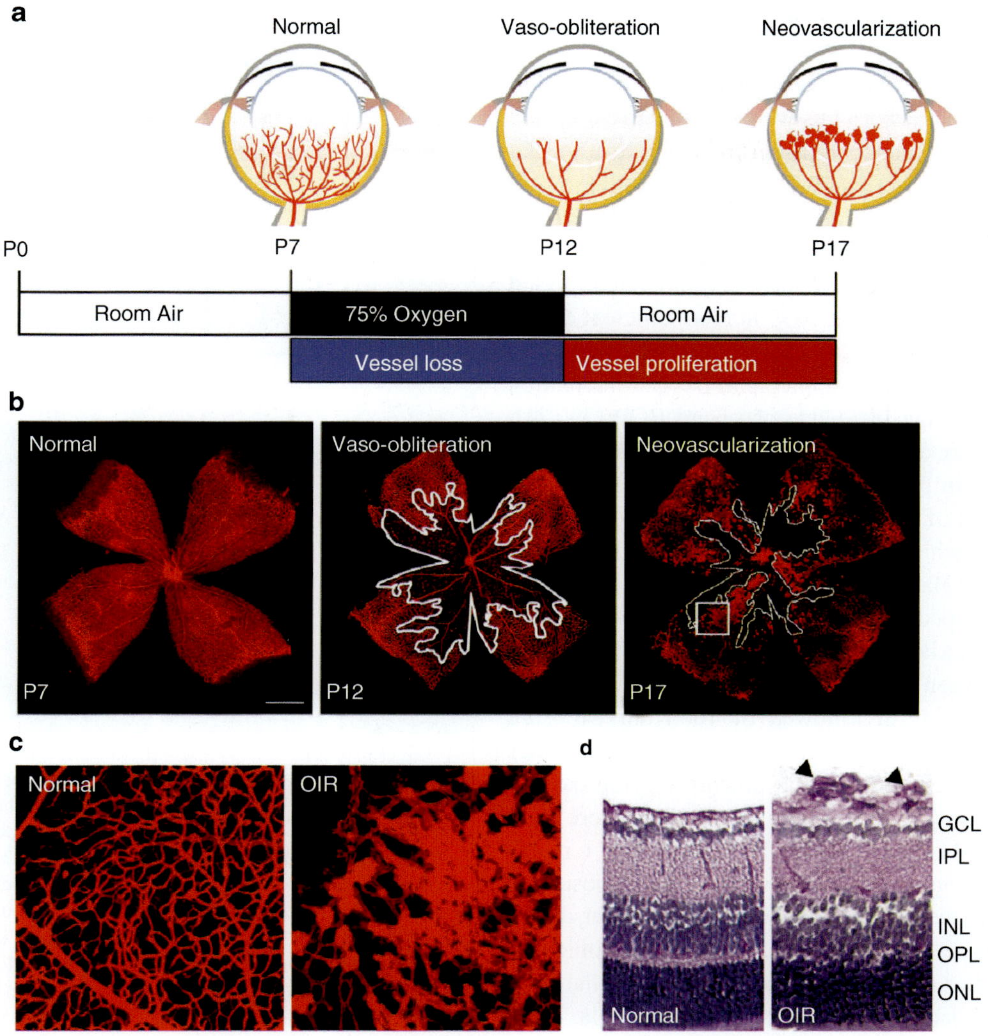

Fig. 2.2 The mouse model of oxygen-induced retinopathy (OIR). (**a**) A schematic diagram illustrates the procedure of mouse OIR. Neonatal litters are exposed to 75% ± 2% oxygen from P7-P12. Hyperoxia suppresses retinal vascular development and leads to the regression of existing immature retinal vessels, resulting in a central zone of vaso-obliteration. At P12, mice are returned to room air, and the relative hypoxia triggers vessel regrowth toward the vaso-obliteration zone as well as pathological neovascularization at the border between the vascular and avascular areas. The levels of neovascularization reach maximum severity at P17. (**b**) Representative images of retinal flat mounts with isolectin staining (red) in the normoxic and OIR retinas show the normal retinal vasculature at P7 (left panel), vaso-obliteration at P12 (middle panel; the area of vessel loss is outlined in white), and pathologic neovascularization at P17 (right panel; the vessel loss area is outlined with a white dashed line). Scale Bar: 1 mm. (**c**) Magnified images of isolectin-stained retinal flat mounts show the normal vasculature (left panel) from normoxia mice and pathological neovessels in the OIR mouse at P17. Right panel image was enlarged from the rectangular region in (**b**). (**d**) Cross-sections of mouse retinas with normoxia (left panel) and OIR (right panel) at P17. The sprouting neovascular tufts (arrows) in the OIR mouse arise from the superficial retinal vascular layer and protrude into the vitreous. GCL, ganglion cell layer; INL, inner nuclear layer; IPL, inner plexiform layer; ONL, outer nuclear layer; OPL, outer plexiform layer. Figure was adapted and reprinted with permission from Liu et al. [36]

VEGF's role in retinopathy. By utilizing the mouse OIR model, previous pioneering studies demonstrated that VEGF induces pathologic retinal neovascularizaion [49] and that inhibition of VEGF suppresses retinal neovascularization in the OIR mouse eyes [48]. This work, together with studies in other ocular angiogenesis animal models [63–66], laid the experimental foundation for developing current anti-VEGF therapies to treat neovascular age-related macular degeneration and ROP. Besides VEGF, other angiogenic factors, such as EPO [47, 50, 67] and additional signaling pathways, are extensively studied in the OIR model. In addition, factors critical in the third trimester and deficient after preterm birth, such as insulin-like growth factors and omega-3 polyunsaturated fatty acids [18, 19], have also been evaluated utilizing the mouse OIR model (which demonstrated that supplementing these factors is beneficial).

2.2.3 The Rat Model of OIR

The rat model of ROP was first demonstrated by Patz [16] in 1954. In that study, newborn rats were exposed to a constant level of high oxygen concentration (60–80%), resulting in preretinal neovascularization [16]. Subsequent studies using rats exposed to hyperoxia conditions also demonstrated abnormal vaso-proliferation with varying inconsistencies [68, 69]. Over the years, investigators explored and revised protocols for modeling human ROP in more efficient experiment settings [70–72]. Clinical studies revealed that, besides continuous oxygen supplement, oxygen fluctuation also contributes to the incidence of severe ROP [73, 74]. The partial pressure of dissolved arterial oxygen may fluctuate very quickly in premature infants, leading to the alternating occurrence of severe and extended hyperoxemia and hypoxemia [73], which in turn may lead to a higher risk of developing ROP. Based on these observations, Penn and colleagues developed the current rat model, which utilizes alternating hyperoxia–hypoxia cycles, in which the oxygen levels cycle between 50% and 10% every 24 hours for the first 14 days after birth followed by room air exposure through P20 [8, 11, 75] (Fig. 2.3). This rat model recreates oxygen tension fluctuation, which mirrors varying oxygen levels measured in preterm infants developing severe ROP [11], whereas in the mouse model the oxygen level remains constant during continuous oxygen exposure. Exposure to cycling levels of oxygen retards the retinal vascular development, leading to a peripheral avascular zone mimicking human ROP. After returning to room air, neovascular tufts grow at the boundary between vascular and avascular areas in the mid-peripheral retina. One main advantage of the rat OIR model lies in its clinically relevant feature of ROP—delayed development of retinal vasculature followed by pathologic neovascularization. The vaso-obliteration phenotype in the rat OIR model is highly reminiscent of the peripheral avascular zone observed in human ROP, whereas in the mouse model it is the central retinal vessels that are obliterated [76, 77]. Disadvantages of the rat model include lack of genetically modified animals, stain-dependent variation in response, and relatively inconsistent and low levels of neovascularization, which together limit its use in evaluating antiangiogenic therapies.

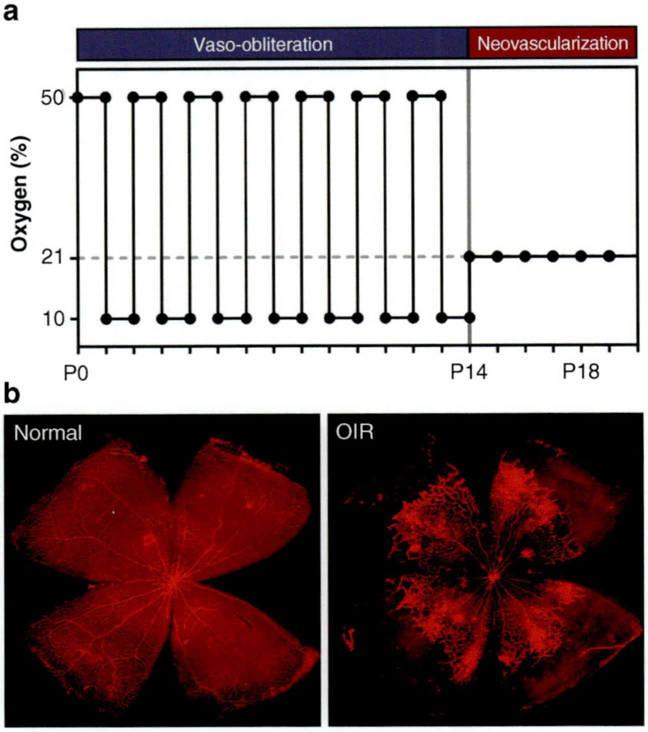

Fig. 2.3 The rat model of oxygen-induced retinopathy (OIR). (**a**) A schematic illustrates the rat OIR regimen, the 50/10 model. This model exposes neonatal rat litters to alternating 24-hour periods of 50% and 10% oxygen from P0 to P14. After 14 days of variable oxygen, rats are returned to room air (21% oxygen), inducing the development of neovascularization. (**b**) Representative retinal flat mount images of normoxic and the 50/10 OIR rat retinas. Retinas were collected from P18 normal (left panel) and OIR (right panel) rats followed by isolectin-staining to visualize the vasculature. Rat retinas with OIR show delayed vascular development in the peripheral area with a vaso-obliterated zone and neovascularization at the boundary of vascular and avascular areas. Panel b: Image courtesy of Dr. James D. Akula, Boston Children's Hospital, Harvard Medical School, Boston, MA, USA

2.2.4 The Zebrafish Model

The zebrafish, albeit not directly relevant for clinical ROP, is an alternative model for studying angiogenesis-dependent ocular diseases and drug screening [78]. An adult zebrafish model of hypoxia-induced retinopathy was generated [30, 79], utilizing blood vessel-specific stable fluorescent reporter transgenic zebrafish [80, 81]. When placed in a hypoxic aquarium with 10% air saturation (820 parts per billion) for 3–12 days, new retinal vessel sprouts reached a plateau of maximal angiogenic responses at day 12 [30, 79]. Subsequently, an embryonic model of ROP was also developed using hypoxia-inducing chemical agents to stimulate abnormal retinal angiogenesis in zebrafish embryos [82].

2.2.5 Hyperglycemia-Associated ROP Models

Neonatal hyperglycemia, common in extremely preterm infants, has been recognized as an ROP risk factor [20–23]. Neonatal hyperglycemia often occurs in preterm infants receiving glucose infusion and is related to incomplete suppression of hepatic glucose production after infusion, inadequate pancreatic beta-cell response, and insulin insensitivity [83–86]. A hyperglycemia-associated retinopathy model was generated in neonatal rats by using a single injection of streptozotocin (STZ) at P1 [24]. Sustained hyperglycemia was induced rapidly from P2/3 to P6, and retinal angiogenesis is inhibited, with associated inflammatory response and inner retinal neuron degeneration within 2 weeks postnatally [24]. Recently, a similar mouse model of hyperglycemia-associated ROP was developed with daily injections of STZ from P1 to P9. Hyperglycemia was induced at P8, followed by delayed deep layer retinal vessel growth and photoreceptor dysfunction [25]. Together these models recapitulate delayed vascular development of ROP and may help elucidate the mechanisms of hyperglycemia-induced retinal damage in ROP.

2.3 Summary

ROP remains a leading cause of visual impairment and a challenge in neonatology worldwide. Animal models of ROP have evolved over the past several decades with vast amounts of research efforts directed toward better understanding of the pathogenesis of ROP, especially in the mechanisms governing retinal angiogenesis. The establishment of different experimental models allows investigators to explore the roles that many influencing factors (e.g., oxygen, light conditions, and hyperglycemia) play in ROP development. For instance, studies from the early feline, canine, and murine models of ROP provided compelling evidence that high levels of oxygen promoted obliteration of blood vessels in the developing retina [29, 69], suggesting the importance of titrating and close monitoring of exogenous oxygen administration to the preterm infants. Insights on an essential role of VEGF in ROP development were also derived from studies in OIR models, which facilitated the development of current anti-VEGF therapies.

Among several different species, the mouse model of OIR is the most representative model for studying ROP and other ocular diseases involving hypoxia-induced angiogenesis. As of December 2018, there are more than 700 PubMed publications using the mouse OIR model of ROP. These studies reflect the broad value of the mouse OIR model for studying mechanisms underlying pathological angiogenesis in retinal and tissue ischemia, including the roles of growth factors, fatty acids, inflammation, signaling cascades, metabolic and transcriptional regulation, and regulatory non-coding RNAs on ROP. In addition, the mouse OIR model, with its fast induction of consistent neovascularization, is also extensively used in evaluating antiangiogenic drugs, to facilitate the development of new therapies for ROP and other vascular eye disorders.

References

1. Terry TL. Fibroblastic overgrowth of persistent tunica vasculosa lentis in infants born prematurely: II. Report of cases-clinical aspects. Trans Am Ophthalmol Soc. 1942;40:262–84.
2. Coats DK. Retinopathy of prematurity: involution, factors predisposing to retinal detachment, and expected utility of preemptive surgical reintervention. Trans Am Ophthalmol Soc. 2005;103:281–312.
3. Hess JH. Oxygen unit for premature and very young infants. Am J Dis Chil. 1934;47:916–7.
4. Silverman WA. Retrolental fibroplasia: a modern parable. New York: Grune & Stratton; 1980.
5. Campbell K. Intensive oxygen therapy as a possible cause of retrolental fibroplasia; a clinical approach. Med J Aust. 1951;2:48–50.
6. Patz A, Hoeck LE, De La Cruz E. Studies on the effect of high oxygen administration in retrolental fibroplasia I. Nursery observations. Am J Ophthalmol. 1952;35:1248–53.
7. Kinsey VE. Retrolental fibroplasia; cooperative study of retrolental fibroplasia and the use of oxygen. AMA Arch Ophthalmol. 1956;56:481–543.
8. Penn JS, Tolman BL, Lowery LA. Variable oxygen exposure causes preretinal neovascularization in the newborn rat. Invest Ophthalmol Vis Sci. 1993;34:576–85.
9. Smith LE, et al. Oxygen-induced retinopathy in the mouse. Invest Ophthalmol Vis Sci. 1994;35:101–11.
10. Chen J, Smith LE. Retinopathy of prematurity. Angiogenesis. 2007;10:133–40.
11. Hartnett ME, Penn JS. Mechanisms and management of retinopathy of prematurity. N Engl J Med. 2012;367:2515–26.
12. Hellstrom A, Smith LE, Dammann O. Retinopathy of prematurity. Lancet. 2013;382:1445–57.
13. Hardy P, et al. Oxidants, nitric oxide and prostanoids in the developing ocular vasculature: a basis for ischemic retinopathy. Cardiovasc Res. 2000;47:489–509.
14. Schaffer DB, The Cryotherapy for Retinopathy of Prematurity Cooperative Group, et al. Prognostic factors in the natural course of retinopathy of prematurity. Ophthalmology. 1993;100:230–7.
15. Foos RY. Chronic retinopathy of prematurity. Ophthalmology. 1985;92:563–74.
16. Patz A. Oxygen studies in retrolental fibroplasia. IV. Clinical and experimental observations. Am J Ophthalmol. 1954;38:291–308.
17. Stahl A, et al. The mouse retina as an angiogenesis model. Invest Ophthalmol Vis Sci. 2010;51:2813–26.
18. Connor KM, et al. Increased dietary intake of omega-3-polyunsaturated fatty acids reduces pathological retinal angiogenesis. Nat Med. 2007;13:868–73.
19. Smith LE, et al. Regulation of vascular endothelial growth factor-dependent retinal neovascularization by insulin-like growth factor-1 receptor. Nat Med. 1999;5:1390–5.
20. Garg R, Agthe AG, Donohue PK, Lehmann CU. Hyperglycemia and retinopathy of prematurity in very low birth weight infants. J Perinatol. 2003;23:186–94.
21. Blanco CL, Baillargeon JG, Morrison RL, Gong AK. Hyperglycemia in extremely low birth weight infants in a predominantly Hispanic population and related morbidities. J Perinatol. 2006;26:737–41.
22. Kaempf JW, et al. Hyperglycemia, insulin and slower growth velocity may increase the risk of retinopathy of prematurity. J Perinatol. 2011;31:251–7.
23. Mohamed S, Murray JC, Dagle JM, Colaizy T. Hyperglycemia as a risk factor for the development of retinopathy of prematurity. BMC Pediatr. 2013;13:78.
24. Kermorvant-Duchemin E, et al. Neonatal hyperglycemia inhibits angiogenesis and induces inflammation and neuronal degeneration in the retina. PLoS One. 2013;8:e79545.

25. Fu Z, et al. Photoreceptor glucose metabolism determines normal retinal vascular growth. EMBO Mol Med. 2018;10:76–90.
26. Ashton N, Ward B, Serpell G. Effect of oxygen on developing retinal vessels with particular reference to the problem of retrolental fibroplasia. Br J Ophthalmol. 1954;38:397–432.
27. McLeod DS, Brownstein R, Lutty GA. Vaso-obliteration in the canine model of oxygen-induced retinopathy. Invest Ophthalmol Vis Sci. 1996;37:300–11.
28. Flower RW, Blake DA. Retrolental fibroplasia: evidence for a role of the prostaglandin cascade in the pathogenesis of oxygen-induced retinopathy in the newborn beagle. Pediatr Res. 1981;15:1293–302.
29. Patz A, Eastham A, Higginbotham DH, Kleh T. Oxygen studies in retrolental fibroplasia. II. The production of the microscopic changes of retrolental fibroplasia in experimental animals. Am J Ophthalmol. 1953;36:1511–22.
30. Cao R, Jensen LD, Soll I, Hauptmann G, Cao Y. Hypoxia-induced retinal angiogenesis in zebrafish as a model to study retinopathy. PLoS One. 2008;3:e2748.
31. Phelps DL, Rosenbaum AL. Effects of marginal hypoxemia on recovery from oxygen-induced retinopathy in the kitten model. Pediatrics. 1984;73:1–6.
32. Kimura T, Chen CH, Patz A. Light and electron microscopic studies of intravitreal proliferative tissues in human and puppy eyes (author's transl). Nippon Ganka Gakkai Zasshi. 1979;83:255–65.
33. McLeod DS, Crone SN, Lutty GA. Vasoproliferation in the neonatal dog model of oxygen-induced retinopathy. Invest Ophthalmol Vis Sci. 1996;37:1322–33.
34. McLeod DS, Lutty GA. Targeting VEGF in canine oxygen-induced retinopathy – a model for human retinopathy of prematurity. Eye Brain. 2016;8:55–65.
35. Young RW. Cell differentiation in the retina of the mouse. Anat Rec. 1985;212:199–205.
36. Liu CH, Wang Z, Sun Y, Chen J. Animal models of ocular angiogenesis: from development to pathologies. FASEB J. 2017;31:4665–81.
37. Chen J, Liu CH, Sapieha P. Anti-angiogenic therapy. In: Stahl A, editor. Ophthalmology. Cham: Springer; 2016. p. 1–19.
38. Fruttiger M. Development of the retinal vasculature. Angiogenesis. 2007;10:77–88.
39. Hartnett ME. Pediatric retina. London: Lippincott Williams & Wilkins; 2013.
40. Ito M, Yoshioka M. Regression of the hyaloid vessels and pupillary membrane of the mouse. Anat Embryol (Berl). 1999;200:403–11.
41. Gyllensten LJ, Hellstrom BE. Retrolental fibroplasia; animal experiments: the effect of intermittingly administered oxygen on the postnatal development of the eyes of fullterm mice. Acta Paediatr. 1952;41:577–82.
42. Gerschman R, Nadig PW, Snell AC Jr, Nye SW. Effect of high oxygen concentrations on eyes of newborn mice. Am J Phys. 1954;179:115–8.
43. Curley FJ, Habegger H, Ingalls TH, Philbrook FR. Retinopathy of immaturity in the newborn mouse after exposure to oxygen imbalances. Am J Ophthalmol. 1956;42:377–92.
44. Connor KM, et al. Quantification of oxygen-induced retinopathy in the mouse: a model of vessel loss, vessel regrowth and pathological angiogenesis. Nat Protoc. 2009;4:1565–73.
45. Lange C, et al. Kinetics of retinal vaso-obliteration and neovascularisation in the oxygen-induced retinopathy (OIR) mouse model. Graefes Arch Clin Exp Ophthalmol. 2009;247:1205–11.
46. Gu X, et al. Effects of sustained hyperoxia on revascularization in experimental retinopathy of prematurity. Invest Ophthalmol Vis Sci. 2002;43:496–502.
47. Chen J, Connor KM, Aderman CM, Smith LE. Erythropoietin deficiency decreases vascular stability in mice. J Clin Invest. 2008;118:526–33.
48. Aiello LP, et al. Suppression of retinal neovascularization in vivo by inhibition of vascular endothelial growth factor (VEGF) using soluble VEGF-receptor chimeric proteins. Proc Natl Acad Sci U S A. 1995;92:10457–61.
49. Pierce EA, Avery RL, Foley ED, Aiello LP, Smith LE. Vascular endothelial growth factor/vascular permeability factor expression in a mouse model of retinal neovascularization. Proc Natl Acad Sci U S A. 1995;92:905–9.
50. Chen J, et al. Suppression of retinal neovascularization by erythropoietin siRNA in a mouse model of proliferative retinopathy. Invest Ophthalmol Vis Sci. 2009;50:1329–35.
51. Stahl A, et al. Computer-aided quantification of retinal neovascularization. Angiogenesis. 2009;12:297–301.
52. Vahatupa M, et al. Lack of R-Ras Leads to Increased Vascular Permeability in Ischemic Retinopathy. Invest Ophthalmol Vis Sci. 2016;57:4898–909.
53. Chen J, Stahl A, Hellstrom A, Smith LE. Current update on retinopathy of prematurity: screening and treatment. Curr Opin Pediatr. 2011;23:173–8.
54. Fulton AB, et al. Retinal degenerative and hypoxic ischemic disease. Doc Ophthalmol. 2009;118:55–61.
55. Xu Q, Qaum T, Adamis AP. Sensitive blood-retinal barrier breakdown quantitation using Evans blue. Invest Ophthalmol Vis Sci. 2001;42:789–94.
56. Chan CK, et al. Differential expression of pro- and antiangiogenic factors in mouse strain-dependent hypoxia-induced retinal neovascularization. Lab Investig. 2005;85:721–33.
57. Ritter MR, et al. Myeloid progenitors differentiate into microglia and promote vascular repair in a model of ischemic retinopathy. J Clin Invest. 2006;116:3266–76.
58. Wallace DK, Kylstra JA, Phillips SJ, Hall JG. Poor postnatal weight gain: a risk factor for severe retinopathy of prematurity. J AAPOS. 2000;4:343–7.
59. Allegaert K, et al. Perinatal growth characteristics and associated risk of developing threshold retinopathy of prematurity. J AAPOS. 2003;7:34–7.
60. Lofqvist C, et al. Longitudinal postnatal weight and insulin-like growth factor I measurements in the prediction of retinopathy of prematurity. Arch Ophthalmol. 2006;124:1711–8.
61. Stahl A, et al. Postnatal weight gain modifies severity and functional outcome of oxygen-induced proliferative retinopathy. Am J Pathol. 2010;177:2715–23.
62. Gole GA, Browning J, Elts SM. The mouse model of oxygen-induced retinopathy: a suitable animal model for angiogenesis research. Doc Ophthalmol. 1990;74:163–9.
63. Miller JW, et al. Vascular endothelial growth factor/vascular permeability factor is temporally and spatially correlated with ocular angiogenesis in a primate model. Am J Pathol. 1994;145:574–84.
64. Shima DT, et al. Cloning and mRNA expression of vascular endothelial growth factor in ischemic retinas of *Macaca fascicularis*. Invest Ophthalmol Vis Sci. 1996;37:1334–40.
65. Adamis AP, et al. Inhibition of vascular endothelial growth factor prevents retinal ischemia-associated iris neovascularization in a nonhuman primate. Arch Ophthalmol. 1996;114:66–71.
66. Krzystolik MG, et al. Prevention of experimental choroidal neovascularization with intravitreal anti-vascular endothelial growth factor antibody fragment. Arch Ophthalmol. 2002;120:338–46.
67. Watanabe D, et al. Erythropoietin as a retinal angiogenic factor in proliferative diabetic retinopathy. N Engl J Med. 2005;353:782–92.
68. Brands KH, Hofmann H, Klees E. Not Available. Geburtshilfe Frauenheilkd. 1958;18:805–14.
69. Ashton N, Blach R. Studies on Developing Retinal Vessels Viii. Effect of Oxygen on the Retinal Vessels of the Ratling. Br J Ophthalmol. 1961;45:321–40.
70. Ricci B, Calogero G. Oxygen-induced retinopathy in newborn rats: effects of prolonged normobaric and hyperbaric oxygen supplementation. Pediatrics. 1988;82:193–8.

71. Penn JS, Tolman BL, Lowery LA, Koutz CA. Oxygen-induced retinopathy in the rat: hemorrhages and dysplasias may lead to retinal detachment. Curr Eye Res. 1992;11:939–53.
72. Ventresca MR, Gonder JR, Tanswell AK. Oxygen-induced proliferative retinopathy in the newborn rat. Can J Ophthalmol. 1990;25:186–9.
73. York JR, Landers S, Kirby RS, Arbogast PG, Penn JS. Arterial oxygen fluctuation and retinopathy of prematurity in very-low-birth-weight infants. J Perinatol. 2004;24:82–7.
74. Cunningham S, Fleck BW, Elton RA, McIntosh N. Transcutaneous oxygen levels in retinopathy of prematurity. Lancet. 1995;346:1464–5.
75. Penn JS, Rajaratnam VS, Collier RJ, Clark AF. The effect of an angiostatic steroid on neovascularization in a rat model of retinopathy of prematurity. Invest Ophthalmol Vis Sci. 2001;42:283–90.
76. Madan A, Penn JS. Animal models of oxygen-induced retinopathy. Front Biosci. 2003;8:d1030–43.
77. Grossniklaus HE, Kang SJ, Berglin L. Animal models of choroidal and retinal neovascularization. Prog Retin Eye Res. 2010;29:500–19.
78. Rezzola S, Paganini G, Semeraro F, Presta M, Tobia C. Zebrafish (*Danio rerio*) embryo as a platform for the identification of novel angiogenesis inhibitors of retinal vascular diseases. Biochim Biophys Acta. 2016;1862:1291–6.
79. Cao Z, et al. Hypoxia-induced retinopathy model in adult zebrafish. Nat Protoc. 2010;5:1903–10.
80. Alvarez Y, et al. Genetic determinants of hyaloid and retinal vasculature in zebrafish. BMC Dev Biol. 2007;7:114.
81. Weinstein BM, Stemple DL, Driever W, Fishman MC. Gridlock, a localized heritable vascular patterning defect in the zebrafish. Nat Med. 1995;1:1143–7.
82. Wu YC, et al. Hypoxia-induced retinal neovascularization in zebrafish embryos: a potential model of retinopathy of prematurity. PLoS One. 2015;10:e0126750.
83. Cowett RM, Rapoza RE, Gelardi NL. The contribution of glucose to neonatal glucose homeostasis in the lamb. Metabolism. 1998;47:1239–44.
84. Mitanchez-Mokhtari D, et al. Both relative insulin resistance and defective islet beta-cell processing of proinsulin are responsible for transient hyperglycemia in extremely preterm infants. Pediatrics. 2004;113:537–41.
85. Cowett RM, Oh W, Schwartz R. Persistent glucose production during glucose infusion in the neonate. J Clin Invest. 1983;71:467–75.
86. Sunehag A, Gustafsson J, Ewald U. Very immature infants (< or = 30 Wk) respond to glucose infusion with incomplete suppression of glucose production. Pediatr Res. 1994;36:550–5.

Evolution of Major Clinical Trials in ROP

3

Supalert Prakhunhungsit and Audina M. Berrocal

Abstract

Retinopathy of prematurity (ROP) is a vasoproliferative disorder occurring in premature infants' retinas. With the advances in neonatal care in recent years, ophthalmologists are increasingly encountering premature babies, who have higher risks of developing ROP. The occurrence and severity of ROP depend on several factors, which have been reported by various clinical trials. This chapter demonstrates the evolution of several aspects of major clinical trials in ROP, including its treatment, the role of oxygen in ROP development, and the roles of light and nutrients in ROP.

Keyword

Retinopathy of prematurity · Clinical trials · Treatment Oxygen · Light

3.1 Major Clinical Trials: ROP Treatment (Summary in Table 3.1)

3.1.1 The Multicenter Trial of Cryotherapy for ROP (CRYO-ROP) [1–5]

CRYO-ROP was one of the major trials in ROP, and most of the current clinical understanding of ROP derives from that study. This multicenter, randomized control trial of cryotherapy for the treatment of ROP aimed to evaluate the efficacy and safety of the treatment in preventing serious sequelae of ROP in very-low-birth-weight infants. The study registered 9751 infants with a birth weight of less than 1251 g. The patients were then screened for the development of threshold disease; this was defined as five or more contiguous, or eight cumulative, clock hours of stage 3 ROP in zone 1 or 2, in the presence of plus disease. In all, 291 patients were included in the final cohort. Two hundred and forty eyes were classified as symmetric cases, in which both eyes developed threshold ROP. In this group, one eye was randomized to receive cryotherapy while the other eye was observed as a control. The remaining 51 eyes were in the asymmetric group, and only the eyes that developed threshold ROP were included in the study and randomized to either cryotherapy or observation.

If cryotherapy was assigned, it was performed within 72 h and prior to the development of stage 4A ROP. Usually, a conjunctival incision was not required. Cryotherapy was then started at the ora serrata, followed by more-posterior applications. The cryotherapy applications were contiguous and single, with an endpoint of the sudden whitening of the retina; this equated to approximately 2–3 s of freeze time. All avascular retina anterior to the ROP ridge was treated. When there were skipped or untreated areas with a persistence of plus disease, retreatment was performed. The outcomes were measured by the development of unfavorable outcomes (posterior retinal detachment, retinal fold involving macula, or retrolental tissue).

Overall, approximately 82% of the patients had a symmetric disease, and 11 cases needed retreatment with cryotherapy. In the third month after treatment, 31.1% of the eyes that received treatment developed unfavorable outcomes, versus 51.4% of the control eyes; this represented a risk reduction of approximately 40%. No major complications were found. As this result supported the efficacy of cryotherapy in reducing the risk of unfavorable outcomes from threshold ROP, cryotherapy was subsequently recommended for both eyes with stage 3+ ROP in zone 1. The report of CRYO-ROP at 5.5 years was the first study from CRYO-ROP to demonstrate the functional outcomes of

S. Prakhunhungsit
Ophthalmology Department, Faculty of Medicine Siriraj Hospital, Mahidol University, Bangkok, Thailand

Bascom Palmer Eye Institute, University of Miami, Miller School of Medicine, Miami, FL, USA

A. M. Berrocal (✉)
Bascom Palmer Eye Institute, University of Miami, Miller School of Medicine, Miami, FL, USA
e-mail: aberrocal@med.miami.edu

W.-C. Wu, W.-C. Lam (eds.), *A Quick Guide to Pediatric Retina*, https://doi.org/10.1007/978-981-15-6552-6_3

Table 3.1 Summary of the major clinical trials in retinopathy of prematurity

Clinical trials	Objective	Criteria	Number enrolled	Intervention	Endpoint	Outcome measurement	Outcomes
CRYO-ROP (1986–2003)	To evaluate efficacy and safety of cryotherapy compared to observation	BW < 1251 g; survived to 28 days; and no major ocular or systemic congenital anomalies	291; 240 symmetric cases, and 51 asymmetric cases; one eye treated with cryotherapy, and the fellow eye as control; 247 patients followed and analyzed at year 10	Trans-scleral cryotherapy	Reports: Preliminary; 3 months; and 1, 3, 5.5, and 10 years	Structural unfavorable outcomes: Posterior retinal detachment, retinal folds involving macula, retrolental mass; visual function	At 3 mos: 31.3% cryo vs. 51.4% control had unfavorable outcomes. At 5.5 y: 47.1% cryo vs. 61.7% control had VA < 20/200; 26.9% cryo vs. 45.4% control had unfavorable structural outcomes. At 15.5 y: 44.7% cryo vs. 64.3% control had VA < 20/200; 30% vs. 51.9% had unfavorable structural outcomes.
ETROP (1999–2002)	To evaluate visual and structural outcomes of high-risk prethreshold ROP compared to threshold ROP	BW < 1251 g, and prethreshold ROP	828 prethreshold. 401 high risk (type 1) were randomized; 317 bilateral, and 84 asymmetric	Retinal ablation: Laser photocoagulation (cryotherapy allowed)	9 mos postmenstrual age	Visual function at 6 and 9 mos; structural outcomes at 9 mos.	Unfavorable VA; 19.5% threshold vs. 14.5% prethreshold (P = 0.01) and unfavorable structural outcomes; 15.6% threshold vs. 9.1% prethreshold (P < 0.001). Type 2: Wait-and-watch.
Laser compared to cryotherapy	Compare laser to cryo at 10 years for threshold ROP	Threshold ROP	118 eyes from 66 patients for treatment; 44 eyes from 25 patients were examined at 10 years	(1) laser vs. cryotherapy (2) refraction	10 years	(1) BCVA vs. retinal dragging (2) spherical equivalent	(1) mean BCVA: 20/66 laser vs. 20/182 cryo (P = 0.015); 7.2 times more retinal dragging in cryo eyes (95% CI, 1.54–3.36). (2) SE: −4.88 laser vs. -7.65 cryo (P = 0.019); lens power contributes to myopia.
BEAT-ROP (2008–2010)	To evaluate efficacy of bevacizumab for stage 3+ in zone I and posterior zone II	BW < 1500 g; GA < 30 weeks; and stage 3+ ROP in zone I or posterior zone II	150 infants (67 with zone I, and 83 with posterior zone II); 7 died; 75 laser, and 75 intravitreal injection	Intravitreal bevacizumab vs. laser	54 weeks postmenstrual age	Recurrence of ROP requiring treatment in either eye	4% bevacizumab vs. 22% laser (P = 0.002).

STOP-ROP (1994–1999)	Supplemental oxygen to reduce progression of prethreshold to threshold and need for retinal ablation	Prethreshold, and < 94% oxygen saturation in room air	325 conventional vs 324 supplemental	Conventional, SaO_2 89%–94% vs. supplemental, SaO_2 96%–99%	3 mos	Threshold ROP requiring treatment	Progression to threshold: 48% conventional vs. 41% supplemental. OR for progression after ROP baseline adjustment, 0.72 (95% CI, 0.52–1.01). Use of supplemental oxygen did not reduce ROP requiring treatment.
HOPE-ROP (1996–1999)	Compare to infants from STOP-ROP (SaO_2 < 94%)	Prethreshold in one eye, and median SaO_2 > 94%	136 infants vs. 229 STOP-ROP	None	Progressed to threshold ROP or resolved	Number of progressions	Progression to threshold: 25% HOPE-ROP vs. 46% STOP-ROP (OR, 0.607; 95% CI, 0.359–1.026); not statistically significant.
SUPPORT (2005–2009)	Compare target of oxygen saturation	GA 24 wks to 27.6 wks; decision for full resuscitation; and no major anomalies.	1316 infants; 654 (lower group) vs. 662 (higher group)	Target oxygen saturation: 85%–89% vs 91%–95%	36 wks postmenstrual age or did not need ventilator for 72 h, whichever first	Composite outcomes of severe ROP (threshold; need intervention or intravitreal injection), death, or both	No significant difference between the two groups in terms of composite outcomes ($P = 0.21$). Death excluded, the lower group: Less cases of severe ROP ($P < 0.001$). More deaths before discharge in the lower group ($P = 0.04$).
LIGHT-ROP (1995–1997)	Assess the effects of lighting conditions on the incidence in high-risk infants	BW < 1251 g, and GA < 31 wks	188 with goggles, and 173 in control	Goggles	Postconceptional age of 31 weeks or 4 weeks after birth	Any ROP	ROP development: 54% with goggles vs. 58% control ($P = 0.50$).
Vitamin E (1978–1981)	Increased serum vitamin E reduced stage 3+ ROP	BW ≤ 1500 g.	1414 VLBW infants; 704 vitamin E vs. 714 controls	Vitamin E prophylaxis	Stage 3+ ROP	Incidence of ROP stage 3+	Stage 3+ incidence: 2.4% vitamin E vs. 5.3% control ($P < 0.02$). 52% reduction in the incidence of stage 3+ ROP. Unable to assess adverse effects.

Abbreviations: *cryo* cryotherapy, *BCVA* best-corrected visual acuity, *BW* birth weight, *CI* confidence interval, *GA* gestational age, *OR* odds ratio, *ROP* retinopathy of prematurity, SaO_2 oxygen saturation, *SE* spherical equivalent, *VA* visual acuity, *VLBW* very low birth weight these groups of patients. The data revealed that the eyes that were treated with cryotherapy were much less likely to be blind; instead, they tended to have visual acuity ranging from 20/60 to 20/200. The risk of unfavorable functional outcomes was decreased from 61.7% in the control eyes to 47.1% in the treated eyes ($P < 0.005$). Anatomically, the outcomes showed a reduction in the unfavorable outcomes in the treated versus control eyes (26.9% vs 45.4%, respectively; $P < 0.001$). In the tenth year after treatment, 247 patients were being monitored. Functionally, 44.4% of the treated eyes had a visual acuity of 20/200 or worse, compared to 62.1% for the control eyes ($P < 0.001$). In addition, the total retinal detachment rate remained the same as the 5-year result (22.0%). In the fifteenth year, 30% of the treated eyes developed unfavorable structural outcomes, compared with 51.9% of the control eyes ($P < 0.001$). Unfavorable visual acuity outcomes were found in 44.7% of the treated group, compared to 64.3% of the control eyes.

In conclusion, the CRYO-ROP results support the long-term efficacy and safety of cryotherapy in the treatment of threshold ROP. However, the treated patients still experienced a high rate of unfavorable functional and structural outcomes after treatment with cryotherapy when the patients were monitored to the last follow-up point.

3.1.2 Cryotherapy Versus Laser Photocoagulation [6, 7]

Randomized control trials were conducted by Connolly et al. and included 118 eyes from 66 patients with threshold ROP, who were treated with either cryotherapy or laser treatment. At 10 years post-treatment, the laser group had better visual outcomes, with a mean of the best-corrected visual of 20/66, whereas the cryotherapy group had a mean of 20/182 ($P = 0.015$). Moreover, the laser-treated eyes were 5.2 times more likely than the cryotherapy eyes to have a best-corrected visual acuity of 20/50 or better. Structurally, the eyes treated with cryotherapy developed 7.2 times more retinal dragging than the laser-treated patients, which was consistent with the poorer visual outcomes of the cryotherapy group [6]. In terms of refraction, Ng et al. reported the same group of patients that cryotherapy eyes were significantly more myopic than those that received laser treatment. The mean of the spherical equivalent for the laser-treated patients was −4.48 diopters while the cryotherapy patients had a mean spherical equivalent of −7.65 diopters ($P = 0.019$). Interestingly, a longer axial length was observed in the laser group (laser group, 22.9 mm. vs. cryotherapy group, 22.7 mm; $P = 0.024$). However, the cryotherapy patients had greater lens thickness (cryotherapy, 4.33 vs laser, 3.95; $P = < 0.001$). Therefore, the lens component, from the lens thickness and crystalline lens power, seemed to be a predominant part of the greater myopic progression in the cryotherapy eyes [7].

3.1.3 Early Treatment for Retinopathy of Prematurity Randomized Trial (ETROP) [8, 9]

Despite adequate treatment with cryotherapy in threshold ROP in the CRYO-ROP study, the treated patients still experienced a high rate of unsatisfactory outcomes both in visual acuity and retinal structure. At the last follow-up of the CRYO-ROP, 44.4% of the treated patients ultimately developed a poor visual acuity (worse than 20/200), and 30% of the treatment group experienced an unfavorable retinal structure. The need for an effort to identify earlier treatment criteria was raised by the ETROP study; this would result in the earlier treatment of eyes at risk of developing threshold ROP or unfavorable outcomes if left untreated.

The study included patients who had a birth weight of less than 1251 grams and had survived at least 28 days, and who were located at 26 participating centers. The patients were first screened for ROP at the chronological age of 6 weeks and they were followed from 1 to 2 weeks. The risk of developing high-risk prethreshold was subsequently calculated by the coordinating center using the Risk Model for Retinopathy of Prematurity 2, a risk model analysis program based on longitudinal data acquired by the CRYO-ROP study. The high-risk prethreshold eyes (defined as those that reached 15% or more of developing unfavorable outcomes by the model) were assigned at random to ablative treatment within 48 h. Only the high-risk patients were randomized because a significant number of eyes undergo spontaneous ROP resolution. The other eyes in the bilateral cases were observed as control and treated only when they developed threshold disease, in accordance with the standard of care derived from CRYO-ROP at that time. Generally, the main ablative treatment was laser treatment, but cryotherapy was also allowed in the study. Infants with threshold ROP (as defined by the CRYO-ROP study) before the randomization process were excluded from the study.

A total of 828 infants developed prethreshold ROP in at least one eye. Of the cohort, 401 eyes were at high-risk prethreshold disease and were enrolled for randomization. At the corrected age of 9 months, visual acuity was assessed; it revealed that the early treatment resulted in a reduction in unfavorable outcomes from 19.5% to 14.5% ($P = 0.01$). The unfavorable structural outcomes were also reduced from 15.6% to 9.1% ($P < 0.001$). A further analysis of the study also recommended the use of ablative treatment in cases with type 1 ROP, which was defined as:

- Zone I, any stage ROP with plus disease
- Zone I, stage 3 ROP without plus disease or
- Zone II, stage 2 or 3 ROP with plus disease

Furthermore, from the analysis, it was recommended that no ablative treatment be applied for type 2 ROP unless it progresses to type 1 ROP or threshold disease. In other words, a wait-and-watch approach was recommended for those type 2 ROP infants.

Later, the ETROP study reported the final visual acuities of the patients at the age of 6 years, with comparisons between the early treatment and the conventional treatment groups. The results demonstrated the benefits of early treatment for type 1 ROP but not for type 2 ROP (25.1% vs 32.8% unfavorable outcomes; P = 0.02). Therefore, the data supported the use of the early treatment scheme for type 1 ROP, but not type 2, because as many as 52% of type 2 ROP (low-risk prethreshold) spontaneously regressed without requiring treatment.

3.1.4 Efficacy of Intravitreal Bevacizumab for Stage 3+ Retinopathy of Prematurity (BEAT-ROP) [10, 11]

BEAT-ROP was a prospective, randomized, multicenter study that compared the efficacy of standard laser-therapy treatment with intravitreal bevacizumab as monotherapy treatment for stage 3 ROP with plus disease in zone I or posterior zone II. The 150 infants in the trial had a birth weight of 1500 grams or less, a gestational age of 30 weeks or less, and stage 3+ ROP in zone I or posterior zone II; a total of 300 eyes were studied. The first eye examination started at 4 weeks of chronological age or 31 weeks of postmenstrual age, whichever came later. The enrolled infants with stage 3+ ROP in zone I or posterior zone II were randomized to a bevacizumab injection (0.625 mg in 0.025 ml) versus a conventional laser. Fundus imaging of all infants was performed with a RetCam camera before and after the treatment, and the images were sent to a BEAT-ROP reading center for interpretation. The primary outcome was the recurrence of retinopathy that occurred before the postmenstrual age of 54 months and that required treatment in one or both eyes.

By 54 weeks of postmenstrual age, only 143 eyes were left for analysis. Before then, seven infants (five in the bevacizumab group, and two in the laser-therapy group) had died and were not included in the primary outcome analyses. The statistically significant result was a decreased rate of recurrent retinopathy in the bevacizumab-group infants with stage 3+ in zone I compared to those in the conventional laser-treatment group (laser group, 42% vs. bevacizumab group, 6%; odds ratio [OR] with bevacizumab, 0.09; 95% confidence interval [CI], 0.02–0.43; P = 0.003), whereas it was not significantly different for disease in posterior zone II (P = 0.27). The time to recurrence was 16.0 ± 4.6 weeks (mean ± SD) for six eyes from the bevacizumab group, compared with 6.2 ± 5.7 weeks for 32 eyes from the conventional laser group. This emphasized the need for careful follow-up of infants treated with an intravitreal injection. Moreover, the study also demonstrated the advantages of the intravitreal injection over laser treatment in terms of retinal vessel growth; the progression of retinal vessels was observed beyond the previous stage III ridge, with regression of the extraretinal neovascularization after the intravitreal injection of bevacizumab. However, the number of participants in this study was too small to assess the safety of the intravitreal injection therapy.

In conclusion, the intravitreal bevacizumab monotherapy showed a significant benefit for stage 3+ ROP in zone I, but not in posterior zone II, disease. The peripheral retinal vessels developed without interruption after the treatment with intravitreal bevacizumab.

3.2 Major Clinical Trials: The Role of Oxygen

3.2.1 Supplemental Therapeutic Oxygen for Prethreshold Retinopathy of Prematurity (STOP-ROP) [12]

Retinal hypoxia from the peripheral avascular retina in ROP contributes to neovascularization. Therefore, supplemental oxygen might be beneficial in reducing the hypoxic environment and downregulating the hypoxia-induced neovascularization in the premature infants' eyes. The STOP-ROP study undertook an evaluation of the efficacy and safety of the use of supplemental oxygen for the treatment of prethreshold ROP in order to decrease the chance of progression to threshold disease and to reduce the need for subsequent ablative treatment. Infants with prethreshold ROP in at least one eye and with an oxygen saturation below 94% were enrolled from 30 centers over the 5-year period. They were randomized into two groups: a control group, which targeted a pulse oximetry of 89% to 94%, and a supplemental group, which aimed for 96% to 99% for at least 2 weeks. The patients were followed to the endpoint of the study, which was determined to be either full vascularization to the retinal periphery or regression of ROP into zone III.

The results showed that 48% of infants in the control arm ultimately reached the disease threshold, whereas only 41% in the supplemental oxygen arm did. However, after adjustment for baseline characteristics, the supplemental oxygen strategy failed to demonstrate the chance of a reduction in the threshold ROP development (OR, 0.72; 95% CI, 0.52–1.01). Also, the use of supplemental oxygen was unable to reduce the number of patients who finally underwent subsequent ablative treatment. Not only did the trial fail to prove the efficacy of supplemental oxygen, but it also showed the risk of adverse pulmonary events, such as pneumonia and chronic lung disease exacerbation. The use of supplemental oxygen was no longer considered as an ROP treatment strategy.

3.2.2 High Oxygen Percentage in Retinopathy of Prematurity Study (HOPE-ROP Study) [13]

HOPE-ROP, the parallel study of STOP-ROP, included a patient who had an arterial oxygen saturation by pulse oximetry above 94% in room air at the time of the prethreshold diagnosis which was excluded from STOP-ROP. A comparison was made between patients who had an oxygen saturation above 94% (HOPE-ROP patients) versus below 94% (STOP-ROP patients) to determine the rate of progression from prethreshold ROP to threshold disease. The results revealed a difference in baseline characteristics, including a greater gestational age and a greater postmenstrual age in the 136 HOPE-ROP infants. Consequently, 25% of the HOPE-ROP infants developed threshold ROP at the endpoint, while 46% of the STOP-ROP infants did. Unfortunately, after baseline-characteristics adjustment, the study failed to show clinical significance for the targeted high oxygenation use on prethreshold ROP babies (OR, 0.61; 95% CI, 0.359–1.026).

3.2.3 Target Ranges of Oxygen Saturation in Extremely Preterm Infants (the Surfactant, Positive Pressure, and Oxygenation Randomized Trial (SUPPORT) [14]

The SUPPORT study aimed to clarify the optimal range of oxygen saturation to minimize the risk of ROP development without increasing the adverse outcomes. The study was a controlled multicenter trial with a 2-by-2 factorial design, and it compared two oxygen saturation targets and two ventilation approaches. It included 1316 extremely preterm infants (defined as a gestational age between 24 weeks and 27 weeks 6 days). The lower-oxygen-saturation group was defined as a targeted oxygen saturation 85%–89%, whereas the higher-oxygen-saturation group was between 91 and 95%. The primary outcome was the composite of severe retinopathy, death before discharge, or both. The severe retinopathy included threshold ROP, a need for surgical intervention, or bevacizumab use.

The outcomes showed no significant differences between the two groups in terms of the composite outcome; severe retinopathy or death (lower-oxygen-saturation group, 28.3%, and higher-oxygen-saturation group, 32.1%; relative risk [RR], 0.90; 95% CI, 0.76–1.06; P = 0.21). However, when death is excluded from the composite outcome, the lower-oxygen-saturation group had a lower incidence of severe ROP development (8.6% vs. 17.9%; RR, 0.52; 95% CI, 0.37–0.73; P < 0.001). In contrast, the lower-oxygen-saturation group experienced a larger number of deaths before hospital discharge (19.9% of infants vs. 16.2%; RR, 1.27; 95% CI, 1.01–1.60; P = 0.04). In conclusion, the study showed a large reduction in the incidence of severe ROP among infants who survived, but there was an increased rate of mortality that would be of concern if the strategy of a low-oxygen-saturation target for preterm infants was implemented.

3.2.4 Systematic Review and Meta-analysis

A recent meta-analysis of 67 studies, which included 21,819 ROP infants, revealed a 14% reduction in the risk of overall ROP development in the lower oxygen saturation group, as defined by each study (RR, 0.86; 95% CI, 0.77–0.97). Moreover, there was a 42% risk reduction in the severe ROP or ROP requiring treatment group (RR, 0.58; 95% CI, 0.45–0.74). However, the lower oxygen saturation increased the mortality rate (RR, 1.15; 95% CI, 1.04–1.29) [15]. However, a different conclusion was reached by another meta-analysis that included the results of five clinical trials. The rate of ROP development was similar for two groups with different oxygen saturation targets (restricted group with oxygen saturation, 85%–89%, versus liberal group with oxygen saturation, 91%–95%). The differences in the conclusion of these studies could result from different assessments of the quality of each outcome and bias. However, in the restricted oxygen saturation group, a significant mortality rate before hospital discharge was found (RR, 1.18; 95% CI, 1.03–1.36) [16]. Overall, the ideal oxygen saturation strategy for ROP still remains uncertain. Many other factors need to be considered for the best ocular and systemic-result outcomes.

3.3 Major Clinical Trial: The Role of Light

3.3.1 Lack of Efficacy of Light Reduction in Preventing Retinopathy of Prematurity (LIGHT-ROP) [17]

Light exposure was considered as one of the causes of ROP in the past. Without adequate support from studies, however, the hypothesis that exposure of infants' eyes to light resulted in the generation of free radicals was doubted. LIGHT-ROP was a prospective, randomized, and multicenter study that was designed to assess the effects of the ambient-lighting conditions of neonatal intensive care nurseries on the incidence of retinopathy of prematurity in high-risk infants. The study included premature infants with a birth weight less than 1251 grams and a gestational age less than 31 weeks. The infants were randomized to two groups; goggles were placed on the infants in the first group, whereas the infants in the other group were exposed to the conventional lighting conditions in an intensive care unit, without the use of goggles. The goggles were placed on the infants within 24 h of their birth; they were retained until the postconceptional age of 31 weeks or 4 weeks after birth. The babies were then examined for the incidence of ROP by ophthalmologists who were masked to the treatment of the individual infants. The results showed similar baseline characteristics of the patients in both groups. In the case of the goggles group, 54% of the patients were diagnosed with ROP, which was slightly less than the figure of 58% for the control group (RR, 0.9; 95% CI, 0.8–1.1; P = 0.50). It was concluded that the reduction in the light exposure levels did not alter the incidence of ROP.

3.4 Major Clinical Trial: The Role of Nutrients

3.4.1 Vitamin E Prophylaxis to Reduce Retinopathy of Prematurity: A Reappraisal of Published Trial [18]

The role of vitamin E as an anti-oxidant in influencing the clinical course of ROP is in doubt. Many clinical trials have studied the role of vitamin E as a prophylaxis treatment for ROP. This particular meta-analysis study included a total of six trials. Together, they enrolled 1414 very-low-birth-weight infants (704 in the vitamin E prophylaxis group, and 714 in the control group). Overall, the total incidence of ROP development in the two groups was similar. However, the incidence of stage 3+ ROP was lower in the group receiving vitamin E (vitamin E group, 2.4% vs. control, 5.3%). The study reported a 52% overall reduction in the incidence of stage 3+ ROP after receiving vitamin E. However, the study had some limitations. Firstly, the number of clinical trials included, six, gave low power to detect homogeneity for analysis. In addition, many neonatal care practices were not uniformly controlled, which could be a confounding factor for ROP development.

References

1. Cryotherapy for Retinopathy of Prematurity Cooperative Group. Multicenter trial of cryotherapy for retinopathy of prematurity. Preliminary results. Arch Ophthalmol. 1988;106:471–9.
2. Cryotherapy for Retinopathy of Prematurity Cooperative Group. Multicenter trial of cryotherapy for retinopathy of prematurity. Three-month outcome. Arch Ophthalmol. 1990;108:195–204.
3. Cryotherapy for Retinopathy of Prematurity Cooperative Group. Multicenter trial of cryotherapy for retinopathy of prematurity. One year outcome-structure and function. Arch Ophthalmol. 1990;108:1408–16.
4. Cryotherapy for Retinopathy of Prematurity Cooperative group. Multicenter trial of cryotherapy for retinopathy of prematurity: natural history ROP: ocular outcome at 5 1/2 years in premature infants with birth weight less than 1251 g. Arch Ophthalmol. 2002;120:595–9.
5. Cryotherapy for Retinopathy of Prematurity Cooperative Group. Multicenter trial of cryotherapy for retinopathy of prematurity: ophthalmological outcomes at 10 years. Arch Ophthalmol. 2001;119:1110–8.
6. Ng EY, Connolly BP, McNamara JA, Regillo CD, Vander JF, Tasman W. A comparison of laser photocoagulation with cryotherapy for threshold retinopathy of prematurity at 10 years: part 1. Visual function and structural outcome. Ophthalmology. 2002 May 1;109(5):928–34.
7. Connolly BP, Ng EY, McNamara JA, Regillo CD, Vander JF, Tasman W. A comparison of laser photocoagulation with cryotherapy for threshold retinopathy of prematurity at 10 years: part 2. Refractive outcome. Ophthalmology. 2002 May 1;109(5):936–41.
8. Good WV, Early Treatment for Retinopathy of Prematurity Cooperative Group. Final results of the early treatment for retinopathy of prematurity (ETROP) randomized trial. Trans Am Ophthalmol Soc. 2004;102:233–48.
9. Early Treatment for Retinopathy of Prematurity Cooperative Group, Good WV, Hardy RJ, Dobson V, Palmer EA, Phelps DL, Tung B, Redford M. Final visual acuity results in the early treatment for retinopathy of prematurity study. Arch Ophthalmol. 2010 Jun;128(6):663–71.
10. Mintz-Hittner HA, Ronal RK Jr. Intravitreal injection of bevacizumab (Avastin) for treatment of stage 3 retinopathy of prematurity in zone I or posterior zone II. Retina. 2008 Jun 1;28(6):831–8.
11. Mintz-Hittner HA, Kennedy KA, Chuang AZ. Efficacy of intravitreal bevacizumab for stage 3+ retinopathy of prematurity. N Engl J Med. 2011 Feb 17;364(7):603–15.
12. STOP-ROP Multicenter Study Group. Supplemental therapeutic oxygen for prethreshold retinopathy of prematurity (STOP-ROP), a randomized, controlled trial. I: primary outcomes. Pediatrics. 2000 Feb 1;105(2):295–310.
13. McGregor ML, Bremer DL, Cole C, McClead RE, Phelps DL, Fellows RR, Oden N, HOPE-ROP Multicenter Group. High oxygen percentage in retinopathy of prematurity study. Retinopathy of prematurity outcome in infants with prethreshold retinopathy of prematurity and oxygen saturation > 94% in room air: the high oxygen percentage in retinopathy of prematurity study. Pediatrics. 2002;110(3):540–4.
14. SUPPORT Study Group of the Eunice Kennedy Shriver NICHD Neonatal Research Network. Target ranges of oxygen saturation in extremely preterm infants. N Engl J Med. 2010 May 27;362(21):1959–69.
15. Fang JL, Sorita A, Carey WA, Colby CE, Murad MH, Alahdab F. Interventions to prevent retinopathy of prematurity: a meta-analysis. Pediatrics. 2016 Apr 1;137(4):e20153387.
16. Manja V, Lakshminrusimha S, Cook DJ. Oxygen saturation target range for extremely preterm infants: a systematic review and meta-analysis. JAMA Pediatr. 2015 Apr 1;169(4):332–40.
17. Reynolds JD, Hardy RJ, Kennedy KA, Spencer R, Van Heuven WA, Fielder AR. For the light reduction in retinopathy of prematurity (LIGHT-ROP) cooperative group. Lack of efficacy of light reduction in preventing retinopathy of prematurity. N Engl J Med. 1998;338(22):1572–6.
18. Raju TN, Langenberg P, Bhutani V, Quinn GE. Vitamin E prophylaxis to reduce retinopathy of prematurity: a reappraisal of published trials. J Pediatr. 1997 Dec 1;131(6):844–50.

4 Diagnosis and Classification of ROP

Anna L. Ells

Abstract

Retinopathy of prematurity (ROP) is a vasoproliferative disease that affects those infants born of the smallest weight and lowest gestational ages. The disease is characterized by its morphology and described as the International Classification of Retinopathy of Prematurity (ICROP). Zone, stage, presence of pre-plus or plus disease and aggressive posterior disease, define the morphology possibly seen during the acute phase of ROP.

Keywords

Retinopathy of prematurity (ROP) · International classification of ROP (ICROP) · Zone · Stage · Plus disease · Aggressive posterior ROP

4.1 Introduction

Retinopathy of prematurity (ROP) is a vasoproliferative disease that affects those infants born of the smallest weight and lowest gestational ages [1]. The disease is characterized by its morphology and described in the International Classification of Retinopathy of Prematurity (ICROP) [2–4]. ICROP is used by all ophthalmologists to document the severity of the ROP seen on clinical examination.

4.2 Diagnosis

Premature infants are examined in the neonatal intensive care unit (NICU). Visualization of the premature retina is performed using an indirect ophthalmoscope and a 25 or 28 diopter condensing lens [5]. Digital imaging systems can also be used to identify, photograph, and document the ROP [6, 7]. In some tertiary centers, fluorescein angiography may be performed for additional diagnostic purposes [8].

Most countries have their own national evidence-based recommended ROP screening guidelines that are used as a protocol for screening [9, 10]. In the United States, infants with a birth weight of less than 1500 g or a gestational age of less than 31 weeks require an ROP screening examination [11]. Also, infants of less than 2000 g with an unstable clinical course may be referred for an ROP examination [11, 12]. It is important to note that premature infants requiring ROP examinations in developing countries are larger in weight and have older gestational ages [10].

The first exam is at 4 to 6 weeks after birth but this can be dramatically earlier in infants born in developing countries [10, 11, 13]. Subsequent ROP examinations intervals are determined by the examining ophthalmologist and will be every 1 or 2 weeks unless treatment is required. Treatment is recommended within 48–72 hours of diagnosis of Type I ROP, defined as: zone I, any stage ROP with plus; zone I with stage 3, with or without plus and zone II with stage 2 or 3, with plus disease [13, 14].

Ongoing retinal ROP examinations are required until the retina is vascularized into zone III and the infant is at least 37 weeks of post-menstrual age. If ROP is still present, examinations should continue until there are at least two consecutive exams without ROP and vessels are in zone III.

4.3 Classification

The classification system is based on the morphology of the vasoproliferative disease present at the time of examination.

4.4 Location of Disease

The location of ROP is defined by anteroposterior zones, in three concentric rings.

A. L. Ells (✉)
University of Calgary, Calgary, AB, Canada

W.-C. Wu, W.-C. Lam (eds.), *A Quick Guide to Pediatric Retina*, https://doi.org/10.1007/978-981-15-6552-6_4

Zone I is centered on the optic disc with a radius of twice the distance from the center of the optic disc to the center of the fovea. This zone is the most posterior and ROP located within this zone is predicted to be the most severe form of the disease [4].

Zone II defines the area of the retina from the border of zone I to the nasal ora serrata.

Zone III is the crescent of retina adjacent to the temporal border of zone II (Fig. 4.1).

4.5 Clinical Approach to Localization the Zone of ROP

If using indirect ophthalmoscopy to perform the ROP clinical examination, the extent of zone I can be defined by using a 25 or 28 diopter condensing lens and placing the nasal edge of the optic disc at one end of the physician's field of view, then the retina that is visualized will be within zone I (Fig. 4.2). [5]. If wide-field digital imaging systems are used,

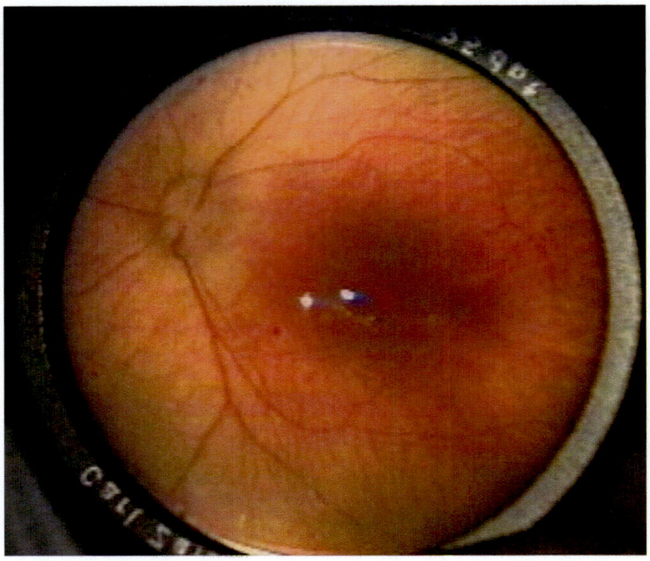

Fig. 4.2 Indirect ophthalmoscopy image through a 25 diopter condensing lens, may be used to clinically approximate the extent of zone I [4]. © International Committee for the Retinopathy of Prematurity

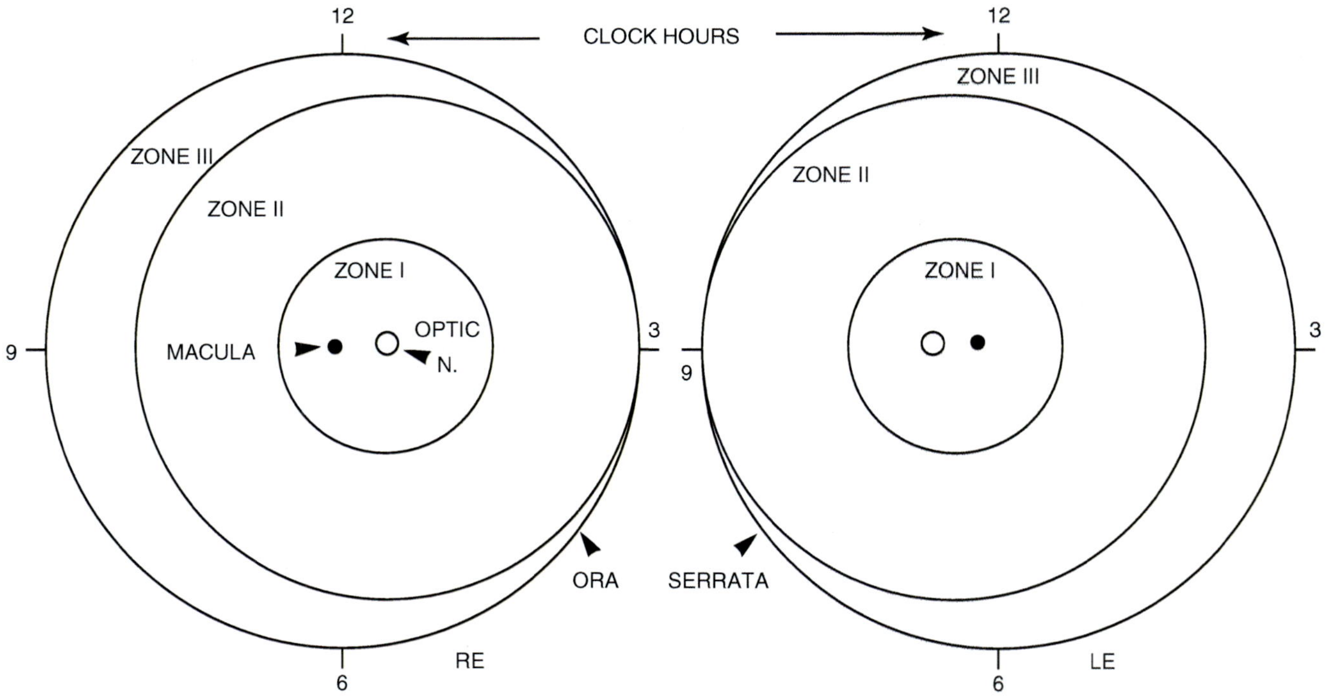

Fig. 4.1 This figure illustrates the position of the concentric zones, with zone I and II, centered around the optic disc. Clock hours are also used to localize the ROP lesions [4]. © International Committee for the Retinopathy of Prematurity

the physician must identify the fovea (which may be underdeveloped and difficult to identify), in order to define zone I limits [15–17].

4.5.1 Key Points About Zones

1. Zones define the geography and location of the ROP.
2. Zones I and II are concentric rings centered around the optic disc.
3. Zone I is most posterior and the predictor of the most severe ROP.

4.6 Staging of the Disease

The five stages of the disease describe the morphology of the ROP as seen on clinical examination or on digital imaging. One or more stages of disease can be present at any time in the eye (Fig. 4.9). The stages are documented according to how many clock hours they occupy in the retina. Retinal vascularization may initially be incomplete but no ROP is present, and this is referred to as immature retina (Fig. 4.3).

- Stage 1: defined by a demarcating intra-retinal structure or line that divides the vascularized retina from the avascularized retina (Fig. 4.4).

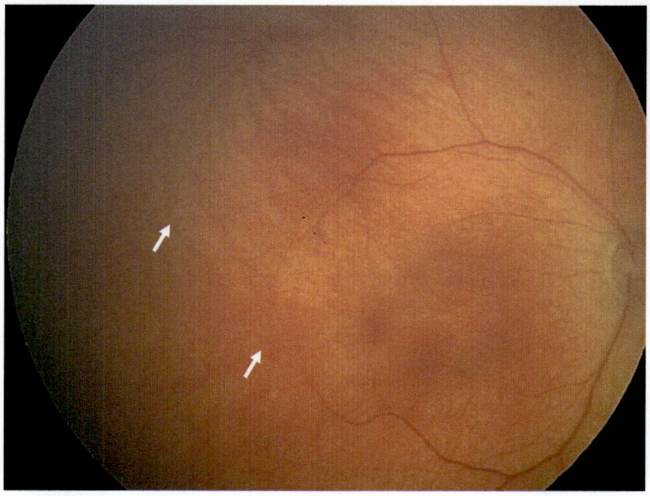

Fig. 4.3 Immature retina. This image demonstrates the immature retinal vessels (arrows) located in posterior zone II without the presence of ROP. © International Committee for the Retinopathy of Prematurity

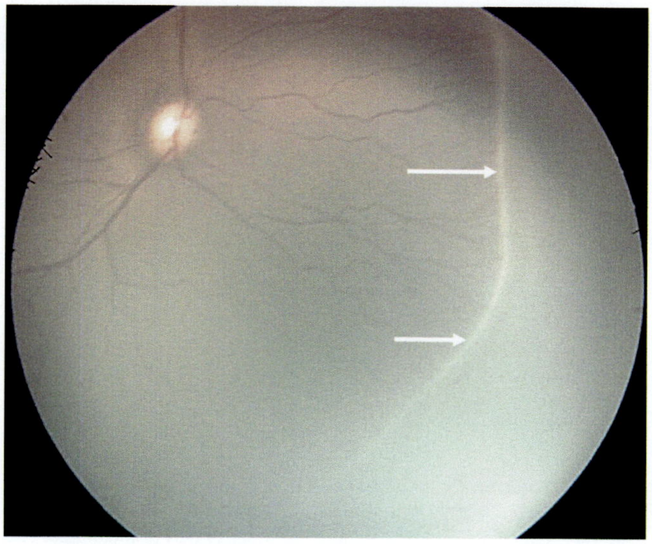

Fig. 4.4 Stage 1 ROP. Arrows are at the demarcating line between vascularized and non-vascularized retina. © International Committee for the Retinopathy of Prematurity

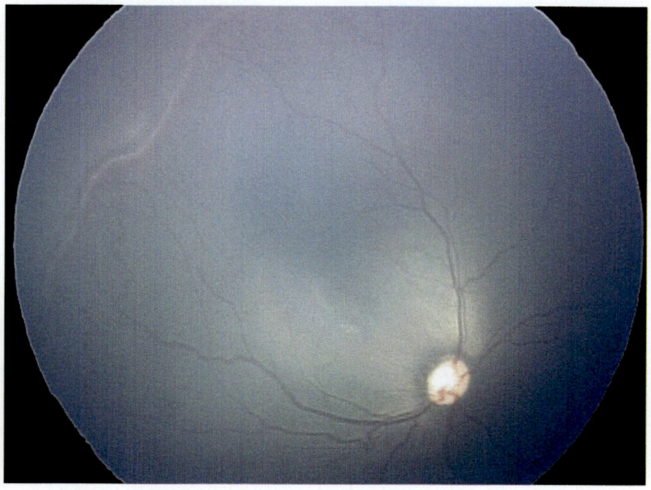

Fig. 4.5 Stage 2 ROP. The ridge can be seen between vascularized and non-vascularized retina. © International Committee for the Retinopathy of Prematurity

- Stage 2: defined by a ridge structure that has height and width and develops from the demarcating line as the disease progresses (Fig. 4.5).
- Stage 3: defined by extraretinal fibrovascular proliferation or neovascularization that extends from the ridge structure into the vitreous (Figs. 4.6, 4.7, 4.8, and 4.9).
- Stage 4A: extrafoveal retinal detachment (Fig. 4.10).

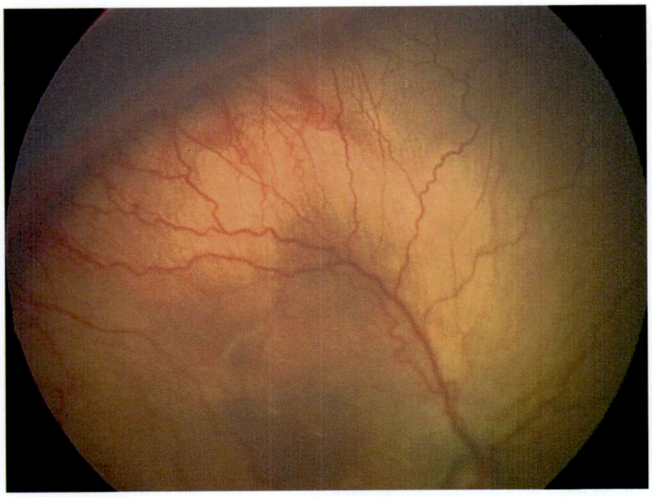

Fig. 4.6 Stage 3 ROP can be seen in the superior part of the image. The ridge is elevated and there is neovascularization on the surface of the ridge. Note the arborization of vessels just posterior to the ridge. © International Committee for the Retinopathy of Prematurity

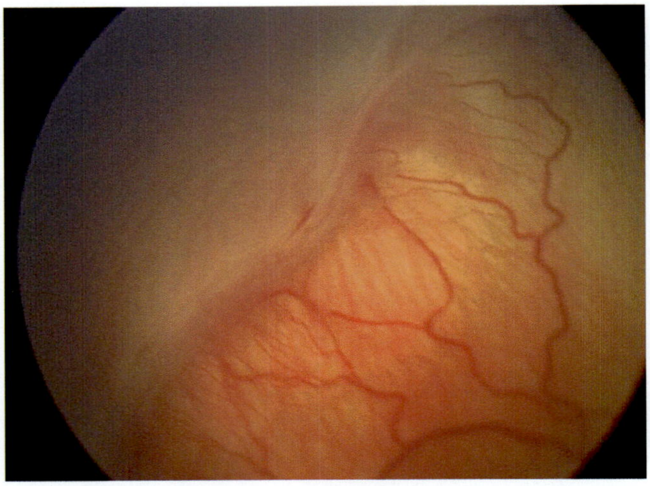

Fig. 4.7 High magnification of Stage 3. © International Committee for the Retinopathy of Prematurity

- Stage 4B: foveal retinal detachment (Fig. 4.11).
- Stage 5: total retinal detachment that is usually tractional, concave, or funnel in shape (Fig. 4.12).

4.6.1 Key Points About Stages of ROP

1. Stages describe the morphology and severity of the ROP.
2. Include stages 1–5.
3. There may be one or more stages within an eye concurrently.

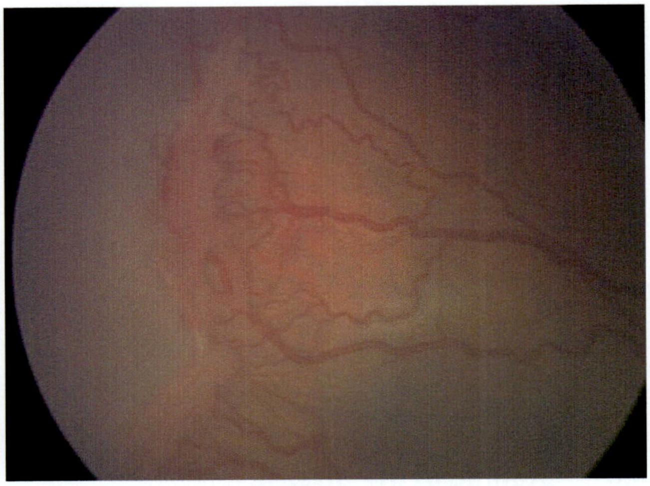

Fig. 4.8 High magnification of stage 3 fibrovascular proliferation at the junction between vascularized retina and non-vascularized retina. © International Committee for the Retinopathy of Prematurity

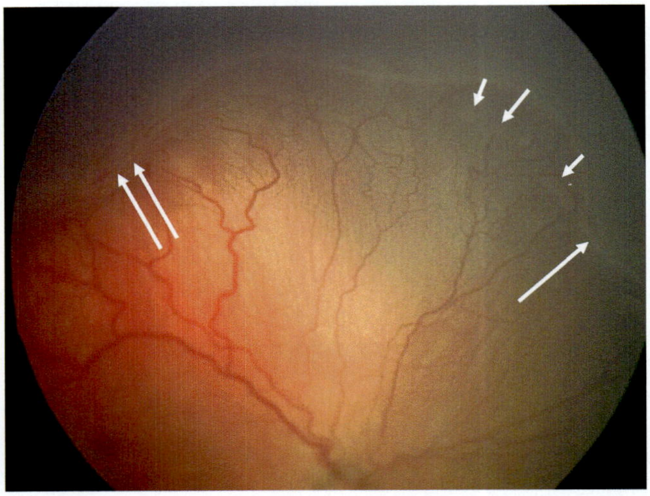

Fig. 4.9 Multiple stages of ROP may be concurrently present in the eye. Note stage 2 (long, single arrow), stage 3 (double arrows), and "popcorn" (short arrows) which are small regressing buds of neovascularization. There is also plus disease. © International Committee for the Retinopathy of Prematurity

4.7 Pre-plus and Plus Disease

In addition to the abnormal proliferation of retinal vasculature that is described in the stages of ROP, the existing arteries and veins of the retina may undergo changes as the severity of the ROP increases over time which include both dilation and tortuosity. Iris vascular engorgement may also occur. Mild dilation and tortuosity of the posterior pole vessels is called "pre-plus" disease and is defined as changes

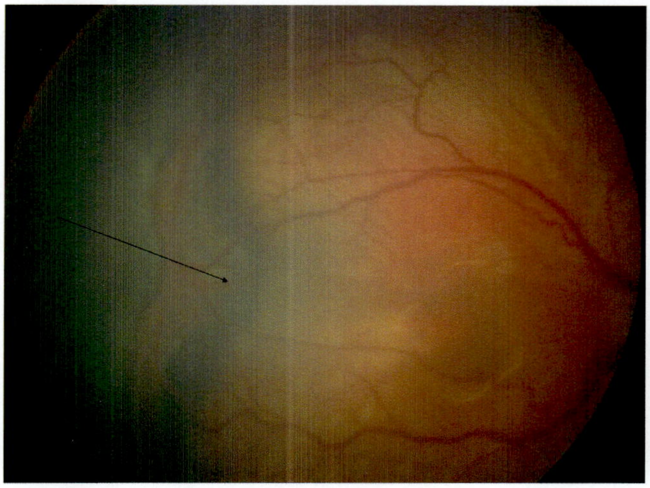

Fig. 4.10 Stage 4A. Widefield digital retinal image of 4A retinal detachment in ROP. Note the shallow temporal retinal detachment that does not involve the fovea (arrow). © International Committee for the Retinopathy of Prematurity

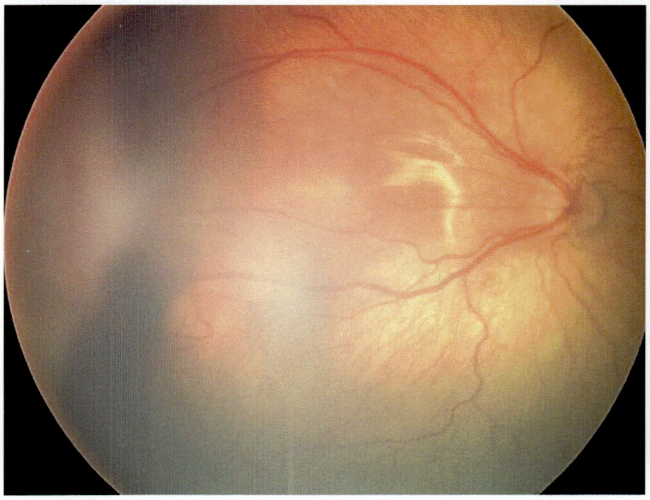

Fig. 4.11 Stage 4B. Widefield retinal image of stage 4B retinal detachment in ROP. Note the foveal involvement. © International Committee for the Retinopathy of Prematurity

that are insufficient for the diagnosis of plus disease but are not normal (Fig. 4.13). These vascular changes may progress over time to become "plus disease" or they may regress to more normal caliber vessels as the ROP regresses. Plus disease is defined as venous and arterial dilation and tortuosity in at least two quadrants that met a minimum amount of abnormality that was originally defined by a photograph of the posterior pole in the original classification publication in 1984 (Fig. 4.14). [2] The clinical diagnosis of pre-plus and plus disease may vary between examiners either at the bedside during the clinical exam or in the evaluation of wide-field retinal digital images [6]. Automated retinal vessel computerized software is currently being researched and developed which may assist in the quantification of vascular changes so that the diagnosis of pre-plus and plus disease can be standardized between examiners [18–20]. The presence of plus disease almost always determines the need to treat an infant's eye with ROP therefore the standardization of this important clinical manifestation of ROP is critical [7].

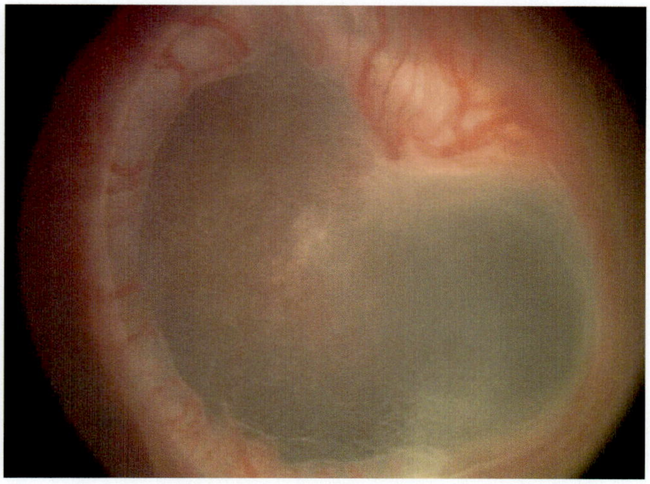

Fig. 4.12 Image of stage 5 ROP with an open funnel, total retinal detachment. © International Committee for the Retinopathy of Prematurity

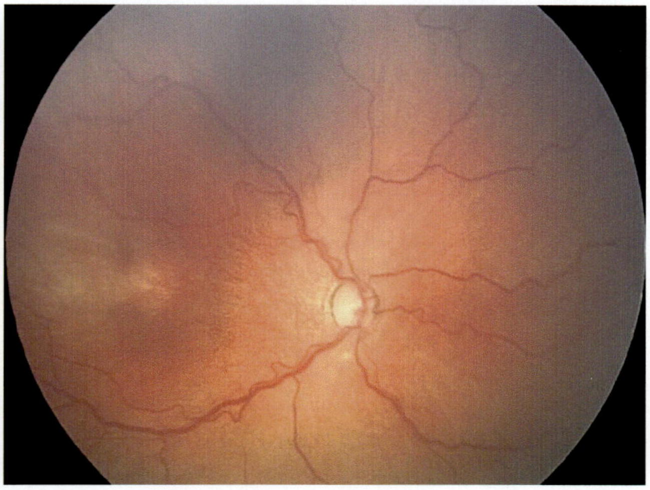

Fig. 4.13 Pre-plus disease. Image of pre-plus disease in ROP. There is a greater than normal amount of vascular dilation and tortuosity but insufficient for the diagnosis of plus disease. © International Committee for the Retinopathy of Prematurity

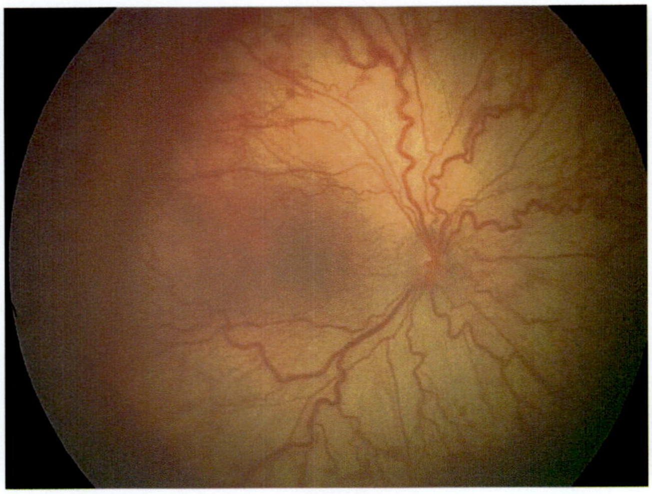

Fig. 4.14 Plus disease. Widefield digital retinal image of plus disease. Note extensive dilation and tortuosity in all four quadrants in the posterior pole. Venules are more dilated than the arterioles. It is difficult to see the temporal stage 3 present. © International Committee for the Retinopathy of Prematurity

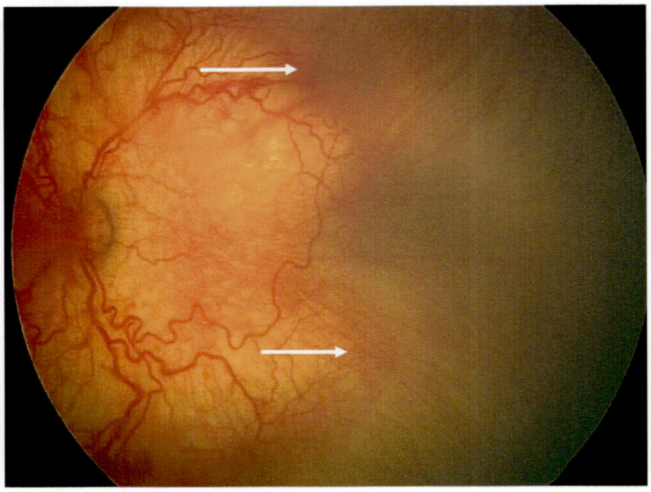

Fig. 4.15 Aggressive posterior ROP. © International Committee for the Retinopathy of Prematurity

4.7.1 Key Points About Pre-plus and Plus Disease

1. Pre-plus vascular changes are insufficient for the diagnosis of plus disease.
2. Plus disease requires at least two quadrants of abnormal dilation and tortuosity of posterior pole vessels.
3. The presence of plus disease almost always indicates the need to treat the eye.

4.8 Aggressive Posterior ROP (AP-ROP)

Aggressive posterior ROP is a rare but most severe form of ROP that is seen in extremely premature and low weight infants or in infants with prematurity and associated co-morbidities of prematurity such as sepsis, pulmonary disease, and necrotizing enterocolitis [21, 22]. This virulent form of ROP is called aggressive posterior ROP and is characterized by its posterior location, usually zone I, relatively flat and extensive stage 3 neovascularization, and massive plus disease in all four quadrants (Figs. 4.15 and 4.16). An important feature of AP-ROP is that it does not usually progress through the stages of ROP but develops a flat network of neovascularization early on in the disease without the preexisting ridge.

4.8.1 Key Points About AP-ROP

1. AP-ROP is the most virulent and aggressive form of ROP.

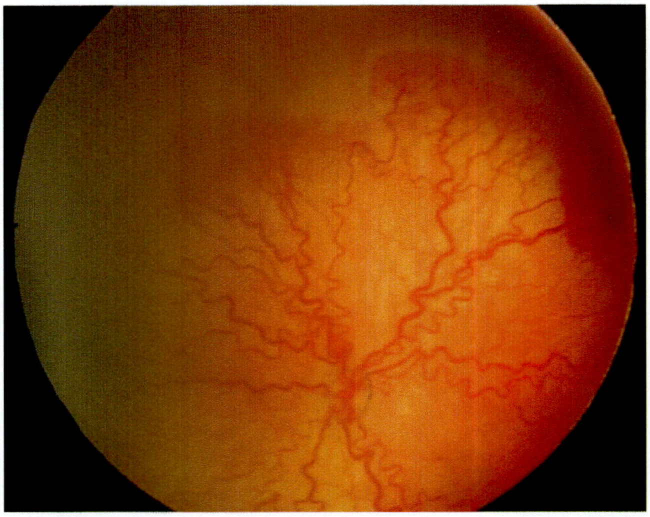

Fig. 4.16 Image of aggressive posterior ROP. Note the posterior location of zone I, the flat neovascularization (arrows), and the extensive plus disease present. © International Committee for the Retinopathy of Prematurity

2. Features massive plus disease, flat neovascularization, and usually zone I.
3. Lacks the classic stages of 1, 2, and 3. Often there is no ridge seen.

4.9 Regression of ROP

Acute ROP either progresses to a point that requires treatment, or it spontaneously regresses. Often the failure of one stage to progress to the next stage is an indication of regression. Signs of regression occur at the junction between vascularized and non-vascularized retina and retinal vessels usually advance slowly toward the ora serrata. [23] The most peripheral retina may remain avascular as was noted in the 1987 ICROP publication on regression and retinal detachment [3]. It is extremely important to continue retinal examinations after treatment (regardless of treatment modality) or spontaneous regression to ensure adequate vascularization into zone III without reactivation of neovascularization. Failure to detect inadequately regressed ROP or significant persistent peripheral avascular retina over time may lead to cicatricial ROP causing visual loss or blindness. [24].

4.10 Summary

1. Clinical examination of the premature infant's retina is performed using an indirect ophthalmoscope or digital imaging systems to identify or photograph and document the ROP.
2. Evidence-based screening guidelines have been published for many countries and it is important to note that developing countries have very different birthweights and gestational ages of at-risk infants for Type I ROP.
3. ICROP is an international classification system, based on the morphology of the disease. The unifying principle of this classification is the more posterior the disease and the greater the amount of involved retinal vascular tissue, the more serious the disease. The presence of plus disease is critical to identify, as it almost always indicates the need for treatment.
4. Careful description, documentation, and photography may lead to more timely and accurate treatment of ROP.

Acknowledgments All figures are reprinted from the International Classification of Retinopathy of Prematurity Revisited, Arch Ophthalmol/Vol. 123, July 2005, with permission from the ICROP committee.

References

1. Quinn GE, Barr C, Bremer D, Fellows R, Gong A, Hoffman R, Repka MX, Shepard J, Siatkowski RM, Wade K, Ying GS. Changes in course of retinopathy of prematurity from 1986 to 2013: comparison of three studies in the United States. Ophthalmology. 2016;123(7):1595–600. https://doi.org/10.1016/j.ophtha.2016.03.026. Epub 2016 Apr 12
2. Committee for the Classification of Retinopathy of Prematurity. An international classification of retinopathy of prematurity. Arch Ophthalmol. 1984;102:1130–4.
3. ICROP Committee for Classification of Late Stages ROP. An international classification of retinopathy of prematurity, II: the classification of retinal detachment. Arch Ophthalmol. 1987;105:906–12.
4. International Committee for the Classification of Retinopathy of Prematurity. The international classification of retinopathy of prematurity revisited. Arch Ophthalmol. 2005 Jul;123(7):991–9.
5. Vander JF, Handa J, McNamara JA, Trese M, Spencer R, Repka MX, Rubsamen P, Li H, Morse LS, Tasman WS. Early treatment of posterior retinopathy of prematurity: a controlled trial. Ophthalmology. 1997;104(11):1731–5. discussion 1735-6
6. Ells AL, Holmes JM, Astle WF, Williams G, Leske DA, Fielden M, Uphill B, Jennett P, Hebert M. Telemedicine approach to screening for severe retinopathy of prematurity: a pilot study. Ophthalmology. 2003 Nov;110(11):2113–7.
7. Quinn GE, Ying GS, Daniel E, E-ROP Cooperative Group, et al. Validity of a telemedicine system for the evaluation of acute-phase retinopathy of prematurity. JAMA Ophthalmol. 2014;132(10):1178–84.
8. Lepore D, Quinn GE, Molle F, Orazi L, Baldascino A, Ji MH, Sammartino M, Sbaraglia F, Ricci D, Mercuri E. Follow-up to age 4 years of treatment of type 1 retinopathy of prematurity intravitreal bevacizumab injection versus laser: fluorescein angiographic findings. Ophthalmology. 2018 Feb;125(2):218–26.
9. Gilbert C, Foster A. Childhood blindness in the context of VISION 2020—the right to sight. Bull World Health Organ. 2001;79:227–32.
10. Gilbert C, Fielder A, Gordillo L, et al. Characteristics of infants with severe retinopathy of prematurity in countries with low, moderate, and high levels of development: implications for screening programs. Pediatrics. 2005;115:e518–25.
11. American Academy of Pediatrics Section on Ophthalmology, American Academy of Ophthalmology, American Association for Pediatric Ophthalmology and Strabismus, American Association of Certified Orthoptists. Screening examination of premature infants for retinopathy of prematurity. Pediatrics. 2013;131:189.
12. Hartnett ME, Penn JS. Mechanisms and management of retinopathy of prematurity. N Engl J Med. 2012;367(26):2515–26.
13. Good W, On behalf of the ETROP Cooperative Group. Final results of the early treatment for retinopathy of prematurity (ETROP) randomized trial. Trans Am Ophthalmol Soc. 2004;102:233–50.
14. Early Treatment for Retinopathy of Prematurity Cooperative Group. Revised indications for the treatment of retinopathy of prematurity: results of the early treatment for retinopathy of prematurity randomized trial. Arch Ophthalmol. 2003;121:1684–94.
15. Chiang MF, Thyparampil PJ, Rabinowitz D. Interexpert agreement in the identification of macular location in infants at risk for retinopathy of prematurity. Arch Ophthalmol. 2010 Sep;128(9):1153–9.
16. Hendrickson AE, Yuodelis C. The morphological development of the human fovea. Ophthalmology. 1984;91(6):603–12.
17. Isenberg SJ. Macular development in the premature infant. Am J Ophthalmol. 1986;101(1):74–80.
18. Wallace DK, Zhao Z, Freedman SF. A pilot study using "ROPtool" to quantify plus disease in retinopathy of prematurity. J AAPOS. 2007;11:381–7.
19. Chiang MF, Gelman R, Martinez-Perez ME, et al. Image analysis for retinopathy of prematurity diagnosis. J AAPOS. 2009;13:438–45.
20. Campbell JP, Ataer-Cansizoglu E, Bolon-Canedo V, Bozkurt A, Erdogmus D, Kalpathy-Cramer J, Patel SN, Reynolds JD, Horowitz J, Hutcheson K, Shapiro M, Repka MX, Ferrone P, Drenser K, Martinez-Castellanos MA, Ostmo S, Jonas K, Chan RV, Chiang MF, Imaging and Informatics in ROP (i-ROP) Research Consortium. Expert diagnosis of plus disease in retinopathy of prematurity from computer-based image analysis. JAMA Ophthalmol. 2016 Jun 1;134(6):651–7.
21. Lundgren P, Lundberg L, Hellgren G, Holmström G, Hård AL, Smith LE, Wallin A, Hallberg B, Hellström A. Aggressive posterior retinopathy of prematurity is associated with multiple infectious episodes and thrombocytopenia. Neonatology. 2017;111(1):79–85.
22. Drenser K, Trese M, Capone A. Aggressive posterior retinopathy of prematurity. Retina. 2010 April;30(4):S37–40.
23. Ying-Qin NI, Huang X, Xue K, Yu J, Ruan L, Shan H-D, Xu G-Z. Natural involution of acute retinopathy of prematurity not requiring treatment: factors associated with the time course of involution. Investig Ophthal Visual Sci. 2014 May;55:3165–70.
24. Hu J, Blair M, Shapiro M, Lichtenstein S, Galasso J, Kapur R. Reactivation of retinopathy of prematurity after bevacizumab injection. Arch Ophthalmol. 2012;130:1000.

5 Differential Diagnosis of ROP

G. Caputo

Abstract

History of prematurity mainly sustains the diagnosis of retinopathy of prematurity. The features of ROP are retinal ischemia, exudation, and neovascularization responsible for secondary tractional retinal detachment. The differential diagnosis of ROP to consider are diseases that feature similar clinical presentations such as FEVR, incontinentia pigmenti, Coats' disease, and persistent fetal vascularization. Family history, genetic testing, and wide-angle angiography allow to clarify these conditions.

Keywords

Retinal ischemia · Retinal exudation · Retinal folds Retinal detachment · FEVR · ROP · Incontinentia pigmenti · Coats disease · Persistent fetal vasculature (PFV)

Various conditions can simulate retinopathy of prematurity at different stages of the disease.

ROP is characterized by the development of extraretinal neovascular proliferation secondary to nonperfusion of large retinal territories.

Early stages of ROP and their specific clinical features ease the differential diagnosis. In the case of advanced stages of ROP complicated by retinal detachment, the latter can be more controversial since each clinical feature is seen in several diseases; many congenital or vascular retinal diseases can present with retinal ischemia, subretinal exudation, retinal detachment, retinal dragging, and retinal folds.

G. Caputo (✉)
Rothschild Hospital Foundation, Paris, France

5.1 Medical History

Past medical history of prematurity is the main answer to differential diagnosis of ROP. According to the country of birth, gestational age, and birth weight at risk for developing severe retinopathy of prematurity can vary; developed countries have different thresholds than developing regions. In Nepal, babies less than 2000 g at birth and born at 36 WG or less have a 3,8% rate of stage 3 or more disease [1].

5.1.1 Genetic Background

Differential diagnosis of ROP involves retinal diseases with a common genetic background concerning the WNT signaling pathway. Mutations in the NDP gene, present in Norrie disease can be shared with some cases of familial exudative vitreoretinopathy (FEVR) [2]. Norrin by its interaction with the product of FZD4 is implicated in the Wnt signaling pathway, essential to angiogenesis. Mutations in FZD4, LRP5, TSPAN12, or ZNF408 genes are responsible for FEVR, and no clear phenotype–genotype correlation has been established [3]. In rare cases of Coats' disease and ROP, a mutation in the FZD4 gene has been reported [4]. Mutations in the FZD4 gene that could explain surprising evolutions of the disease are present in up to 3% of severe cases of ROP [5, 6].

5.2 Clinical Observations

5.2.1 Retinal Ischemia

5.2.1.1 Familial Exudative Vitreoretinopathy

Peripheral retinal ischemia is characteristic of ROP and is also present in familial exudative vitreoretinopathy (FEVR). In the latter, peripheral retinal ischemia develops during childhood responsible for extraretinal neovascularization; tractional and exudative retinal detachment are present in the late stages of the disease; ischemia is predominant in the

W.-C. Wu, W.-C. Lam (eds.), *A Quick Guide to Pediatric Retina*, https://doi.org/10.1007/978-981-15-6552-6_5

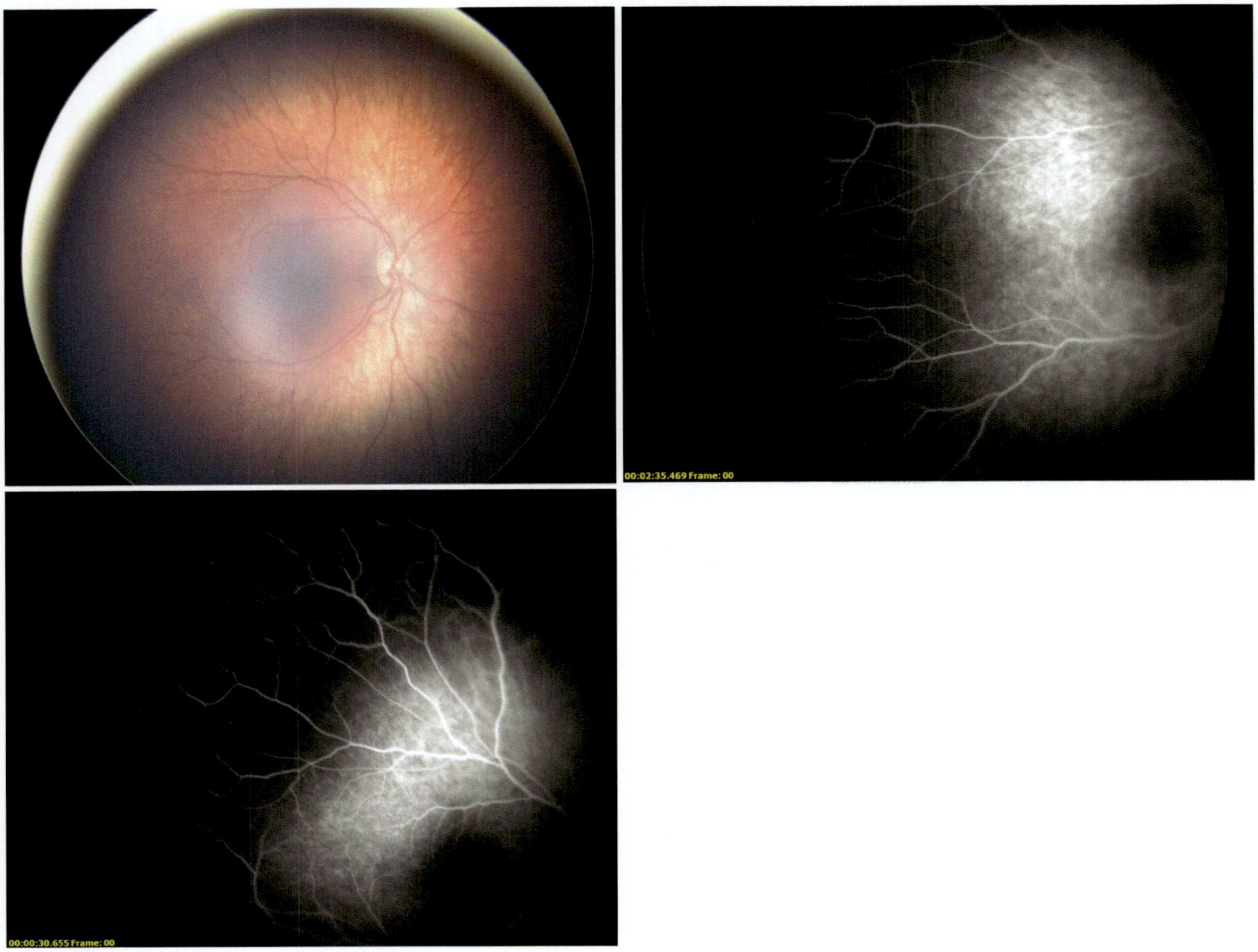

Fig. 5.1 Retinal ischemia in FEVR patient. Fundus photograph is unremarkable and wide-angle angiography shows peripheral retinal ischemia

temporal retina, associated to thin peripheral vascular arborization and capillary drop-out (Fig. 5.1). Dominant, recessive, or X-linked transmission is encountered in FEVR and no history of prematurity is noted. Mutations affect FRZL4, LRP5, Norrie, TSPAN12, or ZNF408 genes [7].

In young babies with advanced stages of FEVR, the exudative component is often predominant in the retinal detachment.

5.2.1.2 Incontinentia Pigmenti

Incontinentia pigmenti is a dominant genetic disease linked to chromosome X; it is lethal for boys. Retinal ischemia is observed during the first year of life. The presentation is quite asymmetrical and usually affects one eye because of the lionization of chromosome X (Fig. 5.2). The dermatological lesions are specific features of this disease; they consist of pigmented lesions of the skin on the legs, only visible during the first months of life [8].

5.2.1.3 Shaken Baby Syndrome

Peripheral ischemia and secondary neovascularization have been described in shaken baby syndrome; they could be due to the shearing effect of the trauma on the retinal vessels (Fig. 5.3) [9].

5.2.2 Subretinal Exudation

Subretinal exudation is less common in ROP, but can be observed in advanced stage 4 or 5 of the disease with active plus presentation.

This feature can be predominant in FEVR because of the presence of large anastomosis of the peripheral vessels.

Vascular dilation of capillaries, rarefaction of capillary meshwork, and retinal exudation leading to total retinal detachment is observed in Coats' disease (Figs. 5.4 and 5.5) [10]. Eighty-five percent of the cases concern boys [11].

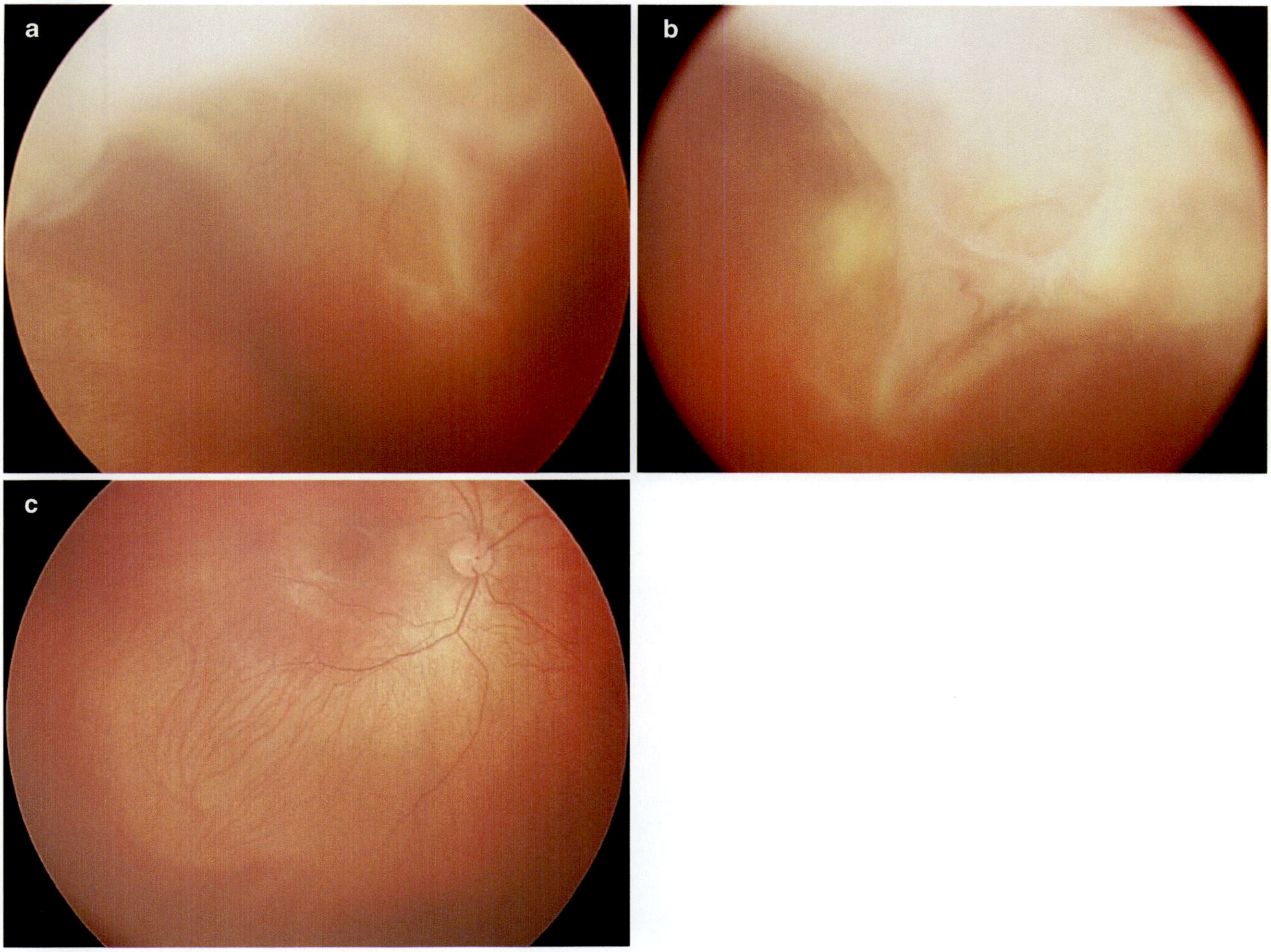

Fig. 5.2 Retinal ischemia and preretinal neovascularization in incontinentia pigmenti (**a**, **b**). Controlateral fundus photography showing mild vascular changes but inferio-temporal ischemia (**c**)

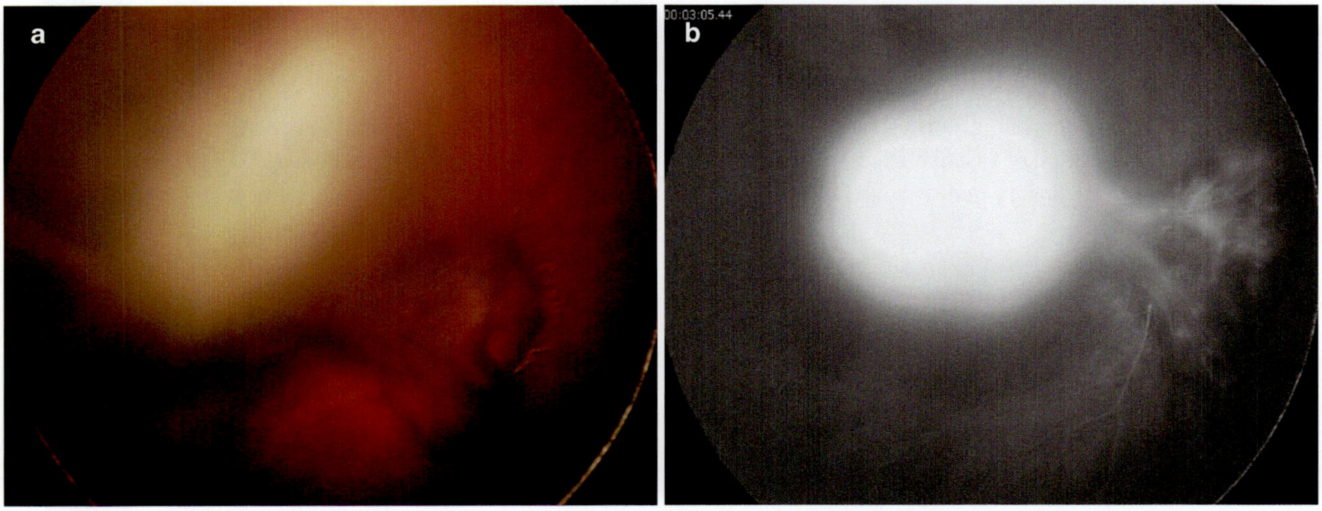

Fig. 5.3 Partial retinal detachment in a case of shaken baby syndrome: fundus photography (**a**), fluorescein angiogram showing extensive retinal ischemia (**b**)

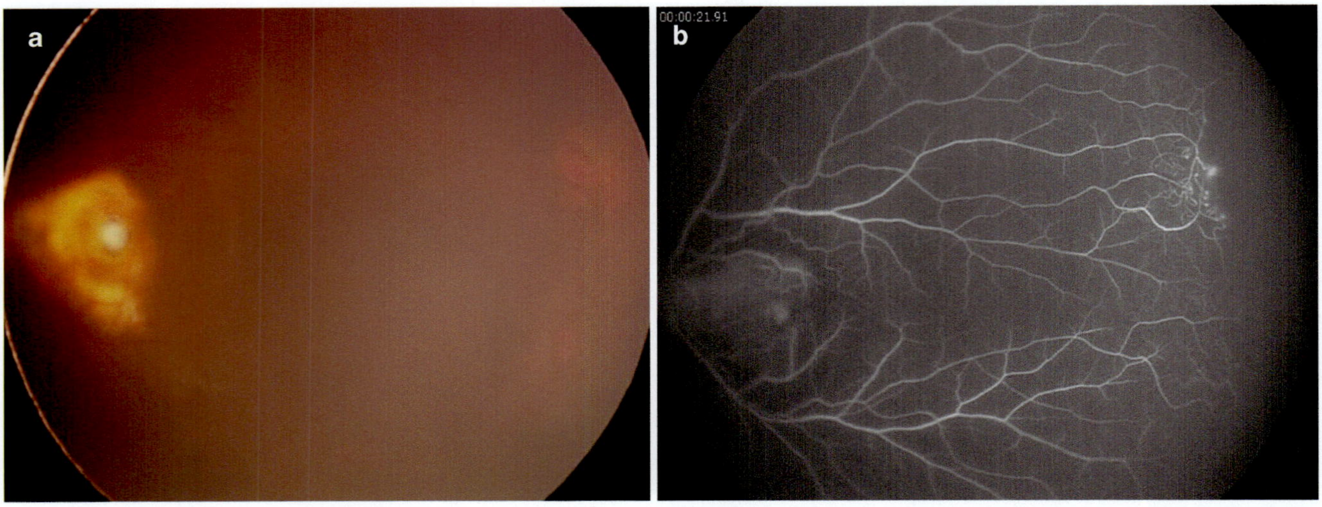

Fig. 5.4 Example of retinal exudation in Coats' disease. Fundus photography (**a**), fluorescein angiography (**b**)

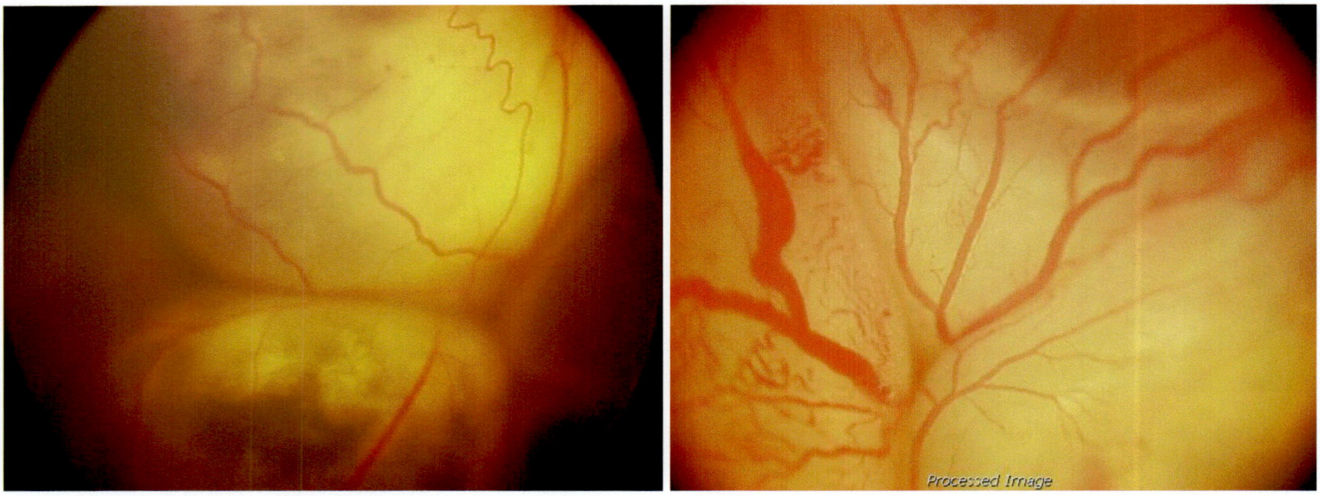

Fig. 5.5 Two cases of retinal detachment due to Coat's disease. Note the exudative nature of the detachment and the absence of vitreous involvement

Vitreous is not implicated initially in Coats' disease; extensive laser photocoagulation of vascular aneurysms can induce retinal ischemia and secondary neovascularization [12].

5.2.3 Retinal Detachment

Retinal detachment is present in stage 4 and 5 ROP. The vascular component of the preretinal neovascularization regresses in the late phases of these detachments, and the fibrous tissue is responsible for the tractional detachments are characterized by total retinal detachment is observed in advanced stages of FEVR (Fig. 5.6). Infants can also be affected, but the mean age of retinal detachment in this disease is young infancy or adolescence. Subretinal exudation is often observed in FEVR.

A wide variety of clinical observations can be present in Persistent fetal vascularization (PFV) according to the amount of fibrovascular tissue remnants. Severe cases will have a total retinal detachment; the absence of vascular disease in the fellow eye will confirm the diagnosis; peripheral retinal ischemia is eliminated by wide-angle angiography.

In retinal dysplasia, ocular lesions similar to PFV are bilateral (Fig. 5.7) [13]. Norrie disease is a genetic disease, an X-linked disease affecting boys; hearing impairment and autistic disorder are often associated.

5.2.4 Macular Ectopia

Retinal dragging by the temporal extraretinal neovascularization is responsible for macular ectopia and can be observed

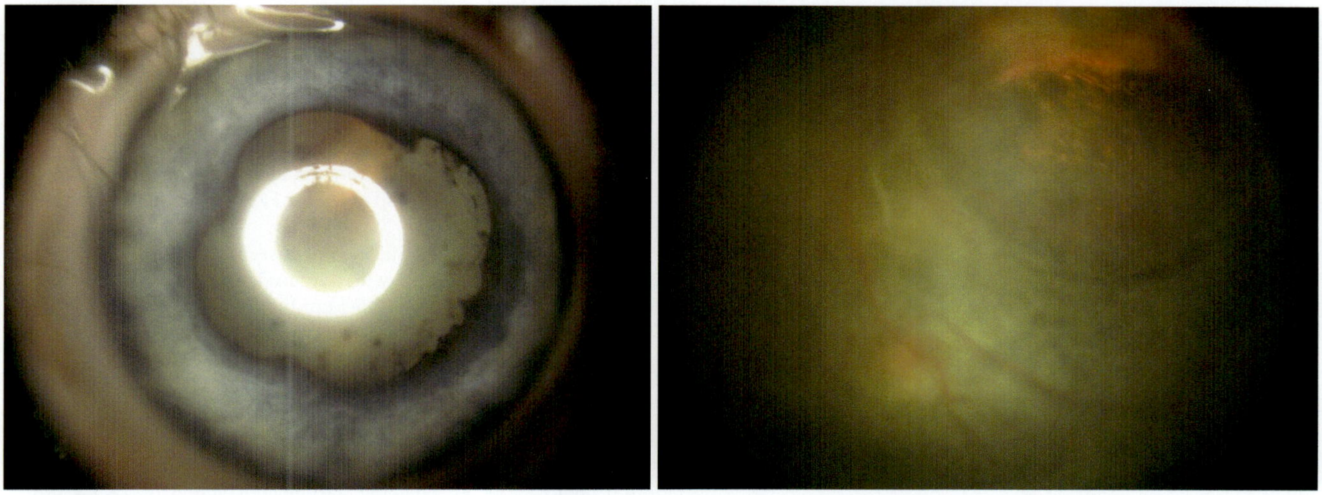

Fig. 5.6 A case of unilateral total retinal detachment in FEVR comparable to stage 5 ROP

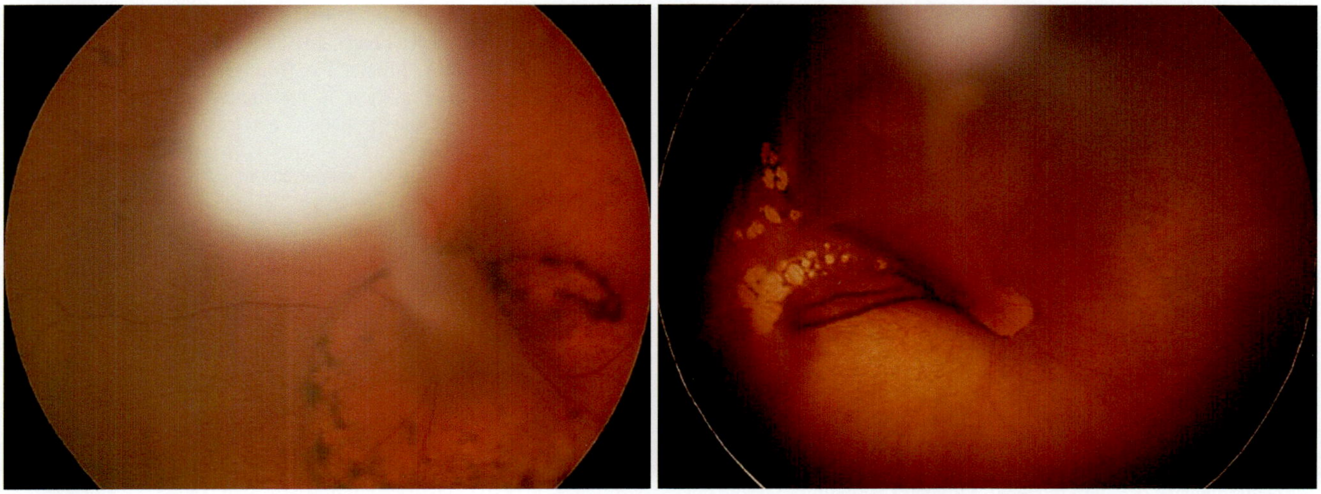

Fig. 5.7 Retinal dysplasia associated bilateral retinal fold. Note the pigmentary subretinal changes that help recognizing diagnosis

in ROP and FEVR. Retinal temporal vessels develop a straight pattern instead of their natural curvature.

5.2.5 Retinal Folds

Retinal folds are observed in the cicatricial form of stage 4A and 4B ROP. Progressive temporal fibrous tissue contraction leads to a localized macular fold. FEVR, PFV, Norrie disease, and retinal dysplasia can present with a similar clinical presentation [14] (Fig. 5.8).

Vessels in the fold are more commonly seen in FEVR and ROP (the absence of vessels and heavy epiretinal alterations are more common features of PFV and retinal dysplasia) (Fig. 5.9).

In summary, differential diagnosis of ROP is easy when medical history is well known; it can be difficult in case of

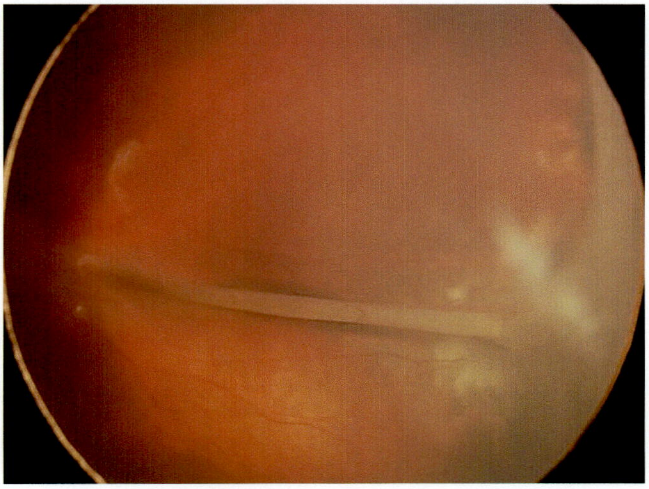

Fig. 5.8 A case of unilateral retinal fold in FEVR: note the subretinal exudates and extraretinal fibrovascular proliferation

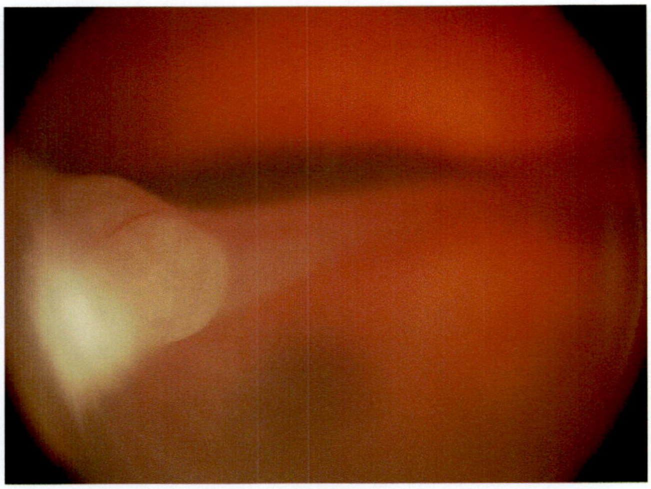

Fig. 5.9 Unilateral retinal fold due to persistent fetal vasculature

mild prematurity in countries where the standard of care does not reach the one in developed regions. Many diseases can simulate some clinical features of ROP, and a thorough analysis of the clinical presentation associated with wide-angle angiography allows doing the right diagnosis. All these differential diagnoses share some common genetic background with the Norrie/FZD4 Wnt signaling pathway implicated in angiogenesis. Understanding and analyzing these mechanisms will help diagnose and classify these vascular retinal diseases.

References

1. Shrestha JB, et al. Incidence of retinopathy of prematurity in a neonatal intensive care unit in Nepal. J Pediatr Ophthalmol Strabismus. 2010;47(5):297–300.
2. Dickinson JL, et al. Mutations in the NDP gene: contribution to Norrie disease, familial exudative vitreoretinopathy and retinopathy of prematurity. Clin Exp Ophthalmol. 2006;34(7):682–8.
3. Wu WC, et al. Retinal phenotype-genotype correlation of pediatric patients expressing mutations in the Norrie disease gene. Arch Ophthalmol. 2007;125(2):225–30.
4. Drenser KA, et al. Clinical presentation and genetic correlation of patients with mutations affecting the FZD4 gene. Arch Ophthalmol. 2009;127(12):1649–54.
5. Shastry BS, et al. Identification of missense mutations in the Norrie disease gene associated with advanced retinopathy of prematurity. Arch Ophthalmol. 1997;115(5):651–5.
6. Ells A, et al. Severe retinopathy of prematurity associated with FZD4 mutations. Ophthalmic Genet. 2010;31(1):37–43.
7. Gilmour DF. Familial exudative vitreoretinopathy and related retinopathies. Eye (Lond). 2015;29(1):1–14.
8. Holmstrom G, Thoren K. Ocular manifestations of incontinentia pigmenti. Acta Ophthalmol Scand. 2000;78(3):348–53.
9. Caputo G, et al. Ischemic retinopathy and neovascular proliferation secondary to shaken baby syndrome. Retina. 2008;28(3 Suppl):S42–6.
10. Morris B, Foot B, Mulvihill A. A population-based study of coats disease in the United Kingdom I: epidemiology and clinical features at diagnosis. Eye (Lond). 2010;24(12):1797–801.
11. Daruich A, Matet A, Munier FL. Younger age at presentation in children with coats disease is associated with more advanced stage and worse visual prognosis: a retrospective study. Retina. 2018;38(11):2239–46.
12. Sigler EJ, et al. Current management of coats disease. Surv Ophthalmol. 2014;59(1):30–46.
13. Walsh MK, et al. Early vitrectomy effective for Norrie disease. Arch Ophthalmol. 2010;128(4):456–60.
14. Nishina S, et al. Clinical features of congenital retinal folds. Am J Ophthalmol. 2012;153(1):81–7 e1.

Aggressive Posterior Retinopathy of Prematurity (APROP)

6

Michael P. Blair, Sarah Hilkert Rodriguez,
Sidney A. Schechet, and Michael J. Shapiro

Abstract

In this chapter, we will discuss the definition APROP, optimal treatment regimen, and provide example photographs for pattern recognition.

Keywords

Retinopathy of prematurity (ROP) · Aggressive posterior retinopathy of prematurity (APROP) · Plus disease Neovascularization · Oxygen-induced retinopathy Bevacizumab · Laser photocoagulation · International classification of ROP

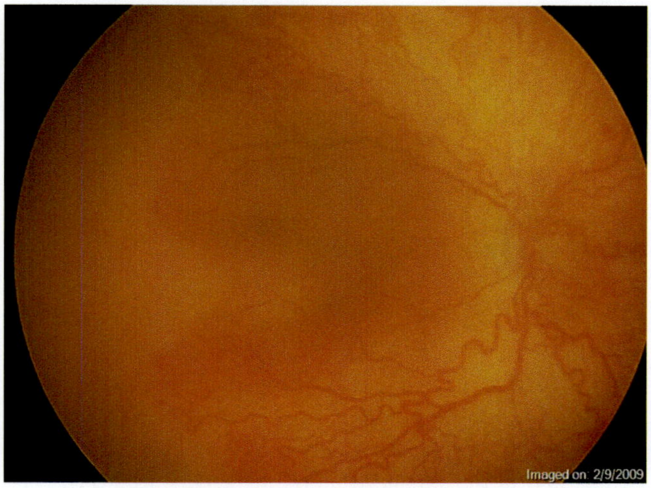

Fig. 6.1 APROP. Note prominent plus disease, out of proportion to perceived retinopathy due to lack of fibrotic elements. However, note the temporal anastomotic vessels and blush from fine neovascularization that obscures the underlying vessels

6.1 What is APROP?

Aggressive Posterior Retinopathy of Prematurity (APROP) is an uncommon form of ROP that can rapidly lead to retinal detachment and blindness if untreated or treated late [1]. *APROP is generally a posterior disease in Zone I or posterior Zone II. APROP displays stage 3 as a flat neovascularization without a detectable fibrotic component. This neovascularization is often invisible with standard techniques. Therefore, APROP is currently defined as prominent plus disease with an ill-defined retinopathy or out of proportion to the observed retinopathy* (Fig. 6.1). This is because APROP does not contain the classic ROP (CROP) fibrotic features, i.e., the stage 1 demarcation line, stage 2 ridge, or fibrotic extraretinal proliferation of stage 3.

6.2 Importance of APROP Recognition: Poor Response to Treatment

One factor in the worse outcomes for APROP may be late treatment. Since the neovascularization does not contain fibrotic elements (which provide a sharp contrast to the normally developing retina) it is much harder to recognize. Careful examination with low ambient light and increased magnification (e.g., 20 diopter lens) are critical. If the "naked" neovascularization is missed repeatedly, then the eye may be called immature and given a 2–3 weeks exam interval that is too long and leads to sudden severe disease. The disease will advance to include fibrotic elements which will contract, lead to tractional retinal detachment (TRD), and given the posterior location, rapidly involve most of the

M. P. Blair (✉)
Department of Ophthalmology and Visual Science, University of Chicago, Chicago, IL, USA

Retina Consultants, Ltd., Des Plaines, IL, USA

S. H. Rodriguez · S. A. Schechet
Department of Ophthalmology and Visual Science, University of Chicago, Chicago, IL, USA

M. J. Shapiro
Retina Consultants, Ltd., Des Plaines, IL, USA

W.-C. Wu, W.-C. Lam (eds.), *A Quick Guide to Pediatric Retina*, https://doi.org/10.1007/978-981-15-6552-6_6

posterior pole, including the macula. One major contribution of the revised International Classification of ROP [1] definition of APROP was to increase its awareness among ROP screeners. With increased disease recognition treatment has been performed earlier in the disease course. Specifically, in our catchment locale, rates of referral for TRD from untreated APROP declined dramatically after publication of this definition.

Even when treated promptly the failure rates are higher for APROP than for CROP [2–5]. Rates of progression to TRD despite laser photocoagulation range from 20 to 50% [2–4, 6, 7] whereas rates of anatomic failure after laser are generally around 10% [8]. Response to treatment with anti-VEGF or combination treatment of laser photocoagulation and anti-VEGF have been reported to be better, with a failure rate of less than 5% [9]. Since early treatment of APROP and modification of the treatment regime may be helpful in ensuring better outcomes, early recognition of this disease is critical.

6.3 Formal ICROP Definition

ICROP [1, 3] defined APROP as a special form of ROP which we will present below. Prior to the publication of the revised ICROP [1] with its improved photographic documentation of disease examples, this severe posterior ROP was variously termed Rush Disease, Fulminate ROP, Zone I ROP, and in the Japanese literature Type 2 ROP [10, 11]. The term APROP has supplanted this prior terminology in the literature.

ICROP defines APROP as follows: "The characteristic features of this type of ROP are its posterior location, prominence of plus disease, and the ill-defined nature of the retinopathy." Although the descriptors "posterior location" and "prominence of plus disease" may be helpful in distinguishing CROP from APROP, describing it as an "ill-defined retinopathy" is less helpful. Since ETROP criteria for treatment are basically driven by the presence of plus disease, even cases of unrecognized APROP (e.g., posterior plus without CROP demarcation/fibrosis) qualify for treatment. This relatively earlier treatment of APROP that otherwise may not have been recognized until late in the course (i.e., after it evolved to severe fibrosis and TRD) has decreased blindness from APROP. However, as discussed above, the response to conventional treatment of APROP remains worse than CROP. Therefore, identification of APROP may allow modification of the treatment regimen to allow for better outcomes, whether with anti-VEGF, earlier laser treatment, or other strategies. However, the examiner must be able to positively identify APROP, potentially at an earlier timepoint. Stage 3 neovascularization of APROP qualifies for treatment under ETROP guidelines even before the development of plus disease, when in Zone I. We will discuss features that allow positive identification of APROP below.

6.4 Positive Features of APROP

ICROP does further describe some positive features of APROP that are helpful in its identification including: (1) Posterior vessels show increased dilation and tortuosity out of proportion to the peripheral disease; (2) Shunting occurs from posterior to the vascular–avascular junction; (3) Difficulty in distinguishing between arterioles and venules because of the shunting, dilation, and tortuosity; (4) Hemorrhages at the junction between the vascularized and avascular retina; (5). APROP typically is accompanied by circumferential vessels; (6) Lack of progression through CROP stage 1–3; and (7) APROP may appear as a flat network of neovascularization at the deceptively featureless junction between vascularized and non-vascularized retina (Fig. 6.2).

This last feature, in the opinion of the authors, is the most specific finding of APROP: neovascularization without fibrosis. Neovascularization is the purely vascular form of fibrovascular proliferation (stage 3). This differentiates CROP from APROP. Since there are no accompanying fibrotic (i.e., white) elements (which are present in CROP stage 1–3) the vascular–avascular junction appears "featureless." Additionally, there may be a blush of flat neovascular tissue that obscures the underlying retinal vessels (Fig. 6.3).

Additional features that may point to APROP are lack of anterior growth of posterior immature vessels, rapid progression of plus disease, and persistence of tunica vasculosa lentis (Fig. 6.4). Indeed, the inability to achieve sufficient dilation due to tunica is a poor prognostic sign.

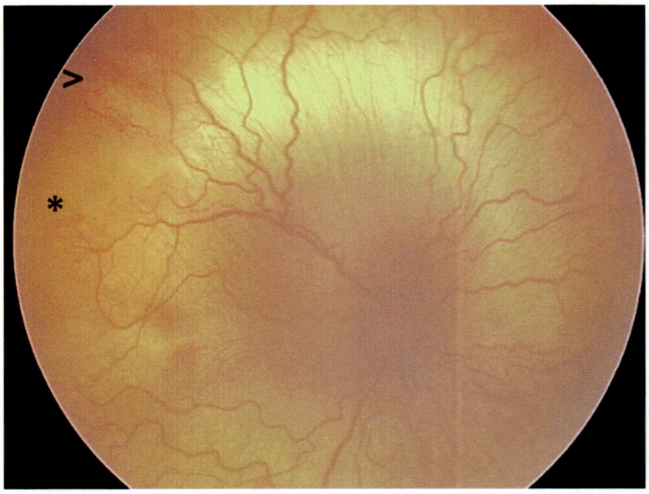

Fig. 6.2 This is an example of APROP. Plus disease is out of proportion to perceived retinopathy. Note the fine, flat network of neovascularization (*) and shunt vessel (>)

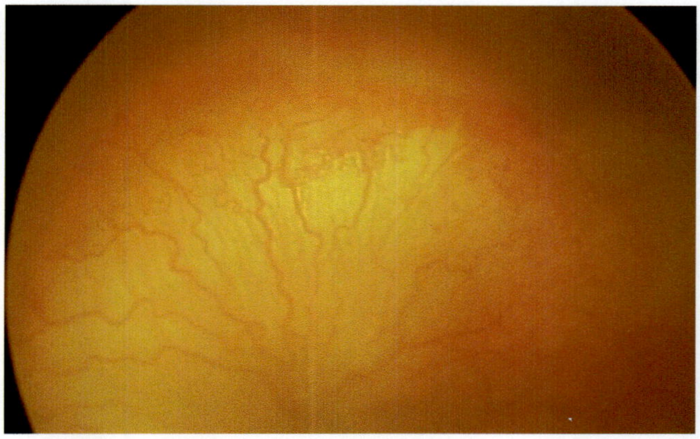

Fig. 6.3 APROP. There is a prominent plus disease despite lack of fibrosis. Note the prominent tangle of naked neovascularization just out of the plane of the retina superiorly that obscures the retinal vessels as they approach the vascular–avascular junction. There is a slight halo superiorly but no corresponding structure (This is a Mach Band due to change in contrast. A Mach band is an illusion of a line at the exaggerated border of two adjoining subtle, yet distinct, shades of a color by triggering edge-detection in the visual system. For further discussion on Mach Band, please see our chapter in Retinopathy of Prematurity: Current Diagnosis and Management by Kychenthal and Dorta [5]

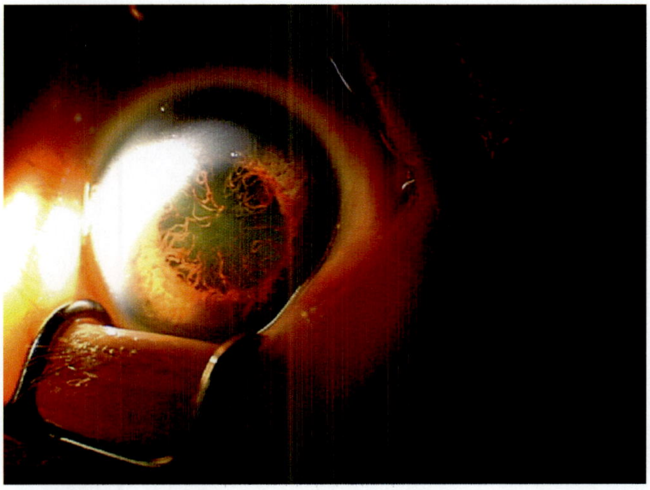

Fig. 6.4 Persistent dilated tunica vasculosa lentis

6.5 Toward Updating the Definition of APROP

The practical objective is to diagnose eyes destined to reach APROP using these positive features that can lead to suspicion of APROP development and thus closer examination even in the absence of plus disease. Strategies during examination to allow detection of difficult to see features such as fine neovascularization include optimizing pupillary dilation, media clarity, magnification (e.g., 20 diopter lens

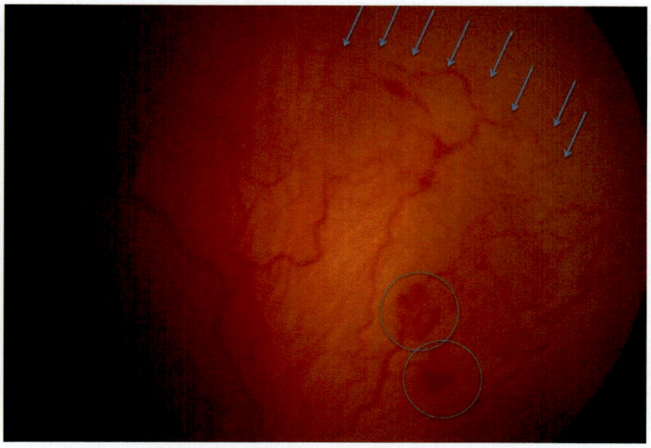

Fig. 6.5 Arrows show terminal vascular shunt, which can be seen in early APROP. Circles demonstrate neovascularization posteriorly

instead of 28), improved focus, glare reduction, and control of movement of the infant's head.

In order to aid in early detection of APROP, we would like to redefine APROP including subclassification of stages, ignoring plus disease for the moment.

Early APROP Vascular shunts. These may be circumferential vessels at the vascular–avascular junction or posterior to the junction (Fig. 6.5). Dilation and tortuosity may be present. This is equivalent to CROP stage 2. Eyes with early APROP but without plus disease need to be monitored closely (at least weekly examination) to allow for timely treatment if progression occurs. If plus disease is present this should be treated, per ETROP criteria.

It is not obvious that a CROP stage 1 equivalent exists in APROP as there is an absence of fibrosis, but this may be the absence of anterior growth of vessels when the vascular–avascular junction is posterior. In practice, this may be difficult to distinguish from simply immature vessels without photographic documentation of lack of anterior growth. Importantly, however, lack of anterior progression should prompt a closer examination schedule, i.e., weekly examination rather than every other week.

Moderate APROP Flat neovascularization, usually in a tangle (Fig. 6.5). This is equivalent to CROP stage 3. This may be associated with (1) annular, C-shaped, or arc-shaped hemorrhages, which may help highlight the otherwise difficult to detect flat neovascular frond without fibrosis (Fig. 6.6); (2) blush of pink/red at vascular termination which is the fine neovascularization (Fig. 6.7); and (3) disappearance of details of retinal vessels as they approach the vascular–avascular junction, since they may be covered by a thin tangle of neovascularization (Fig. 6.8). This is the stage at which the dilation and tortuosity is likely to be out of proportion to the

Fig. 6.6 Annular hemorrhage is visible near temporal vascular termination. Extraretinal vessels are likely present in the center

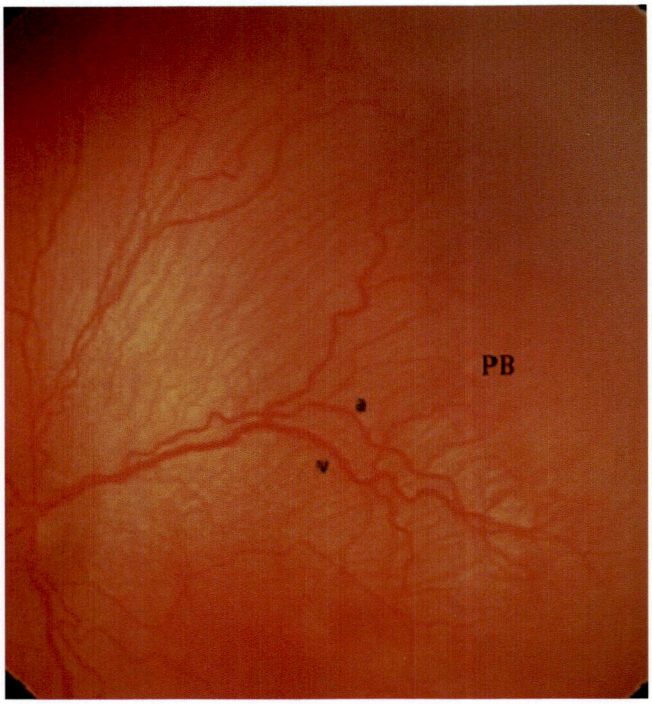

Fig. 6.7 Pink blush (PB) is seen at the vascular termination. This likely represents fine extraretinal vessels. "a" indicates artery and "v" indicates vein

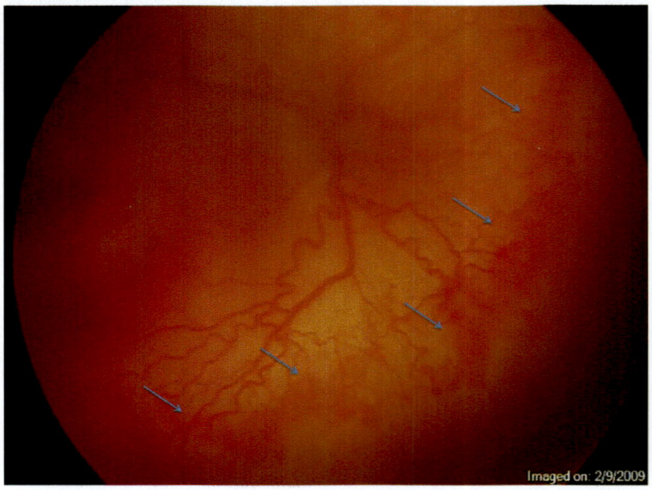

Fig. 6.8 Retina vessels that lose detail or disappear as they approach the avascular retina. They are covered by the blush of "naked" neovascularization. There is no fibrosis present, as would be the case with classic ROP. There is, however, a halo temporally but it has no definitive structure

perceived retinopathy, but this should be the signal to look closer for fine vessels that do explain the dilation and tortuosity. Moderate APROP should be treated. If plus disease is present, then treatment should be done per ETROP recommendation. Similarly, Zone I neovascularization (even without fibrosis since it is stage 3) should be treated even in the absence of plus disease. Moderate APROP in Zone II without plus does not technically meet treatment criteria of ETROP, but treatment should be strongly considered as APROP may progress to late stages quickly.

Late APROP Fibrosis. At first glance, this may look like CROP stage 3 but over time did not progress through the series of conventional stages 1–3 ridges. Instead, the fibrosis developed from the previously "naked" neovascularization, similar to that seen in proliferative diabetic retinopathy. However, once the naked vessels become fibrotic, they frequently contract without treatment (Fig. 6.9). Treatment with anti-VEGF can lead to "crunch" [12]. This "crunch" phenomenon in ROP after anti-VEGF has only been seen by the present authors in the few cases that were sent late for examination and treatment. These eyes have a high rate of progression to tractional retinal detachment with laser as well. With improved awareness and early recognition based on the previous features described, ideally, eyes would not reach this stage.

Very Late APROP Tractional retinal detachment. This is CROP stages 4 and 5. Detachment can occur quickly and

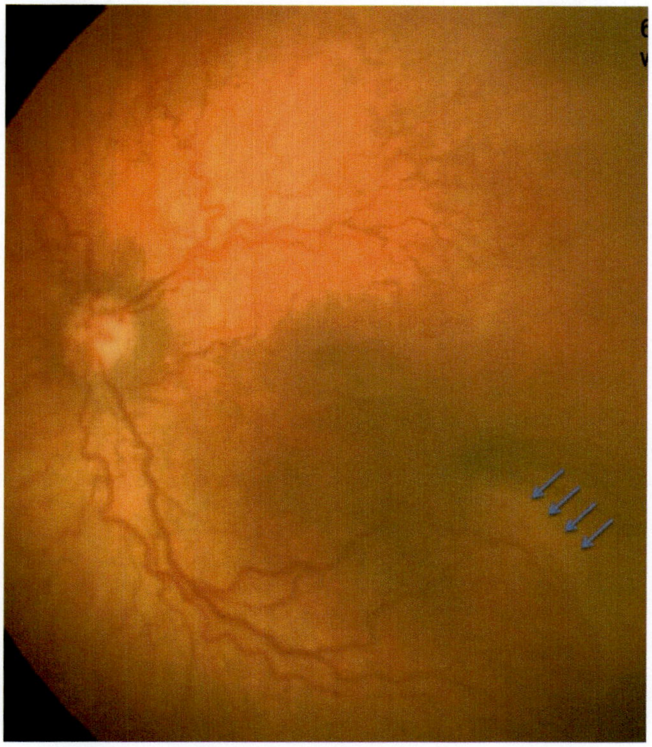

Fig. 6.9 Note the dilation and tortuosity out of proportion to apparent peripheral findings. The central macula has not vascularized. Neovascular tangles are present superotemporally. The fibrotic band demarcated by the arrows is not classic ROP but rather contracted APROP causing localized retinal detachment

should be treated with vitrectomy, although on rare occasions other treatments may be successful, such as scleral buckle [13] or anti-VEGF alone. If the vascularity is quite active, then decreasing anti-VEGF drive before surgery is warranted with anti-VEGF and/or laser. Active vascularity can lead to intraoperative and postoperative bleeding that may complicate surgery and postoperative evaluation.

6.6 Suspected Pathophysiology

The pathophysiologically distinct origin of APROP as opposed to CROP has not been proven but is possibly related to the distinction between vasculogenesis and angiogenesis [14]. In vasculogenesis, retinal vessels form de-novo from mesenchymal cells, whereas in angiogenesis they arise via budding from existing vessels. According to this distinction, CROP forms from the vascular termination where angiogenesis is normally occurring and creates a circumferential ridge. In contradistinction, APROP forms in a more haphazard manner in a posterior location de novo from mesenchymal cells (vasculogenesis). This may explain why foveal formation does not seem to be inhibited by anti-VEGF medications. [15] Alternatively, APROP may be due to extremely high levels of VEGF which cause neovascularization at away from the vascular–avascular junction.

6.7 Special Forms of APROP: Oxygen Induced

This involves obliteration of capillary beds and creates abnormal shunts both at vascular–avascular junction and posterior to it. This occurs in larger babies, usually in less developed nations where oxygen regulation may not be as tight. This, in our view, is not primary APROP but a secondary APROP that results from a later intervention, excessive oxygen or free radical damage. It is probably useful to recognize this pattern for interaction with neonatology about oxygen monitoring. In the literature, this may be called oxygen-induced retinopathy (OIR) or may be labeled as APROP, particularly in areas where it is more common [16]. Reasons that we believe it to be a distinct form of APROP include:

1. It occurs in situations of systemic stress, most commonly the use of unblended, unmonitored, and uncontrolled oxygen supplementation.
2. It occurs among much older infants with a mean gestational age of 28 weeks (median 30 weeks), who often have birth weights above 1250 g.
3. The vascular findings are often well into Zone II, whereas APROP usually is a posterior disease.
4. The angiogram shows a special pattern of an ablative retinopathy with loss of capillary perfusion with retention of larger arterioles and venules which have a looping appearance (Fig. 6.10).

This last pattern indicates vascular damage rather than a primary defect of vascular growth.

6.8 Special Forms of APROP: Recurrence/Reactivation after anti-VEGF

This is an area of interest as descriptors are needed for patterns of ROP reactivation after anti-VEGF. Anterior vascular development may occur and may undergo secondary arrest with shunting and dilated terminal structures (Fig. 6.11). Recurrent extraretinal neovascularization may occur without fibrosis at anterior or posterior locations. Vessels that grow out of the retina at a posterior location seem to do so in areas of prior vascular arrest and extraretinal neovascularization. This seems to recapitulate APROP. Chen et al. describe plus disease as an early sign of reactivation of ROP after anti-VEGF treatment [17]. This again seems to mimic APROP where plus is out of proportion to perceived ROP (Figs. 6.12 and 6.13).

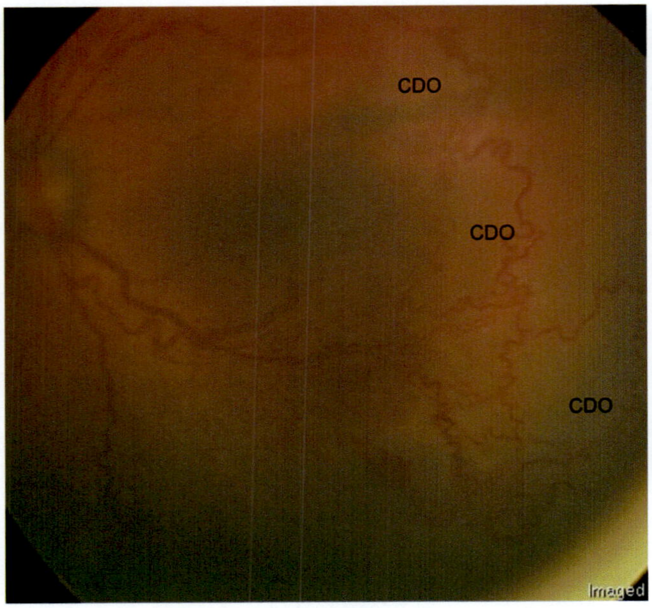

Fig. 6.10 An example of oxygen-induced retinopathy. Large looping vessels are seen surrounding areas of capillary drop out (CDO)

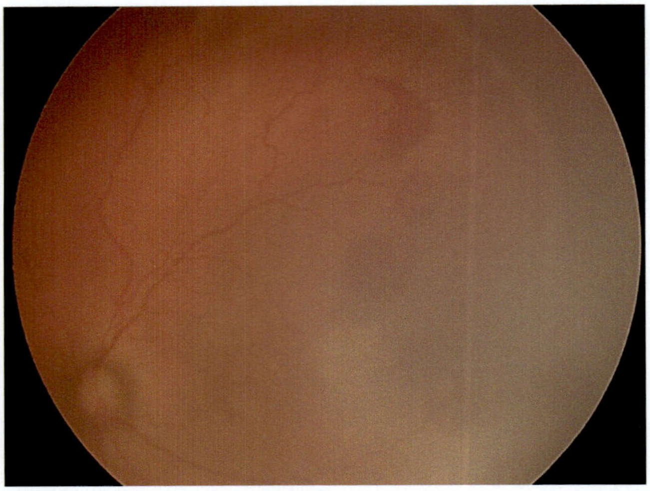

Fig. 6.12 This eye was treated originally with bevacizumab. C-shaped hemorrhages are seen at the area of original neovascularization and a partially fibrotic demarcation ridge is seen temporally at the vascular–avascular junction. The C (or reverse C) shape is due to hemorrhage around a center of extraretinal vessels. In an eye without apparent active ROP, this sign should alert the examiner to the presence of extraretinal neovascularization and possible APROP

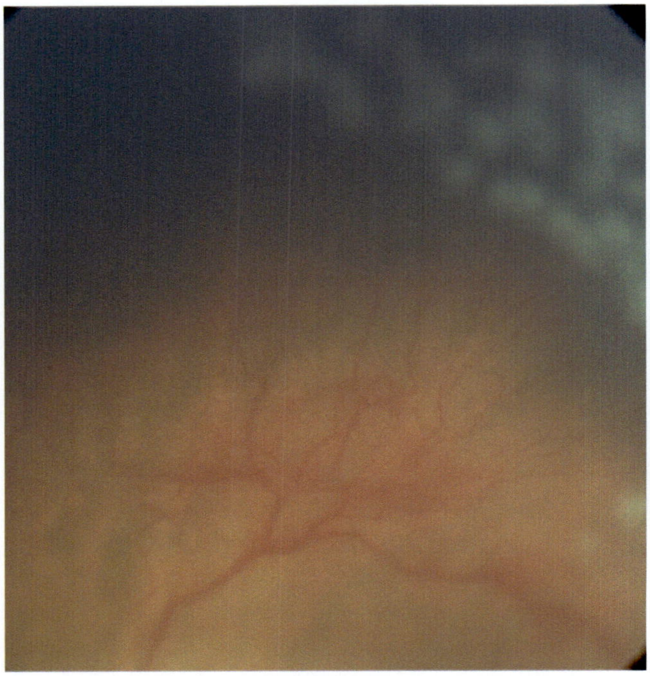

Fig. 6.11 The eye was originally treated with bevacizumab and then subsequently was treated with laser to avascular retina after reactivation. Note fine extraretinal vessels at the posterior location of original neovascularization

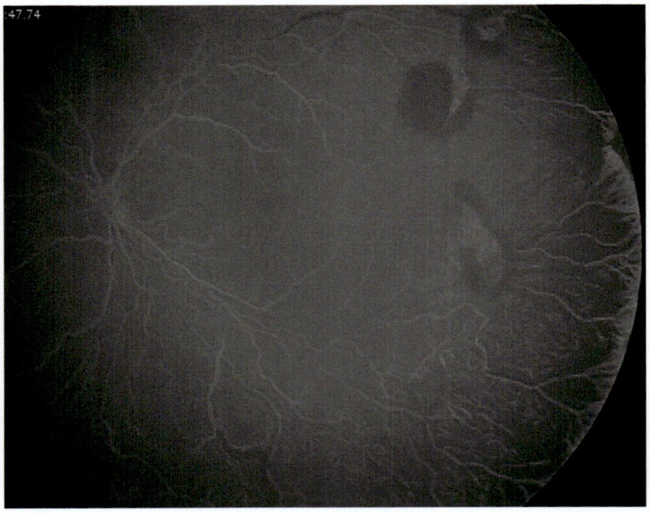

Fig. 6.13 Fluorescein angiography of eye in Fig. 6.12. Perfused vessels are demonstrated at the center of the C-shaped hemorrhages. Capillary dropout is also present, which can be seen in APROP and OIR

6.9 Present State of APROP Detection and Treatment Options

APROP is currently detected by clinical examination looking for the signs described above. If flat extraretinal neovascularization without fibrosis is seen, then APROP is present. Plus disease out of proportion to perceived retinopathy, hemorrhages at the border of the vascular–avascular junction, lack of anterior migration, rapid progression of disease, and persistence of fetal vessels, such as tunica vasculosa lentis and hyaloid artery remnant, should prompt a search for APROP, perhaps switching to increased magnification with 20 diopter lens.

It should be noted that similar to known disagreement among experts in plus disease diagnosis, APROP diagnosis may not be agreed upon using photographs [18, 19]. It is our hope that in the future imaging technology may better standardize this difficult diagnosis.

Fluorescein angiography at the bedside may be helpful in diagnosing APROP. Image processing to increase contrast may be helpful in identifying fine neovascularization [20]. Similarly, OCT and OCTA may help aid its detection, but these need to be demonstrated with further studies [21].

6.10 Treatment of APROP: Laser or Anti-VEGF

There is controversy of the role of anti-VEGF in the treatment of ROP in general and this extends to APROP. The controversy is due to a lack of high-level data comparing treatment options, but in general, there is more agreement that APROP responds poorly to laser and better to anti-VEGF treatment. We will review the rationale and available data for treatment preference.

APROP, like ROP in general, is a disease of non-perfusion, ischemia, proliferation, hemorrhage, and traction retinal detachment. The proliferative retinopathy is driven by VEGF. The essence of effective management is the timely reduction of VEGF. In order to achieve this with laser, treatment must include the entire avascular retina including any avascular zones that are under the neovascularization. Since VEGF is largely produced just anterior to the vascularized retina, posterior skip areas have particularly bad outcomes in all cases of ROP—especially APROP.

Barriers to complete laser photocoagulation include:

1. A persistent pupillary membrane (often called a "persistent tunica vasculosa lentis") that obscures the retina. As discussed above, this is more common in APROP.
2. Limited field of view from iris rigidity and small pupil due to poor dilation and intraoperative constriction.
3. Broad areas of neovascularization may camouflage an underlying area of ischemic retina.
4. Fine neovascularization may be obscured by hazy media.
5. A large area of treatment due to posterior disease may increase the risk of laser complications such as inflammation, exudative detachment, ocular ischemia, and cataract.
6. A longer treatment duration to complete the extensive laser required for APROP and overall more fragile systemic status of infants who are likely to develop APROP may increase the risks of anesthesia. On occasion, these challenges make a complete laser ablation of the avascular retina impossible. Ultimately, incomplete treatments greatly increase the risk of failure and unfavorable outcomes.

Anti-VEGF injection also removes VEGF from the vitreous reservoir immediately whereas laser only stops its production by ischemic retina, allowing already present VEGF to modulate vessels until its vitreal levels decline spontaneously. Another reason for the difficulty treating APROP is that the levels of VEGF in APROP eyes are likely higher than CROP as evidenced by the decreased efficacy of a reduced dose of bevacizumab. Lorenz et al. showed that 0.312 mg bevacizumab induced regression in 100% of Zone II CROP eyes, 80% of Zone I eyes, but only 25% of APROP eyes [22]. It is likely that larger areas of persistent avascular retina found in APROP than CROP after bevacizumab contribute to the likely higher VEGF load [23–25].

In our recent retrospective study [9] of patients treated for APROP at the University of Chicago Comer Children's Hospital, with minimum follow-up to 80 weeks PMA, APROP responded better to bevacizumab than laser photocoagulation. TRD occurred in 1 of 22 eyes with treated with bevacizumab and in 5 of 14 eyes in the laser group ($p = 0.002$). However, reactivation requiring treatment was common in both groups, 9/22 after bevacizumab and 6/14 after laser (NS). The mean gestational age was 24.5 weeks with a mean birth weight of 632 g in the bevacizumab group and 24.7 weeks and 777 g in the laser group. Most eyes in the bevacizumab group did receive treatment completion laser after 60 weeks PMA to reduce the chance of late reactivation of ROP (described below).

In addition to a lower rate of TRD after bevacizumab compared to laser in our recent study, the lower rate of TRD also compares favorably to prior reports of laser treatment for APROP. Drenser [2] reported progression to retinal detachment in 8 of 44 eyes with APROP and Pandya [4] described 3 of 6 eyes with APROP progressing to detachment despite laser. Sanghi reported 17% of APROP eyes progressed to detachment after laser [3]. Gunn reported 2 of 11 APROP eyes progressing to detachment [26]. Ahn et al. found a 15% failure rate of laser for APROP [27]. There are reports of vitrectomy after laser failure for APROP [6].

Most studies comparing the efficacy of bevacizumab to laser for APROP are from outside the United States, and results may be different when infants are larger. Nonetheless, outcomes after bevacizumab are generally more favorable. In a study from Turkey, Gunay reported 0 of 25 APROP eyes progressing to detachment after bevacizumab while 2 of 15 APROP eyes detached after laser [28]. The mean birth weight of infants in the bevacizumab group was 900 g. Nicoara similarly found improved regression of APROP after bevacizumab (94%) versus laser (83%) in a Romanian population with a mean birth weight over 1 kg [29]. Outcomes for the smaller infants treated for APROP in our recent study [9], with a mean birth weight of 632 g in the bevacizumab group, might have been expected to be worse given the lower birth weight. However, the single detachment out of 22 eyes that received initial bevacizumab compares favorably.

With respect to the selection of an anti-VEGF medication, bevacizumab has the most experience worldwide and appears to work well for Type 1 ROP in general and APROP in particular. Ranibizumab use is increasing due to systemic safety concerns (discussed below) but appears to have a higher rate of reactivation, ranging from 26 to 64% for ROP in general, not just APROP [30–37]. Moreover, Chuluunblat found an 18% rate of non-responsiveness [36]. The lack of efficacy may be related to a shorter half-life and therefore early reactivation. Treatment failure for APROP is likely higher. Sukgen and Kocluk [34] found an approximately 50% rate of reactivation of APROP after ranibizumab treatment. Given the lack of concrete data on adverse systemic safety issues, the possibility of blindness due to suboptimal anti-VEGF must be considered. The use of aflibercept [38] and conbercept [39] for ROP have been reported but experience, particularly with APROP, is limited.

With regard to systemic safety concerns regarding anti-VEGF, it is known that the medication reaches systemic circulation and suppresses systemic VEGF and that this effect is longer for bevacizumab than for ranibizumab [40]. The implications of this VEGF suppression, and even optimal levels in preterm neonates [41], are not known. Nonetheless, concerns regarding adverse effects on neurodevelopment continue to limit the use of anti-VEGF, particularly after work by Morin et al. [42]. That data was gathered retrospectively and was unfortunately fraught with bias [43]. The first bias was for the treatment of sicker infants with anti-VEGF, which is demonstrated by SNAP-II scores that measure the severity of systemic illness. The second was for the treatment of infants with more severe ROP with anti-VEGF. Also, 11 patients in the laser arm had mild enough disease to not even meet the usual criteria for treatment. There were no such patients in the bevacizumab arm. The study included infants treated before more wide-spread use of anti-VEGF (after the publication of BEAT-ROP [44]) when bevacizumab was reserved for children not well enough for laser or for salvage treatment. Importantly, both sicker systemic disease and worse ROP are known risk factors for poorer neurodevelopment [45–48]. The study also suffers from significant loss to follow-up of 28% of patients. Among infants that did have sufficient follow-up, nine patients in the laser arm were excluded for inability to perform testing for reasons such as poor cooperation, development delay, blindness, and deafness, whereas only one such patient was excluded from the bevacizumab arm. These patients should have been included as having poor neurodevelopment. Recalculating neurodevelopmental outcomes with the above patients included as having severe delay changes the difference in severe developmental delay to be nonsignificant. Indeed, other studies have failed to find a difference in neurodevelopment between children whose ROP was treated with laser or bevacizumab. [49–52].

To date, no good data exists from unbiased clinical investigations that anti-VEGF causes harmful systemic effects. Given the favorable ocular effect of bevacizumab over laser, and likely ranibizumab, for APROP, the real risk of blindness from retinal detachment must be weighed against the unproven, theoretical risk of neurodevelopment in neonates.

6.11 Reactivation After Anti-VEGF

Due to known late reactivation of ROP after bevacizumab injection [25, 53–57], our standard protocol is to perform fluorescein angiography after 60 weeks PMA to identify and ablate persistent avascular retina with laser. We term this "treatment completion" to emphasize that initial treatment with bevacizumab may have a temporary effect. If these eyes had been treated initially with laser, areas of avascular retina would be considered "skip areas" and these untreated areas would generally be treated to prevent reactivation of disease. The delay in the timing of laser treatment completion reduces anesthesia risk [58, 59] and allows anterior growth of retinal vessels.

We remain vigilant after the use of anti-VEGF because it has a limited blockade effect and a risk of reactivation. Larger areas of persistent avascular retina may explain why APROP is more likely to reactivate than CROP. In a recent study, Mintz-Hittner found 6/6 eyes with APROP reactivated [60]. Dikci et al. found that 5 out of 10 APROP eyes treated with bevacizumab 0.5 mg needed laser to treat recurrence [61]. Our recent study [9] found a 41% reactivation rate for eyes with APROP. The difference in morphology of APROP may point to a meaningful difference in the molecular environment that is related to the increased reactivation rate. Therefore, APROP may behave differently than CROP in the same zone in terms of response to initial treatment and rate of reactivation.

Based on naturally regressed ROP and FEVR, we suspect that reactivation may occur years or even decades later. Therefore, our approach is to treat the acute disease with anti-VEGF and residual peripheral ischemic retina with laser at a later date.

The choice of the term ROP "reactivation" over "recurrence" takes into account several observations. First, bevacizumab binds VEGF to suppress neovascularization but does not prevent its continued production. Second, the pathologic avascular retina is the most essential part of ROP as this retina produces VEGF that drives ROP. Third, treatment that leaves a pathologic ischemic zone of the retina has not cured the ROP and is incomplete. Fourth, pathologic neovascularization after the period of VEGF suppression in the face of ischemia should be expected rather than surprising. Finally, as long as there is pathologic avascular retina the disease is manifestly persistent, and the progression is therefore not a recurrence. The idea of reactivation is that ROP persisted (in a dormant state) and then became active again—progressing to neovascularization or worse, to tractional retinal detachment.

It must be remembered that late retinal detachment can occur up to (and likely past) 3 years of age [25, 53, 54]. Most eyes that received bevacizumab in our recent study [9] as initial treatment for APROP underwent treatment completion fluorescein angiography and laser treatment completion to persistent avascular retina to prevent late retinal detachment. Indeed, the only eye that progressed to detachment in this group did not receive prophylactic late laser and has been described elsewhere [25]. Although we believe bevacizumab to be superior to laser in the treatment of APROP, late prophylactic laser is recommended. Only after this final laser do we consider the treatment complete since it treats the residual avascular area. We expect that the long-term quiescence after late laser prophylaxis will also mimic the outcome of conventional laser treatment. This is consistent with our observations after one decade of anti-VEGF use. However, ROP remains a life-long disease.

References

1. International Committee for the Classification of Retinopathy of, P. The international classification of retinopathy of prematurity revisited. Arch Ophthalmol. 2005;123(7):991–9.
2. Drenser KA, Trese MT, Capone A Jr. Aggressive posterior retinopathy of prematurity. Retina. 2010;30(4 Suppl):S37–40.
3. Sanghi G, et al. Aggressive posterior retinopathy of prematurity: risk factors for retinal detachment despite confluent laser photocoagulation. Am J Ophthalmol. 2013;155(1):159–64. e2
4. Pandya HK, et al. Macular development in aggressive posterior retinopathy of prematurity. Biomed Res Int. 2015;2015:808639.
5. Shapiro MJ, et al. Aggressive posterior retinopathy of prematurity (APROP). In: Andres KB, Paola Dorta S, editors. Retinopathy of prematurity: current diagnosis and management, vol. 1. 1st ed; 2017. p. 49–70.
6. Tereshchenko AV, Belyy YA, Sidorova YA, Trifanenkova IG, Tereshchenkova MS, Yudina YA. Vitrectomy technique in aggressive posterior retinopathy of prematurity. Vestn oftalmol. 2018;134(1):32–7.
7. Early Treatment for Retinopathy of Prematurity Cooperative Group, Good WV, Hardy RJ, Dobson V, Palmer EA, Phelps DL, Tung B, Redford M. Final visual acuity results in the early treatment for retinopathy of prematurity study. Arch Ophthalmol. 2010 Jun;128(6):663–71.
8. Early Treatment for Retinopathy of Prematurity Cooperative Group. Revised indications for the treatment of retinopathy of prematurity: results of the early treatment of retinopathy of prematurity randomized trial. Arch Ophthalmol. 2003;121:1684–94.
9. Blair M, Gonzalez JMG, Snyder L, Schechet S, Greenwald M, Shapiro M, Rodriguez SH. Bevacizumab or laser for aggressive posterior retinopathy of prematurity. Taiwan J Ophthalmol. 2018 Oct-Dec;8(4):243–8.
10. Shah PK, Narendran V, Saravanan VR, Raghuram A, Chattopadhyay A, Kashyap M, Devraj S. Fulminate type of retinopathy of prematurity. Indian J Ophthalmol. 2004 Dec;52(4):319–20.
11. Fetus and Newborn Committee, Canadian Paediatric Society. Retinopathy of prematurity: A systematic review of the literature. Paediatr Child Health. 1998 May;3(3):173–80.
12. Yonekawa Y, Wu WC, Nitulescu CE, Chan RVP, Thanos A, Thomas BJ, Todorich B, Drenser KA, Trese MT, Capone A Jr. Progressive retinal detachment in infants with retinopathy of prematurity treated with intravitreal bevacizumab or ranibizumab. Retina. 2018 Jun;38(6):1079–83.
13. Shah RJ, Garcia-Gonzalez JM, Blair MP, Galasso J, Shapiro MJ. Concurrent scleral buckle and intravitreal bevacizumab for advanced retinopathy of prematurity-related retinal detachment. Retin Cases Brief Rep. 2016 Spring;10(2):183–6.
14. Flynn JT, Chan-Ling T. Retinopathy of prematurity: two distinct mechanisms that underlie zone 1 and zone 2 disease. Am J Ophthalmol. 2006 Jul;142(1):46–59.
15. Garcia Gonzalez JM, et al. Foveal development after use of bevacizumab for aggressive posterior retinopathy of prematurity. Ophthalmic Surg Lasers Imaging Retina. 50(6):e185–7.
16. Martinez-Castellanos MA, Velez-Montoya R, Price K, Henaine-Berra A, García-Aguirre G, Morales-Canton V, Cernichiaro-Espinosa LA. Vascular changes on fluorescein angiography of premature infants with low risk of retinopathy of prematurity after high oxygen exposure. Int J Retina Vitreous. 2017 Jan 16;3:2.
17. Chen TA, Shields RA, Bodnar ZH, Callaway N, Schachar IH, Moshfeghi DM. A spectrum of regression following intravitreal bevacizumab in retinopathy of prematurity. Am J Ophthalmol. 2018;198:63–9.
18. Woo R, Chan RV, Vinekar A, Chiang MF. Aggressive posterior retinopathy of prematurity: a pilot study of quantitative analysis of vascular features. Graefes Arch Clin Exp Ophthalmol. 2015 Feb;253(2):181–7.
19. Shapiro MJ, Blair MP, Garcia-Gonzalez JM. Experts contradict established classification. Graefes Arch Clin Exp Ophthalmol. 2016 Jan;254(1):199.
20. Jayadev C, Vinekar A, Mohanachandra P, Desai S, Suveer A, Mangalesh S, Bauer N, Shetty B. Enhancing image characteristics of retinal images of aggressive posterior retinopathy of prematurity using a novel software, (RetiView). Biomed Res Int. 2015;2015:898197.
21. Vinekar A, Chidambara L, Jayadev C, Sivakumar M, Webers CA, Shetty B. Monitoring neovascularization in aggressive posterior retinopathy of prematurity using optical coherence tomography angiography. J AAPOS. 2016 Jun;20(3):271–4.
22. Lorenz B, et al. Retinal vascular development with 0.312 MG intravitreal bevacizumab to treat severe posterior retinopathy of prematurity: a longitudinal fluorescein angiographic study. Retina. 2017;37(1):97–111.
23. Garcia Gonzalez JM, et al. Prophylactic peripheral laser and fluorescein angiography after bevacizumab for retinopathy of prematurity. Retina. 2017;38(4):764–72.
24. Toy BC, et al. Chronic vascular arrest as a predictor of bevacizumab treatment failure in retinopathy of prematurity. Ophthalmology. 2016;123(10):2166–75.
25. Snyder LL, et al. Very late reactivation of retinopathy of prematurity after monotherapy with intravitreal bevacizumab. Ophthalmic Surg Lasers Imaging Retina. 2016;47(3):280–3.
26. Gunn DJ, Cartwright DW, Gole GA. Prevalence and outcomes of laser treatment of aggressive posterior retinopathy of prematurity. Clin Exp Ophthalmol. 2014;42(5):459–65.
27. Ahn YJ, Hong KE, Yum HR, Lee JH, Kim KS, Youn YA, Park SH. Characteristic clinical features associated with aggressive posterior retinopathy of prematurity. Eye (Lond). 2017 Jun;31(6):924–30.
28. Gunay M, et al. Evaluation of 2-year outcomes following intravitreal bevacizumab (IVB) for aggressive posterior retinopathy of prematurity. Arq Bras Oftalmol. 2015;78(5):300–4.

29. Nicoara SD, et al. Regression rates following the treatment of aggressive posterior retinopathy of prematurity with bevacizumab versus laser: 8-year retrospective analysis. Med Sci Monit. 2016;22:1192–209.
30. Ells AL, Wesolosky JD, Ingram AD, Mitchell PC, Platt AS. Low-dose ranibizumab as primary treatment of posterior type I retinopathy of prematurity. Can J Ophthalmol. 2017 Oct;52(5): 468–74.
31. Huang Q, Zhang Q, Xu Y, Ji X, Fei P, Peng J, Li YA, Zhao P. Asymmetric outcomes of type 1 retinopathy of prematurity after bilateral intravitreal ranibizumab treatment. J Ophthalmol. 2017;2017:1741386.
32. Hu Q, Bai Y, Chen X, Huang L, Chen Y, Li X. Recurrence of retinopathy of prematurity in zone II stage 3+ after ranibizumab treatment: a retrospective study. J Ophthalmol. 2017;2017:5078565.
33. Huang Q, Zhang Q, Fei P, Xu Y, Lyu J, Ji X, Peng J, Li YA, Zhao P. Ranibizumab injection as primary treatment in patients with retinopathy of prematurity: anatomic outcomes and influencing factors. Ophthalmology. 2017 Aug;124(8):1156–64.
34. Sukgen EA, Koçluk Y. The vascularization process after intravitreal ranibizumab injections for aggressive posterior retinopathy of prematurity. Arq Bras Oftalmol. 2017 Jan-Feb;80(1):30–4.
35. Lyu J, Zhang Q, Chen CL, Xu Y, Ji XD, Li JK, Huang QJ, Zhao PQ. Recurrence of retinopathy of prematurity after intravitreal ranibizumab monotherapy: timing and risk factors. Invest Ophthalmol Vis Sci. 2017 Mar 1;58(3):1719–25.
36. Chuluunbat T, Chan RV, Wang NK, Lien R, Chen YP, Chao AN, Chen KJ, Chen TL, Hwang YS, Lai CC, Wu WC. Nonresponse and recurrence of retinopathy of prematurity after intravitreal ranibizumab treatment. Ophthalmic Surg Lasers Imaging Retina. 2016 Dec 1;47(12):1095–105.
37. Zhang G, Yang M, Zeng J, Vakros G, Su K, Chen M, Li H, Tian R, Li N, Tang S, He H, Tan W, Song X, Zhuang R, Shenzhen Screening for Retinopathy of Prematurity Cooperative Group. Comparison of intravitreal injection of ranibizumab versus laser therapy for zone ii treatment-requiring retinopathy of prematurity. Retina. 2017 Apr;37(4):710–7.
38. Vural A, Perente İ, Onur İU, Eriş E, Seymen Z, Hergünsel GO, Salihoğlu Ö, Yiğit FU. Efficacy of intravitreal aflibercept monotherapy in retinopathy of prematurity evaluated by periodic fluorescence angiography and optical coherence tomography. Int Ophthalmol. 2018 Nov 26;39(10):2161–9.
39. Bai Y, Nie H, Wei S, Lu X, Ke X, Ouyang X, Feng S. Efficacy of intravitreal conbercept injection in the treatment of retinopathy of prematurity. Br J Ophthalmol. 2018 Jul 20;103(4):494–8.
40. Wu WC, Shih CP, Lien R, Wang NK, Chen YP, Chao AN, Chen KJ, Chen TL, Hwang YS, Lai CC. Serum vascular endothelial growth factor after bevacizumab or ranibizumab treatment for retinopathy of prematurity. Retina. 2017 Apr;37(4):694–701.
41. Kandasamy Y, Hartley L, Rudd D, Smith R. The association between systemic vascular endothelial growth factor and retinopathy of prematurity in premature infants: a systematic review. Br J Ophthalmol. 2017 Jan;101(1):21–4.
42. Morin J, Luu TM, Superstein R, Ospina LH, Lefebvre F, Simard MN, Shah V, Shah PS, Kelly EN, Canadian Neonatal Network and the Canadian Neonatal Follow-Up Network Investigators. Neurodevelopmental outcomes following bevacizumab injections for retinopathy of prematurity. Pediatrics. 2016 Apr;137(4):e20153218.
43. Blair MP, Shapiro MJ, Ad Hoc Group Concerning Neurodevelopment and antiVEGF. Re: Good: bevacizumab for retinopathy of prematurity: treatment when pathology is embedded in a normally developing vascular system (Ophthalmology. 2016;123:1843-1844). Ophthalmology. 2017 Oct;124(10):e74–5.
44. Mintz-Hittner HA, Kennedy KA, Chuang AZ. BEAT-ROP Cooperative Group. Efficacy of intravitreal bevacizumab for stage 3+ retinopathy of prematurity. N Engl J Med. 2011 Feb 17;364(7):603–15.
45. Msall ME, Phelps DL, DiGaudio KM, Dobson V, Tung B, McClead RE, Quinn GE, Reynolds JD, Hardy RJ, Palmer EA, Behalf of the Cryotherapy for Retinopathy of Prematurity Cooperative Group. Severity of neonatal retinopathy of prematurity is predictive of neurodevelopmental functional outcome at age 5.5 years. Pediatrics. 2000 Nov;106(5):998–1005.
46. Molloy CS, Anderson PJ, Anderson VA, Doyle LW. The long-term outcome of extremely preterm (<28 weeks' gestational age) infants with and without severe retinopathy of prematurity. J Neuropsychol. 2016 Sep;10(2):276–94.
47. Cooke RW, Foulder-Hughes L, Newsham D, Clarke D. Ophthalmic impairment at 7 years of age in children born very preterm. Arch Dis Child Fetal Neonatal Ed. 2004 May;89(3):F249–53.
48. Beligere N, Perumalswamy V, Tandon M, Mittal A, Floora J, Vijayakumar B, Miller MT. Retinopathy of prematurity and neurodevelopmental disabilities in premature infants. Semin Fetal Neonatal Med. 2015 Oct;20(5):346–53.
49. Lien R, Yu MH, Hsu KH, Liao PJ, Chen YP, Lai CC, Wu WC. Neurodevelopmental outcomes in infants with retinopathy of prematurity and bevacizumab treatment. PLoS One. 2016 Jan 27;11(1):e0148019.
50. Kennedy KA, Mintz-Hittner HA, BEAT-ROP Cooperative Group. Medical and developmental outcomes of bevacizumab versus laser for retinopathy of prematurity. JAAPOS. 2018 Feb;22(1):61–65.e1.
51. Araz-Ersan B, Kir N, Tuncer S, Aydinoglu-Candan O, Yildiz-Inec D, Akdogan B, Ekici B, Demirel A, Ozmen M. Preliminary anatomical and neurodevelopmental outcomes of intravitreal bevacizumab as adjunctive treatment for retinopathy of prematurity. Curr Eye Res. 2015 May;40(6):585–91.
52. Kong L, Dinh KL, Schechet SA, Coats DK, Voigt RG, Demny AB, Steinkuller PG. Comparison of ocular and developmental outcomes in laser-and bevacizumab-treated infants with retinopathy of prematurity. Ophthalmol Res. 3(1):13–22.
53. Hajrasouliha AR, et al. Reactivation of retinopathy of prematurity three years after treatment with bevacizumab. Ophthalmic Surg Lasers Imaging Retina. 2017;48(3):255–9.
54. Hu J, et al. Reactivation of retinopathy of prematurity after bevacizumab injection. Arch Ophthalmol. 2012;130(8):1000–6.
55. Hoang QV, et al. Fluorescein angiography of recurrent retinopathy of prematurity after initial intravitreous bevacizumab treatment. Arch Ophthalmol. 2010;128(8):1080–1.
56. Ittiara S, et al. Exudative retinopathy and detachment: A late reactivation of retinopathy of prematurity after intravitreal bevacizumab. J Am Assoc Pediat Ophthalmol Strab. 17(3):323–5.
57. Patel RD, et al. Significant treatment failure with intravitreous bevacizumab for retinopathy of prematurity. Arch Ophthalmol. 2012;130(6):801–2.
58. Walther-Larsen S, Rasmussen LS. The former preterm infant and risk of post-operative apnoea: recommendations for management. Acta Anaesthesiol Scand. 2006;50(7):888–93.
59. Cote CJ, et al. Postoperative apnea in former preterm infants after inguinal herniorrhaphy. A combined analysis. Anesthesiology. 1995;82(4):809–22.
60. Mintz-Hittner HA, Geloneck MM, Chuang AZ. Clinical management of recurrent retinopathy of prematurity after intravitreal bevacizumab monotherapy. Ophthalmology. 2016;123(9):1845–55.
61. Dikci S, Ceylan OM, Demirel S, Yılmaz T. Which dose of bevacizumab is more effective for the treatment of aggressive posterior retinopathy of prematurity: lower or higher dose? Arq Bras Oftalmol. 2018 Jan-Feb;81(1):12–7.

Familial Exudative Vitreoretinopathy or Retinopathy of Prematurity

7

Atchara Amphornphruet and Audina M. Berrocal

Abstract

Retinopathy of prematurity (ROP) and familial exudative vitreoretinopathy (FEVR) can have very similar clinical presentations. Both diseases have abnormal development of retinal vessels and lead to severe vitreoretinopathy which causes blindness in newborn infants. The single most important difference is prematurity. In ROP, the most important risk factors are gestational age and low birth weight. In FEVR, it is the genetic mutation. Identifying the underlying mutations in the causative gene can predict the prognosis of patients with FEVR. ROP tends to resolve naturally or with treatment, but FEVR is a lifelong disease. Even we know that the clinical characteristics and risk factors between both diseases are different; the clinical similarity makes differential diagnosis difficult, especially in FEVR patients who were born prematurely. In such a scenario, patients could exhibit features of FEVR or ROP or both and found to have a discrepancy between birth history and fundus appearance, thus ROPER/fROP was used to describe these patients under such conditions.

Keywords

Familial exudative vitreoretinopathy (FEVR) · FZD4 LRP5 · Retinopathy of prematurity (ROP) · ROPER TSPAN12 · Win pathway · ZNF408

A. Amphornphruet (✉)
Department of Ophthalmology, Rajavithi Hospital, Queen Sirikit National Institute of Child Health, Ministry of Public Health, College of Medicine, Rangsit University, Bangkok, Thailand

A. M. Berrocal
Department of Ophthalmology, Bascom Palmer Eye Institute, Miller School of Medicine, University of Miami, Miami, FL, USA

7.1 Introduction

In regards to eye development, a particular Wnt pathway, Norrin-FZD4, has been identified as playing a major role in retinal angiogenesis. Signaling through this pathway is necessary for the development and maintenance of retinal vasculature [1–4]. Mutations affecting genes of this pathway can result in several pediatric vitreoretinopathies, such as Norrie disease (ND), familial exudative vitreoretinopathy (FEVR), and pseudo-glioma and osteoporosis syndrome [5–8]. Wnt pathway mutations also have been reported in Coats disease and persistent fetal vasculature (PFV) [9–12].

Retinopathy of prematurity (ROP) seldom reports to have an association of genetic mutation. However, some studies have identified Wnt pathway mutations such as FZD4, LRP5, and TSPAN12 in patients with advanced ROP [13–15] Mutations in both the NDP and FZD4 genes have been reported in ROP cases and make Wnt pathway mutations a candidate for developing severe ROP [14]. However, most ROP patients do not show any genetic mutation, in contrast, as high as 50% of FEVR patients are associated with known genetic mutations of the Wnt pathway [16, 17].

FEVR occurs in an X-linked (NDP), autosomal recessive (LRP5), or autosomal dominant inheritance pattern (FZD4, TSPAN12, ZNF408). Most reported cases of autosomal dominant FEVR have been associated with mutations in the FZD4 gene [18]. ROP and FEVR have overlapping phenotypes, and premature birth history makes it difficult to differentiate between both diseases. In the past, ROP is distinguished from FEVR by premature birth and the lack of a family history of retinal diseases (Table 7.1). But as advances in infertility technology and neonatal care improve, so does the survival rate of newborns. Therefore, more cases of premature infants with features of FEVR are recognized. Testing for FEVR genetic mutations is useful in patients with suspected FEVR and ROP. Studies have shown that the [P33S(;)P168S] FZD4 variant is associated with FEVR and ROP [18, 19].

W.-C. Wu, W.-C. Lam (eds.), *A Quick Guide to Pediatric Retina*, https://doi.org/10.1007/978-981-15-6552-6_7

Table 7.1 Characteristic features between FEVR, ROP, and fROP/ROPER

Characteristics	FEVR	ROP	fROP/ROPER
Family history	Familial pattern	Negative family history	Familial pattern
Birth history	Normal birth weight and gestation	Low birth weight and gestation	Mild premature and low birth weight
Progression	Progression after birth in childhood or adulthood	Usually does not progress or recur in childhood	More aggressive progression after birth
Time course	Variable time course, any time period after birth	The disease follows a predictable chronological time course	Acute onset of active diseases after birth and can progress in childhood
Oxygen exposure	Absence of supplementary oxygenation at birth	The cumulative exposure to supplemental oxygen	Absence of premature or positive oxygen exposure among the at-risk group

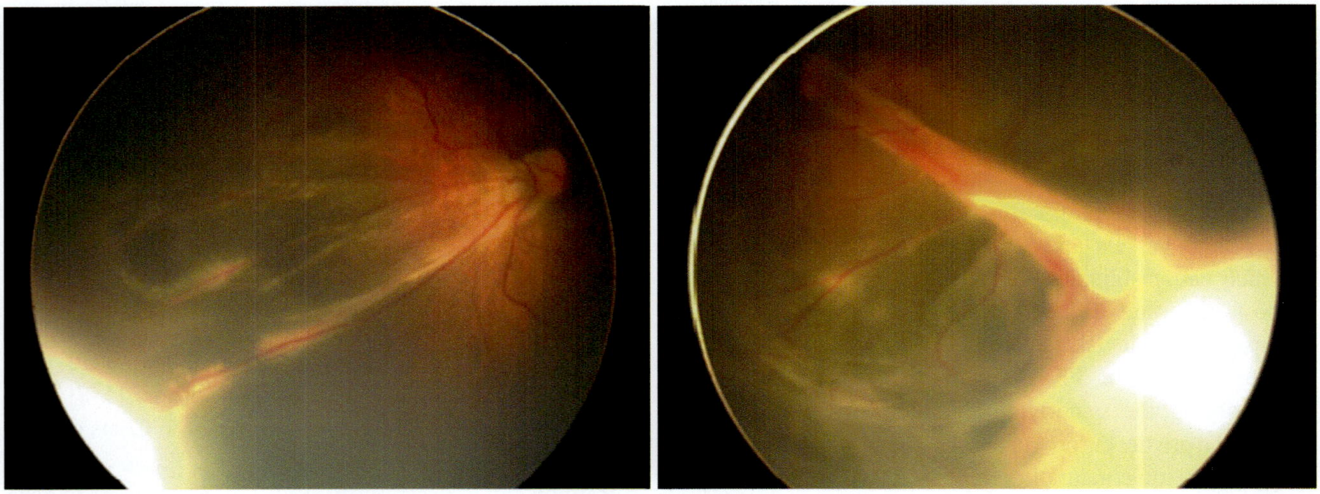

Fig. 7.1 Representative fundus photos of a male infant diagnosed with FEVR but born prematurely at GA 26 weeks, BW 900 g. Photo was taken at PMA 41 weeks, both eyes showing exudation, tractional retinal detachment, vascular anomalies posteriorly, and radial temporal retinal fold in the left eye, which resembled typical features of FEVR

Genetic testing may be beneficial to screen premature infants when we suspect a FEVR mutation [18]. Clinically, identifying the underlying mutations in the causative gene can help us manage the patient and predict the prognosis of the disease. Patients with positive gene mutation tend to have more severe phenotypes that progress and develop recurring retinal detachment. In ROP, acute progression to retinal detachment should be monitored more strictly and the suspicion of ROPER/fROP should be entertained [19–21].

This chapter focuses on FEVR patients who are born *prematurely* and exhibit features of FEVR, ROP, or both. Discrepancies between birth, family history, and fundus appearance should alert to the possible diagnosis of FEVR (Table 7.1 and Fig. 7.1). In such a scenario, ROPER/fROP was postulated to be used to refer to these patients.

Also staging in both diseases was compared in Table 7.2 [22].

From characteristic features, FEVR can be distinguished from ROP by:

- Familial pattern
- Progression after birth in childhood or adulthood

Table 7.2 Staging of FEVR and ROP

Stage	FEVR	ROP
1	Avascular retinal periphery or anomalous intraretinal vascularization 1A: Without exudate or leakage 1B: With exudate or leakage	Demarcation line
2	Avascular retinal periphery with extraretinal vascularization 2A: Without exudate or leakage 2B: With exudate or leakage	Ridge with height and width
3	Extramacular retinal detachment 3A: Without exudate or leakage 3B: With exudate or leakage	Extraretinal fibrovascular proliferation
4	Macula-involving retinal detachment 4A: Without exudate or leakage 4B: With exudate or leakage	Partial retinal detachment 4A: Extrafoveal retinal detachment 4B: Foveal retinal detachment
5	Total retinal detachment 5A: Open funnel 5B: Close funnel	Total retinal detachment

- Absence of severe prematurity (mostly older than 28 weeks)
- Absence of supplementary oxygenation at birth
- Presence of more exudation and trend to reactivate or recur after treatment
- Asymmetric disease

With ROP:

- Mostly occurs as an acute disease after birth; stable after the acute episode.
- Premature with low birth weight/young gestational age.
- The disease follows a predictable chronological time course.
- Usually does not progress or recur in childhood.
- The cumulative exposure to supplemental oxygen.
- Usually symmetrical disease.

In premature infants who are not at risk for ROP, it is easier to identify features associated to FEVR rather than ROP. If the premature infant is at risk of ROP, many of the clinical features associated with FEVR may overlap with those commonly found in ROP, making a definite diagnosis of FEVR challenging (Figs. 7.2 and 7.3).

The management and follow-up of the two disorders are different, and both may lead to severe vitreoretinopathy with tractional detachments and potential blindness. Positive genetic testing results may support the diagnosis of FEVR, but it is important to remember that a negative result or negative family history does not rule out the diagnosis [23, 24] (Table 7.3). In FEVR, 50% of the cases have no known mutation and a negative family history can simply signify a new mutation. Also, the follow up of these patients is quite different. Patients with ROP require very close monitoring, especially at a certain gestational age. FEVR is a lifelong disease

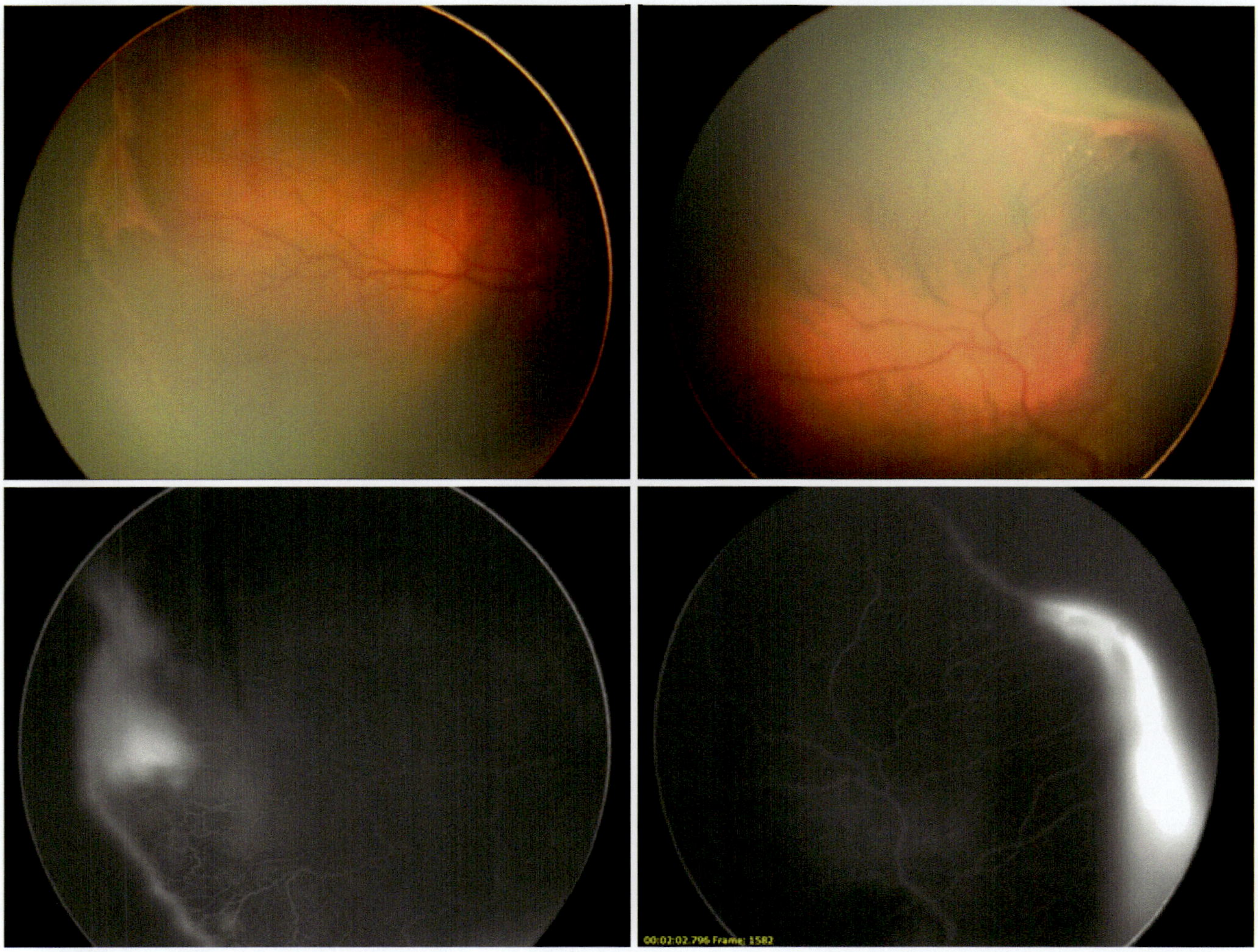

Fig. 7.2 Representative photos of a male infant diagnosed with fROP/ROPER born prematurely at GA 29 weeks, BW 1330 g. Color fundus was taken at PMA 47 weeks. The right eye demonstrated stage 3 ROP. The color fundus showed typical ridge tissue, retinal hemorrhage, and active neovascularization. Fluorescein angiogram demonstrated classic homogenous vascularization pattern at ridge tissue and focal leakage of neovascularization, which are more characteristic of ROP

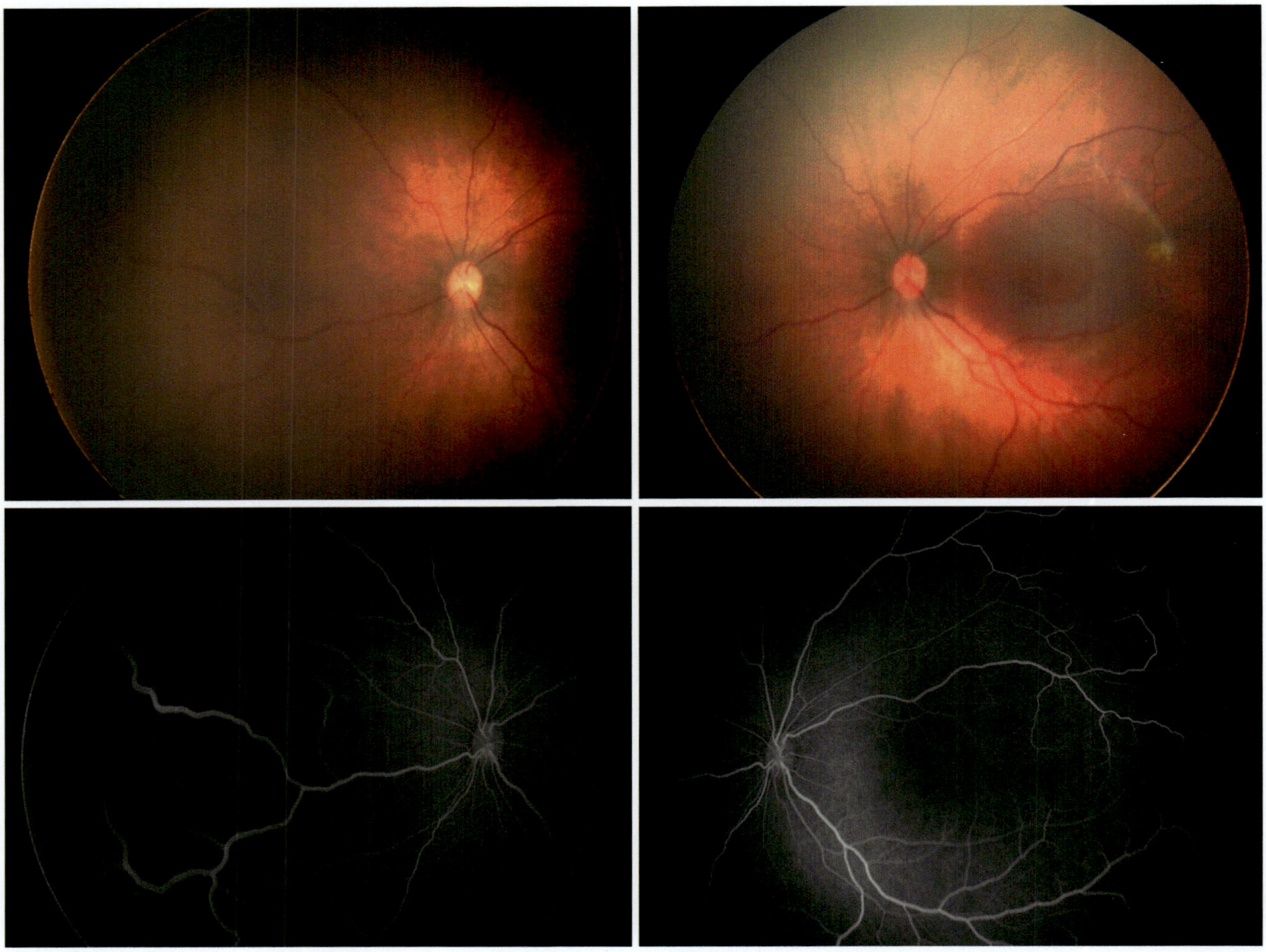

Fig. 7.3 The same patient as Fig. 7.2: The left eye showed anomalous retinal vasculature posteriorly and the anomalous circumferential peripheral vessels, as well as the asymmetry between both eyes, making it more like FEVR. So, this case looks like a hybrid for both ROP and FEVR

Table 7.3 Differential diagnosis of premature infants with FEVR and ROP with fundus appearance

Clinical	FEVR	ROP
Exudation	Any time period in early birth, often during the subsequent progression and reactivation.	Late stage of ROP, which are not signs of progression and reactivation
Retinal vascular change	More variation of vasculature with subretinal fluid, exudates, telangiectasias, and aneurysms.	Mostly follow a pattern of stage by stage progression
Posterior retina vasculature	Dragged appearance with peripheral traction in early active stage leading to advance stage	Dragged appearance in optic nerve and macula may be referred as regression of ROP

that requires lifelong management. ROP is a disease that resolves naturally or with treatment. The management for fROP/ROPER is retinal photocoagulation to the avascular area as is in ROP. Anti-VEGF can be considered as an adjuvant to laser especially in cases when there is generalized leakage in the retinal vessels. Monitoring these cases with wide-field fluorescein angiography (WFA) is essential to diagnose early recurrences or progression of the disease to avoid tractional retinal detachments. If detachment occurs, scleral buckles alone or in combination with vitrectomies may be needed.

In one of the author's centers, Queen Sirikit National Institute of Child Health (QSNICH), Bangkok, 125 cases of FEVR were reported during 2013–2017. Twenty-four patients (20%) were born prematurely, and angiographic testing showed characteristics of FEVR-like changes rather than ROP. In premature infants with FEVR, 9/24 cases (37.5%) were at risk of ROP (GA </= 28 weeks or BW </=1500 g) whose mean GA was 27 weeks and mean birth weight 1460 g; 15/24 cases (62.5%) were not at risk of ROP whose mean GA was 37 weeks and mean birth weight 2300 g. Berrocal et al. had reported 9 FEVR cases who were born prematurely with a mean GA of 30 weeks and mean

birth weight 1226 g and showed these cases to be FEVR in the presence of prematurity. These studies aimed to show a better classification of these cases and the proposed name of ROPER (ROP vs. FEVR) for premature infants who behaved like FEVR cases [25, 26]. Drenser et al. termed this disease "fROP." This subset of fROP/ROPER will have the risks of continual disease activity and will alter the treatment, follow-up, and family counseling [12].

7.2 Widefield Fluorescein Angiography in ROP, FEVR, and fROP/ROPER

Imaging is important for the management of ROP and FEVR. The diagnosis of both FEVR and ROP are based on ophthalmoscopy or color photography findings, and WFA helps in identifying the early or flat neovascularization and more accurately identify the borders between vascular and avascular retina. WFA also allows for early identification of vascular changes that are not seen by ophthalmoscopy or color photography [27–29]. WFA is the best diagnostic tool particularly in eyes with atypical fundus findings in premature infants suspected of having ROPER. It provides additional information by identifying angiographic characteristics of ROP versus FEVR-like syndrome or may contain features of both [29]. WFA is also useful in monitoring disease progression, regression, and treatment planning in pediatric vitreoretinopathies such as ROP and FEVR.

Characteristics of WFA in ROP [27, 28]:

- Vascular tuft formation
- Focal capillary dilatation
- Neovascularization and leakage
- Classic homogenous vascularization pattern at the ridge
- Arteriovenous shunting

Characteristics of WFA in FEVR [22, 23]:

- More vascular branching
- Venous–venous shunting
- Anomalous circumferential peripheral vessels
- Peripheral avascular abnormalities
- Supernumerous vascular abnormalities at the junction
- Central or peripheral telangiectasias
- Late phase disc leakage

Characteristic of WFA in fROP/ROPER [25, 26]:

- Contain features of both ROP and FEVR
- Irregular sprouts vascularization at the junction
- Distinct pruning of vessels
- Pinpoints areas of hyperfluorescence
- Segmental areas of vascular leakage

7.3 Conclusion

Both ROP and FEVR can exhibit dragged disc, ectopic macular, and pseudostrabismus due to fibrovascular tractional lesions from active avascular areas. If patients were born prematurely less than 37 weeks and present with vascular reactivity and demonstrate fresh exudation, leaky vascular areas, or asymmetric retinal findings, then FEVR is the more likely diagnosis. ROP is a disease of prematurity and resolves with time. The fundus features of adults with ROP complications are secondary to persistent avascular area, lattice degeneration, rhegmatogenous components at the edge of treated versus untreated retina, or tractional retinal detachment from vitreous contraction. Patients with fROP/ROPER will continue to progress throughout their lifetime with exudation, neovascularization, vitreous hemorrhage, Coats-like response, tractional retinal detachment, and even vasoproliferative tumor.

When not certain about the diagnosis of fROP/ROPER in premature infants who demonstrate more characteristics of FEVR than ROP in acute diseases, we recommend performing fluorescein angiography and genetic testing. This allows for a better understanding of the clinical presentation of the patient. A definite diagnosis will lead to better management of the patient and the prevention of visual compromise. fROP/ROPER tends to pose a continuing risk of progression and reactivation which is unlike classic ROP that is mostly stable after the resolution of active disease. The best advice is that if it is not behaving like ROP, think of FEVR.

References

1. Wang Y, Rattner A, Zhou Y, et al. Norrin/frizzled 4 signaling in retinal vascular development and blood brain barrier plasticity. Cell. 2012;151:1332–44.
2. Braunger BM, Tamm ER. The different functions of norrin. Adv Exp Med Biol. 2012;723:679–83.
3. Ohlmann A, Tamm ER. Norrin: molecular and functional properties of an angiogenic and neuroprotective growth factor. Prog Retin Eye Res. 2012;31:243–57.
4. Ye X, Wang Y, Nathans J. The norrin/Frizzled4 signaling pathway in retinal vascular development and disease. Trends Mol Med. 2010;16:417–25.
5. Sims KB. NDP-related retinopathies. In: Pagon RA, Adam MP, Ardinger HH, et al., editors. Gene reviews(R). Seattle, WA: University of Washington; 1993.
6. Chamney S, McLoone E, Willoughby CE. A mutation in the Norrie disease gene (NDP) associated with familial exudative vitreoretinopathy. Eye (Lond). 2011;25:1658.
7. Chen ZY, Battinelli EM, Fielder A, et al. A mutation in the norrie disease gene (NDP) associated with X-linked familial exudative vitreoretinopathy. Nat Genet. 1993;5:180–3.
8. Dickinson JL, Sale MM, Passmore A, et al. Mutations in the NDP gene: contribution to norrie disease, familial exudative vitreoretinopathy and retinopathy of prematurity. Clin Experiment Ophthalmol. 2006;34:682–8.

9. Robitaille JM, Wallace K, Zheng B, et al. Phenotypic overlap of familial exudative vitreoretinopathy (FEVR) with persistent fetal vasculature (PFV) caused by FZD4 mutations in two distinct pedigrees. Ophthalmic Genet. 2009;30:23.
10. Black GC, Perveen R, Bonshek R, et al. Coats' disease of the retina (unilateral retinal telangiectasis) caused by somatic mutation in the NDP gene: a role for norrin in retinal angio- genesis. Hum Mol Genet. 1999;8:2031–5.
11. Robitaille JM, Zheng B, Wallace K, et al. The role of frizzled- 4 mutations in familial exudative. Br J Ophthalmol. 95(4):574–9.
12. Drenser KA, Dailey W, Vinekar A, et al. Clinical presentation and genetic correlation of patients with mutations affecting the FZD4 gene. Arch Ophthalmol. 2009;127:1649–54.
13. Kondo H, Kusaka S, Yoshinaga A, et al. Genetic variants of FZD4 and LRP5 genes in patients with advanced retinopathy of prematurity. Mol Vis. 2013;19:476–85.
14. Wu WC, Drenser K, Trese M, et al. Retinal phenotype- genotype correlation of pediatric patients expressing muta- tions in the Norrie disease gene. Arch Ophthalmol. 2007;125:225–30.
15. Hiraoka M, Takahashi H, Orimo H, et al. Genetic screening of Wnt signaling factors in advanced retinopathy of prematurity. Mol Vis. 2010;16:2572–7.
16. Hiroyuki K. Complex genetics of familial exudative vitreoretinopathy and related paediatric retinal detachments. Taiwan J of Ophthalmol. 2015;5:56–62.
17. Mukai S, et al. The Wnt signaling pathway in familial exudative Vitreoretinopathy and Norrie diseases. Sem in Ophthalmology. 2007;22:211–7.
18. Dailey WA, Gryc W, Garg PG, Drenser KA. Frizzled-4 variations associated with retinopathy and intrauterine growth retardation: a potential marker for prematurity and retinopathy. Ophthalmology. 2015;122:1917–23.
19. MacDonald ML, Goldberg YP, Macfarlane J, Samuels ME, Trese MT, Shastry BS. Genetic variants of frizzled-4 gene in familial exudative vitreoretinopathy and advanced retinopathy of prematurity. Clin GenetClin Genet. 2005;67:363e366.
20. Ells A, Guernsey DL, Wallace K, et al. Severe retinopathy of prematurity associated with FZD4 mutations. Ophthalmic Genet. 2010;31:37e43.
21. Drenser KA, Dailey W, Vinekar A, Dalal K, Capone A Jr, Trese MT. Clinical presentation and genetic correlation of patients with mutations affecting the FZD4 gene. Arch Ophthalmol. 2009;127:1649e1654.
22. Kashani AH, Brown KT, Chang E, et al. Diversity of retinal vascular anomalies in patients with familial exudative vitreoretinopathy. Ophthalmology. 2014;121:2220–7.
23. Ranchod TM, Ho LY, Drenser KA, Capone A Jr, Trese MT. Clinical presentation of familial exudative vitreoretinopathy. Ophthalmology. 2011;118(10):2070–5.
24. Liche F, Majji AB. Familial exudative vitreoretinopathy. Ophthalmology. May 2012;119(5):1093.
25. Gologorsky D, Chang JS, Hess DJ, Berrocal AM. Familial exudative vitreoretinopathy in a premature child. Ophthalmic Surg Lasers Imaging Retina. 2013;44:603–5.
26. John VJ, Mc Clintic JI, Hess DJ, Berrocal AM. Retinopathy of prematurity versus familial exudative vitreoretinopathy: report on clinical and angiographic findings. Ophthalmic Surg Lasers Imaging Retina. 2016;47:14–9.
27. Zepeda-Romero LC, Oregon-Miranda AA, Lizarraga-Barrón DS, et al. Early retinopathy of prematurity findings identified with fluorescein angiography. Graefes Arch Clin Exp Ophthalmol. 2013;251:2093–7.
28. Azad R, Chandra P, Khan MA, Darswal A. Role of intravenous fluorescein angiography in early detection and regression of retinopathy of prematurity. J Pediatr Ophthalmol Strabismus. 2008;45:36–9.
29. Ng EYJ, Lanigan B, O'Keefe M. Fundus fluorescein angiography in the screening for and management of retinopathy of prematurity. J Pediatr Ophthalmol Strabismus. 2006;43:85–90.

Telemedicine in Retinopathy of Prematurity

8

Anand Vinekar and Shivani Sinha

Abstract

Telemedicine has been used worldwide in several medical specialties including Ophthalmology. However, its use in infant eye screening especially for Retinopathy of Prematurity (ROP) has been more limited. Ironically, it is for this disease entity wherein telemedicine promises possibly the highest benefit. A short time window of screening, a standard classification of the disease, specially designed infant retinal cameras and lossless image transfer tools make this feasible. Furthermore, the lack of trained experts and the large number of infants that require screening in the outreach make "tele-ROP" an attractive prospect. Yet, its relatively poor adoption can be attributed to several real-world challenges like the cost of the technology, cost of implementation, cost benefit, and medicolegal concerns. Drawing from the experience of over 150,000 infant screening sessions in the "KIDROP-Tele-ROP" program in India, this chapter addresses these challenges and suggests possible solutions for a wider expansion.

Keywords

Retinopathy of prematurity · Tele-medicine · Tele-ROP KIDROP · Wide-field imaging · RetCam shuttle · Neo WISE-ROP · Impact

Telemedicine (TM) is a subset of telehealth aimed to address uneven distribution and shortage of human resources and infrastructure in delivering primary or secondary healthcare. It employs communication networks to provide healthcare services and/or medical education to another geographic location [1]. Telemedicine in radiology is in vogue for over five decades. Its uptake in other fields of medicine has become increasingly popular with the advent of image-based documentation and the ubiquitous internet.

Telemedicine in ophthalmology has been used especially in the screening and management of retinal disorders. A meta-analysis concluded that digital imaging techniques combining mydriasis with wide-field imaging can be effectively used for diabetic retinopathy (DR) screening [2]. It has also been used in the evaluation of the optic nerve, visual fields, and nerve fiber layer analysis. Increasingly, no ophthalmic subspecialty is untouched by telemedicine [3]. In middle-income countries like India, the telemedicine model has been successfully used for DR screening using non-mydriatic fundus photography captured on low-cost, portable, indigenous cameras that provide screening, especially in the rural areas [4, 5]. Telemedicine in pediatric retinal diseases, with a special focus on Retinopathy of prematurity (ROP) has evolved more recently and will be the focus of this chapter.

8.1 Telemedicine in Retinopathy of Prematurity

ROP appears to fulfill the criteria described by Wilson and Jungner [6] for screening a disease of public health importance. These include the fact that it is an important health problem in a defined population subset, with a natural history that is studied, an accepted diagnostic test, treatment, and an agreed policy on who to treat. Importantly, case finding should be a continuous process and not a "once and for all" project.

ROP is one of the leading causes of preventable infant blindness in the world especially plaguing middle-income countries. Indirect ophthalmoscopy was regarded as the gold standard for screening. However, with the increasing number of infants requiring screening and a scarcity of ROP specialists, other models of screening have been suggested and used

Authors have no conflict of interest.

A. Vinekar (✉) · S. Sinha
Department of Pediatric Retina, Narayana Nethralaya Eye Institute, Bangalore, India

W.-C. Wu, W.-C. Lam (eds.), *A Quick Guide to Pediatric Retina*, https://doi.org/10.1007/978-981-15-6552-6_8

around the world. (Table 8.1) [7] There has been an evolution from "proof of concept" regarding the use of telemedicine in ROP to real-world scenarios. A report by the American Association of Ophthalmologists AAO concluded that wide-angle digital fundus photography can complement standard ROP care. It provides objective documentation of clinical examination findings, improved recognition of disease progression by comparing previous photographs and opportunities for education and research [8, 9].The advantages of telemedicine in ROP are listed in (Table 8.2).

Telemedicine for ROP uses remote digital fundus imaging (RDFI). The concept was first proposed in 1999 [10]. It used the store and forward, "hub and spoke" model. The images were obtained from the neonatal intensive care unit (NICU) and stored and then uploaded via the Internet. The images were then received and interpreted by the grader. Multiple NICU served as the spoke while the reader serves as the hub [11]. Ells et al. defined two important concepts for RDFI, i.e., "standardized fundus imaging" and "referral warranted ROP." The standardized fundus images consisted of five images captured for each eye; these included posterior pole, temporal, nasal, superior, and inferior retinal fields. Referral-warranted ROP (RW-ROP) was defined as: any ROP in zone 1, the presence of plus disease, or the presence of any stage 3 ROP [12]. The PHOTO ROP trial gave another set of six standard images used widely [13, 14]. Six images consisted of five images from the study of Ells et al. and one external iris photograph. Lorenz et al. used the term "suspected treatment-requiring ROP" (STR- ROP) which included threshold ROP zone II, pre-threshold ROP zone I (type-1 ROP according to ETROP). Importantly, some ROP requiring treatment are not reliably gradable from the images [15]. Comparing both RW-ROP and STR-ROP eyes that finally received laser therapy, a different referral pattern emerged. In the study by Ells et al., only 43.5% of eyes with RW-ROP (10/23 eyes) received laser therapy compared to 88.2% of the eyes with STR-ROP in the study by Lorenz et al. (30/34). The wider definition of RW-ROP by Ells ensures a higher level of safety but considerably lowers the positive predictive value as to STR-ROP.

The KIDROP model is an example of a highly successful RDFI tele-ROP model in a middle-income country [16–18]. The model employs accredited nonphysicians to image, grade, and report ROP while in NICU. The reporting based on triage using a decision-based algorithm of "red," "orange," and "green" groups which represent patients requiring treatment, needing follow-up, or fit for discharge, respectively. These are based on the ETROP classification and creates a wider safety net. Images captured are uploaded on the cloud and are accessible on the smartphones of ROP specialists located remotely. Another layer in the safety net is that infants are discharged from screening only if "mature retina" appears, i.e., the vascularization noted up to the ora serrata is documented in two successive visits between 41 and 45 weeks postmenstrual age. The KIDROP model differed from other programs in: (1) non- physicians are allowed to report and analyze the images as the first point of contact, thereby providing the diagnosis and decision to the rural mother before she leaves the center; (2) indirect ophthalmoscopy is not mandated before an infant can be discharged from screening; and (3) the program aims at detecting any stage, not just treatment-requiring disease. This differs from other programs that used referral-warranted or treatment requiring ROP as their end-point [12, 15]. Table 8.3 compares various RDFI model. However, currently, telemedicine techniques amount to only 21% of ROP screening services [25].

Table 8.1 Traditional and emerging models of ROP screening (adapted from: The National Health and Medical Research Council (NHMRC, Australia) report based on the Center for Disease Control (CDC) guidelines) [7]

	Pros	Cons
Tele-imaging model	Works well for a large number of at-risk population Imaging and reporting possible with non-physicians	Camera cost Technological restraints Administrative support needed to protect the imaging staff and the infant
Ophthalmologist-led model in district hospitals	Has been the standard examination for many years cost-effective	Insufficient ROP specialists Evidence to show it works well in large-population settings is limited Not a compliant model, as shown in the Mexican experience
Pediatrician-led model (Gilbert et al.)	Images can be taken by the resident nurses or doctors Ensures all infants are screened	Every neonatal unit requires its own camera and a leader to take charge. Needs multidisciplinary coordination

Table 8.2 Advantages of telemedicine in ROP

Photo-documentation allows:

1. Objective evaluation
2. Longitudinal comparison
3. Second opinion
4. Evaluating response to treatment
5. Easy and effective counseling of parents/guardians
6. Educational opportunities
7. Leveraging the trained ophthalmologist for treatment requiring ROP
8. Medicolegal protection

Table 8.3 Summary of region-wise tele-ROP programs across the world

Country	Year(s)	Program	Camera /devices	Infants recruited	Imagers/graders	Reporting	Outcome recorded	Results
North & South America								
Canada (Alberta)	2000–2001	Ells A et al. [12] Canada	One Retcam 120	44	ROP specialist	ROP specialist who imaged. Indirect Ophthalmoscopy and RetCam imaging was done on each baby each time	Referral warranted disease (RW-ROP)	Sensitivity 100%, specificity 96% Positive predictive value 92% and negative predictive value 100%
United States (Montana)	2007 to 2011	Weaver DT & Murdock TJ [19]	One Retcam II in a single NICU	137	Registered nurse and a neonatal nurse practitioner	Pediatric Ophthalmologists (Retrospective analysis)	Referral warranted ROP	Sensitivity of 100% and a specificity of 96.3% for detecting type 1 ROP. The positive predictive value of detecting type 1 ROP was 61.5%. The negative predictive value was 100%.
United States (Stanford)	2005 to 2010	SUNDROP program Fijalkowski N et al. [20]	RetCam imaging in 3 NICUs	511	NICU nurse	ROP specialist Every infant received indirect ophthalmoscopy examinations until termination criteria were achieved or until treatment.	(1) Treatment-warranted ROP (TW-ROP) (2) ETROP type 1 and (3) Adverse anatomical events.	No TW-ROP was missed and no adverse outcome noted TW-ROP had 100% sensitivity, 99.8% specificity, 93.8% positive predictive value, and 100% negative predictive
United States and Canada	2011 to 2013	Quinn GE et al. [21] E-ROP	Each (13) center had their own RetCam and ROP specialist	1257	Twenty-five certified non-physicians	Two remote, non-physician readers, who were study certified. Every baby had Retcam imaging along with clinical examination by study ROP specialist	Referral warranted ROP	Remote grading of images of an eye at a single session had sensitivity of 81.9% and specificity of 90.1%. When both eyes were considered for RW-ROP, the sensitivity was 90.0%, specificity of 87.0%, negative predictive value of 97.3%, and positive predictive value of 62.5%
Chile, South America	2012–2015	Ossandon et al. [22]	RetCam Shuttle	1024	Five trained neonatology nurse midwife or ophthalmic technician.	ROP experts (same day)	Severity of ROP image quality	98% agreement between imaging and clinical judgment of treatment requiring ROP

(continued)

Table 8.3 (continued)

Country	Year(s)	Program	Camera /devices	Infants recruited	Imagers/graders	Reporting	Outcome recorded	Results
Europe								
Germany (East Bavaria)	2001–2007	Lorenz B et al. 15	RetCam 120 5 units	1222	Senior Resident, General Ophthalmologist or Pediatric Ophthalmologist Ophthalmologists continued to perform indirect ophthalmoscopy on site	Same day or next day by remote pediatric ophthalmologist. Report sent via email	(1) Clinically relevant ROP (2) Suspected treatment requiring ROP (3) Treatment requiring ROP	Sensitivity for ST-ROP was 100% Positive predictive value for TR-ROP was 82.4%
Australia & New Zealand								
New Zealand	13 months period ? 2012–2013 (Date not provided)	Shah SP et al. [23]	One RetCam shuttle traveling between 2 NICU (20 kms apart)	64	Specialist ROP nurse	Nurse imaged, graded and proposed follow-up which was compared with a ROP expert	(1) Any stage ROP (2) Referral warranted ROP	Agreement of plan in 84.8% of cases. Sensitivity, specificity, positive predictive value, and negative predictive value of ROP grading were 91.7%, 80.6%, 45.8%, and 98.2%, respectively
Asia								
India (Multicenter, rural & urban)	2008 to date	Vinekar A et al KIDROP [16–18, 24]	127 Rural NICUs 600–800 km radius in Karnataka state using RetCam Shuttle & "3Nethra Neo" ROP Camera (Forus Health, India)	40,230 (as on 1.1.2019)	Five- teams with Level 3 technician and project manager each traveling within respective zones	The respective imaging technicians onsite. Images reported onsite and viewed and validated remotely by ROP expert	(1) Any stage ROP (2) Treatment grade ROP (3) Decision to discharge from ROP screening	Technicians validated as per KIDROP algorithm Government vs Private hospital, regional variations discussed

8.2 Challenges in Tele-ROP

The challenges in the promotion of Tele-ROP screening in ROP have been summarized in Table 8.4 and have been addressed below:

1. **Cost of the implementation of an ROP program** involves: (a) the cost of the camera and the viewing software and the maintenance of the equipment; (b) human resource training; (c) salaries of the imaging and grading teams; (d) recurrent transport costs of the device and team; and (e) cost of the consumables.

(a). **Cost of the camera:** Cameras currently available for telemedicine screening in ROP are relatively expensive. Most tele-ROP programs have used the RetCam family of products, most commonly the RetCam Shuttle (Formerly Clarity Medical Systems, USA, now Natus, USA). More recently, the "3Nethra Neo" developed in India is a more affordable option [26]. The "Neo" is a wide-field camera providing a 120-degree field of view and has some advancements in the liquid lens system to dynamically focus the image, an LED light source, and an integrated lens hand piece. The image resolution is better at 2040 × 2040 pixels when compared to 1800 × 1600 of the RetCam Shuttle. The images are a "square" which provides an extra arc of the superior and inferior retina which are lost in images from the RetCam's rectangular images. The "Neo" has been evaluated as an ROP screening tool by comparing it with images from the RetCam. Sensitivity of 97–99% and specificity of 75–81% were reported for diagnosis and decision from a cohort of preterm infants [27]. The systemic and ophthalmic safety of the camera have been established [26]. A novel smartphone-based fundus camera with the ability to image peripheral retina has been reported to be useful in imaging infants with ROP [28]. Comparison of the three camera systems is summarized in Table 8.5.

(b). **Cost-effectiveness:** Besides the cost of the camera, other recurrent costs include training and certification of the imagers, costs involved in data capture, storage and transfer while adhering to HIPAA and other regulatory requirements, financial compensation of the imagers and the cost of transport which would vary depending on the number of centers and the size of the geographic zones.

Table 8.4 Challenges in tele-ROP programs

Cost of implementation
Logistics of screening in the NICU
Quality and resolution of images
Training and accreditation of imagers
Medicolegal aspects and regulations
Government and legislative support

Table 8.5 Comparison of commercially available ROP cameras

	Retcam shuttle (Natus, Pleasanton, CA)	3Nethra Neo (Forus Health, India)	MII Ret Cam
Cost	120,000 (in India)	22,000 USD (in India)	USD 350
Portability	Can be transported in a vehicle	More portable, needs a smaller vehicle	Portable
Resolution	1800 × 1600	2040 × 2040	Variable
Field of imaging	130	120	Can image wide-field
Weight of hand piece/ device	Depends on the lens used	310 gm (handpiece with integrated lens)	150 gm (device)
Mydriatic/ Non mydriatic camera	Mydriatic camera	Mydriatic camera	Mydriatic camera
Capability	Integrated into tele-ROP programs	Integrated into tele-ROP programs	Useful in image documentation
Certification	FDA & CE	FDA & CE	Not available

Telemedicine pricing has normalized costs across geographic areas. Pricing variation in the local market tends to normalize when the number of service providers increases and compete among themselves. The availability of more affordable ROP cameras in the last 5 years is an example in this regard.

NICUs often have contracts with local ophthalmologists to perform ROP screening using indirect ophthalmoscopy. The cost of hiring includes being paid for work and also for the perceived risk of medicolegal liability. With the increasing trend in the latter, there has been a decline in the number of specialized ophthalmologists willing to screen. A survey indicated that there was difficulty in retaining or maintaining screeners for ROP in NICU [25]. A survey by the AAO reported that only 76% of the specialists providing ROP screening services intended to continue forward [29]. This leads to failure of the NICU to hire screening specialists. In developing countries like India, there are less than 200 ROP specialists to screen an overwhelming number of preterm infants [30]. This leads to an inefficient screening model which is both time consuming for the screening physician and expensive to the service provider.

The cost-effectiveness of the tele-screening model over indirect ophthalmoscopy has been established previously [31]. A Hungarian tele-screening program concluded that bedside screening with remote interpretation was more cost-saving than transport-based screening with indirect ophthalmoscopy from the perspective of the service provider and also the return on initial (ROI) investment recovered within 5 years after the project initiation [32].

(c). **Image quality and resolution:** Image quality plays a very important role in grading of ROP effectively and reliably. Ungradable images ranged from 8% to 21% among the published studies [13, 33].

Factors affecting the image quality are small palpebral fissure, suboptimal pupil dilatation, darkly pigmented fundi, poor contrast, corneal and vitreous haze due to extreme prematurity, cataract, vitreous hemorrhage, hyaloid reminant, retinal pigment epithelium thickness, choroidal blood vessels, and motion artifacts. Better image quality and a large number of images have been found to be associated with greater sensitivity for detecting RW-ROP. Repeated imaging or referral for standard ROP examination was suggested when less than four acceptable quality images were obtained [34]. Newer ROP cameras have better resolution of 2040 × 2040 compared to previously available RetCams [26].

Another method to improve image quality is by image enhancement. RetiView is a noninvasive and inexpensive method of customized image enhancement [35]. It helps to detect clinically difficult characteristics in APROP images and can influence treatment planning. Various image processing techniques like Gabor filter, Canny's method, and geometrical methods, study changes in the characteristics of the major temporal arcade and provides good accuracy in computer-aided diagnosis of plus disease [36] especially useful in APROP [37].

(d). **Training and accreditation of imagers:** Non-physician imagers form the backbone of any tele-ROP program. Reports suggest that non-physician graders after being trained and certified can detect ROP with good intra-grader and inter-grader consistency and minimal temporal drift. Various successful programs have used imaging personnel ranging from physician to non-physician imagers are summarized in Table 8.3. The KIDROP STAT (Score for Training and Accreditation of Technicians) was developed to train and certify imagers. This comprises of three levels (I, II, and III) and has a 20 point score, which tests the knowledge, skill, and practice patterns of the imager in their native setting. On average, training a new imager can take between 30 and 90 working days. The training period has been considerably shortened after the introduction of online training. The online platform "WISE-ROP" (Wide-field Imaging for Screening and Education for ROP) has several training modules based on the onsite training curriculum [38, 39]. Imagers read and undergo self-assessment quizzes at the end of each module. Video sessions and viva voce to correct the technique and practical difficulties are scheduled with an assigned mentor. Skill is graded as per the STAT-Score levels and tested before a completion certificate is awarded [16, 39].

(e). **Medicolegal liability and regulation:** Medicolegal liability assumes importance in telemedicine in ROP where compensation awarded runs in millions of dollars [40]. In India, US$350,000 has been awarded as a compensation against a government tertiary hospital for not providing "timely ROP screening." To date, no lawsuit related to tele-ROP screening has been reported. But with increasing telemedicine practice, the risks are bound to increase. The laws governing telemedicine are poorly defined and differs widely among countries. The regulations regarding the duties and responsibilities of ophthalmologists in telemedicine are also not defined. The joint technical report by the American Academy of Paediatrics, the American Academy of Ophthalmology, and the American Academy of Certified Orthoptists have outlined relevant practical and risk management considerations that should be followed when including imaging-based ROP care [9]. The obligation of the ophthalmologists interpreting images for a reading center but not providing ROP care at the hospital is also not defined. Tracking and follow-up of these infants must be a joint responsibility between the pediatrician and ophthalmologist until the acute screening and/or treatment is completed. The National Health and Medical Research Council (NHMRC, Australia) report based on the Center for Disease Control (CDC) guidelines [7] on the KIDROP program noted that "regressing back from the current model of tele-imaging to indirect ophthalmoscopy performed by inadequately trained ophthalmologists is fraught with the danger of sub-optimal management of ROP care." [7] This underlines the importance of accreditation and validation of ROP caregivers.

(f). **Government and financial support**: To maintain a successful tele-ROP model regulatory, logistic and financial support from the government are important. Unfortunately, not many tele-ROP programs are supported by the government. The KIDROP model in India is an example of public–private partnership. The national telemedicine network for retinopathy of prematurity screening in Chile has been funded by the government [22]. National Task Force of ROP in India is an apex body that regulates and promotes such activities. In India, the operational guidelines for ROP from the National Task force (2018) for the first time recommend image-based screening as a viable alternative for ROP screening to indirect ophthalmoscopy. More participation is needed from the state and federal government to promote ROP care in the public health delivery system.

The Future of Tele-ROP Artificial intelligence (AI) appears as a relatively cost-effective alternate accessible screening modality that is being explored in ophthalmology. FDA has recently approved the first autonomous AI system to provide a diagnostic decision independent of human graders and also checks the image quality [41]. Remidio AI-based software can make the diagnosis of sight-threatening diabetic retinopathy with high sensitivity [42].

It is intuitive to expect that AI in ROP has a good potential. ROP compared to DR is relatively limited by retinal findings but the complexity lies in the urgency of intervention in type 1 ROP and in the management of systemic comorbidity in a neonate compared to adults with DR. Deep convoluted neural network (CNN) models to identify plus disease have already been investigated [43]. Recently CNN models accurately assessed retinal fundus image quality in ROP in a manner comparable with the experts [44]. The i-ROP deep learning (DL) system has been found to accurately identify diagnostic categories and overall disease severity in an automated fashion. This iROP DL system has only been trained on posterior pole vascular morphology [45]. The data provides a proof of concept that a deep learning system can be used in an automated fashion to diagnose ROP.

A significant advantage of ROP screening with imaging, rather than indirect ophthalmoscopy lies in the documentation of other non-ROP conditions. In a study of 1450 preterm infants screened by the KIDROP program, 7.7% had a diagnosis other than ROP, which included conditions as severe as retinoblastoma [46]. Furthermore, the program has expanded to provide "universal screening," for full-term, healthy infants consistent with the government's universal health coverage program. In a study of 1021 term infants imaged within 3 days of birth showed that 4.7% had an abnormality, 1.6% required medical or surgical intervention [47].

Impact of Tele-ROP An impact assessment of scaling up the image-based tele-ROP program in India showed that in the 10 high-risk ROP states, with a population of roughly 680 million, over 35,000 infants would be detected with ROP and over 1200 need treatment annually. The financial saving in "blind-person-year" (BPY) is estimated at USD 108 million [24]. The United Nations Development Program (UNDP) report on the tele-imaging program [48] and the National Health and Medical Research Council (NHMRC, Australia) report based on the Center for Disease Control (CDC) guidelines [7] on the KIDROP program, strongly suggest that wide-field imaging is likely to become the new gold standard in ROP screening for Indian and other nations with similar ROP demographics.

References

1. Sood S, Mbarika V, Jugoo S, Dookhy R, Doarn CR, Prakash N, Merrell RC. What is telemedicine? A collection of 104 peer-reviewed perspectives and theoretical underpinnings. Telemed J E Health. 2007;13:573–90.
2. Shi L, Wu H, Dong J, Jiang K, Lu X, Shi J. Telemedicine for detecting diabetic retinopathy: a systematic review and meta-analysis. Br J Ophthalmol. 2015;99:823–31.
3. Newton MJ. The promise of telemedicine. Surv Ophthalmol. 2014;59:559–67.
4. Rani PK, Bhattarai Y, Sheeladevi S, ShivaVaishnavi K, Ali MH, Babu JG. Analysis of yield of retinal imaging in a rural diabetes eye care model. Indian J Ophthalmol. 2018;66:233–7.
5. Gadkari S. Innovative model for telemedicine-based screening for diabetic retinopathy in the developing world. Can J Ophthalmol. 2016;51:e109–11.
6. Wilson JMG, Jungner G. Principles and practice of screening for disease. WHO_PHP_34. (1968). Available at http://apps.who.int/iris/handle/10665/37650 Accessed 16 Oct 2017.
7. CDC. Developing an effective evaluation report. Available from: http://www.paediatrics.uwa.edu.au/__data/assets/pdf_file/0008/2816783/KIDROP-report-2015.pdf. (2013). Accessed 24 Apr 2020.
8. Chiang MF, Melia M, Buffenn AN, Lambert SR, Recchia FM, Simpson JL, Yang MB. Detection of clinically significant retinopathy of prematurity using wide-angle digital retinal photography: a report by the American Academy of Ophthalmology. Ophthalmology. 2012;119:1272–80.
9. Fierson WM, Capone JA. Telemedicine for evaluation of retinopathy of prematurity. Pediatrics. 2015;135:e238–54.
10. Lorenz B, Bock M, Muller HM, et al. Telemedicine based screening of infants at risk for retinopathy of prematurity. Stud Health Technol Inform. 1999;64:155–63.
11. Hartnett ME, editor. Pediatric retina. London: Lippincott Williams & Wilkins; 2005. p. 523–32.
12. Ells AL, Holmes JM, Astle WF, et al. Telemedicine approach to screening for severe retinopathy of prematurity: a pilot study. Ophthalmology. 2003;110:2113–7.
13. Photographic Screening for Retinopathy of Prematurity (Photo-ROP) Cooperative Group. The photographic screening for retinopathy of prematurity study (Photo-ROP): primary outcomes. Retina. 2008;28:S47–54.
14. Vinekar A, Trese MT, Capone A Jr, Photographic Screening for Retinopathy of Prematurity (PHOTO-ROP) Cooperative Group. Evolution of retinal detachment in posterior retinopathy of prematurity: impact on treatment approach. Am J Ophthalmol. 2008;145:548–55.
15. Lorenz B, Spasovska K, Elflein H, et al. Wide-field digital imaging based telemedicine for screening for acute retinopathy of prematurity (ROP). Six-year results of a multicentre field study. Graefes Arch Clin Exp Ophthalmol. 2009;247:1251–62.
16. Vinekar A, Gilbert C, Dogra M, Kurian M, Shainesh G, Shetty B, Bauer N. The KIDROP model of combining strategies for providing retinopathy of prematurity screening in underserved areas in India using wide-field imaging, tele-medicine, non-physician graders and smart phone reporting. Indian J Ophthalmol. 2014;62:41.
17. Vinekar A, Jayadev C, Mangalesh S, Shetty B, Vidyasagar D. Role of tele-medicine in retinopathy of prematurity screening in rural outreach centers in India–a report of 20,214 imaging sessions in the KIDROP program. Semin Fetal Neonatal Med. 2015;20:335–45.
18. Vinekar A, Jayadev C, Bauer N. Need for telemedicine in retinopathy of prematurity in middle-income countries: e-ROP vs KIDROP. JAMA Ophthalmol. 2015;133:360–1.

19. Weaver DT, Murdock TJ. Telemedicine detection of type 1 ROP in a distant neonatal inten- sive care unit. J AAPOS. 2012;16:229–33.
20. Fijalkowski N, Zheng LL, Henderson MT, et al. Stanford University network for diagnosis of retinopathy of prematurity (SUNDROP): five years of screening with telemedicine. Ophthalmic Surg Lasers Imaging Retina. 2014;45:106–13.
21. Quinn GE, Ying G, Daniel E, et al. Validity of a telemedicine system for the evaluation of acute-phase retinopathy of prematurity. JAMA Ophthalmol. 2014;132:1178–84.
22. Ossandón D, Zanolli M, Stevenson R, Agurto R, Ortiz P, Dotan G. A national telemedicine network for retinopathy of prematurity screening. J AAPOS. 2018;22:124–7.
23. Shah SP, Wu Z, Iverson S, et al. Specialist nurse screening for retinopathy of prematurity: a pilot study. Asia Pac J Ophthalmol (Phila). 2013;2:300–4.
24. Vinekar A, Mangalesh S, Jayadev C, Gilbert C, Dogra M, Shetty B. Impact of expansion of telemedicine screening for retinopathy of prematurity in India. Indian J Ophthalmol. 2017;65:390.
25. Vartanian RJ, Besirli CG, Barks JD, Andrews CA, Musch DC. Trends in the screening and treatment of retinopathy of prematurity. Pediatrics. 2017;139(1):e20161978.
26. Vinekar A, Rao SV, Murthy S, Jayadev C, Dogra MR, Verma A, Shetty B. A novel, low-cost, wide-field, infant retinal camera, "neo": technical and safety report for the use on premature infants. Transl Vis Sci Technol. 2019;8(2):2.
27. Vinekar A, Dogra MR, Jayadev C, Murthy S, Rao SV, Shetty B. Evaluation of a new, low-cost, portable, wide-field, digital, retinal camera,"Neo" for screening infants for retinopathy of prematurity–a prospective, multi-center, validation report in Asian Indian infants. Invest Ophthalmol Vis Sci. 2016;57:11–20.
28. Sharma A. Emerging simplified retinal imaging. In: Bandello F, editor. Management of Diabetic Retinopathy, vol. 60. Basel: S. Karger; 2017. p. 56–62.
29. Roach L. ROP crisis near, survey says. News in review. EyeNet 2006.
30. Vinekar A, Azad R, Dogra MR, Narendran V, Jalali S, Bende P. The Indian retinopathy of prematurity society: a baby step towards tackling the retinopathy of prematurity epidemic in India. Ann Eye Sci. 2017;2:6.
31. Jackson KM, Scott KE, Zivin JG, Bateman DA, Flynn JT, Keenan JD, Chiang MF. Cost-utility analysis of telemedicine and ophthalmoscopy for retinopathy of prematurity management. Arch Ophthalmol. 2008;126:493–9.
32. Kovacs G, Somogyvári Z, Maka E, Nagyjánosi L. Bedside ROP screening and telemedicine interpretation integrated to a neonatal transport system: Economic aspects and return on investment analysis. Early Hum Dev. 2017;106:1–5.
33. Wu C, Petersen RA, Vanderveen DK. Retcam imaging for retinopathy of prematurity screening. J AAPOS. 2006;10:107–11.
34. Bothun ED, Morrison D, Ying GS, Daniel E, Baumritter A, Quinn G. Impact of number and quality of retinal images in a telemedicine screening program for ROP: results from the e-ROP study. J AAPOS. 2016;20:e11–2.
35. Jayadev C, Vinekar A, Mohanachandra P, Desai S, Suveer A, Mangalesh S, Bauer N, Shetty B. Enhancing image characteristics of retinal images of aggressive posterior retinopathy of prematurity using a novel software,(RetiView). Biomed Res Int. 2015;2015:898197.
36. Oloumi F, Rangayyan RM, Casti P, Ells AL. Computer-aided diagnosis of plus disease via measurement of vessel thickness in retinal fundus images of preterm infants. Comput Biol Med. 2015;66:316–29.
37. Rajashekar D, Srinivasa G, Vinekar A. Comprehensive retinal image analysis for aggressive posterior retinopathy of prematurity. PLoS One. 2016;11:e0163923.
38. Vinekar A. A Novel Online Retinopathy Of Prematurity (ROP) Training Model For Rural India–"WISEROP. COM". Best Free Papers
39. Vinekar A, Bhende P. Innovations in technology and service delivery to improve Retinopathy of Prematurity care. Community Eye Health. 2018;31:S20.
40. Reynolds JD. Malpractice and the quality of care in retinopathy of prematurity (an American Ophthalmological Society thesis). Trans Am Ophthalmol Soc. 2007;105:461.
41. Abràmoff MD, Lavin PT, Birch M, Shah N, Folk JC. Pivotal trial of an autonomous AI-based diagnostic system for detection of diabetic retinopathy in primary care offices. Npj Digit Med. 2018;1:39.
42. Rajalakshmi R, Subashini R, Anjana RM, Mohan V. Automated diabetic retinopathy detection in smartphone-based fundus photography using artificial intelligence. Eye. 2018;32:1138–44.
43. Brown JM, Campbell JP, Beers A, Chang K, Ostmo S, Chan RP, Dy J, Erdogmus D, Ioannidis S, Kalpathy-Cramer J, Chiang MF. Automated diagnosis of plus disease in retinopathy of prematurity using deep convolutional neural networks. JAMA Ophthalmol. 2018;136:803–10.
44. Brown JM, Campbell JP, Beers A, Chang K, Donohue K, Ostmo S, Chan RP, Dy J, Erdogmus D, Ioannidis S, Chiang MF. Fully automated disease severity assessment and treatment monitoring in retinopathy of prematurity using deep learning. In Medical Imaging 2018: Imaging Informatics for Healthcare, Research, and Applications. 2018;10579:105790Q. International Society for Optics and Photonics.
45. Redd TK, Campbell JP, Brown JM, Kim SJ, Ostmo S, Chan RV, Dy J, Erdogmus D, Ioannidis S, Kalpathy-Cramer J, Chiang MF. Evaluation of a deep learning image assessment system for detecting severe retinopathy of prematurity. Br J Ophthalmol. 2018; https://doi.org/10.1136/bjophthalmol-2018-313156.
46. Jayadev C, Vinekar A, Bauer N, Mangalesh S, Mahendradas P, Kemmanu V, Mallipatna A, Shetty B. Look what else we found-clinically significant abnormalities detected during routine ROP screening. Indian J Ophthalmol. 2015;63:373.
47. Vinekar A, Govindaraj I, Jayadev C, Kumar AK, Sharma P, Mangalesh S, Simaldi L, Avadhani K, Shetty B, Bauer N. Universal ocular screening of 1021 term infants using wide-field digital imaging in a single public hospital in India–a pilot study. Acta Ophthalmol. 2015;93:e372–6.
48. Good Practices Resource Book: Niti Ayog & UNDP. 2015. Last accessed 9 Apr 2019. http://www.niti.gov.in/writereaddata/files/human-development/Resource_Book_on_Good_Practices.pdf

Optical Coherence Tomography in Retinopathy of Prematurity

9

Xinxin Zhang and Lejla Vajzovic

Abstract

Retinopathy of prematurity is a vasoproliferative condition characterized by abnormal vascularization of the retina which may lead to tractional retinal detachment. Timely screening and treatment with laser and/or anti-vascular endothelial growth factor agents help prevent blindness. While bedside indirect ophthalmoscopy remains the gold standard for screening, optical coherence tomography has emerged as a new modality for understanding the pathogenesis of retinopathy of prematurity, providing in-vivo monitoring, and evaluating subclinical findings. This chapter provides an overview of optical coherence tomography in retinopathy of prematurity, including available models and adjustments in the neonatal population, differences between preterm, term and adult foveal anatomy, current usages of optical coherence tomography in retinopathy of prematurity as well as descriptions of popcorn retinopathy, macular edema, vitreous bands on imaging.

Keywords

Retinopathy of prematurity · Spectral-domain optical coherence tomography · Preretinal tissue · Plus disease · Vitreous bands · Macular edema of prematurity

9.1 Introduction

Retinopathy of prematurity (ROP) is a disease of premature and/or low birth weight infants, characterized by incomplete retinal vascularization, retinal ischemia, subsequent abnormal neovascularization, and eventually tractional retinal detachment if left untreated. Given timely screening, treatment with laser photocoagulation and/or anti-vascular endothelial growth factor agents prevent blindness.

Grading of disease depends on the location or zone of involvement, severity, or stage of disease, extent of disease, and presence or absence of plus disease [1]. The location of pathology is described as zones I, II, or III (Fig. 9.1). Zone I consists of a circular area with the optic disc as the center and a radius of twice the distance between the optic disc and the macula center. Zone II is an extension of Zone I to the nasal ora serrata. Zone III consists of the remainder of the temporal retina. The severity of disease is described in stages from stage 0 to stage 5.

Stage 1 consists of a demarcation line that distinguishes the vascular retina from the avascular retina. Stage 2 shows the formation of a ridge, and small isolated extraretinal neovascular tufts may be present. Stage 3 is characterized by extraretinal fibrovascular proliferation that grows from the ridge into the vitreous. Stage 4 involves partial retinal detachment that is either extrafoveal (4A) or fovea-involving (4B). Stage 5 shows a total retinal detachment. The extent of disease is the number of clock hours involved. Plus disease con-

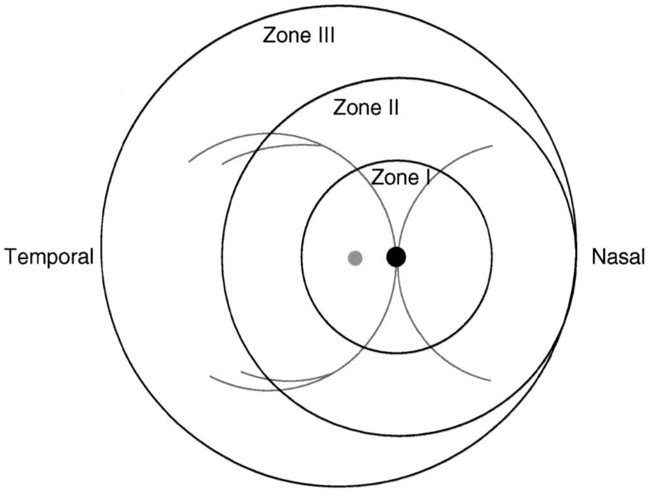

Fig. 9.1 Diagram of zones I, II, and III of retinopathy of prematurity. Images courtesy of Dr. Xi Chen

X. Zhang · L. Vajzovic (✉)
Department of Ophthalmology, Duke University Eye Center, Durham, NC, USA
e-mail: lejla.vajzovic@duke.edu

W.-C. Wu, W.-C. Lam (eds.), *A Quick Guide to Pediatric Retina*, https://doi.org/10.1007/978-981-15-6552-6_9

sists of venous dilation and arteriolar tortuosity in at least two quadrants [1].

The gold standard for screening is bedside indirect ophthalmoscopy, though other modalities such as fundus photography can be useful supplements. Current screening criteria for ROP includes all infants with a birth weight below 1500 g or gestational age of less than 30 weeks. Infants with birth weights between 1500 g and 2000 g or gestational age greater than 30 weeks who have had unstable clinical courses or additional risk factors should also be screened [2].

Screening for ROP begins at either 4 to 6 weeks after delivery or 31 to 33 weeks postmenstrual age, whoever interval comes later [2]. Follow-up time intervals range from less than 1 week to 3 weeks depending on the severity of the disease found [2]. Screening may cease when full retinal vascularization close to the ora for 360 degrees has been achieved, the patient has reached a postmenstrual age of 50 weeks without detection of prethreshold disease or worse ROP, there is regression of ROP, or if there is vascularization of zone III without previous zone I or II ROP [2].

9.2 SD-OCT

Spectral-domain optical coherence tomography (SD-OCT) uses light interference to produce a cross-sectional image of the anatomy of interest. Various table-top and portable SD-OCTs are available; however, there is logistical and physical difficulty in examining uncooperative young patients and unstable neonates in the intensive care unit [3]. The Envisu (Bioptigen, NC, USA) model is a handheld device that can be used in the office, in the unit, and in the operating room. The advantages of SD-OCT include lack of contact, short imaging time, and the ability to evaluate without anesthesia. Adjustments of imaging protocols such as using shorter scan lengths for shorter axial length, reducing the number of A-scans to avoid unnecessary light exposure, and correcting reference arm position to avoid excessive magnification can all help produce higher quality images in the neonatal population [3]. Maldonado et al provides a reference table for age-specific corrections in neonates and infants to improve image quality [4]. Specific protocols have been proposed to reduce imaging time and patient discomfort [4].

9.3 OCT Difference Between Adult, Term and Preterm Infants

There are a number of differences between the eyes of adults, term infants, and preterm infants found on OCT imaging (Fig. 9.2). As the eye develops, the inner retinal cells migrate outward from the fovea, photoreceptor layers grow inward toward the fovea and the foveal photoreceptor layer thickens [5, 6]. Compared to term infants, preterm infants have delayed development of photoreceptor inner and outer segments, specifically delayed appearance of the ellipsoid zone in the foveal center and a greater mean distance between the foveal center to the ellipsoid zone [7]. Compared to adults, preterm infants have shallower foveal depression, persistent inner retinal layers, and shorter foveal photoreceptors [6, 8].

Pathology discovered on SD-OCT in infants may prognosticate subsequent visual outcomes. For instance, Rothman et al. found that children who had macular edema on SD-OCT in infancy had worse visual outcomes compared to those who were not found to have macular edema on SD-OCT in infancy [9].

9.4 OCT in ROP

SD-OCT allows for in vivo, cross-sectional analysis and can provide subclinical details undetected by indirect ophthalmoscopy. For instance, Lee et al. performed SD-OCT during routine bedside ROP screenings and found macular cystoid structures in 39% and epiretinal membranes in 32%, none of which were apparent on indirect ophthalmoscopy [10]. Advanced image processing techniques such as segmentation allows for detailed analysis of specific retinal layers [11]. While SD-OCT does not replace gold standard bedside indirect ophthalmoscopy for evaluation of ROP, particularly in more peripheral disease, OCT has advanced the understanding of subclinical disease processes in ROP and enabled in-vivo monitoring of microstructure evolution that has previously only been detectable on histopathology [3, 10].

The hallmarks of each stage of ROP development have been described in greater detail using OCT. In stage 1 disease, the posterior vascular retina shows three inner layers on OCT whereas the anterior avascular retina has one hyperreflective layer [12]. The ridge in stage 2 disease can be seen on OCT as a homogenous thickening of the inner hyperreflective band, with occasional small elevated tufts of preretinal tissue that is likely early pathologic proliferation [12]. Stage 3 disease shows significant thickening of the hyperreflective band and more marked preretinal elevations, sometimes with inner retinal split and focal vitreous traction [12].

OCT can also be used to monitor treatment response, similar to adult disease processes like neovascular age-related macular degeneration. OCT before and after anti-VEGF injection in stage 3 disease showed reduced thickness of inner retinal layers, decreased neovascular elevations, and further extension of three-layered inner retina [12]. OCT can also detect subtle progression despite treatment, such as early tractional retinoschisis in progressive ROP despite laser photocoagulation [13].

A number of specific subclinical SD-OCT changes have been found in infants during ROP screening, including cys-

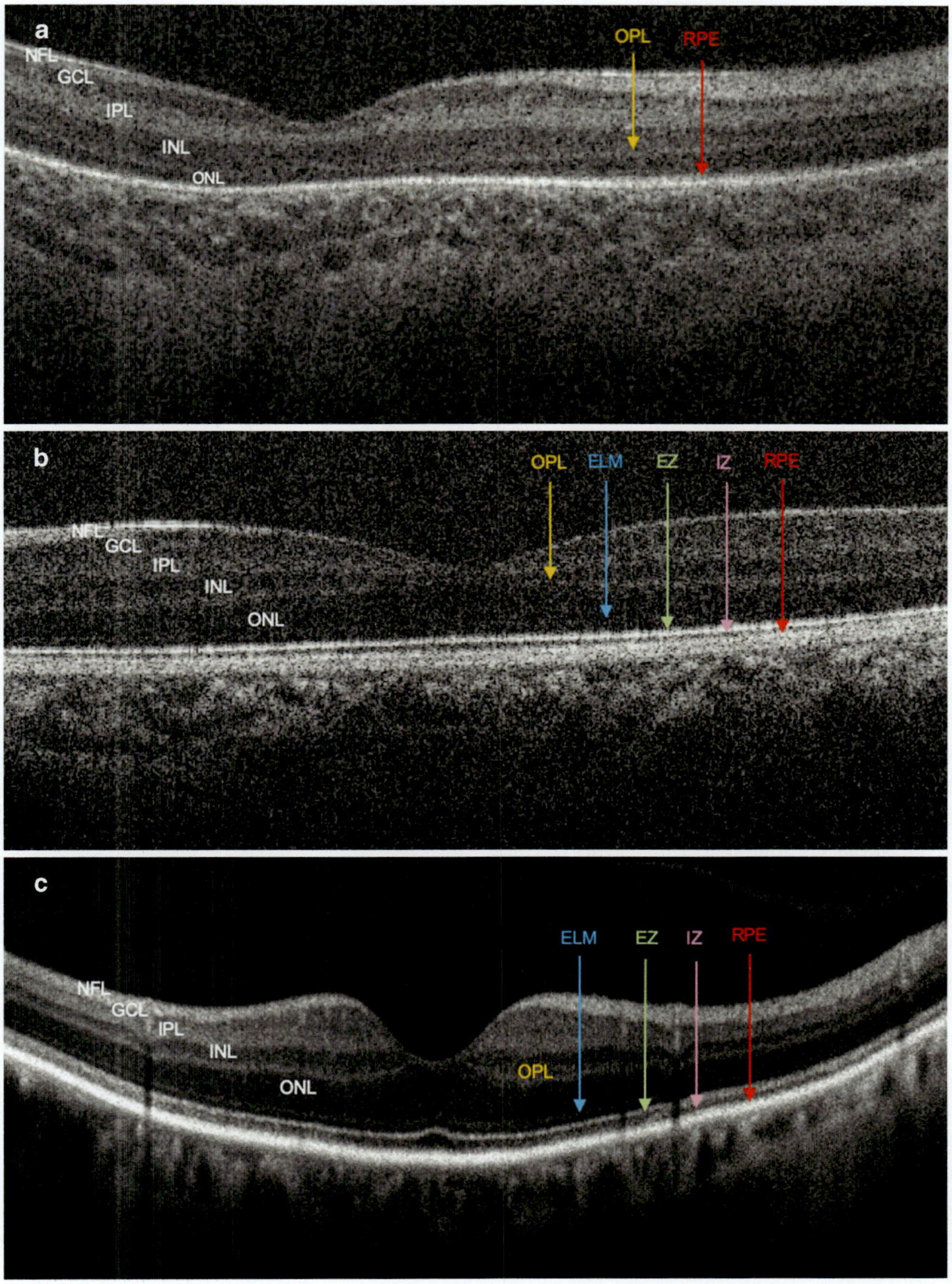

Fig. 9.2 SD-OCT images showing normal foveal anatomy of a premature neonate, full-term neonate, and an adult. (**a**) shows foveal anatomy of a 31 weeks postmenstrual age neonate. Note the persistent, distinct nerve fiber layer, ganglion cell layer, and inner plexiform layers at the foveal center. The photoreceptors structures, including the external limiting membrane, inner segment/outer segment junction, and outer segments are not seen. The foveal depression is more shallow and the inner retinal layers are thicker compared to the outer retinal layers. With development, the ganglion cell layer, inner plexiform, and inner nuclear layers migrate centrifugally whereas the photoreceptors migrate centripetally. (**b**) shows the foveal anatomy of a 40-weeks postmenstrual age neonate. Compared to (**a**), the ellipsoid zone is developed in the periphery, and in the foveal center, the inner retinal cells are migrating centrifugally from the foveal center, and the foveal depression is deepened. The inner retinal layers now appear thinner than the outer retinal layers at the foveal center. The fovea continues to mature over the next decade as continual cone packing and elongation at the foveal center occurs. (**c**) shows the foveal contour of a 72-year-old adult. The foveal contour is deep and the inner retinal layers are thin and indistinguishable at the foveal center. Abbreviations: *NFL* nerve fiber layer, *GCL* ganglion cell layer, *IPL* inner plexiform layer, *INL* inner nuclear layer, *OPL* outer plexiform layer, *ONL* outer nuclear layer, *ELM* external limiting membrane, *EZ* ellipsoid zone, *IZ* interdigitation zone, *RPE* retinal pigment epithelium. Images courtesy of Dr. Xi Chen

toid macular changes, vitreous changes, preretinal tissue and plus disease vascular changes [3, 12, 14, 15]. Each entity is described in detail below.

9.4.1 Macular Edema

Hyporeflective cystoid spaces at the inner nuclear layer level is a frequent finding in premature infants and infants with ROP (Fig. 9.3) [16–18]. This entity has been termed macular edema of prematurity (MEOP), as it is not typically found in full-term infants, though there may be some racial variation [19, 20]. Of the multiple phenotypes found, vertically elongated cysts with a "bulging" foveal contour is common [16]. Vinekar et al. characterize this dome-shaped bulging fovea with intraretinal cystoid spaces separated by vertical septae as "pattern A," and also describe a "pattern B" cystoid macular edema which shows multiple confluent hyporeflective spaces with a more preserved foveal depression [21]. The presence of MEOP has not been found to be associated with ROP outcomes and does not appear to be correlated with the ROP stage [18]. However, eyes with plus disease, stage 3 ROP, and the need for laser treatment have been found to have increased central foveal thickness which is induced by the macular edema [16]. Furthermore, very preterm infants who had cystoid macular edema were found to have poorer motor and language skills compared to those who did not [22]. It has been hypothesized that since the retina represents an extension of the CNS, cellular and developmental events occurring elsewhere in the CNS may manifest in the neuroretinal tissue [22].

9.4.2 Vitreous Pathology

Tractional vitreous bands may be visualized in advanced ROP during vitrectomies. Zepeda et al. used handheld OCT during ROP screenings and found hyperreflective vitreous opacities or vitreous bands in 71% of participants [15]. Vitreous band presence is associated with hyperreflective opacities (Fig. 9.4) [23]. They found an association between the presence of vitreous bands and the presence of epiretinal membranes as well as cystoid macular edema, which suggests a tractional component in the pathogenesis of these entities. There was no association between vitreous band detection and ROP severity [15].

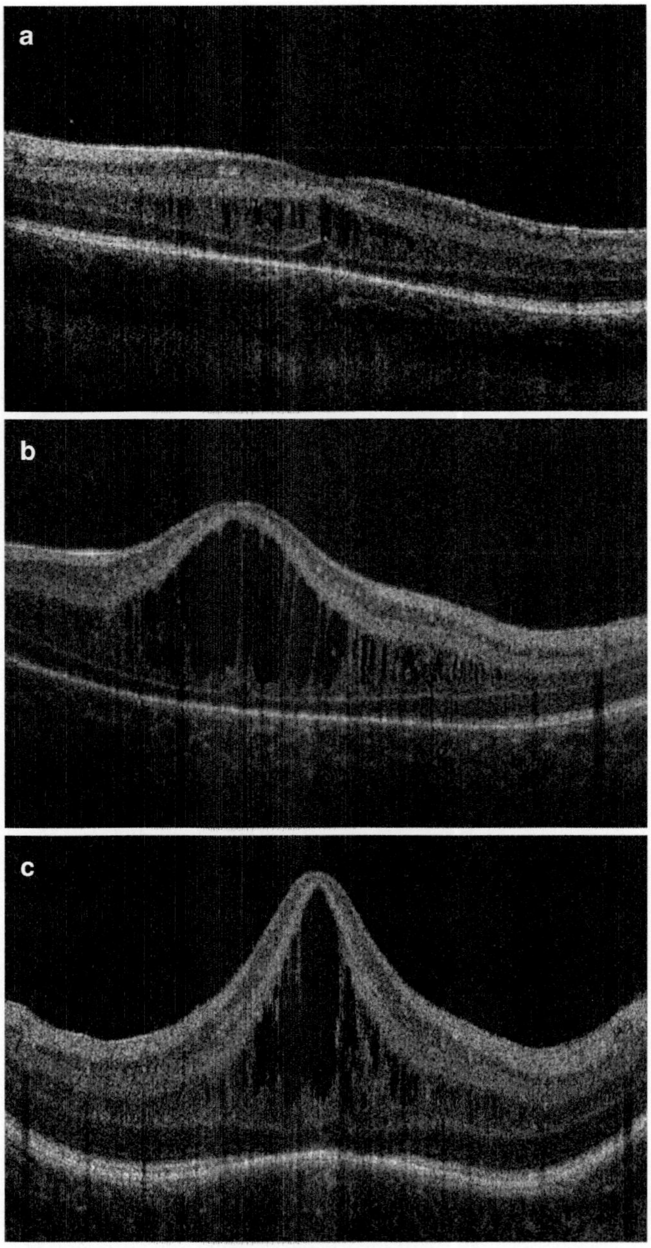

Fig. 9.3 SD-OCT images showing varying degrees of cystoid macular edema in approximately 38-weeks postmenstrual age infants. (**a**) shows mild cystoid macular edema with hyporeflective cystic spaces in the inner nuclear layer with vertical hyperreflective septae, with minimal changes to foveal contour. (**b**) shows moderate cystoid macular edema with vertical elongation of cystic spaces and "bulging" foveal contour. (**c**) shows severe cystoid macular edema with marked bulging of the foveal center. Images courtesy of Dr. Xi Chen

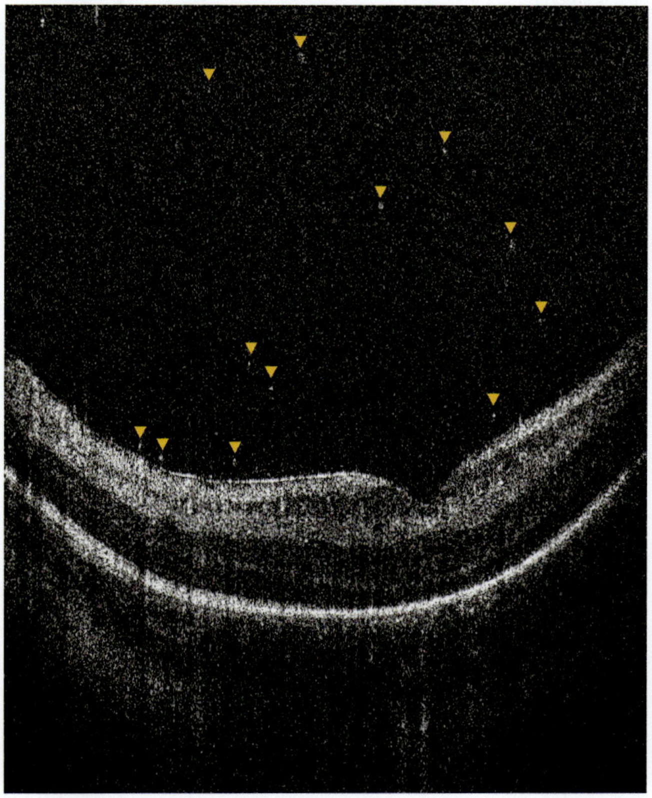

Fig. 9.4 SD-OCT image showing hyperreflective vitreous opacities (yellow arrows) in a 39-weeks postmenstrual age infant. Images courtesy of Dr. Xi Chen

9.4.3 Popcorn Retinopathy/Extraretinal Tissue

The International Classification of ROP makes note of isolated neovascular tufts on the retinal surface found close to the ridge in stage 2 ROP [1], which has been confirmed on OCT (Fig. 9.5) [12, 24]. The presence of these isolated tufts (also known as "popcorn") has been associated with increased risk of zone II, stage 2 disease progressing to stage 3, as well as the development of plus disease and requirement of laser treatment [14]. SD-OCT provides a monitoring modality for these lesions.

9.4.4 Plus Disease

The presence of plus disease is an indication for laser treatment, and the presence of pre-plus disease (a lesser degree of vascular dilation and tortuosity) is associated with the progression of disease requiring laser. However, there is a degree of subjectivity even among experienced examiners [25]. OCT can provide anatomical details of vessel changes in plus and pre-plus disease and possibly aid in more objective differentiation between these clinical entities [3]. OCT is able to evaluate vessel elevation, hyporeflective vessels, and scalloped retinal layers which were significantly associated with plus disease (Fig. 9.5) [26]. Maldonado et al. describes a Vascular Abnormality Score by OCT (VASO) which weighs these characteristics based on common versus uncommon features, and found significantly higher VASO in premature infants with plus disease compared to those with ROP but without plus disease [26].

Moreover, traditional evaluation of plus disease depends on the *en face* view of the posterior pole by indirect ophthalmoscopy or photography, whereas cross-sectional SD-OCT images allow an additional dimension of analysis. For instance, anterior to posterior vessel dilation and tortuosity may be better appreciated on continuous cross-sections [26].

9.4.5 Foveal Involvement

SD-OCT also aids in the differentiation between stage 4A (extrafoveal) and 4B (foveal-involvement) ROP. Foveal abnormalities may impact outcomes in patients with 4A disease and impact treatment outcomes despite anatomic success of detachment repair [27].

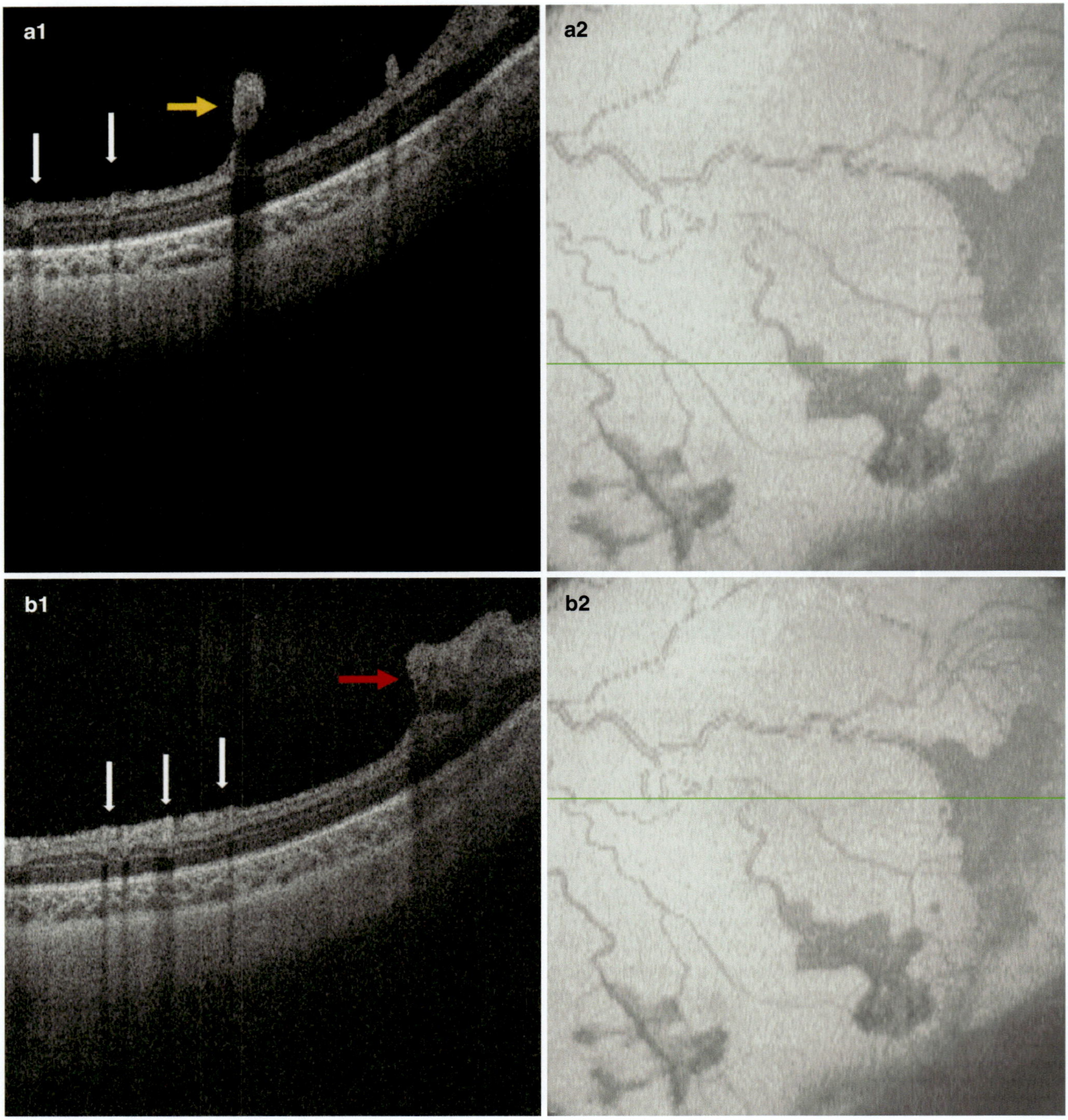

Fig. 9.5 SD-OCT (left) and en face OCT SVP images (right) of a 43-week-old postmenstrual age infant showing plus disease with dilation and tortuosity and peripheral neovascularization with plaque formation confirming stage 3 ROP. The green line on en face OCT SVP in the right column indicates slice location of SD-OCT on the left. (**a1**) shows vessels (white arrows) and "popcorn retinopathy" (yellow arrow). This preretinal neovascular tissue may be present in stage 2 ROP. (**b1**) shows vessels (white arrows) and preretinal neovascular plaques (red arrow) indicative of stage 3 ROP. (**c1**) shows dilated, elevated vasculature (white arrows) with hollow surrounding and continuation of the same plaque shown in **b1** (red arrow). The vessels are elevated with subsequent distortion of the retinal layers, which produces a scalloped appearance of the retinal layers. In **c2** at the green line, the vessel of interest appears more dilated compare to surrounding vessels. The VASO score proposed by Maldonado et al. takes into account vessel characteristics including mild versus severe elevation, retinal layer scalloping involving the inner plexiform layer versus outer plexiform layer, any presence of hyporeflective vessels, and any presence of retinal spaces to give a unified score of vessel abnormality. Images courtesy of Dr. Xi Chen

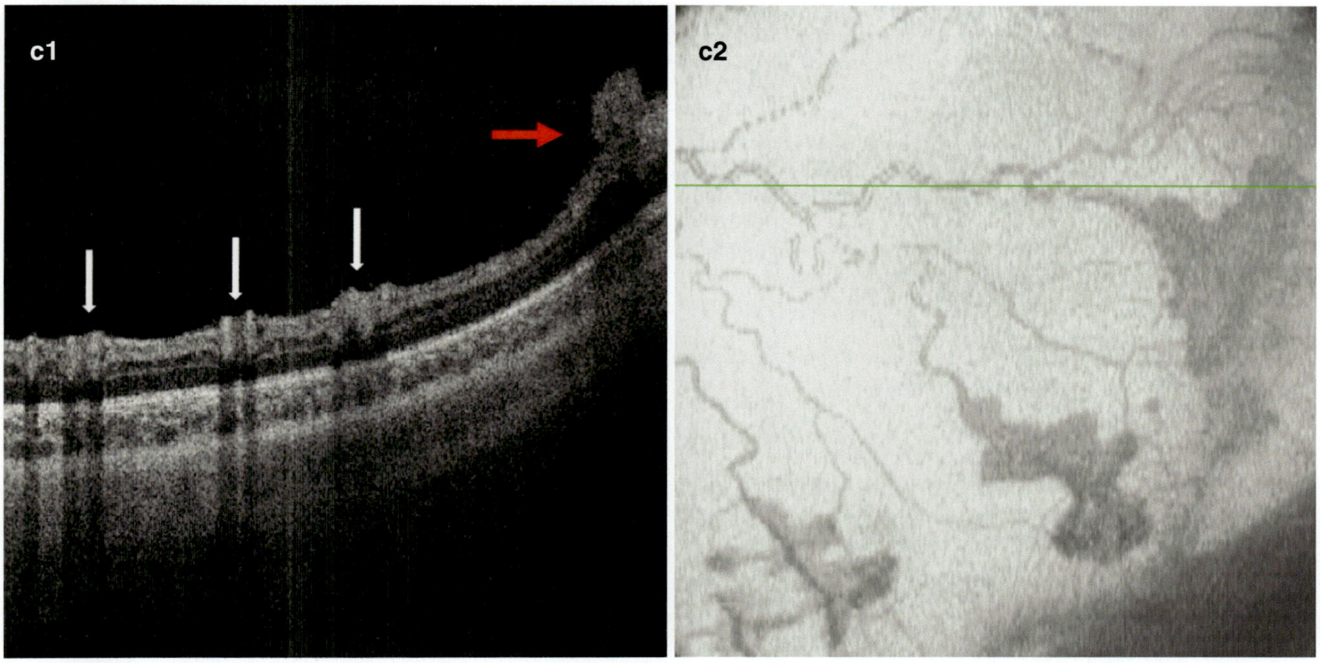

Fig. 9.5 (continued)

9.5 Conclusion

SD-OCT offers in vivo monitoring of retinal structure over time and can identify subclinical details not visible on indirect ophthalmoscopy in ROP. Adapted models and techniques improve the ease and efficacy of imaging in the neonatal population.

References

1. The International Classification of Retinopathy of Prematurity Revisited. Arch Ophthalmol. 2005;123(7):991–9. https://doi.org/10.1001/archopht.123.7.991.
2. American Academy of Ophthalmology. Retinopathy of prematurity. In: Basic and clinical science course, vol. 12. San Francisco: American Academy of Ophthalmology; 2019. p. 155–88.
3. Maldonado RS, Toth CA. Optical coherence tomography in retinopathy of prematurity. Clin Perinatol. 2013;40(2):271–96. https://doi.org/10.1016/j.clp.2013.02.007.
4. Maldonado RS, Izatt JA, Sarin N, et al. Optimizing hand-held spectral domain optical coherence tomography imaging for neonates, infants, and children. Invest Ophthalmol Vis Sci. 2010;51(5):2678–85. https://doi.org/10.1167/iovs.09-4403.
5. Vinekar A, Mangalesh S, Jayadev C, Maldonado RS, Bauer N, Toth CA. Retinal imaging of infants on spectral domain optical coherence tomography. Biomed Res Int. 2015;2015:782420. https://doi.org/10.1155/2015/782420.
6. Hendrickson A, Possin D, Vajzovic L, Toth CA. Histologic development of the human fovea from midgestation to maturity. Am J Ophthalmol. 2012;154(5):767–778.e2. https://doi.org/10.1016/j.ajo.2012.05.007.
7. Vajzovic L, Rothman AL, Tran-Viet D, Cabrera MT, Freedman SF, Toth CA. Delay in retinal photoreceptor development in very preterm compared to term infants. Invest Ophthalmol Vis Sci. 2015;56(2):908–13. https://doi.org/10.1167/iovs.14-16021.
8. Vajzovic L, Hendrickson AE, O'Connell RV, et al. Maturation of the human fovea: correlation of spectral-domain optical coherence tomography findings with histology. Am J Ophthalmol. 2012;154(5):779–789.e2. https://doi.org/10.1016/j.ajo.2012.05.004.
9. Rothman AL, Tran-Viet D, Vajzovic L, et al. Functional outcomes of young infants with and without macular edema. Retina Phila Pa. 2015;35(10):2018–27. https://doi.org/10.1097/IAE.0000000000000579.
10. Lee AC, Maldonado RS, Sarin N, et al. Macular features from spectral-domain optical coherence tomography as an adjunct to indirect ophthalmoscopy in retinopathy of prematurity. Retina Phila Pa. 2011;31(8):1470–82. https://doi.org/10.1097/IAE.0b013e31821dfa6d.
11. Chiu SJ, Li XT, Nicholas P, Toth CA, Izatt JA, Farsiu S. Automatic segmentation of seven retinal layers in SDOCT images congruent with expert manual segmentation. Opt Express. 2010;18(18):19413–28. https://doi.org/10.1364/OE.18.019413.
12. Chen X, Mangalesh S, Dandridge A, et al. Spectral-domain OCT findings of retinal vascular-avascular junction in infants with retinopathy of prematurity. Ophthalmol Retina. 2018;2(9):963–71. https://doi.org/10.1016/j.oret.2018.02.001.

13. Muni RH, Kohly RP, Charonis AC, Lee TC. Retinoschisis detected with handheld spectral-domain optical coherence tomography in neonates with advanced retinopathy of prematurity. Arch Ophthalmol Chic Ill 1960. 2010;128(1):57–62. https://doi.org/10.1001/archophthalmol.2009.361.
14. Wallace DK, Kylstra JA, Greenman DB, Freedman SF. Significance of isolated neovascular tufts ("popcorn") in retinopathy of prematurity. J AAPOS Off Publ Am Assoc Pediatr Ophthalmol Strabismus. 1998;2(1):52–6.
15. Zepeda EM, Shariff A, Gillette TB, et al. Vitreous bands identified by handheld spectral-domain optical coherence tomography among premature infants. JAMA Ophthalmol. 2018;136(7):753–8. https://doi.org/10.1001/jamaophthalmol.2018.1509.
16. Maldonado RS, O'Connell R, Ascher SB, et al. Spectral-domain optical coherence tomographic assessment of severity of cystoid macular edema in retinopathy of prematurity. Arch Ophthalmol Chic Ill 1960. 2012;130(5):569–78. https://doi.org/10.1001/archopthalmol.2011.1846.
17. Bondalapati S, Milam RW, Ulrich JN, Cabrera MT. The characteristics and short-term refractive error outcomes of cystoid macular edema in premature neonates as detected by spectral-domain optical coherence tomography. Ophthalmic Surg Lasers Imaging Retina. 2015;46(8):806–12. https://doi.org/10.3928/23258160-20150909-04.
18. Dubis AM, Subramaniam CD, Godara P, Carroll J, Costakos DM. Subclinical macular findings in infants screened for retinopathy of prematurity with spectral-domain optical coherence tomography. Ophthalmology. 2013;120(8):1665–71. https://doi.org/10.1016/j.ophtha.2013.01.028.
19. Cabrera MT, O'Connell RV, Toth CA, et al. Macular findings in healthy full-term Hispanic newborns observed by hand-held spectral-domain optical coherence tomography. Ophthalmic Surg Lasers Imaging Retina. 2013;44(5):448–54. https://doi.org/10.3928/23258160-20130801-01.
20. Cabrera MT, Maldonado RS, Toth CA, et al. Subfoveal fluid in healthy full-term newborns observed by handheld spectral-domain optical coherence tomography. Am J Ophthalmol. 2012;153(1):167–175.e3. https://doi.org/10.1016/j.ajo.2011.06.017.
21. Vinekar A, Avadhani K, Sivakumar M, et al. Understanding clinically undetected macular changes in early retinopathy of prematurity on spectral domain optical coherence tomography. Invest Ophthalmol Vis Sci. 2011;52(8):5183–8. https://doi.org/10.1167/iovs.10-7155.
22. Rothman AL, Tran-Viet D, Gustafson KE, et al. Poorer neurodevelopmental outcomes associated with cystoid macular edema identified in preterm infants in the intensive care nursery. Ophthalmology. 2015;122(3):610–9. https://doi.org/10.1016/j.ophtha.2014.09.022.
23. Shariff A, Hahn L, Tarczy-Hornoch K, Cabrera MT. Vitreomacular bands in premature infants screened for retinopathy of prematurity as detected by handheld spectral domain optical coherence tomography. J Am Assoc Pediatr Ophthalmol Strabismus. 2017;21(4):e45. https://doi.org/10.1016/j.jaapos.2017.07.160.
24. Chavala SH, Farsiu S, Maldonado R, Wallace DK, Freedman SF, Toth CA. Insights into advanced retinopathy of prematurity using handheld spectral domain optical coherence tomography imaging. Ophthalmology. 2009;116(12):2448–56. https://doi.org/10.1016/j.ophtha.2009.06.003.
25. Chiang MF, Jiang L, Gelman R, Du YE, Flynn JT. Interexpert agreement of plus disease diagnosis in retinopathy of prematurity. Arch Ophthalmol Chic Ill 1960. 2007;125(7):875–80. https://doi.org/10.1001/archopht.125.7.875.
26. Maldonado RS, Yuan E, Tran-Viet D, et al. Three-dimensional assessment of vascular and perivascular characteristics in subjects with retinopathy of prematurity. Ophthalmology. 2014;121(6):1289–96. https://doi.org/10.1016/j.ophtha.2013.12.004.
27. Joshi MM, Trese MT, Capone A. Optical coherence tomography findings in stage 4A retinopathy of prematurity: a theory for visual variability. Ophthalmology. 2006;113(4):657–60. https://doi.org/10.1016/j.ophtha.2006.01.007.

FA in ROP

10

Noriyuki Azuma

Abstract

Fundus fluorescein angiography is useful to evaluate the advancement and effect of treatment of ROP. The findings to focus on are: position and extent of pathologic vascular proliferation, activity of fibrovascular proliferation, angioplany of the retina, absence of capillary network of the retina, extent of photocoagulation, and stabilizing of the vascular activity after treatments.

Keywords

Fluorescein angiography · Pathological new vessel · Plus disease · Retinal detachment · Aggressive posterior ROP · Photocoagulation · Vitrectomy

Because retinopathy of prematurity is a vascular disease, fundus fluorescein angiography (FFA) is an essential tool to evaluate the condition of the disease. Pathological new vessels, retinal capillary network, and circulation dynamics are much more accurately observed with FFA than routine ophthalmoscopy and fundus photography. Minimal new vessel, capillary dropout, activity, or stabilization of vascular proliferation are often determined by only FFA.

Advantages and points to be evaluated with FFA are as follows:

- Position and extent of pathologic vascular proliferation
- Activity of pathologic vascular proliferation, identified by leakage of fluorescein dye
- Vascular pattern of the retina, including abnormal branching, anastomosis, shunt, tortuosity, circulation speed
- Capillary network of the retina, which is absent not only in the non-vascularized retina but often partially in the vascularized retina
- Extent of photocoagulation already applied and spanning area

Use of wide-field digital imaging system is recommended to observe the periphery of the retina. 0.1 ml/kg body weight of 10% fluorescein dye is intravenously injected. Consecutive intravenous injection with 1 ml saline facilitates to put a small amount of dye into the systemic circulation. The intelligibility of images is adjusted by the photographic sensitivity of the CCD image sensor. Monitoring of vital signs by neonatologists or anesthesiologists is necessary during the examination (Fig. 10.1).

To determine the early stage of ROP, vascular shunt and pathological proliferation of primitive vessels in the retina cannot be identified without FFA. Vascular tufts, early intravitreal budding of pathologic new vessels also are easily identified (Figs. 10.2, 10.3, and 10.4). When ROP progresses, the range and extent of fibrovascular proliferation increase (Figs. 10.5, 10.6, 10.7, and 10.8). At an advanced stage, plus disease, tortuosity, and dilation of retinal vessels suggests insufficient retinal circulation. The partial absence of capillary network of retinal vessels is also seen in the retina already vascularized, which needs excessive photocoagulation (Fig. 10.8). When retinal detachment begins to occur, early sign is stretching and tractional elevation of retinal vessels due to dragging of the retina by fibrovascular tissues (Figs. 10.9 and 10.10). Distinctly different from classical ROP that processes in a sequence order of stage 1–4, aggressive posterior ROP rashly develop to stage 4 and 5, which needs early and extensive intervention of photocoagulation and vitreoretinal surgery (Fig. 10.11). Intraretinal vascular proliferation and dropout of the capillary network are important early signs of aggressive posterior ROP (Fig. 10.12). Stabilization of vascular activity in ROP, even spontaneously or after intervention of treatments, is determined by decreasing or disappearance of fluorescein dye leakage (Figs. 10.13 and 10.14).

N. Azuma (✉)
Department of Ophthalmology and Laboratory for Visual Science, National Center for Child Health and Development, Tokyo, Japan
e-mail: azuma-n@ncchd.go.jp

W.-C. Wu, W.-C. Lam (eds.), *A Quick Guide to Pediatric Retina*, https://doi.org/10.1007/978-981-15-6552-6_10

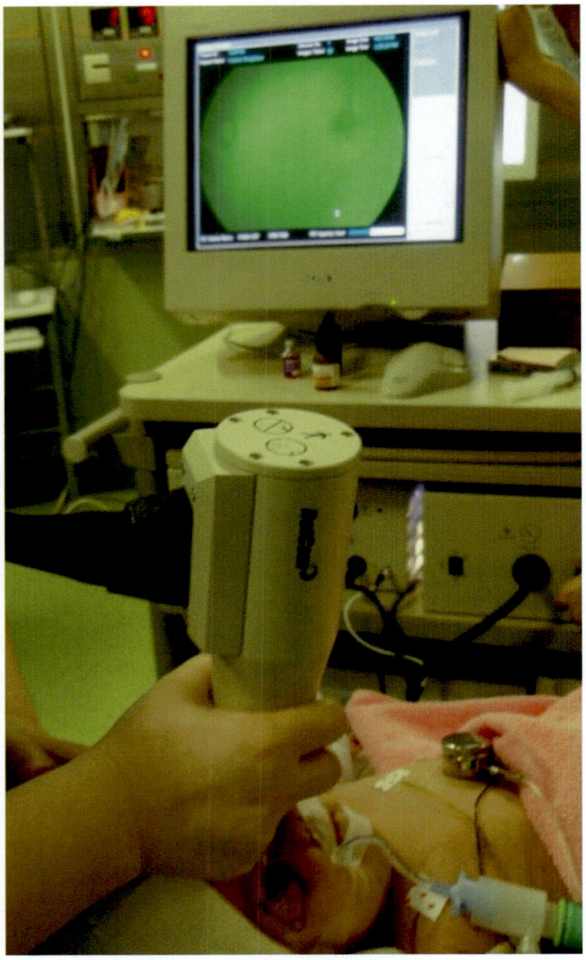

Fig. 10.1 Fundus fluorescein angiography examination for a premature baby using wide-field digital imaging system under general anesthesia

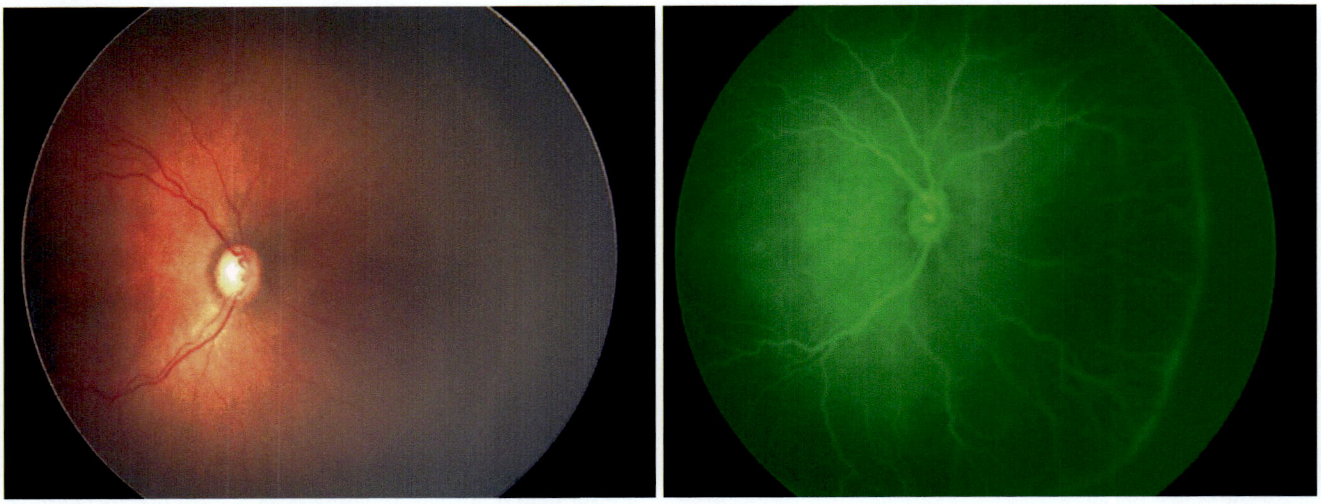

Fig. 10.2 Stage 1 ROP with demarcation line. The demarcation line is formed at the developing end of retinal vessels. Along the demarcation line, circumferential hyperfluorescence is seen at the developing end of the retinal vessels, just posterior to the demarcation line, where immature vessels form shunts. Retinal vessels at the developing end are multi-branched. Fluorescein dye does not leak from the demarcation line

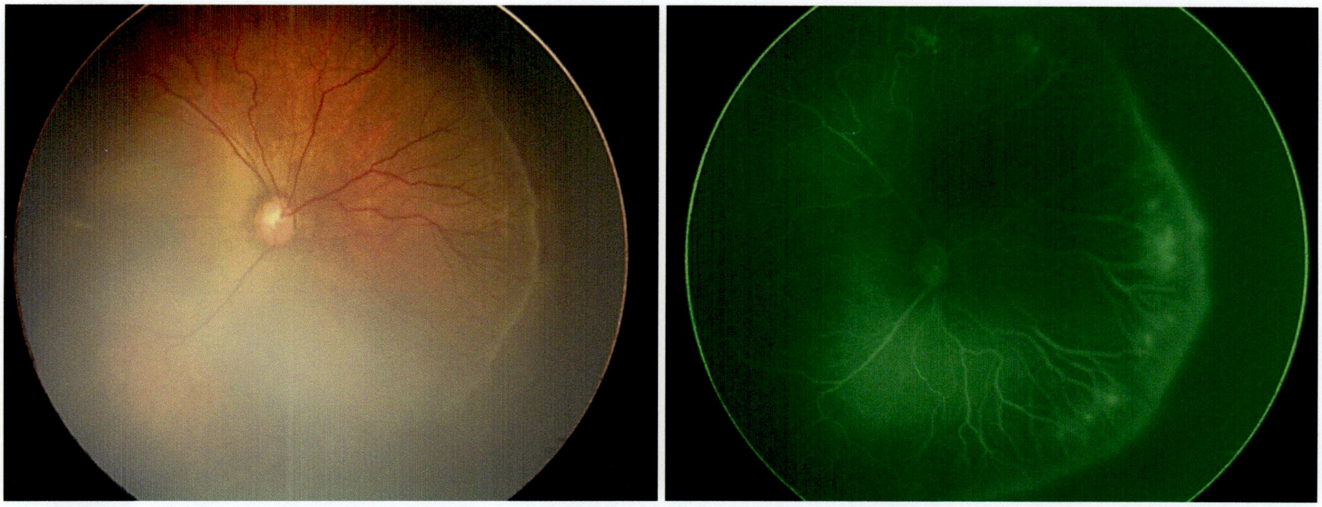

Fig. 10.3 Stage 2 ROP with ridge. Demarcation line changes to a thick ridge with intraretinal proliferation of primitive vascular endothelia. Posterior to the ridge, immature retinal vessels form shunts. Vascular tufts, and small clumps of intravitreal proliferation of pathological new vessels, arise from the retina posterior to the ridge. Leakage of fluorescein dye does not occur from the ridge and vascular shunt but from the vascular tufts

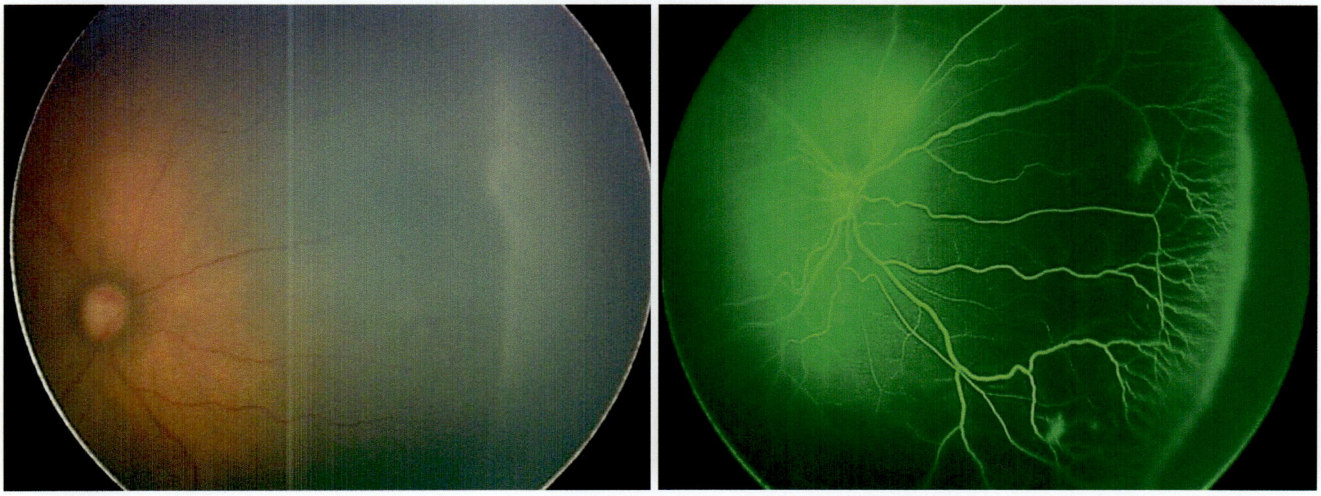

Fig. 10.4 Stage 2 ROP with advanced ridge. Ridge and vascular shunt are diffusely stained by fluorescein dye, probably because of slight dye leakage from immature canal of vascular ends. Dye leakage is clearly seen from the vascular tufts

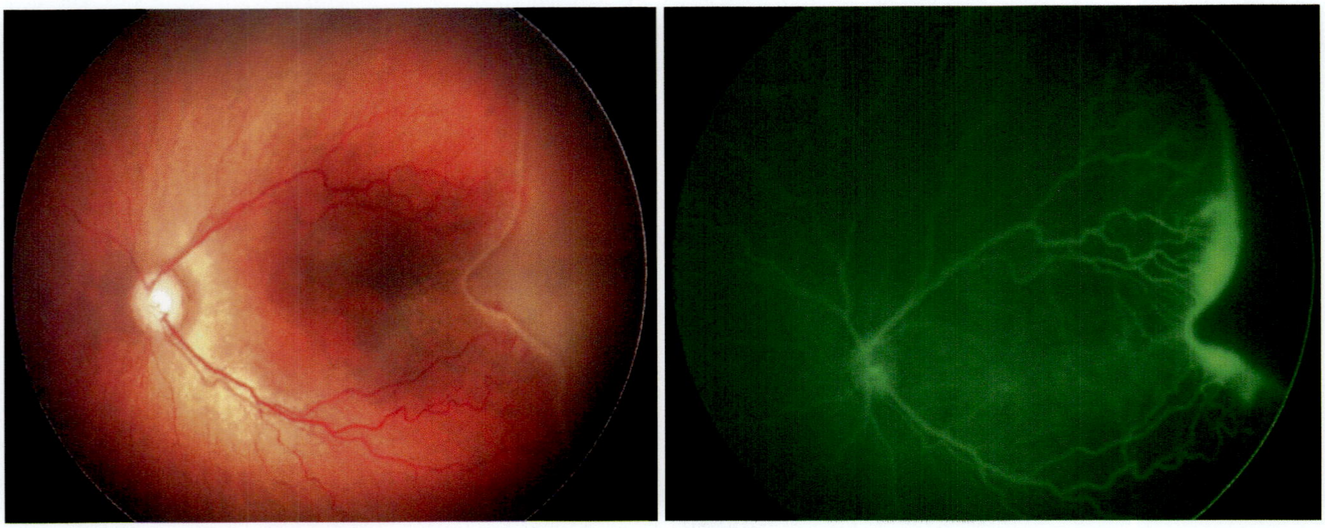

Fig. 10.5 Stage 3 ROP with mild fibrovascular proliferation. Extraretinal proliferation of pathological new vessels occurs along and posterior to the ridge line and begins to fuse circumferentially, which shows fluorescein dye leakage

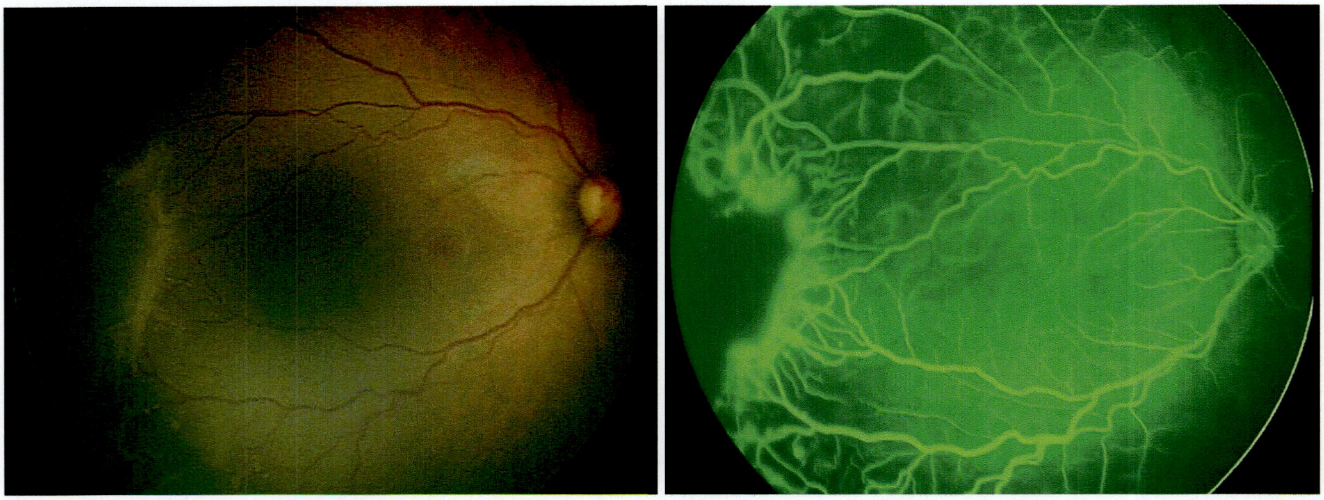

Fig. 10.6 Stage 3 ROP with mild fibrovascular proliferation. Extraretinal proliferation of pathological new vessels along the ridge begins to fuse circumferentially, which shows fluorescein dye leakage

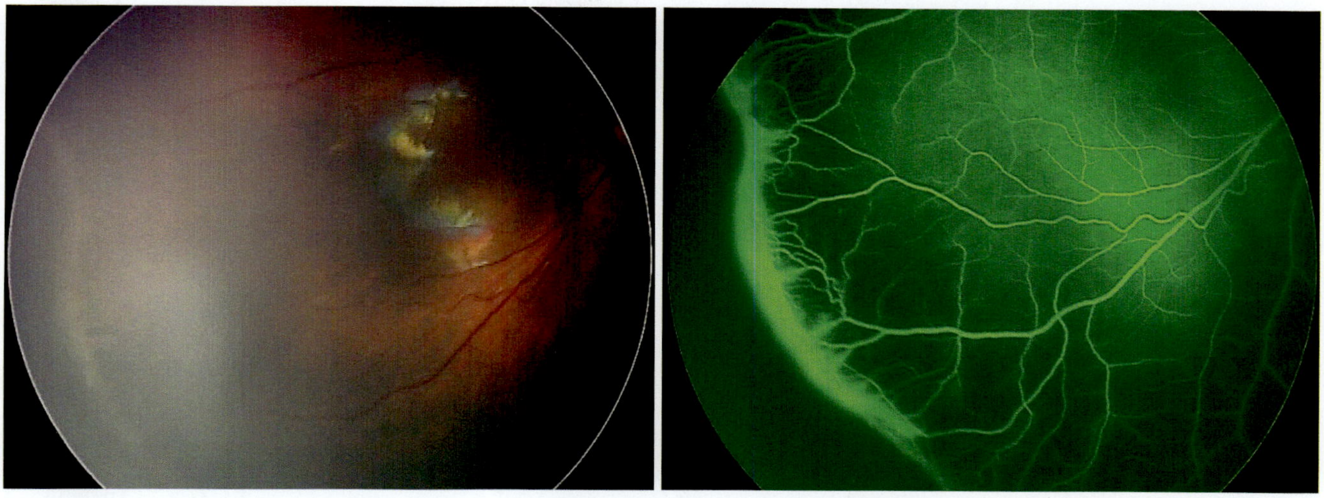

Fig. 10.7 Stage 3 ROP with moderate fibrovascular proliferation. Extraretinal vascular proliferation thickened circumferentially and in antero-posterior direction, where connective tissues begin to be produced pathologically

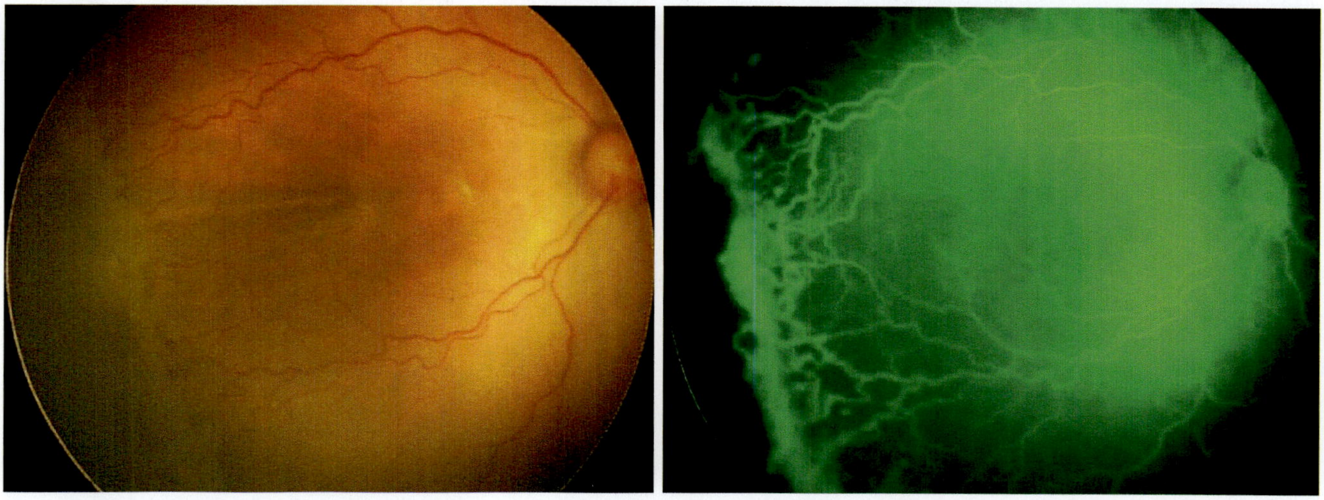

Fig. 10.8 Stage 3 ROP with severe fibrovascular proliferation. Fibrovascular proliferation at the developing end of retinal vessels and also in its posterior portion. Partial dropout of capillary vessels is seen in the vascularized retina. Tortuosity of retinal arteries and dilation of veins indicates plus disease

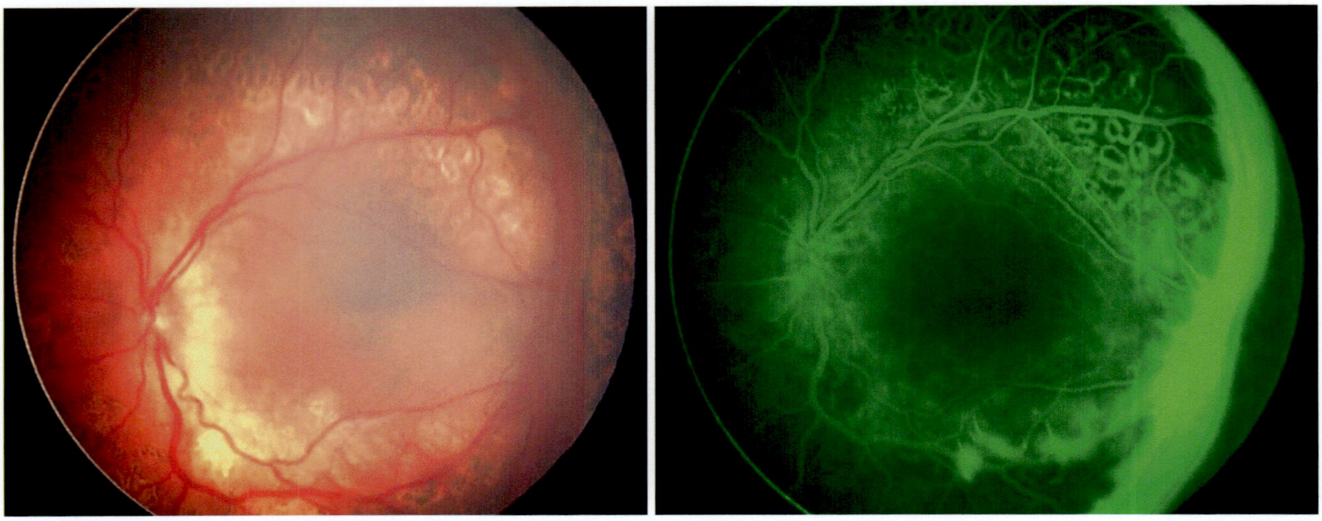

Fig. 10.9 Progression of fibrovascular proliferation after photocoagulation. Fibrovascular tissue that contains numerous pathological new vessels and connective tissues develops even after the application of photocoagulation. Retinal vessels posterior to the fibrous tissues begin to be dragged by contraction of the fibrovascular tissues. Significant leakage of fluorescein dye indicates vascular activity in the fibrovascular tissues. Tortuosity of retinal arteries and dilation of veins are the signs of plus disease, also indicating the activity of ROP. These findings are an indication for vitreoretinal surgery

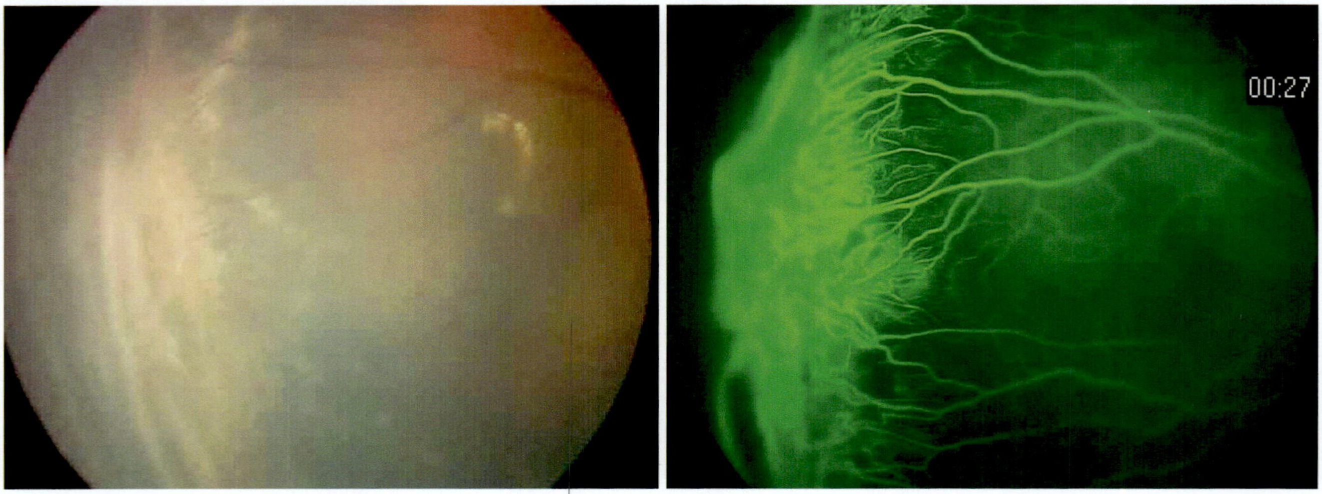

Fig. 10.10 Stage 4A ROP with mild fibrovascular proliferation. Significant fibrovascular proliferation, where connective tissues contract, causing traction retinal detachment, despite the application of photocoagulation. Dragging of the retina by the fibrovascular tissues in anteroposterior and circumferential directions is apprehensible by tractional displacement of retinal vessels

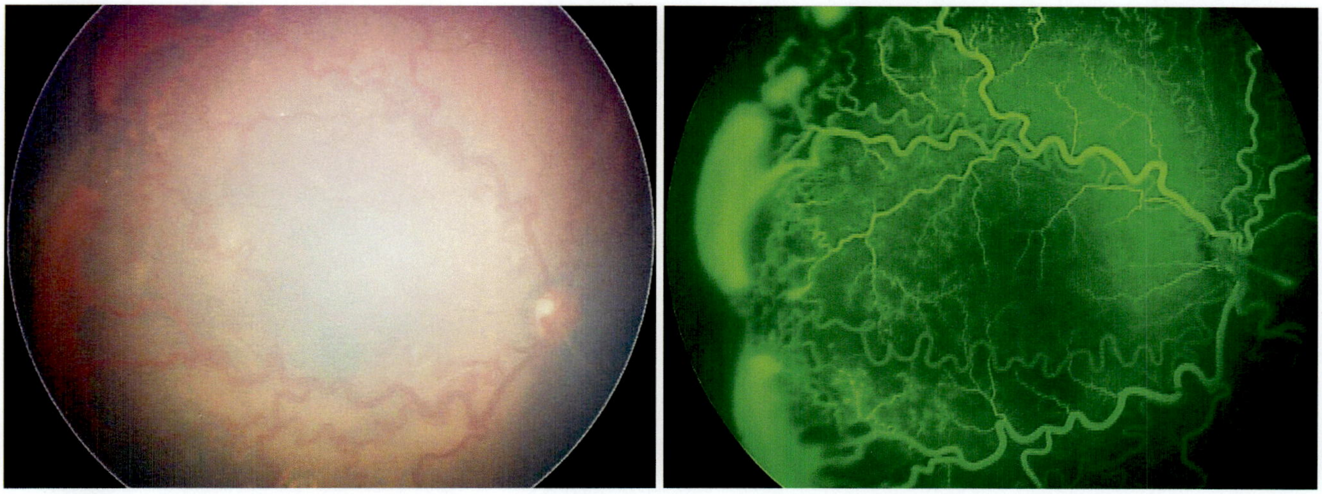

Fig. 10.11 Aggressive posterior ROP. Severe plus disease with prominent tortuosity and dilation of retinal vessels. Vascular proliferation occurs even in the vascularized retina. There are non-perfusion areas of capillary vessels also in the vascularized retina

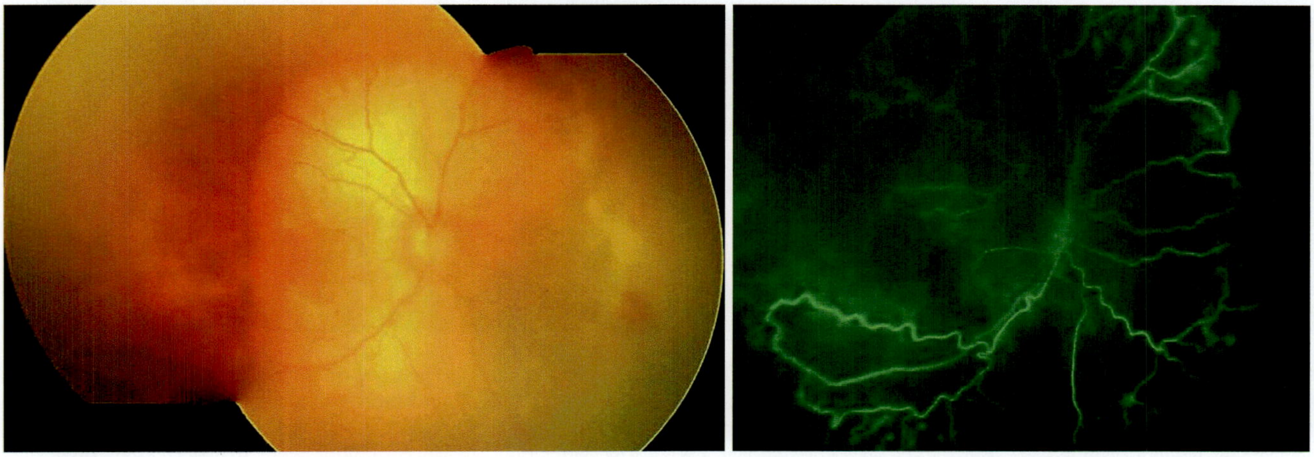

Fig. 10.12 Early phase of aggressive posterior ROP. Although pathological vascular proliferation in the retina is still mild, the capillary network of the retinal vessels is absent in the entire retina, suggesting diffuse obstruction of the capillary vessels. Such finding of severe ischemia is predictive of severe development of vascular proliferation and retinal detachment in the future

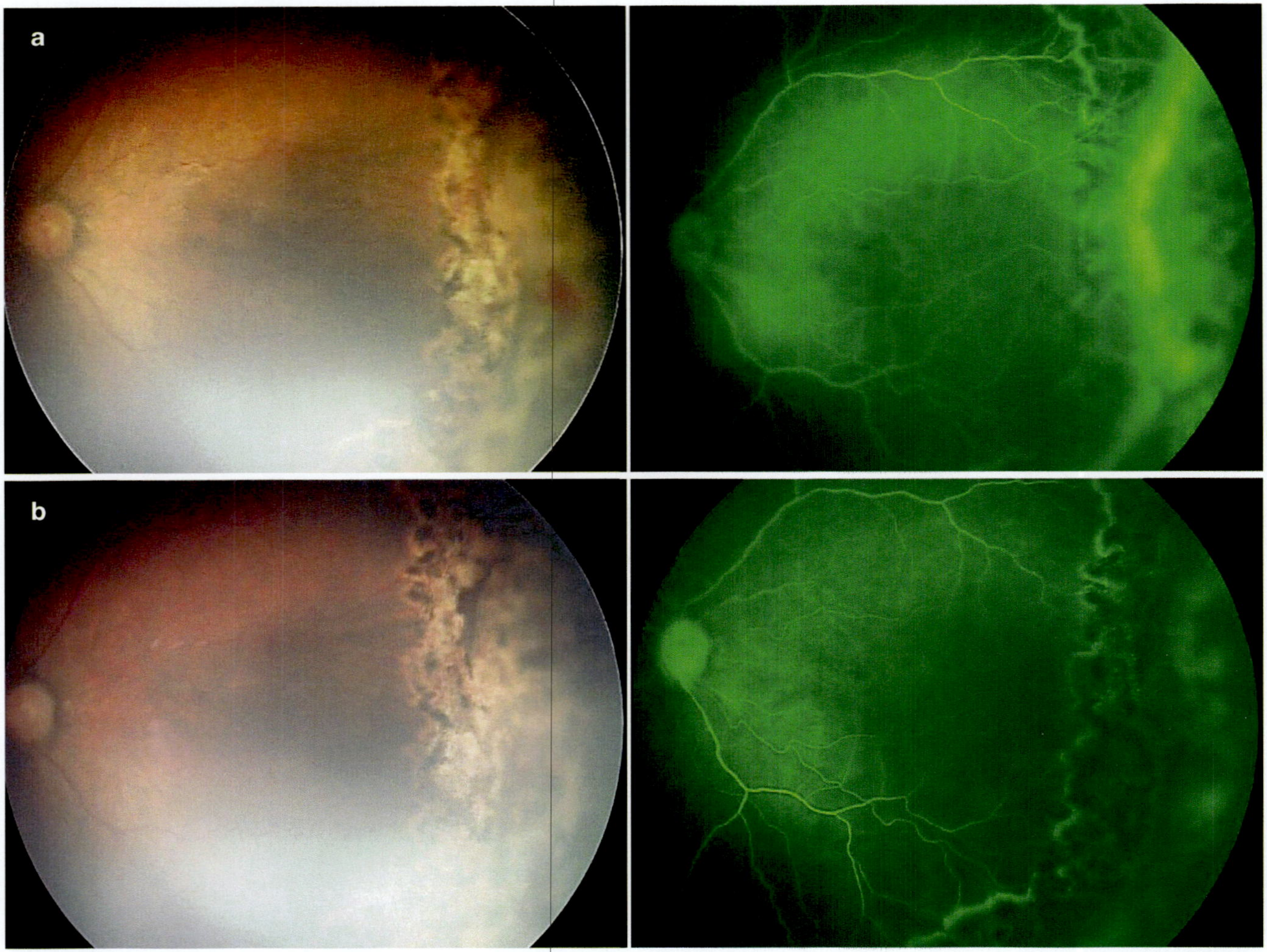

Fig. 10.13 Pre- and post-lens sparing vitrectomy for classic ROP. (**a**) Pre-surgery. Vascular proliferation that shows fluorescein leakage is not stabilized after the application of photocoagulation. Traction retinal detachment has not occurred yet. Born at 23 weeks gestational age, with 495 g body weight. Photocoagulation was applied at 32 weeks corrected gestational age and lens-sparing vitrectomy at 40 weeks. (**b**) Post-surgery. Part of fibrovascular tissues and vitreous gel around them were removed by vitrectomy, and residual tissues regressed 2 weeks after vitrectomy. Leakage of fluorescein dye decreased, suggesting early stabilization of ROP

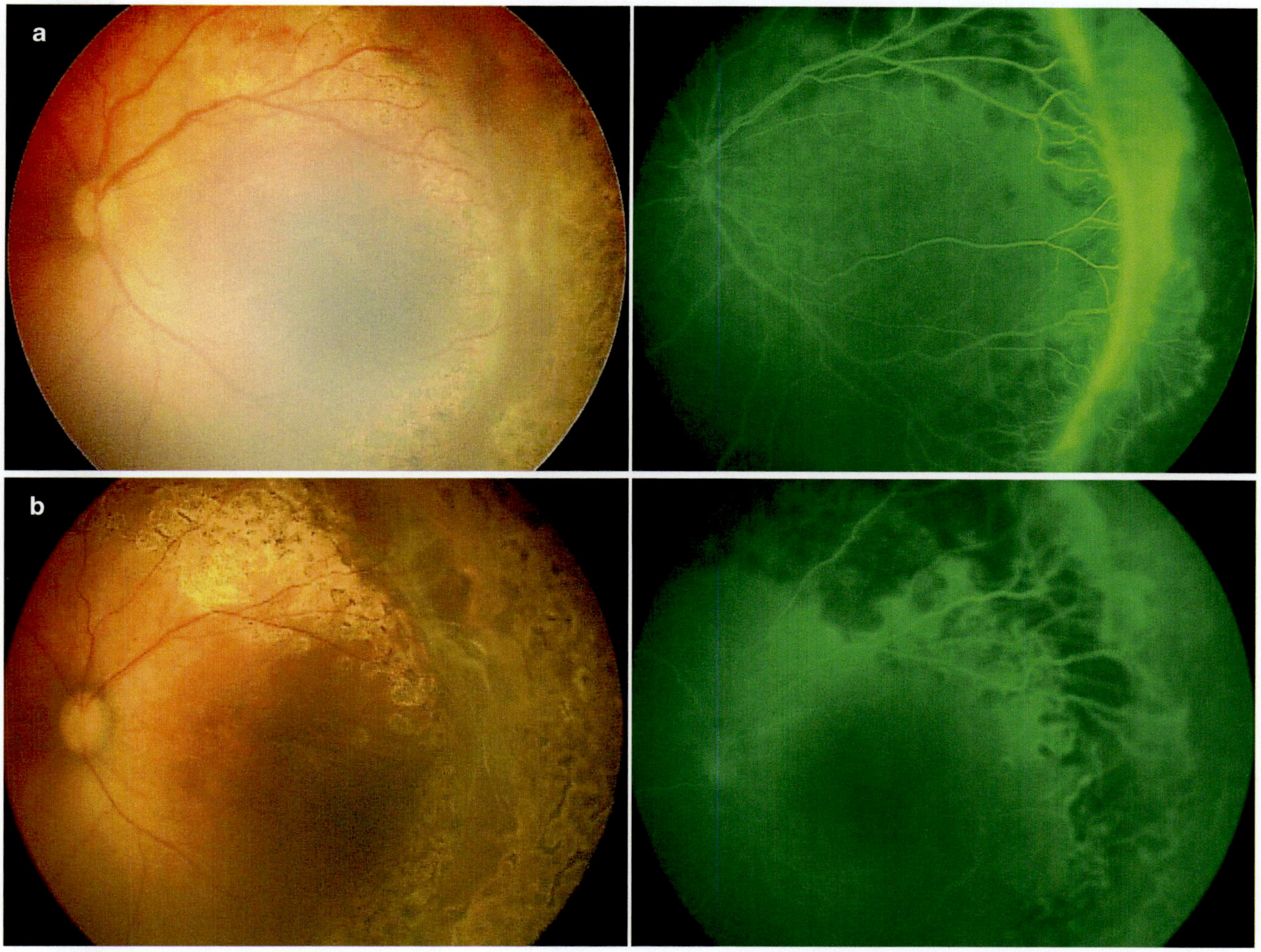

Fig. 10.14 Pre- and post-vitrectomy with lensectomy for aggressive posterior ROP. (**a**) Pre-surgery. Fibrovascular proliferation progresses, which shows prominent leakage of fluorescein dye, even though dense photocoagulation had been applied. Traction retinal detachment occurs underneath the fibrovascular tissues. Dilation of retinal vessels also shows the activity of ROP. Birth at 28 weeks gestational age, with 733gm body weight. Photocoagulation was applied at 33 weeks corrected gestational age and vitrectomy with lensectomy at 36 weeks. (**b**) Post-surgery. Vitreous gel was mostly removed by vitrectomy. Dissection of the fibrous tissues was minimized to avoid bleeding. Because removal of vitreous gel between the fibrovascular tissue and vitreous base was necessary, lensectomy was simultaneously performed. Fibrovascular tissues regressed 2 weeks after surgery, suggested by minimal leakage of fluorescein dye. The retina underneath was reattached. Improvement of retinal vein dilation also suggests regression of ROP

Laser Treatment for Retinopathy of Prematurity

11

Saumya M. Shah and Darius M. Moshfeghi

Abstract

Retinopathy of prematurity (ROP) has been established as the primary cause of visual impairment in premature infants. While cryotherapy used to be a method to treat this condition, laser photocoagulation with indirect ophthalmoscopic delivery has become the gold standard for threshold ROP treatment. This chapter discusses various defining criteria for stages of ROP, conclusions from significant studies such as the ETROP trial, as well as techniques for performing laser photocoagulation and achieving minimal complications. Addressing skip areas using wide-angle photography is a crucial step in ensuring angiogenesis. The next steps, including the role of anti-VEGF (vascular endothelial growth factor) agents in ROP as evident in the BEAT-ROP and RAINBOW trial is promising but requires further results.

Keywords

Retinopathy of prematurity · Skip areas · Angiogenesis Laser photocoagulation · Threshold ROP · Pre-threshold ROP · Diode laser · Anti-VEGF · Cryotherapy · Laser pattern

Retinopathy of prematurity (ROP) has been established as the primary cause of visual impairment in premature infants [1]. With increased survival of extremely low birth weight infants in recent years, it has been reported to be present in more than 84% of survivors born at <28 weeks of gestation [1]. Unlike the normal central to peripheral development of retinal vascularization, phase 1 of the pathogenesis of ROP involves initial vasoconstriction, arrested vessel growth, and relative hyperoxia, followed by phase 2 of relative hypoxia and abnormal vascular proliferation [2]. Supplemental oxygen to improve pulmonary function in premature infants after birth causes postnatal hyperoxemia, which leads to cessation of retinal vasculature maturation and development of a ridge that delineates peripheral avascular and central vascular retinal tissue [1]. The resulting retinal hypoxia induces the release of vascular endothelial growth factors and rapid angiogenesis and the occurrence of ROP [3]. ROP is zoned and staged based on the appearance of vessel at the interface of the vascular and avascular retina [4] Treatment for ROP is most effective during a small time period, making early recognition of disease crucial.

11.1 Cryotherapy

The Multicenter Trial of Cryotherapy for Retinopathy of Prematurity (CRYO-ROP) was one of the first organized attempts to establish the role and efficacy of a therapeutic intervention for ROP. Threshold ROP was defined as at least five contiguous or eight total clock hours of stage 3 disease in zone 1 or 2, or the presence of plus disease [5]. There was an overall 49.3% reduction at 3 months and a 45.8% reduction at 12 months in the rate of unfavorable outcomes in cryotherapy treated versus non-treated eyes (Table 11.1) [5, 6]. With long-term follow-up, the reduction in risk of unfavorable structural outcomes was 43.2% at 10 years and 30% at 15 years [12, 13]. In terms of visual acuity and function, at the 10-year follow-up, 25.2% of treated eyes achieved visual acuity of 20/40 or better, compared to 23.7% of controls [12]. At 15-year follow-up, 44.7% of treated eyes and 64.3% of control eyes had developed unfavorable visual acuity outcomes, emphasizing the need for follow-up of patients with threshold ROP disease on a long-term basis [13].

S. M. Shah
Department of Ophthalmology, Mayo Clinic, Rochester, MN, USA

D. M. Moshfeghi (✉)
Byers Eye Institute, Horngren Family Vitreoretinal Center, Department of Ophthalmology, Stanford University School of Medicine, Palo Alto, CA, USA
e-mail: darius.moshfeghi@stanford.edu

W.-C. Wu, W.-C. Lam (eds.), *A Quick Guide to Pediatric Retina*, https://doi.org/10.1007/978-981-15-6552-6_11

11.2 Laser Photocoagulation

While cryotherapy was extremely efficacious in treating ROP, it proved to be limited in its ability to target posterior areas within the eye. Given its ability to provide targeted treatment without invasive measures to the external eye and need of general anesthesia, laser photocoagulation presented as a more convenient option. The establishment of the laser photocoagulation with indirect ophthalmoscopic delivery as the standard treatment for threshold ROP replaced the role of cryotherapy. Preliminary studies after the introduction of laser photocoagulation as a treatment option for threshold ROP suggested that laser therapy was safe and at least as effective as cryotherapy in treating stage 3+ ROP (Table 11.1) [7, 8, 14, 15]. Comparison of the efficacy of laser photocoagulation and cryotherapy at 7-year and 10-year follow-up showed laser-treated eyes to have a superior mean best-corrected visual acuity (BCVA) of 20/33 and 20/66 compared with 20/133 and 20/182 in cryotherapy-treated eyes, respectively [16, 17]. Eyes treated with cryotherapy were 7.2 times more likely to develop retinal dragging compared with laser treatment [17]. This may have been secondary to the superior ability of the laser to treat more avascular retina in infants with posterior disease, where it is difficult to treat with cryotherapy. Looking at refractive outcome, laser-treated eyes were less myopic with a mean spherical equivalent (SE) of −4.48 D than cryotherapy-treated eyes (mean SE of −7.65 D) [18].

Table 11.1 Summary results for key studies evaluating the success of laser treatment for retinopathy of prematurity

Study name	Year published	Success rate of therapeutic intervention[a]
CRYO-ROP[b]	1990 [6]	78.2% with favorable outcome at 3 months
Argon laser for Stage 3+ ROP[c]	1991 [7]	93.8% (n = 15 of 16) at 3 months
Diode laser for Stage 3+ ROP[d]	1992 [8]	89.3% (n = 25 of 28) at 3 months
ETROP[e]	2004 [9]	85.7% with favorable outcome at 9 months
BEAT-ROP[f]	2011 [10]	74.0% (n = 54 of 73) at 54 weeks
RAINBOW[g]	2008 [11]	66.2% (n = 45 of 68) at 24 weeks

[a]The therapeutic intervention being studied is laser photocoagulation in all studies except CRYO-ROP, which evaluates cryotherapy vs. observation in infants with threshold ROP

[b]The CRYO-ROP study evaluated initial anatomic success of cryotherapy vs. observation at incremental periods of follow-up

[c]This study evaluated the efficacy of argon laser vs. cryotherapy

[d]This study evaluated the efficacy of diode laser vs. cryotherapy

[e]Primary outcome in ETROP was related to visual function. Also, while providers in ETROP had the option to use cryotherapy or laser photocoagulation on patients, all but one patient received laser treatment

[f]The BEAT-ROP studied the rate of recurrence at 54 weeks postmenstrual age as the primary outcome. The above results are for the combined pool of Zone I and Zone II posterior ROP. For Zone I only eyes, the results were 58.0% success (n = 19 of 33 eyes)

[g]The RAINBOW study evaluated the efficacy of two different doses of ranibizumab (0.1 and 0.2 mg) versus laser photocoagulation at maintaining absence of active ROP or absence of unfavorable structural outcomes

Given that a large percentage of infants with ROP continued to face poor visual and structural outcomes despite the developments in treatment, the Early Treatment of ROP (ETROP) trial was conducted to define the role of earlier treatment in infants at high risk of developing threshold ROP or unfavorable structural or visual acuity outcomes. Infants with pre-threshold ROP or considered high risk based on RM-ROP2 analysis were randomized to early peripheral retinal ablation or conventional management of monitoring for progression to threshold ROP [19]. Pre-threshold ROP was defined as any ROP less than threshold in zone I; zone II stage 2 with plus disease; zone II stage 3 without plus disease; or stage 3 with plus disease less than threshold criteria. Unfavorable structural outcomes were reduced from 15.6% to 9.0% ($p < 0.001$) at 9 months, and unfavorable visual acuity outcomes decreased from 19.8% to 14.3% ($p < 0.001$). Based on the findings, type I ROP, defined as zone I, any stage ROP with plus disease; zone I, stage 3 ROP without plus disease; or zone II, stage 2 or 3 with plus disease, were at high risk of developing threshold disease and thus, retinal ablative therapy was recommended. On the other hand, type II ROP, defined as zone I, stage 1 and 2 without plus disease; or zone II, stage 3 without plus disease, could be monitored for progression [9]. The overall anatomic success of laser at 9 months in ETROP was 84.4% (Table 11.1).

A comparison of application with argon green (514 nm) and diode red (810 nm) laser suggested a preference for diode laser given the lower risk of burns to the tunica vasculosa lentis and cataracts with the latter due to deeper retinal lesions. It is important to acknowledge that ablative therapy is associated with acute complications and risks of corneal edema, intraocular hemorrhage, and cataract formation [20]. Initial laser settings often involve a power of 200–300 mW for 0.1–0.2 s, with a targeted burn of whitish-gray color. The laser power is then altered based on the area of treatment; less energy is used for the anterior and superior retina in comparison to the posterior and inferior retina, as well as retinal tissue close to the ridge. Typically, the procedure begins with a demarcation involving one row of laser with ¼ to ½ spot width separations anterior to the ridge and one row posterior to the ora serrata filling in all locations. The nasal and temporal areas over the ciliary artery and nerve utilize 1 to 1½ spot width separations in order to avoid undue damage to these structures. It is essential to treat the entire avascular retina, extending from the ridge (but not including the ridge) to the ora serrata [21]. Performing careful binocular indirect ophthalmoscopy often coupled with wide-angle photography following treatment is helpful to objectively determine if skip areas are present [22]. Any skip areas should be immediately treated and the process of objective photography repeated until no skip areas remain.

As laser photocoagulation became accepted as the standard treatment for threshold ROP, studies focused on optimizing the technique of laser treatment to control disease progression. Banach et al. evaluated the role of the density of laser patterns in the progression of threshold ROP. Compared to the commonly utilized density of 1 to 1.5 burn widths apart, the study found that patients with a near confluent pattern laser treatment (spaced approximately 0.25 burn width apart) had a significantly lower rate of progression of disease to stage 4 or 5 (3.6% overall near confluent vs. 29% overall fixed density, $p = 0.0003$) [23]. Therapeutic ablation of the ischemic avascular retina observed in threshold ROP suppresses the angiogenesis stimulated by vascular endothelial growth factor, which may help with the resolution of ROP. Additionally, the therapy may also promote chorioretinal adhesions, resulting in positive outcomes; however, given that a proportion of eyes with zone 2 disease still progress to retinal detachments [23], this may be a smaller component [24]. A nearly confluent pattern of laser photocoagulation was also found to reduce the rate of re-treatment of the disease (0% of patients with zone 2 disease) [25].

Following laser treatment, it is imperative that a complete viewing of the retina be performed to ensure that no "skip" areas are identified (see Chap. 12, Fig. 4). "Skip" areas may prevent the regression of active vessels and disinhibit the growth of new vasculature, resulting in possible treatment failure. In a retrospective manner, Kang et al. evaluated the most common locations of skip areas as well as the role of using wide-angle digital imaging in training for the treatment of retinopathy of prematurity. The majority of skip areas occurred in the superior and inferior retina, likely due to a more difficult visualization of these regions and differences in the skill level of trainees that participated in the study. Skip areas missed during the initial treatment procedure were easily visualized with wide-angle digital imaging, making it a very helpful tool for ablative treatment related to ROP [22].

The course of ROP subsequent to treatment is of significant importance as complications including retinal detachments leading to subsequent blindness can occur. Coats studied involution patterns of ROP subsequent to laser photocoagulation in detail and the risk of downstream complications in 262 eyes of 132 infants. Complete ROP involution was noted in 80% of eyes within the first 28 days of treatment. Eyes with "clinically important" vitreous organization (defined as two or more dense, contiguous clock hours that significantly reduced visualization of the underlying retina) and vitreous hemorrhage (completely obscuration of retina visualization) were associated with statistically significant increases in the odds of a retinal detachment, making them strong predictive markers. Based on these results, a possible role for preemptive, instead of deferred vitrectomy, in some eyes with clinically important vitreous organization and hemorrhage was suggested [26]. Hartnett and McColm focused their analysis on understanding features that indicated eyes at risk of developing progressive stage 4 ROP requiring surgical intervention after laser treatment for threshold ROP. Absence of clear vitreous, six or more clock hours of ridge elevation, and plus disease in two or more quadrants were all found to be predictive of stage 4 ROP, while neovascularization was not prognostic according to this study. While unclear, the breakdown of the blood–retinal barrier and thickening of the vascular ridge secondary to growth factors such as vascular endothelial growth factor (VEGF) and platelet-derived growth factor may be responsible for the increased vitreous haze and ridge elevation [27].

11.3 Ongoing Treatments

Numerous novel therapeutics are currently under investigation as the pathophysiologic mechanisms behind the occurrence of retinopathy of prematurity become better understood. Given that the ROP is known to develop in two phases of vaso-obliteration followed by neovascularization, ischemia is a major contributor to the disease, recruiting VEGF as a key factor in the process of angiogenesis. As with other diseases involving neovascularization, anti-VEGF therapies may have a promising role in the treatment of ROP. Current anti-VEGF agents such as bevacizumab, ranibizumab, and pegaptanib sodium have all been reported as treatment options in relation to ROP [28–31].

The BEAT-ROP (Bevacizumab Eliminates the Angiogenic Threat of Retinopathy of Prematurity) trial was the first attempt at prospectively study the role of bevacizumab (0.625 mg per 0.025 ml) as primary therapy for ROP, in lieu of laser photocoagulation. The prospective, randomized, unmasked, stratified, multicenter Phase II trial assessed the role of intravitreal bevacizumab as primary therapy for zone I or II posterior stage 3+ ROP. For zone I, stage 3+ disease, the rate of recurrent retinal neovascularization within 54 weeks of treatment to was significantly higher in the group that received laser therapy in comparison to the group that received bevacizumab (42% vs. 6%; 95% CI (0.02 to 0.43), $p = 0.002$). Difference was noted for posterior zone II disease between the two groups, albeit not statistically significant ($p = 0.27$). The time to recurrence for zone I eyes was significantly different between the two groups 19.2 ± 8.6 weeks vs. 6.4 ± 6.7 weeks for bevacizumab and laser, respectively. Overall, laser success was suboptimal at 74.0% in the BEAT-ROP trial (Table 11.1). Based on these results, the authors concluded that bevacizumab was superior to laser for the treatment of zone I, stage 3+ ROP [10]. However, further correspondence subsequent to this study has questioned the safety of bevacizumab in treating ROP, as well as the time of follow-up necessary to account for later recurrence in some infants subsequent to bevacizumab therapy [32–41].

The RAINBOW Phase III study (RAnibizumab Compared With Laser Therapy for the Treatment of INfants BOrn Prematurely With Retinopathy of Prematurity), which is also randomized, open-label, controlled, and multicenter, is being conducted to assess the efficacy and safety of ranibizumab (0.1 and 0.2 mg) in comparison to laser photocoagulation in patients with ROP. Preliminary results indicate the percentage of infants with the absence of active ROP or unfavorable structural outcomes at 24 weeks to be 80% in the ranibizumab 0.2 mg, 75% in the ranibizumab 0.1 mg, and 66.2% in the laser-treated group (p = 0.0254; CI: 0.99 to 4.82) (Table 11.1) [11]. However, further information and analysis of the results is necessary before any conclusions can be made about possible changes in practice.

While anti-VEGF agents show a promising role in future treatment options of ROP—either as primary or adjuvant treatment—a tremendous amount of investigation needs to occur in order to better understand its long-term safety, efficacy, and treatment protocols prior to its acceptance as a mainstay therapy. Along with VEGF inhibitors, therapeutics targeting other mediators involved in the development and progression of ROP, such as EPO and IGF-1 are also under investigation and may offer promising avenues of treatment for ROP [4].

11.4 Conclusions

Since the initial description of retrolental fibroplasia, or ROP in 1942, a significant amount of advancements in the understanding of the pathophysiology of the disease, the incidence, risk factors, and treatment technologies have been made. Utilization of ablative laser photocoagulation in a nearly confluent manner continues to be the gold standard in the treatment of threshold and pre-threshold ROP when coupled with wide-angle photography to objectively evaluate skip areas. Unfortunately, the technicality of the procedure requires significant training and skill development, limiting the number of providers that are able to provide effective treatment. Pediatric retinal surgeons excel at laser technique and with early examinations and frequent monitoring, can prevent the development of complications and progression of disease.

Conflicts of Interest SMS: None.

DMM: 1-800 Contacts (Board of Directors, equity), Alcon (Data Monitoring Committee), Apellis (grant support), Bayer (Grant support), dSentz (Founder, Board of Directors, equity), Iconic Therapeutics (Steering Committee), Grand Legend Technology (equity), Irenix (scientific advisory board), Novartis (CME consultant), Pr3vent (Founder, Board of Directors, equity), Promisight (Founder, Board of Directors, equity), Pykus (Scientific advisory board, equity), Regeneron (CME consultant), Versl (Founder, equity), Vindico (CME consultant), Visunex Medical Systems Co. Ltd. (Founder, equity, consultant).

References

1. Ludwig CA, Chen TA, Hernandez-Boussard T, Moshfeghi AA, Moshfeghi DM. The epidemiology of retinopathy of prematurity in the United States. Ophthalmic Surg Lasers Imaging Retina. 2017;48(7):553–62. https://doi.org/10.3928/23258160-20170630-06.
2. Karna P, Muttineni J, Angell L, Karmaus W. Retinopathy of prematurity and risk factors: a prospective cohort study. BMC Pediatr. 2005;5(1):18. https://doi.org/10.1186/1471-2431-5-18.
3. York JR, Landers S, Kirby RS, Arbogast PG, Penn JS. Arterial oxygen fluctuation and retinopathy of prematurity in very-low-birth-weight infants. J Perinatol. 2004;24(2):82–7. https://doi.org/10.1038/sj.jp.7211040.
4. Houston SK, Wykoff CC, Berrocal AM, Hess DJ, Murray TG. Laser treatment for retinopathy of prematurity. Lasers Med Sci. 2013;28(2):683–92. https://doi.org/10.1007/s10103-011-1021-z.
5. Cryotherapy for Retinopathy of Prematurity Cooperative Group. Multicenter trial of cryotherapy for retinopathy of prematurity. Preliminary results. Arch Ophthalmol (Chicago, Ill 1960). 1988;106(4):471–9.
6. Cryotherapy for Retinopathy of Prematurity Cooperative Group. Multicenter trial of cryotherapy for retinopathy of prematurity. One-year outcome-structure and function. Arch Ophthalmol (Chicago, Ill 1960). 1990;108(10):1408–16.
7. McNamara JA, Tasman W, Brown GC, Federman JL. Laser photocoagulation for stage 3+ retinopathy of prematurity. Ophthalmology. 1991;98(5):576–80. https://doi.org/10.1016/S0161-6420(91)32247-4.
8. McNamara JA, Tasman W, Vander JF, Brown GC. Diode laser photocoagulation for retinopathy of prematurity. Preliminary results. Arch Ophthalmol (Chicago, Ill 1960). 1992;110(12):1714–6.
9. Good WV, Early Treatment for Retinopathy of Prematurity Cooperative Group on behalf of the ET for R of PC. Final results of the early treatment for retinopathy of prematurity (ETROP) randomized trial. Trans Am Ophthalmol Soc. 2004;102:233–48. Discussion 248-50
10. Mintz-Hittner HA, Kennedy KA, Chuang AZ, BEAT-ROP Cooperative Group. Efficacy of intravitreal bevacizumab for stage 3+ retinopathy of prematurity. N Engl J Med. 2011;364(7):603–15. https://doi.org/10.1056/NEJMoa1007374.
11. Clinicaltrials.gov. RAINBOW Study: ranibizumab compared with laser therapy for the treatment of infants born prematurely with retinopathy of prematurity – Study results – ClinicalTrials.gov.
12. Cryotherapy for Retinopathy of Prematurity Cooperative Group. Multicenter trial of cryotherapy for retinopathy of prematurity: ophthalmological outcomes at 10 years. Arch Ophthalmol (Chicago, Ill 1960). 2001;119(8):1110–8.
13. Palmer EA, Hardy RJ, Dobson V, et al. 15-year outcomes following threshold retinopathy of prematurity. Arch Ophthalmol. 2005;123(3):311. https://doi.org/10.1001/archopht.123.3.311.
14. Hunter DG, Repka MX. Diode laser photocoagulation for threshold retinopathy of prematurity: a randomized study. Ophthalmology. 1993;100(2):238–44. https://doi.org/10.1016/S0161-6420(93)31664-7.
15. White JE, Repka MX. Randomized comparison of diode laser photocoagulation versus cryotherapy for threshold retinopathy of prematurity: 3-year outcome. J Pediatr Ophthalmol Strabismus

34(2):83–87.; quiz 121-2. http://www.ncbi.nlm.nih.gov/pubmed/9083952. Accessed 29 Oct 2018.
16. Shalev B, Farr AK, Repka MX. Randomized comparison of diode laser photocoagulation versus cryotherapy for threshold retinopathy of prematurity: seven-year outcome. Am J Ophthalmol. 2001;132(1):76–80.
17. Ng EY, Connolly BP, McNamara JA, Regillo CD, Vander JF, Tasman W. A comparison of laser photocoagulation with cryotherapy for threshold retinopathy of prematurity at 10 years: part 1. Visual function and structural outcome. Ophthalmology. 2002;109(5):928–34. https://doi.org/10.1016/S0161-6420(01)01017-X.
18. Connolly BP, Ng EYJ, McNamara JA, Regillo CD, Vander JF, Tasman W. A comparison of laser photocoagulation with cryotherapy for threshold retinopathy of prematurity at 10 years: part 2. Refractive outcome. Ophthalmology. 2002;109(5):936–41.
19. Clark D, Mandal K. Treatment of retinopathy of prematurity. Early Hum Dev. 2008;84(2):95–9. https://doi.org/10.1016/J.EARLHUMDEV.2007.11.007.
20. Benner JD, Morse LS, Hay A, Landers MB. A comparison of argon and diode photocoagulation combined with supplemental oxygen for the treatment of retinopathy of prematurity. Retina. 1993;13(3):222–9.
21. Jalali S, Azad R, Trehan HS, Dogra MR, Gopal L, Narendran V. Technical aspects of laser treatment for acute retinopathy of prematurity under topical anesthesia. Indian J Ophthalmol. 2010;58(6):509–15. https://doi.org/10.4103/0301-4738.71689.
22. Kang KB, Orlin A, Lee TC, Chiang MF, Chan RVP. The use of digital imaging in the identification of skip areas after laser treatment for retinopathy of prematurity and its implications for education and patient care HHS public access. Retina. 2013;33(10):2162–9. https://doi.org/10.1097/IAE.0b013e31828e6969.
23. Banach MJ, Ferrone PJ, Trese MT. A comparison of dense versus less dense diode laser photocoagulation patterns for threshold retinopathy of prematurity. Ophthalmology. 2000;107(2):324–7. https://doi.org/10.1016/S0161-6420(99)00042-1.
24. Axer-Siegel R, Snir M, Cotlear D, et al. Diode laser treatment of posterior retinopathy of prematurity. Br J Ophthalmol. 2000;84(12):1383–6. https://doi.org/10.1136/BJO.84.12.1383.
25. Rezai KA, Eliott D, Ferrone PJ, Kim RW. Near confluent laser photocoagulation for the treatment of threshold retinopathy of prematurity. Arch Ophthalmol. 2005;123(5):621. https://doi.org/10.1001/archopht.123.5.621.
26. Coats DK. Retinopathy of prematurity: involution, factors predisposing to retinal detachment, and expected utility of preemptive surgical reintervention. Trans Am Ophthalmol Soc 2005;103:281–312. http://www.ncbi.nlm.nih.gov/pubmed/17057808. Accessed 9 Nov 2018.
27. Hartnett ME, McColm JR. Retinal features predictive of progressive stage 4 retinopathy of prematurity. Retina 2004;24(2):237–241. http://www.ncbi.nlm.nih.gov/pubmed/15097884. Accessed 19 Nov 2018.
28. Mintz-Hittner HA. Intravitreal pegaptanib as adjunctive treatment for stage 3+ ROP shown to be effective in a prospective, randomized, controlled multicenter clinical trial. Eur J Ophthalmol. 2012;22(5):685–6. https://doi.org/10.5301/ejo.5000176.
29. Chen S-N, Lian I, Hwang Y-C, et al. Intravitreal anti-vascular Endotherlial growth factor treatment for retinopathy of prematurity: comparison between ranibizumab and bevacizumab. Retina. 2015;35(4):667–74. https://doi.org/10.1097/IAE.0000000000000380.
30. Autrata R, Krejčířová I, Šenková K, Holoušová M, Doležel Z, Borek I. Intravitreal pegaptanib combined with diode laser therapy for stage 3+ retinopathy of prematurity in zone I and posterior zone II. Eur J Ophthalmol. 2012;22(5):687–94. https://doi.org/10.5301/ejo.5000166.
31. Wu W-C, Yeh P-T, Chen S-N, Yang C-M, Lai C-C, Kuo H-K. Effects and complications of bevacizumab use in patients with retinopathy of prematurity: a multicenter study in Taiwan. Ophthalmology. 2011;118(1):176–83. https://doi.org/10.1016/j.ophtha.2010.04.018.
32. Moshfeghi DM, Berrocal AM. Retinopathy of prematurity in the time of bevacizumab: incorporating the BEAT-ROP results into clinical practice. Ophthalmology. 2011;118(7):1227–8. https://doi.org/10.1016/J.OPHTHA.2011.04.028.
33. Moshfeghi DM. Systemic solutions in retinopathy of prematurity. Am J Ophthalmol. 2018;193:xiv–xviii. https://doi.org/10.1016/j.ajo.2018.05.013.
34. Lepore D, Quinn GE, Molle F, et al. Intravitreal bevacizumab versus laser treatment in type 1 retinopathy of prematurity. Ophthalmology. 2014;121(11):2212–9. https://doi.org/10.1016/j.ophtha.2014.05.015.
35. Chen TA, Schachar IH, Moshfeghi DM. Outcomes of intravitreal bevacizumab and diode laser photocoagulation for treatment-warranted retinopathy of prematurity. Ophthalmic Surg Lasers Imaging Retina. 2018;49(2):126–31. https://doi.org/10.3928/23258160-20180129-07.
36. Lepore D, Quinn GE, Molle F, et al. Follow-up to age 4 years of treatment of type 1 retinopathy of prematurity intravitreal bevacizumab injection versus laser: fluorescein angiographic findings. Ophthalmology. 2018;125(2):218–26. https://doi.org/10.1016/j.ophtha.2017.08.005.
37. Garcia Gonzalez JM, Snyder L, Blair M, Rohr A, Shapiro M, Greenwald M. Prophylactic peripheral laser and fluorescein angiography after bevacizumab for retinopathy of prematurity. Retina. 2018;38(4):764–72. https://doi.org/10.1097/IAE.0000000000001581.
38. Hu J, Blair MP, Shapiro MJ, Lichtenstein SJ, Galasso JM, Kapur R. Reactivation of retinopathy of prematurity after bevacizumab injection. Arch Ophthalmol. 2012;130(8):1000. https://doi.org/10.1001/archophthalmol.2012.592.
39. Snyder LL, Garcia-Gonzalez JM, Shapiro MJ, Blair MP. Very late reactivation of retinopathy of prematurity after monotherapy with intravitreal bevacizumab. Ophthalmic Surg Lasers Imaging Retina. 2016;47(3):280–3. https://doi.org/10.3928/23258160-20160229-12.
40. Hajrasouliha AR, Garcia-Gonzales JM, Shapiro MJ, Yoon H, Blair MP. Reactivation of retinopathy of prematurity three years after treatment with bevacizumab. Ophthalmic Surg Lasers Imaging Retina. 2017;48(3):255–9. https://doi.org/10.3928/23258160-20170301-10.
41. Golas L, Shapiro MJ, Blair MP. Late ROP reactivation and retinal detachment in a teenager. Ophthalmic Surg Lasers Imaging Retina. 2018;49(8):625–8. https://doi.org/10.3928/23258160-20180803-11.

Anti-VEGF in ROP

12

Andrés Kychenthal and Paola Dorta

Abstract

In the current management of ROP, anti-VEGF drugs have a very significant role. These drugs can be used in ROP in different clinical situations: as a primary treatment for posterior ROP, for progressing cases after they have been previously treated either with a laser or with an anti-VEGF drug, and as an adjunct in ROP-related vitreoretinal surgery. The beneficial effect of using these drugs for the treatment of ROP is enormous. No significant local or systemic complications attributable to these injections have been detected. The best anti-VEGF drug and dose are still under investigation.

Keywords

Anti-VEGF drugs · Retinopathy of prematurity · ROP
Retinal detachment · Anti-VEGF injection

Antiangiogenics, or anti-VEGF drugs, were introduced more than 10 years ago for the management of Retinopathy of Prematurity (ROP). Notwithstanding very reasonable safety concerns for the use of these types of drugs in developing infants, no complications attributable to these injections have been detected. The beneficial effect of using these drugs for the treatment of ROP is immense. The best anti-VEGF drug and dose for this purpose is still under investigation.

The use of anti-VEGF has proven to be not only effective but less stressful for the infant, as it does not destroy retinal tissue like laser photocoagulation does, and it also induces less myopia (Fig. 12.1).

Anti-VEGF drugs can be used in ROP in different clinical situations. The most relevant are:

A. Kychenthal (✉) · P. Dorta
KYDOFT Foundation, Las Condes, Santiago, Chile
e-mail: akychenthal@kydoft.cl

12.1 Anti-VEGF as a Primary Treatment for ROP

Current indications for the use of anti-VEGF drugs as a primary treatment are zone I and posterior zone II ROP (Fig. 12.2).

12.2 Anti-VEGF for Progressing Cases After They Have Been Previously Treated Either with Laser or with an Anti-VEGF Drug

If there is persistent plus disease in an eye that has received treatment for type 1 ROP, there is a chance of progression with the risk of retinal detachment. Anti-VEGF drugs can play a significant role in inducing ROP regression in some of these cases with the persistence of plus disease.

If a patient underwent laser treatment for zone I ROP and there is persistent plus or reactivation of the disease while vessels are still in zone I, then injecting an anti-VEGF is likely to induce regression. If vessels advance into zone II, then applying more laser should be the first alternative (Fig. 12.3). If there are no skipped areas (Fig. 12.4) and all of the avascular retina is properly filled with laser spots, an anti-VEGF should be injected (Fig. 12.5).

If reactivation or persistent plus disease is observed after an eye was treated for type 1 ROP with laser for a zone II disease, treatment of skipped areas should be performed. If complete laser treatment was given, the use of an intravitreal anti-VEGF drug is indicated (Figs. 12.3 and 12.5).

If the primary treatment was performed with anti-VEGF and there is progression of the ROP, the zone where the vessels are located will determine the secondary treatment. If retinal vessels are still in zone I, a re-injection of anti-VEGF might be more suitable. If vessels are in zone II, then laser photocoagulation seems to be the better alternative (Fig. 12.6).

W.-C. Wu, W.-C. Lam (eds.), *A Quick Guide to Pediatric Retina*, https://doi.org/10.1007/978-981-15-6552-6_12

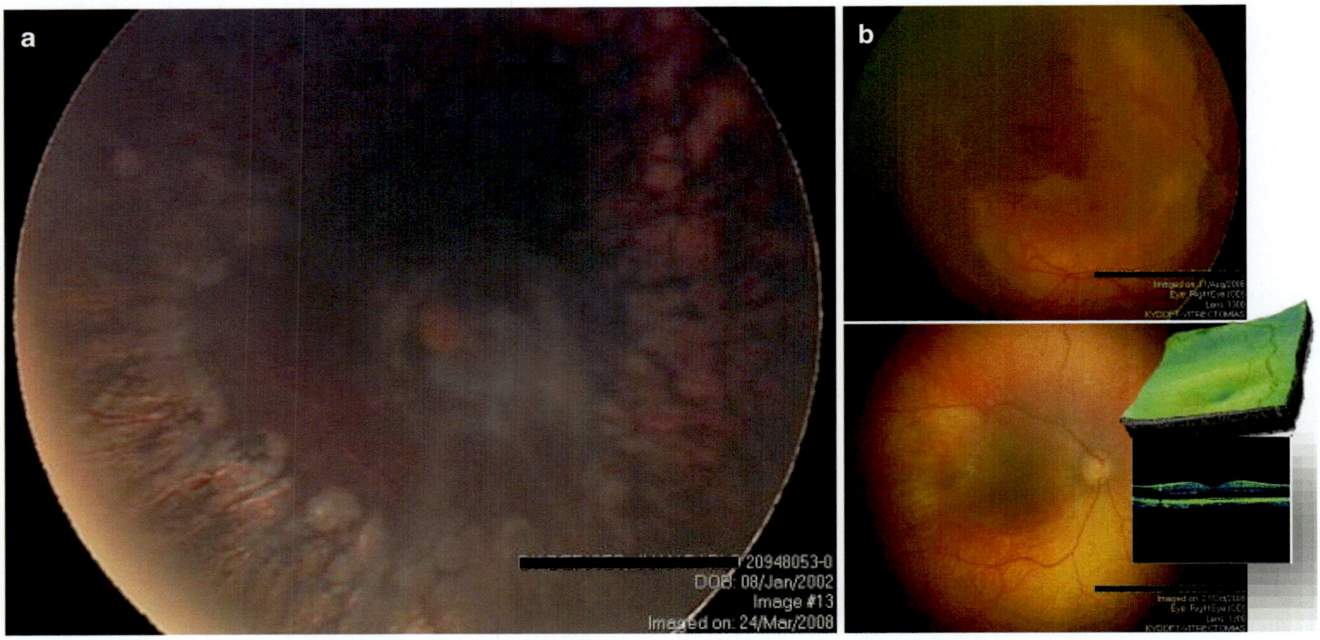

Fig. 12.1 Comparison between laser photocoagulation and anti-VEGF injection for the treatment of posterior zone I ROP. The laser destroys a large area of the retina (**a**). With a single anti-VEGF injection, a normal fundus appearance together with normal macular configurations at the OCT can be obtained in these cases (**b**)

It is very important to consider that reactivation of ROP happens after anti-VEGF treatment with an uncertain risk of progression to retinal detachment. Patterns of regression and recurrence following the use of anti-VEGFs in treatment of ROP are not known; thus, longer follow-ups are needed in these patients than those with laser photocoagulation.

12.3 - Anti-VEGF as an Adjunct in Vitreoretinal Surgery in ROP

The presence of vascular activity is a major problem when operating on an ROP retinal detachment. The risk of bleeding and failure of the surgical procedure are considerably greater in eyes with active vascularity (Fig. 12.7).

Anti-VEGF drugs that can be injected prior to the surgical intervention address this issue by inducing a rapid regression of vascular activity, allowing one to operate on a vascularly inactive or "quiet eye" rather than on an active one (Fig. 12.8).

Especially significant is the fact that this effect allows the surgery to be carried out without the delay of waiting for the natural regression of neovascular activity. Thus, intervention that is performed earlier than previously possible should prevent progression and macular involvement, and offer better visual potential for these eyes.

The right time to inject an anti-VEGF drug and perform the vitrectomy seems especially important when a retinal detachment is already present. A balance between neovascular regression and avoiding the development of fibrous tissue with traction on the retina are essential. Five to seven days after injecting the anti-VEGF drug seems to be an adequate period to perform the surgery. In that period of time, a very significant reduction in vascular activity occurs, allowing for a safe procedure. A longer interval between the injection and the surgery might provoke progression in the detachment or even a rhegmatogenous factor due to traction on the retina induced by the regression and fibrous conversion of the neovascular tissues (Fig. 12.9).

In summary, in the current management of ROP anti-VEGF drugs have a very significant role (Fig. 12.10).

12.4 Injection Technique

Anti-VEGF drugs can be injected in the neonatal intensive care unit or in an operating room with only topical anesthesia or under sedation.

Special attention must be paid to avoid the potential risk of endophthalmitis and to avoid drug delivery problems when managing such small volumes.

The pupils are dilated with tropicamide 1% eye drops. Periocular skin, eyelashes, upper and lower lids are swabbed with povidone-iodine 10%. Proparacaine 0.5% is instilled into the eye. A surgeon, wearing sterile gloves and mask, opens the lids with a sterile speculum. The drug is injected with a 30G insulin syringe temporally (1–1.5 mm from limbus). An antibiotic eye drop use at the end of the procedure is optional.

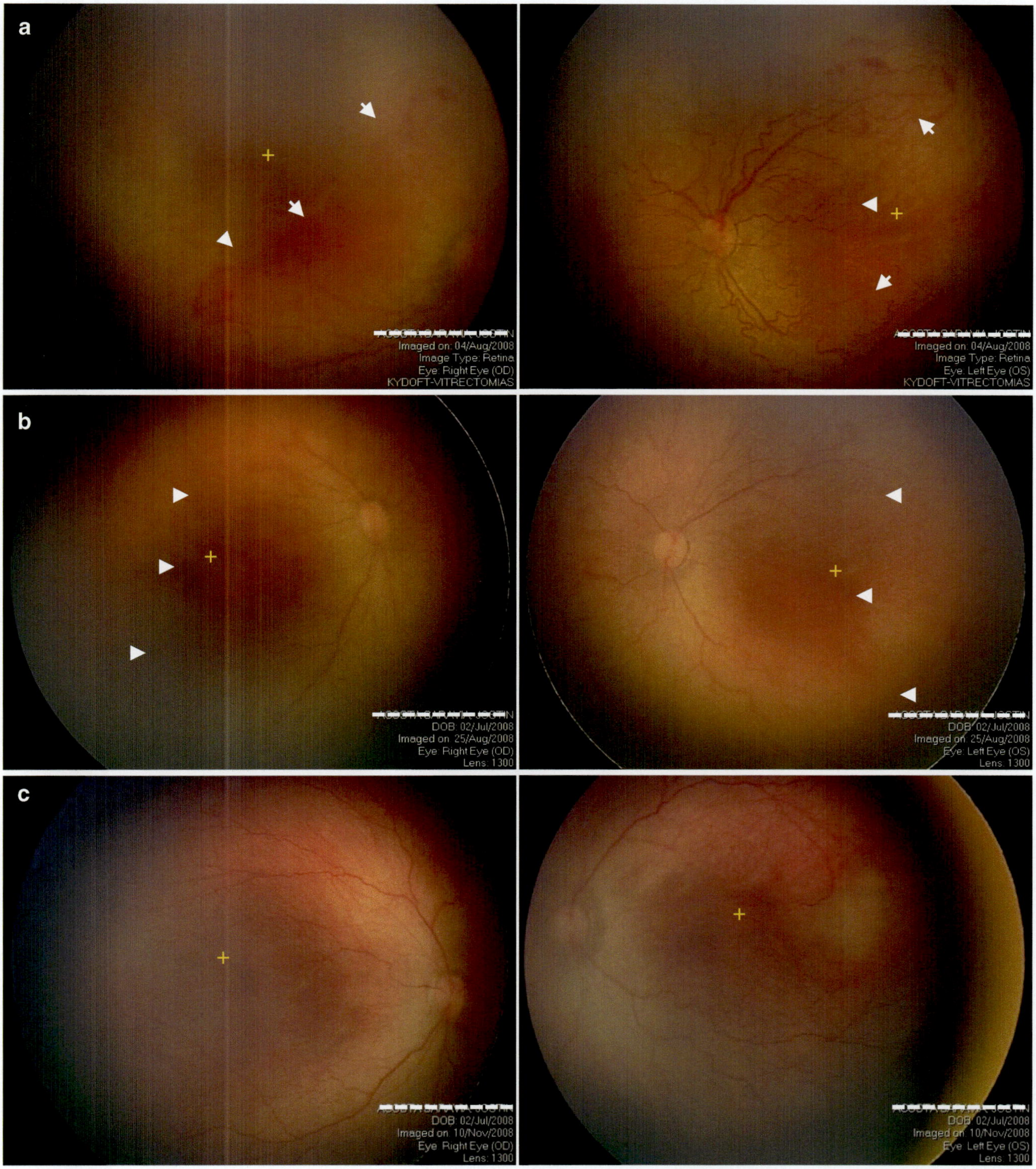

Fig. 12.2 Preterm infant born at 28 weeks with posterior Zone I ROP who developed type I ROP at 32 weeks post menstrual age (PMA), at which time he was treated with a single Avastin® injection. Note that retinal vascularization does not reach the macular area, white arrows (**a**). At 35 weeks PMA, there is no plus disease and retinal vessels are advancing (**b**), reaching zone III by week 46 (**c**)

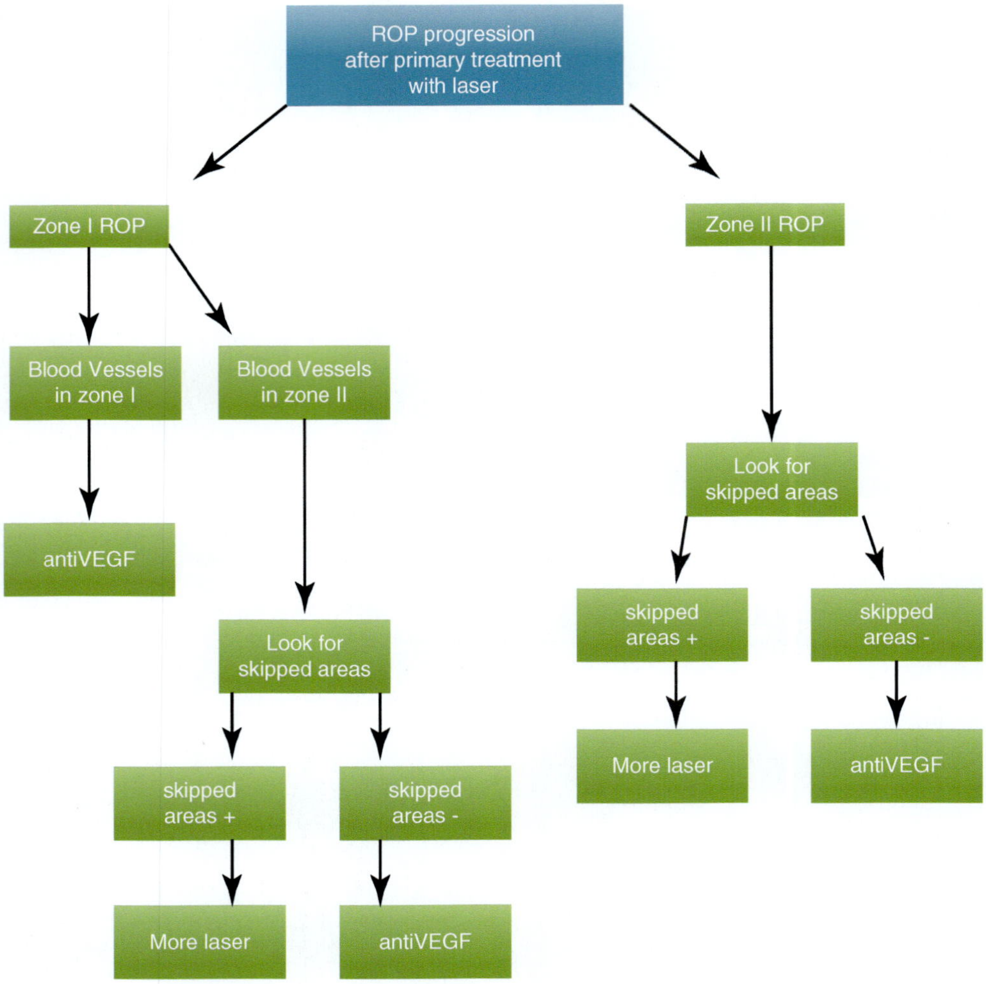

Fig. 12.3 Flowchart showing treatment alternatives for progressing ROP after primary treatment with laser

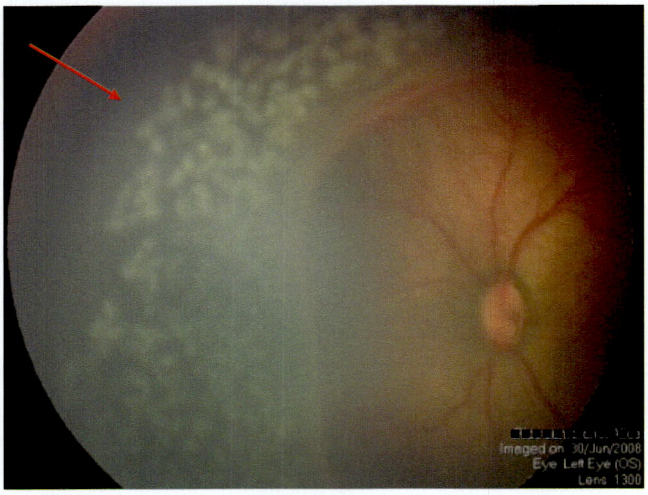

Fig. 12.4 Clinical picture of a case of type 1 ROP that progressed after primary treatment with laser due to incomplete photocoagulation, or "skipped areas," on the avascular retina

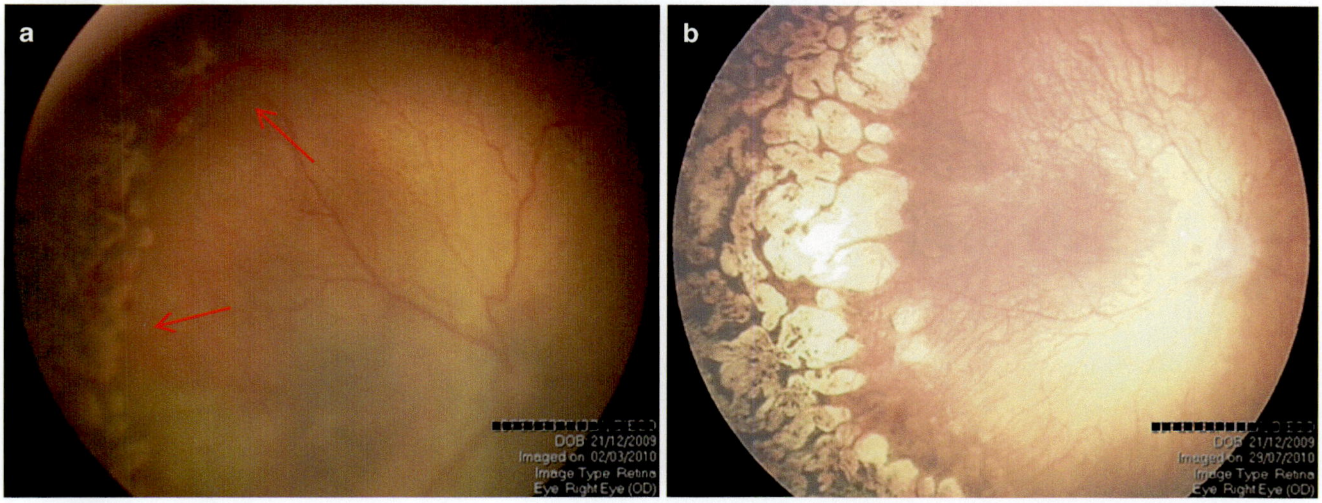

Fig. 12.5 Active neovascular tissue still present in a case adequately treated with laser (**a**). A complete regression of the ROP was obtained after injecting an anti-VEGF (**b**)

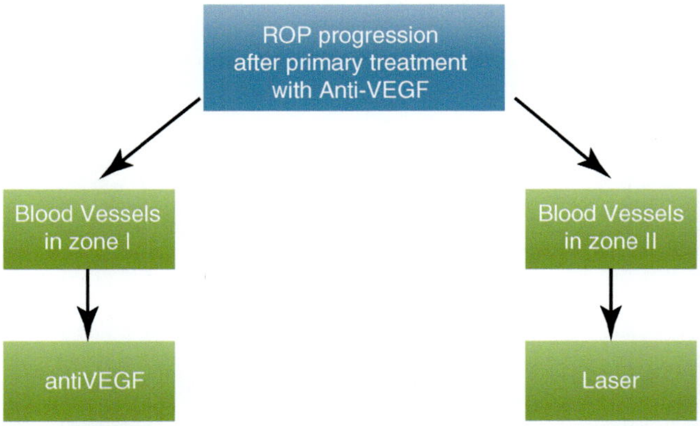

Fig. 12.6 Flowchart showing secondary treatments after primary management of ROP with an anti-VEGF drug

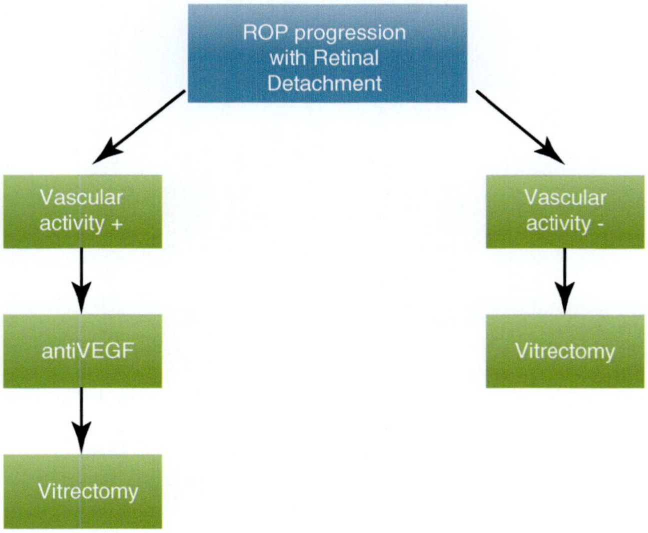

Fig. 12.7 Flowchart showing the management of ROP retinal detachment

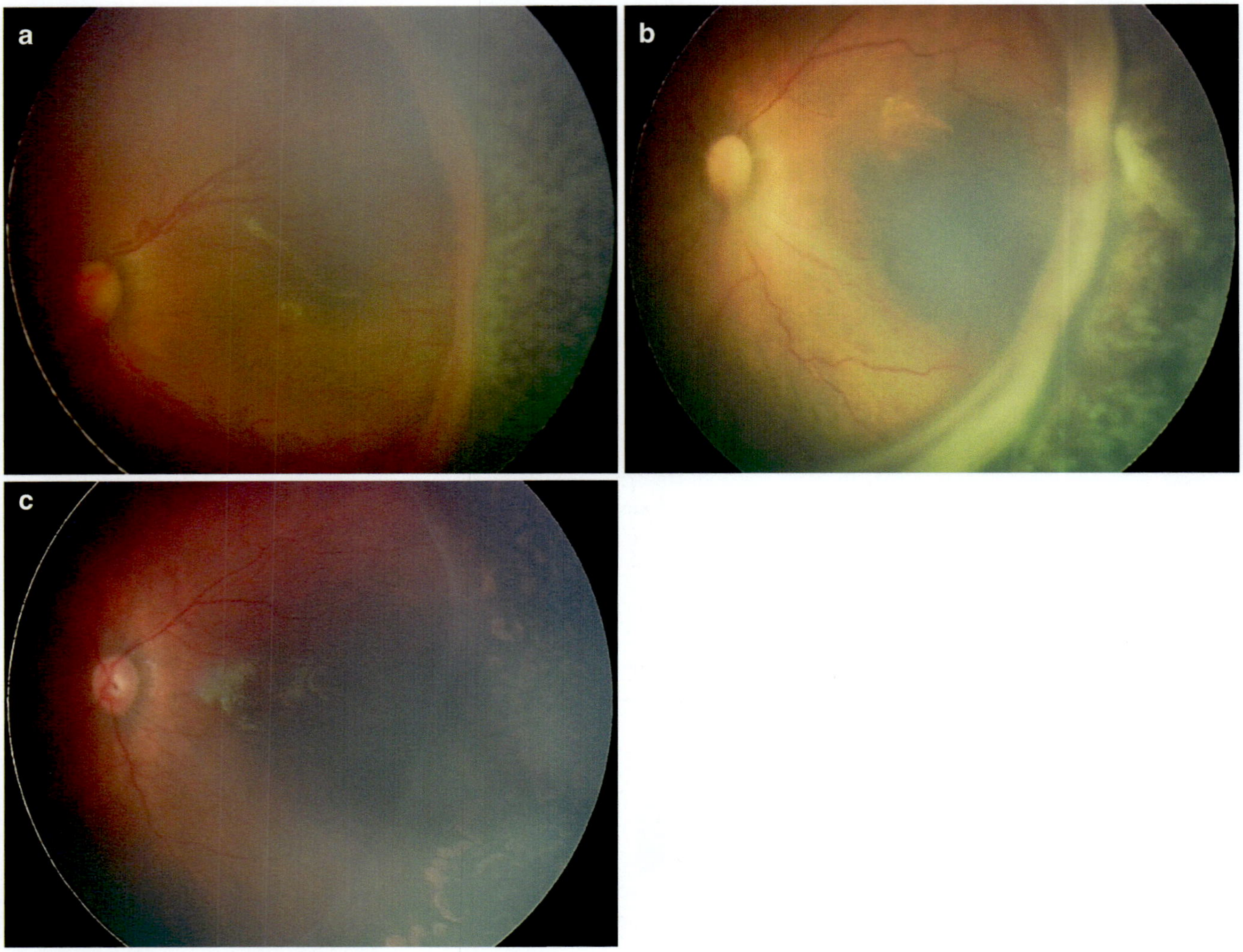

Fig. 12.8 (**a**) Stage 4A retinal detachment present at 37 weeks of gestational age in a preterm infant weighing 760 grams at 24 weeks. Due to the significant vascular activity present, an anti-VEGF drug was injected prior to surgery. (**b**) One week after the anti-VEGF injection, a marked reduction in vascular activity was observed. A 25-gauge lens-sparing vitrectomy was performed at that time. (**c**) Favorable anatomical outcome 9 weeks after surgery. (Permission obtained from Retinopathy of Prematurity, Current Diagnosis and Management; Andrés Kychenthal B., Paola Dorta S. Editors, Springer, 2017 [1])

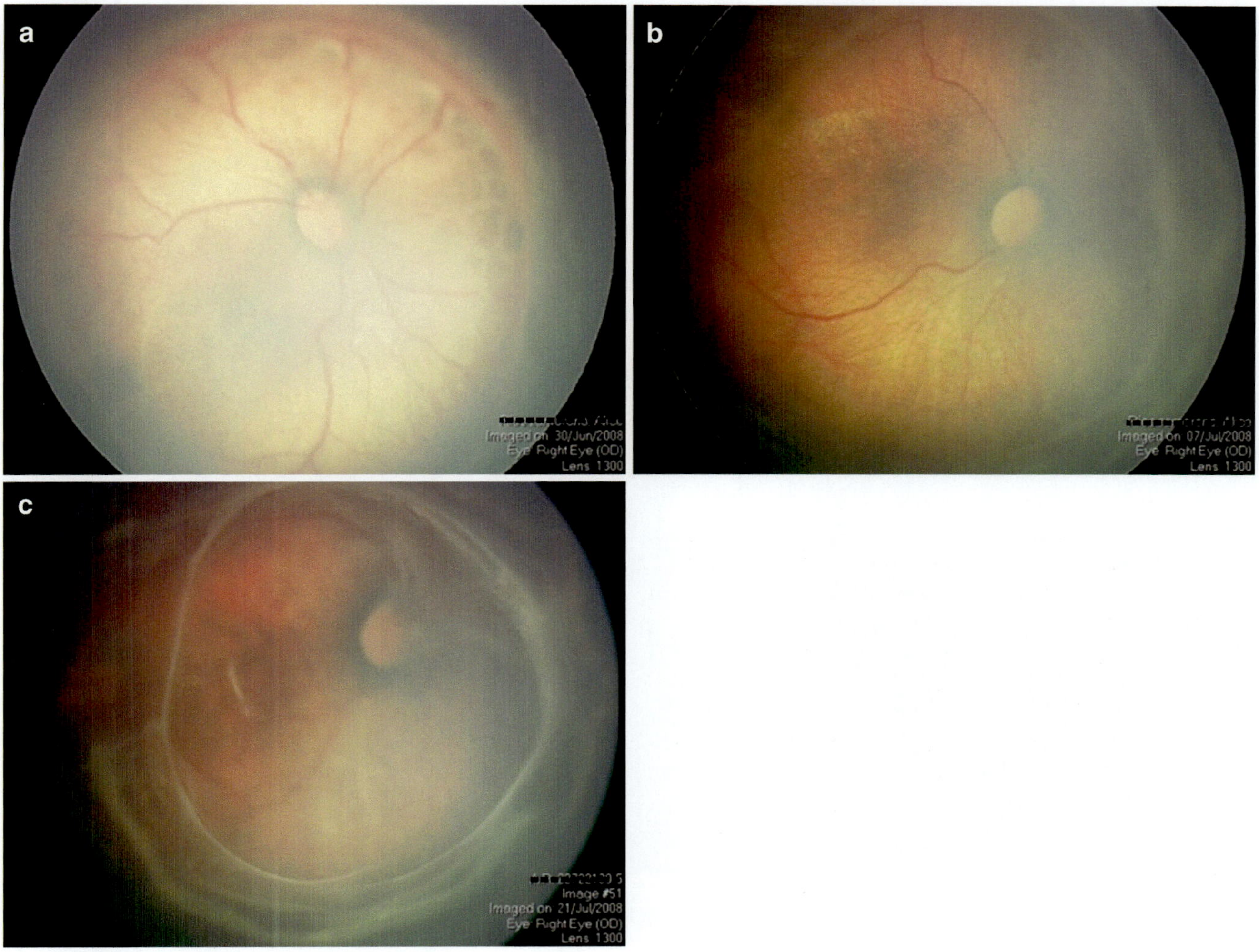

Fig. 12.9 Importance of timing vitreoretinal surgery after injecting an anti-VEGF as an adjunct prior to vitrectomy. Vascularly active ROP retinal detachment (**a**). Five to seven days post injection, there is regression of the vascular activity, signaling the best moment to perform surgery (**b**). After that time, fibrous conversion of the neovascular tissue might induce or promote the progression of the retinal detachment (**c**)

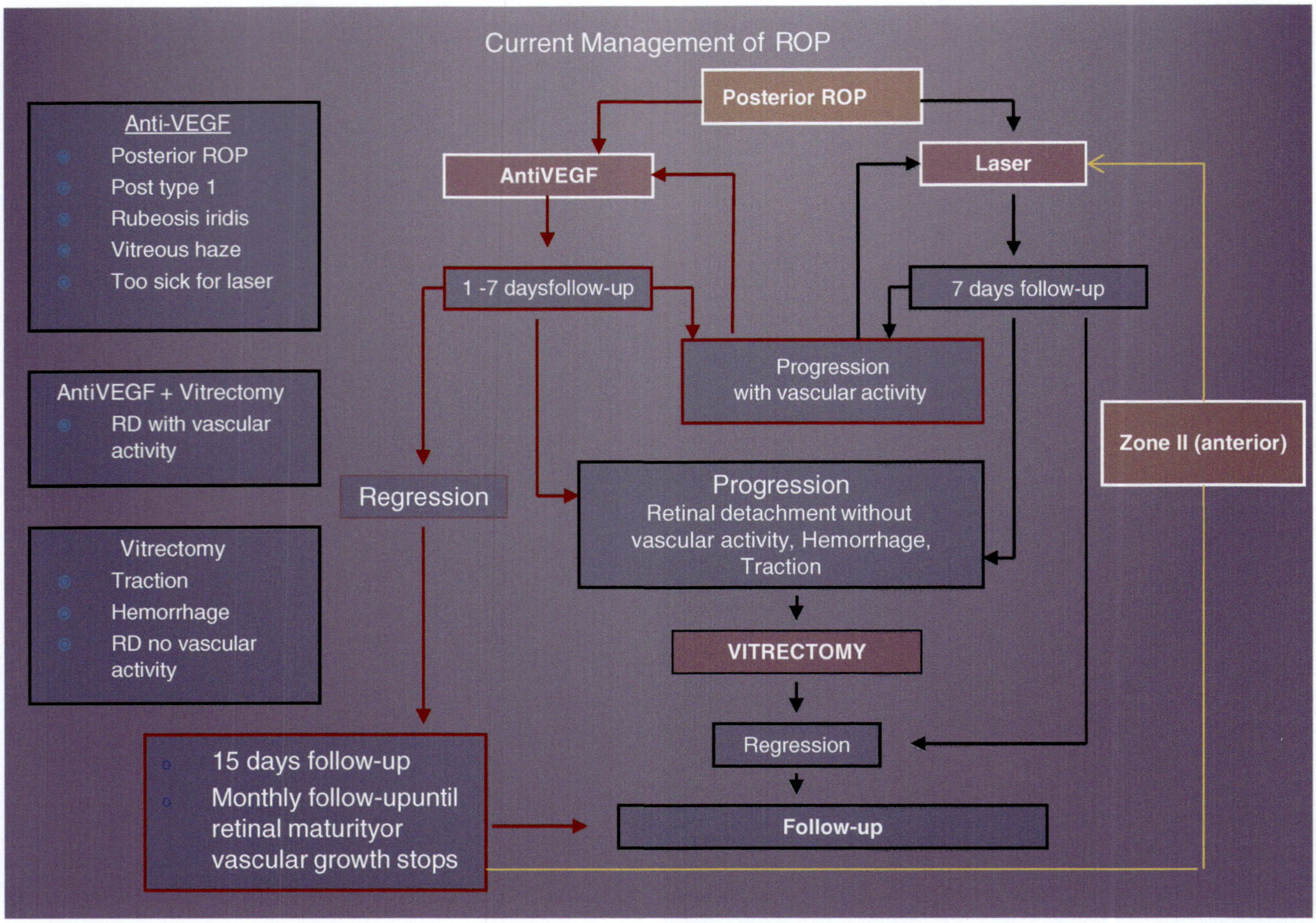

Fig. 12.10 The role of anti-VEGF drugs in the current management of ROP

Reference

1. Andres Kychenthal B, Paola Dorta S, editors. Retinopathy of prematurity, current diagnosis and management. Cham: Springer International Publishing AG; 2017. ISBN: 978-3-319-52188-6, ISBN 978-3-319-52190-9 (e-book)

Surgical Management of Stage 4 ROP

13

Eric Nudleman

Abstract

Although the vast majority of eyes with type 1 ROP successfully regress following treatment, some eyes develop fibrosis. This fibrosis typically occurs along the ridge tissue and can contract, causing traction and resulting in retinal detachment. Over the last 40 years, the surgical approach to repair stage 4 ROP associated retinal detachments have been refined. With an understanding of the vectors of traction, surgery for stage 4 ROP retinal detachments has a high success rate, often with excellent visual outcomes, especially when performed early in the disease process.

Keywords

Retinopathy of prematurity · Pathogenesis of ROP
Cicatricial ROP · Stage 4A ROP · Stage 4B ROP
Lens-sparing vitrectomy

13.1 Epidemiology of Advanced ROP

The incidence of blindness from ROP around the world is variable, largely depending on the level of development that allows for the survival of premature babies. In countries where the infant mortality rate is low and screening programs are established, the rate of blindness from ROP is approximately 10% [1]. In countries with high infant mortality rates, the rate of ROP-related blindness is extremely low, since children are unlikely to survive to the age when ROP develops. In "middle-income" nations, however, ROP is a major cause of childhood blindness, with rates approaching 40% [2]. This is largely due to the absence of screening programs and, although premature infants survive, there is a high rate of progression to stage 5 ROP. In contrast, in the United States, the incidence of any stage of ROP is estimated to be between 1 in 511 and 1 in 820 live births [3, 4]. Among them, roughly 10% require laser photocoagulation, and 0.5% require surgical intervention, the vast majority for stage 4 disease.

13.2 Pathogenesis

The peripheral retinal ischemia in the premature infant drives the expression of high levels of Vascular Endothelial Growth Factor (VEGF). As a result, apoptosis of the hyaloid vessels is delayed, which is clinically visible as persistent tunica vasculosis lentis and rubeosis iridis [5]. In addition, VEGF drives neovascular vessels to proliferate into the vitreous along the vascularized border. Subsequent activation of TGFß1 contributes to excessive scar formation [6–8]. This fibrous proliferation typically follows the aberrant neovascularization, growing along the ridge tissue and extending into the overlying vitreous. The vitreous sheets act as scaffolds for the extension of the fibrotic tissue. Subsequent contraction of the fibrous tissue occurs along various vectors, most commonly toward the center of the eye, as well as posterior toward the optic nerve or anterior toward the lens. Without intervention, the traction will completely detach the neurosensory retina, ultimately leading to blindness.

13.3 Clinical Course

The progression of ROP is relatively predictable. Infants that develop disease, in industrialized nations, are almost all born at <31 weeks gestational age with a birthweight of <1250 g. The earliest manifestations are usually seen at approximately 32 weeks postmenstrual age (PMA), with the conversion to treatment warranted (type 1) disease reached at a mean of 37 weeks PMA [9, 10]. Retinal detachment after appropriate treatment occurs at a mean of 41 weeks PMA [11]. Once the retina begins to detach, it can progress quickly. Within

E. Nudleman (✉)
Shiley Eye Institute, University of California, San Diego, CA, USA

W.-C. Wu, W.-C. Lam (eds.), *A Quick Guide to Pediatric Retina*, https://doi.org/10.1007/978-981-15-6552-6_13

weeks, the detachment can advance from an early Stage 4A to Stage 5, resulting in a far worse prognosis for visual recovery. Therefore, once surgery is determined necessary, earlier intervention is advisable to reduce the progression of the detachment.

A special consideration needs to be given to eyes treated with anti-VEGF therapy for type 1 ROP. Although multiple prospective studies have demonstrated short-term efficacy using these agents [12–14], late reactivation and progression to retinal detachment have been reported long after the traditional screening period. Some reports have identified retinal detachments up to several years following anti-VEGF injections [15–18]. There is increasing evidence that following anti-VEGF therapy, vascular development often remains incomplete, resulting in persistent avascular retina [19, 20]. One potential approach to mitigate the risk of reactivation is sequential therapy. That is, treatment with anti-VEGF to treat acute type 1 ROP, followed by laser to the persistent avascular retina at 50–60 weeks postmenstrual age. This approach has been investigated in one prospective study [21], with additional studies underway. With anti-VEGF therapy now highly prevalent worldwide as a primary therapy for type 1 ROP, strategies to reduce the risk of late detachments are actively being pursued.

13.4 Management

In order to maximize visual potential, the goal in ROP retinal detachment surgery is to normalize anatomy to permit visual development. Surgical success requires an understanding of the tractional vectors present in ROP. Interrupting the traction resulting from fibrous proliferation is the primary surgical goal in ROP detachments. Adequate release of traction can prevent progression, reduce dragging of the macula, and spare visual function. In general, surgical success and visual function is greatest when surgery is performed at the earliest stage of retinal detachment. For this reason, once the decision for surgery is made, it is recommended to proceed as quickly as possible. Successful reattachment has been reported in 74–91% of stage 4A detachments [22–25], 62–92% of stage 4B detachments [22, 24, 26–28], and 22–48% of stage 5 detachments [29–31]. Visual outcomes in successful repair of stage 4A detachment can be expected to be 20/80 or better [22, 32, 33], ambulatory vision following stage 4B repair [28], and form vision following stage 5 repair [34].

13.5 Lens-Sparing Vitrectomy

In general, outcomes are best in ROP surgery when the crystalline lens is retained. Therefore, as long as the anatomy permits adequate space, which is the case in most stage 4A and many stage 4B ROP detachments, a lens-sparing vitrectomy (LSV) is recommended. The surgery is initiated with a partial conjunctival peritomy, primarily to aid in suture closure of the sclerotomies at the conclusion of the case. Since infants have not developed a pars plana, the eye is entered at the pars plicata, approximately 0.5 mm posterior to the limbus (Fig. 13.1). Similar success rates have been reported using a two-port approach, using an infusing light pipe or pic, and three port-approach using a separate infusion line [22, 24]. Attention to the vector of trocar insertion is critical to avoid damage to the lens. The insertion of the trocar should be perpendicular to the iris plane, rather than pointed toward the center of the eye (Fig. 13.1). If using small gauge instruments (23G, 25G, or 27G), the cannula may be too long to allow access to the far periphery in order to segment the peripheral fibrosis. Therefore, it may be helpful to either insert the instruments directly through the sclerotomies or to partially withdraw the cannulas for peripheral maneuvers.

During the core vitrectomy, attention should be directed toward the vectors of traction. Specifically, an effort should be made to transect the transvitreal ridge to ridge tissue (the "drum head"), ridge to periphery, ridge to lens, and optic nerve head to the ridge (Figs. 13.2 and 13.3). Often, the release of traction will be evident with the relaxation of the

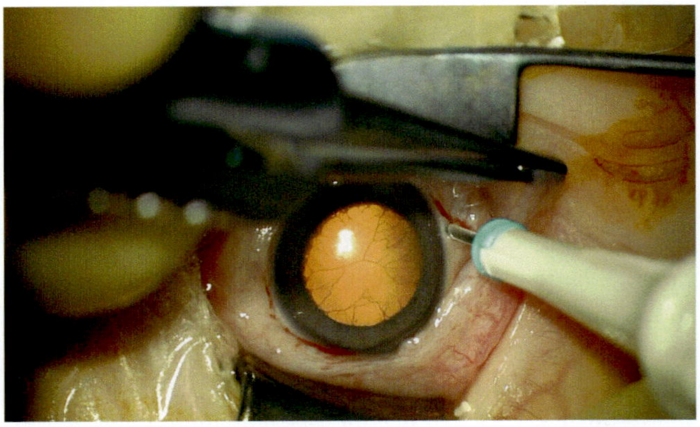

Fig. 13.1 Screen capture demonstrating the location and angle of the trocar insertion. Following a conjunctival peritomy, the trocar is inserted 0.5 mm posterior to the limbus with the angle parallel to the visual axis to avoid trauma to the crystalline lens. Note the persistence of the tunica vasculosis lentis, a common feature of ROP

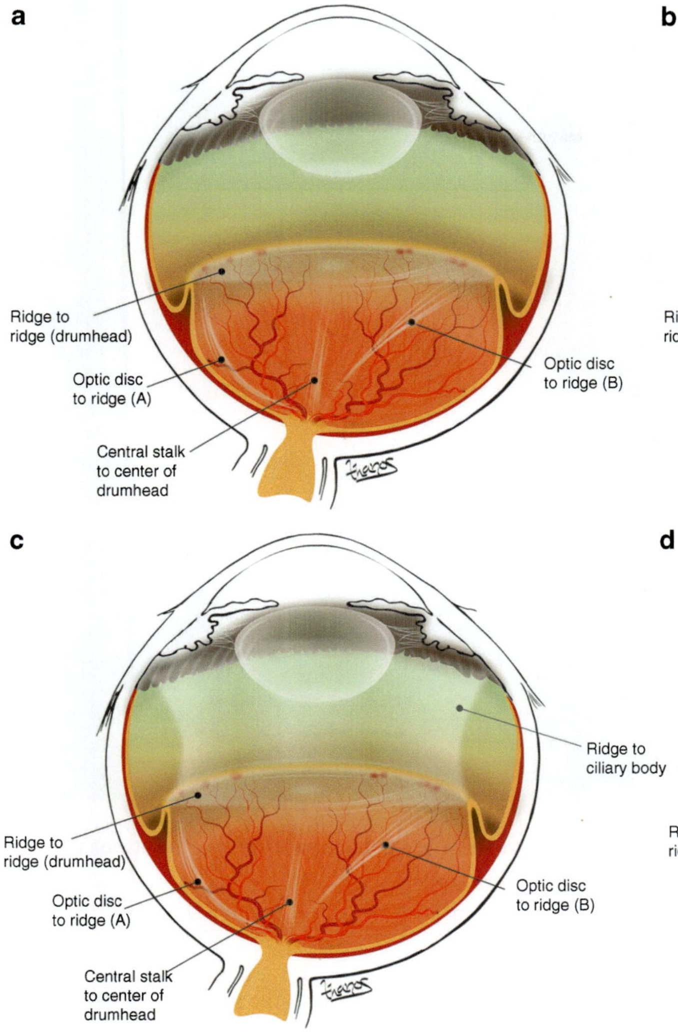

Fig. 13.2 Tractional vectors in ROP. The primary vectors include tissue extending from the optic disc to ridge, and ridge to ridge (**a**), ridge to eye wall (**b**), ridge to ciliary processes (**c**), and ridge to lens (**d**). Successful surgery requires that tractional forces from each of these vectors are adequately transected. Adapted from [35]

tented retina. The vitrector can be used as a pic by gently moving within the vectors of traction without cutting. This will allow the surgeon to see where the traction remains, since the underlying retina will react. These areas should then be addressed until the movement of the underlying retina no longer occurs. Once the dissection is complete, a partial fluid–air exchange is performed to prevent vitreous incarceration into the sclerotomies, and the sclerotomies are sutured. At the conclusion of the case, subretinal fluid is expected, and will reabsorb over the course of weeks to months (Fig. 13.4). During follow-up examinations, the key feature of success is the absence of progression.

In some cases, anterior ridge to ciliary body tissue may create a tight space that risks damage to the crystalline lens by a transvitreal approach. In such instances, an MVR blade can be used to cleave these anterior bands at the time of entry into the eye, an approach described as an *ab interno* incision [36]. The vectors of the initial incision must still be perpendicular to the iris to avoid the lens equator, but can then be turned parallel to the posterior lens capsule to transect the tissue. If the retina is pulled too anterior to safely access the fibrotic tissue bridging between the retina and the lens and ciliary body, then a lensectomy and anterior approach is recommended.

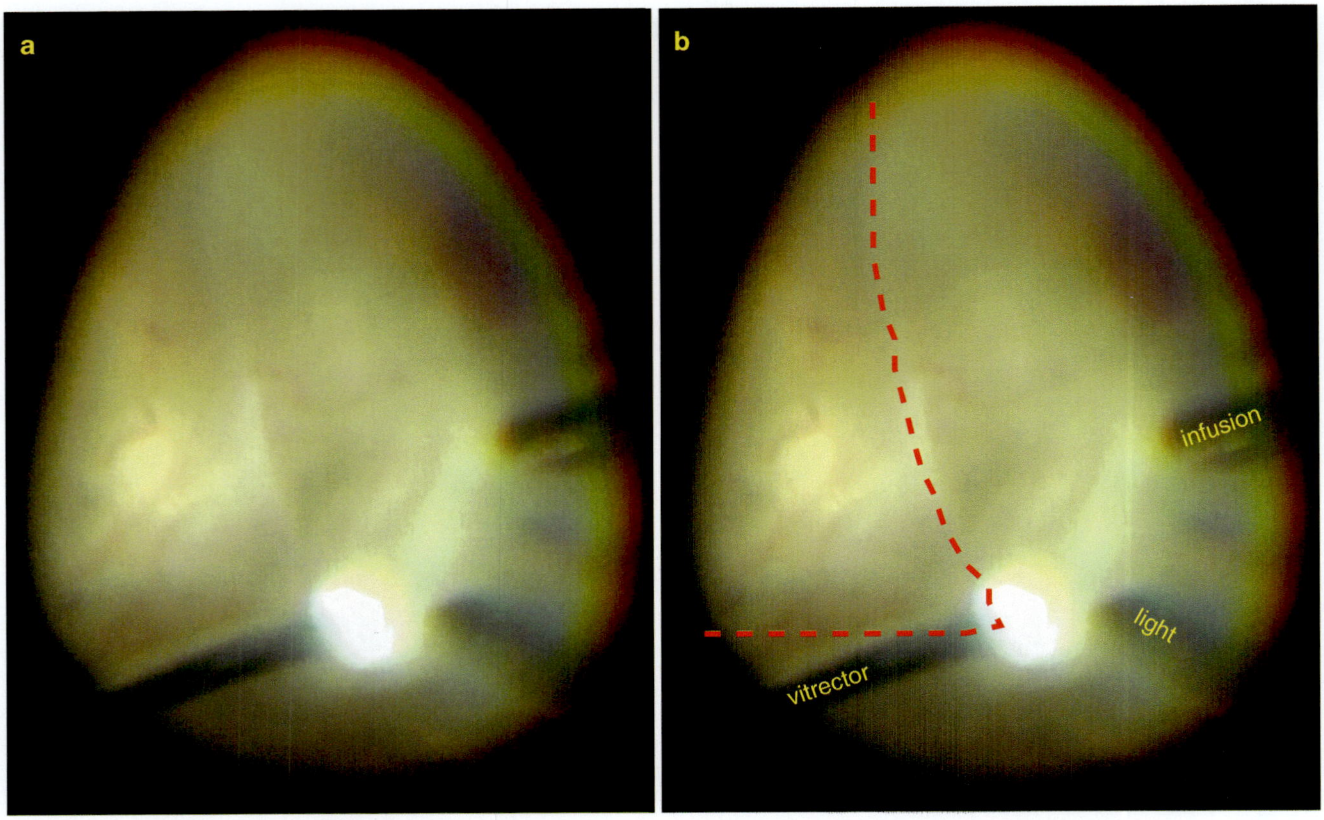

Fig. 13.3 Ridge to eye wall fibrosis. (**a**) Typical intraoperative appearance of ridge to eye wall fibrotic tissue undergoing segmentation using the vitrector. (**b**) Same image, outlining the fibrotic sheet, and the instruments within the eye

13.6 Limbal Approach for Lensectomy and Vitrectomy

Occasionally in Stage 4 ROP, due to anterior fibrosis or a limited view posterior to the lens, a lens-sparing surgery is not possible, necessitating an anterior (translimbal) approach to lensectomy and vitrectomy. In such cases, an inferotemporal or inferior infusion cannula is placed at the limbus, and limbal incisions are then made superonasally and superotemporally. The anterior lens capsule is incised using the trocar blade, and the crystalline lens nucleus and cortex are aspirated with the vitrector. Since the capsule can serve as a scaffold for subsequent fibrosis and traction, which can be very difficult to safely remove, it is recommended the capsule is entirely removed when a lensectomy is performed for ROP surgeries. The edges of the capsule can be easily visualized by externally illuminating through the cornea with the light pipe, and grasping the capsule edge using membrane forceps. Once the zonules are released, the capsule can be removed in a single sheet through the limbal incisions. Once the lens and capsule are removed, the anterior fibrosis can be safely accessed and dissected.

13.7 Minimal Intervention to Achieve Surgical Goals

The goal of Stage 4 ROP surgery is to relieve the vectors of traction. It must be emphasized that aggressive maneuvers during ROP surgery are extremely high risk and should be avoided. Creating an iatrogenic break carries a near certain consequence of massive fibrous proliferation with a devastating outcome. Although it may be tempting to shave close to the retinal surface while addressing fibrosis, such maneuvers are generally unnecessary to achieve surgical goals. In rare cases, a vitrectomy in a child without removing the posterior hyaloid can lead to posterior hyaloid contraction syndrome [37]. Nevertheless, to avoid the risk of iatrogenic breaks, routine removal of the adherent vitreous cortex is not recommended during ROP surgery.

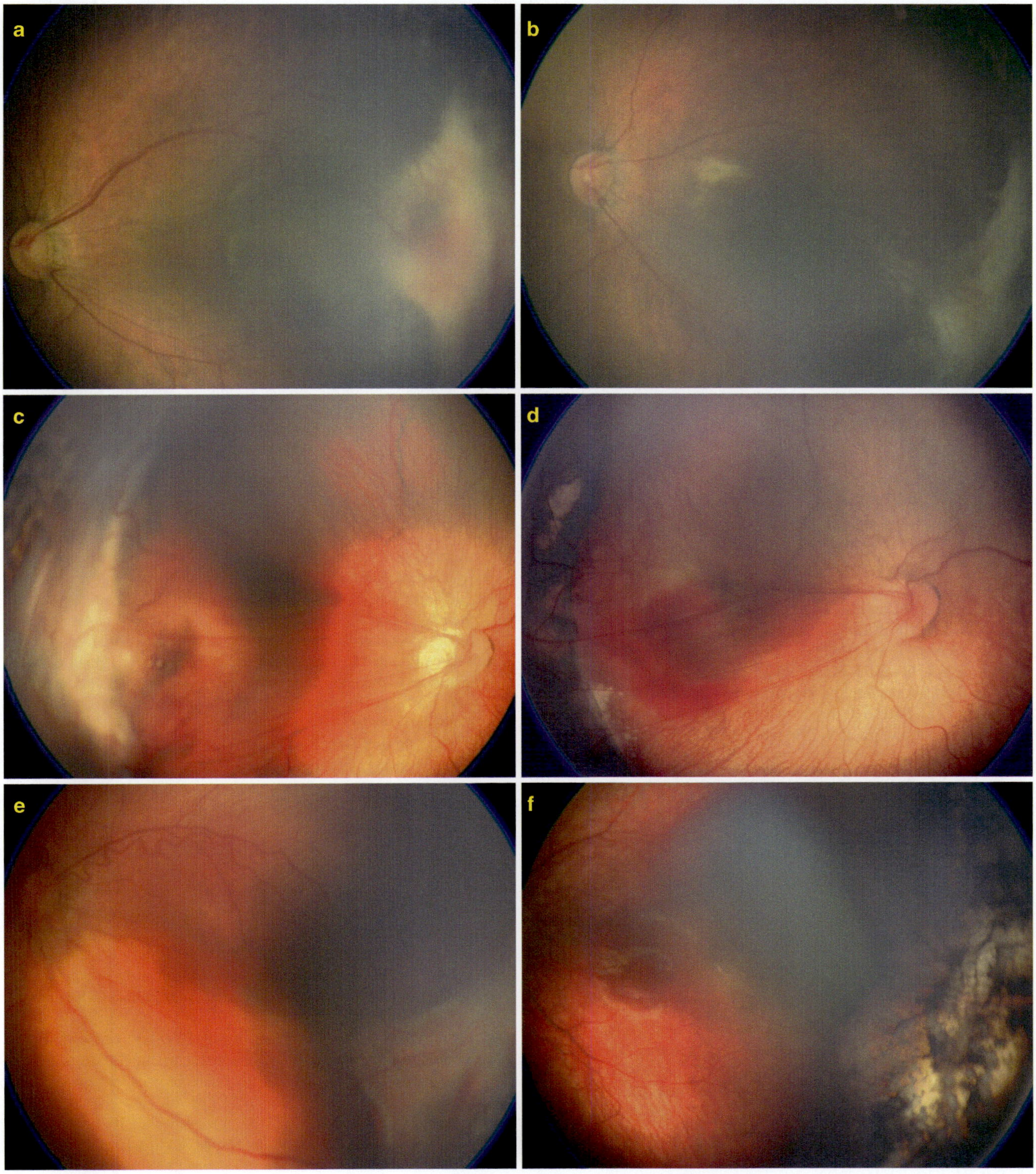

Fig. 13.4 Resolution of subretinal fluid following LSV for Stage 4 ROP at various time intervals. (**a**) Preoperative appearance of Stage 4A ROP. (**b**) Postoperative appearance of the same eye 2 weeks following LSV. The turbid subretinal fluid is improved, but not yet resolved. (**c**) Preoperative appearance of stage 4B ROP, with circumferential traction and subretinal fluid involving the fovea. (**d**) Postoperative appearance 5 weeks following LSV, showing near-complete resolution of subretinal fluid with residual subretinal hemorrhage and temporal dragging. (**e**) Preoperative appearance of Stage 4A ROP. (**f**) Postoperative appearance 10 weeks following LSV showing complete resolution of subretinal fluid

References

1. Gilbert C. Retinopathy of prematurity: a global perspective of the epidemics, population of babies at risk and implications for control. Early Hum Dev. 2008 Feb;84(2):77–82.
2. Gilbert C, Rahi J, Eckstein M, O'Sullivan J, Foster A. Retinopathy of prematurity in middle-income countries. Lancet. 1997 Jul 5;350(9070):12–4.
3. Chiang MF, Arons RR, Flynn JT, Starren JB. Incidence of retinopathy of prematurity from 1996 to 2000: analysis of a comprehensive New York state patient database. Ophthalmology. 2004 Jul;111(7):1317–25.
4. Lad EM, Nguyen TC, Morton JM, Moshfeghi DM. Retinopathy of prematurity in the United States. Br J Ophthalmol. 2008 Feb 26;92(3):320–5.
5. Alon T, Hemo I, Itin A, Pe'er J, Stone J, Keshet E. Vascular endothelial growth factor acts as a survival factor for newly formed retinal vessels and has implications for retinopathy of prematurity. Nat Med. 1995 Oct 1;1(10):1024–8.
6. Flaumenhaft R, Abe M, Mignatti P, Rifkin DB. Basic fibroblast growth factor-induced activation of latent transforming growth factor beta in endothelial cells: regulation of plasminogen activator activity. J Cell Biol. 1992 Aug;118(4):901–9.
7. Sato Y, Rifkin DB. Inhibition of endothelial cell movement by pericytes and smooth muscle cells: activation of a latent transforming growth factor-beta 1-like molecule by plasmin during co-culture. J Cell Biol. 1989 Jul;109(1):309–15.
8. Mandriota SJ, Menoud PA, Pepper MS. Transforming growth factor beta 1 down-regulates vascular endothelial growth factor receptor 2/flk-1 expression in vascular endothelial cells. J Biol Chem. 1996 May 10;271(19):11500.
9. Palmer EA, Flynn JT, Hardy RJ, Phelps DL, Phillips CL, Schaffer DB, The Cryotherapy for Retinopathy of Prematurity Cooperative Group, et al. Incidence and early course of retinopathy of prematurity. Ophthalmology. 1991 Nov;98(11):1628–40.
10. Schaffer DB, Palmer EA, Plotsky DF, Metz HS, Flynn JT, Tung B, The Cryotherapy for Retinopathy of Prematurity Cooperative Group, et al. Prognostic factors in the natural course of retinopathy of prematurity. Ophthalmology. 1993 Feb;100(2):230.
11. Repka MX, Tung B, Good WV, Capone A, Shapiro MJ. Outcome of eyes developing retinal detachment during the early treatment for retinopathy of prematurity study. Arch Ophthalmol. 2011 Sep 12;129(9):1175–9.
12. Mintz-Hittner HA, Kennedy KA, Chuang AZ, BEAT-ROP Cooperative Group. Efficacy of intravitreal bevacizumab for stage 3+ retinopathy of prematurity. N Engl J Med. 2011 Feb 17;364(7):603–15.
13. Stahl A, Krohne TU, Eter N, Oberacher-Velten I, Guthoff R, Meltendorf S, et al. Comparing alternative ranibizumab dosages for safety and efficacy in retinopathy of prematurity: a randomized clinical trial. JAMA Pediatr. 2018 Mar 1;172(3):278–86.
14. Wallace DK, Kraker RT, Freedman SF, Crouch ER, Hutchinson AK, Bhatt AR, et al. Assessment of lower doses of intravitreous bevacizumab for retinopathy of prematurity: a phase 1 dosing study. JAMA Ophthalmol. 2017 Jun 1;135(6):654–6.
15. Lee BJ, Kim JH, Heo H, Yu YS. Delayed onset atypical vitreoretinal traction band formation after an intravitreal injection of bevacizumab in stage 3 retinopathy of prematurity. Eye (Lond). 2012 Jul 1;26(7):903–10.
16. Ittiara S, Blair MP, Shapiro MJ, Lichtenstein SJ. Exudative retinopathy and detachment: a late reactivation of retinopathy of prematurity after intravitreal bevacizumab. J AAPOS. 2013 Jun;17(3):323–5.
17. Snyder LL, Garcia-Gonzalez JM, Shapiro MJ, Blair MP. Very late reactivation of retinopathy of prematurity after monotherapy with intravitreal bevacizumab. Ophthalmic Surg Lasers Imaging Retina. 2016 Mar;47(3):280–3.
18. Hajrasouliha AR, Garcia-Gonzales JM, Shapiro MJ, Yoon H, Blair MP. Reactivation of retinopathy of prematurity three years after treatment with bevacizumab. Ophthalmic Surg Lasers Imaging Retina. 2017 Mar 1;48(3):255–9.
19. Lepore D, Quinn GE, Molle F, Baldascino A, Orazi L, Sammartino M, et al. Intravitreal bevacizumab versus laser treatment in Type 1 retinopathy of prematurity: report on fluorescein angiographic findings. Ophthalmology. 2014 Jul 4;121(11):2212–9.
20. Toy BC, Schachar IH, Tan GSW, Moshfeghi DM. Chronic vascular arrest as a predictor of bevacizumab treatment failure in retinopathy of prematurity. Ophthalmology. 2016 Oct;123(10):2166–75.
21. Yoon JM, Shin DH, Kim SJ, Ham D-I, Kang SW, Chang YS, et al. Outcomes after laser versus combined laser and bevacizumab treatment for type 1 retinopathy of prematurity in Zone I. Retina (Philadelphia, PA). 2017 Jan;37(1):88–96.
22. Hubbard GB, Cherwick DH, Burian G. Lens-sparing vitrectomy for stage 4 retinopathy of prematurity. Ophthalmology. 2004 Dec;111(12):2274–7.
23. Moshfeghi AA, Awner S, Salam GA, Ferrone PJ. Excellent visual outcome and reversal of dragging after lens sparing vitrectomy for progressive tractional stage 4a retinopathy of prematurity retinal detachment. Retina (Philadelphia, PA). 2004 Aug;24(4):615–6.
24. Lakhanpal RR, Sun RL, Albini TA, Holz ER. Anatomic success rate after 3-port lens-sparing vitrectomy in stage 4A or 4B retinopathy of prematurity. Ophthalmology. 2005 Sep;112(9):1569–73.
25. Bhende P, Gopal L, Sharma T, Verma A, Biswas RK. Functional and anatomical outcomes after primary lens-sparing pars plana vitrectomy for Stage 4 retinopathy of prematurity. Indian J Ophthalmol. 2009 Jul;57(4):267–71.
26. Singh R, Reddy DM, Barkmeier AJ, Holz ER, Ram R, Carvounis PE. Long-term visual outcomes following lens-sparing vitrectomy for retinopathy of prematurity. Br J Ophthalmol. 2012 Nov;96(11):1395–8.
27. Choi J, Kim JH, Kim S-J, Yu YS. Long-term results of lens-sparing vitrectomy for stages 4B and 5 retinopathy of prematurity. Korean J Ophthalmol. 2011 Oct;25(5):305–10.
28. Rayes El EN, Vinekar A, Capone A. Three-year anatomic and visual outcomes after vitrectomy for stage 4B retinopathy of prematurity. Retina (Philadelphia, PA). 2008 Apr;28(4):568–72.
29. Gopal L, Sharma T, Shanmugam M, Badrinath SS, Sharma A, Agraharam SG, et al. Surgery for stage 5 retinopathy of prematurity: the learning curve and evolving technique. Indian J Ophthalmol. 2000 Jun;48(2):101–6.
30. Lakhanpal RR, Fortun JA, Chan-Kai B, Holz ER. Lensectomy and vitrectomy with and without intravitreal triamcinolone acetonide for vascularly active stage 5 retinal detachments in retinopathy of prematurity. Retina. 2006 Sep;26(7):736–40.
31. Cusick M, Charles MK, AGR N E, Sangiovanni JP, Ferris FL III, Charles S. Anatomical and visual results of vitreoretinal surgery for stage 5 retinopathy of prematurity. Retina. 2006 Sep;26(7):729–35.
32. Prenner JL, Capone A, Trese MT. Visual outcomes after lens-sparing vitrectomy for stage 4A retinopathy of prematurity. Ophthalmology. 2004 Dec;111(12):2271–3.
33. Lakhanpal RR, Sun RL, Albini TA, Coffee R, Coats DK, Holz ER. Visual outcomes after 3-port lens-sparing vitrectomy in

stage 4 retinopathy of prematurity. Arch Ophthalmol. 2006 May;124(5):675–9.
34. Trese MT, Droste PJ. Long-term postoperative results of a consecutive series of stages 4 and 5 retinopathy of prematurity. Ophthalmology. 1998 Jun;105(6):992–7.
35. Thanos A, Drenser KA, Capone A. Retinopathy of prematurity. In: Yanoff M, Duker JS, editors. Ophthalmology, vol. 1. New York: Mosby; 2018. p. 542.
36. Ho LY, Ranchod TM, Drenser KA, Capone A, Trese MT. Ab interno incision for pediatric vitreoretinal surgery. Retina (Philadelphia, PA). 2010 Oct;30(9):1542–3.
37. Joshi MM, Ciaccia S, Trese MT, Capone A Jr. Posterior hyaloid contracture in pediatric vitreoretinopathies. Retina. 2006 Sep;26(Supplement):S38–41.

14 Surgical Management of Stage 5 Retinopathy of Prematurity

Shunji Kusaka

Abstract

Retinopathy of prematurity (ROP) is a leading cause of childhood blindness worldwide. Proper eye screening and interventions, such as laser ablation and/or anti-vascular endothelial growth factor therapy, are useful in reducing disease activity and preventing blindness. Some eyes are refractory to these treatments and develop tractional retinal detachment, which requires vitrectomy. Vitrectomy for stage 5 ROP is beneficial in preventing total blindness in some eyes; however, its anatomical and functional results are unsatisfactory.

Keywords

Retinopathy of prematurity · Vitrectomy · Lensectomy
Lens-sparing vitrectomy · Retinal detachment · Stage 5

14.1 Introduction

With the introduction of laser ablation therapy, the prognosis of retinopathy of prematurity (ROP) has significantly improved. Since more than a decade ago, the indication for laser ablation has been changed from threshold retinopathy to prethreshold retinopathy, leading to a decrease in the rate of unfavorable functional outcomes from 19.5% to 14.5% and structural outcomes from 15.6% to 9.1% [1]. However, using laser ablation alone, approximately 10% of patients still present with severe vision loss due to the development of retinal folds, retinal detachment, or retrolental fibroplasia [1].

More recently, anti-vascular endothelial growth factor (VEGF) therapy, which comprises intravitreal injection of an anti-VEGF agent as an off-label treatment, has been introduced [2–4] because VEGF may play a major role in the pathogenesis of ROP [5–7]. Anti-VEGF therapy is effective in reducing disease activity and is likely to lead to better ROP treatment outcomes particularly in severe ROP cases, such as zone 1 plus ROP or aggressive posterior ROP [4]. The number of eyes with ROP that progresses from stage 4 to 5 seems to be decreasing using anti-VEGF therapy. In addition, recent improvements in neonatal care have helped decrease ROP in patients, particularly in advanced countries. However, some patients still require vitrectomy for tractional retinal detachment (TRD) even after laser ablation and/or anti-VEGF therapy; the reasons may include improper screening or treatment. Sometimes, despite proper treatment, the patients' condition progresses to TRD due to excessive prematurity. Therefore, surgical treatment for ROP is still required, particularly in developing countries.

14.2 Stage 5 ROP

Fibrovascular membranes develop along the ridge and grow into various directions, including the ridge to the lens, the ridge to the ciliary body, the ridge to the peripheral retina, the ridge to the ridge (circumferential), and the ridge to the posterior retina. In eyes with stage 5 ROP, the retina is totally detached in a complex manner due to these traction forces. The surgical treatment releases these tractions as much as possible, most likely not completely, without creating an iatrogenic retinal break. Because surgery for stage 5 ROP remains extremely challenging and the anatomical and functional results are generally disappointing, surgical treatment should be considered not for stage 5 but for stage 4A ROP (partial retinal detachment without involvement of the macula).

The author has no proprietary interest in any of the products described in this chapter.

S. Kusaka (✉)
Department of Ophthalmology, Kindai University Faculty of Medicine, Osaka, Japan
e-mail: kusaka-ns@umin.net

W.-C. Wu, W.-C. Lam (eds.), *A Quick Guide to Pediatric Retina*, https://doi.org/10.1007/978-981-15-6552-6_14

14.3 Surgical Technique

Scleral buckling alone has been attempted for stage 5 ROP as it is safer than vitrectomy. However, complex retinal detachment caused by various traction forces cannot be effectively alleviated enough to reattach the retina in several cases [8, 9]. Meanwhile, vitrectomy can help effectively relieve the forces by directly cutting the fibrous membranes. In most eyes with stage 5 ROP, lensectomy is required to approach the retrolental fibrous membranes. The locations where surgical entry would be made should be carefully determined preoperatively. If the retrolental fibrous membranes are located adjacent to the ciliary body, the surgical entry should be made at the limbus to avoid an iatrogenic retinal break or ora dialysis. If there is a space between the ciliary body and the membranes, sclerotomies may be made 0.5–1 mm from the limbus, which allows for better visibility and easier manipulation during vitrectomy. In addition, a mixture of limbal (for infusion) and pars plicata (for other two ports) incisions can be used depending on the space between the ciliary body and the membranes. Lensectomy should be meticulously performed and should include the entire lens capsule because its remnants can adhere to the iris and/or remaining retrolental membrane after surgery. If the anterior chamber is shallow and the iris cannot be dilated due to posterior synechiae (Fig. 14.1), which is caused by the anterior displacement of the lens due to contraction of the retrolental fibrous membrane, viscoelastic material can be injected through the limbal wound to provide some space for an infusion cannula and a vitreous cutter. Then, a vitreous cutter is used to remove the lens and the iris of the pupillary margin (Figs. 14.2 and 14.3). Alternatively, instruments that can dilate the iris, such as an iris retractor, can be used.

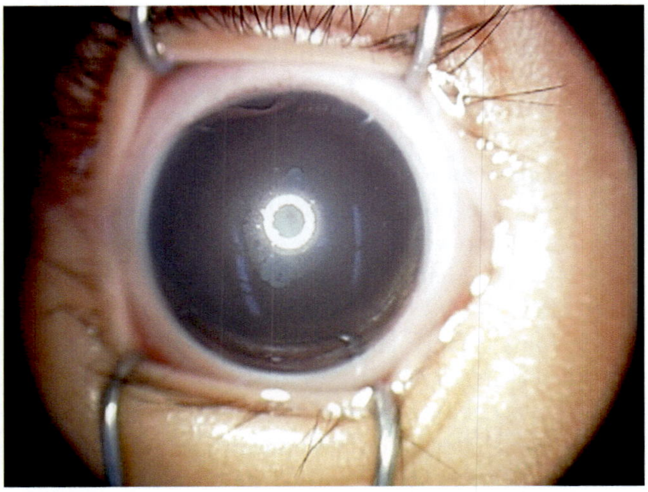

Fig. 14.1 Preoperative image of an eye with stage 5 retinopathy of prematurity. A shallow anterior chamber with posterior synechiae and peripheral anterior synechiae was observed

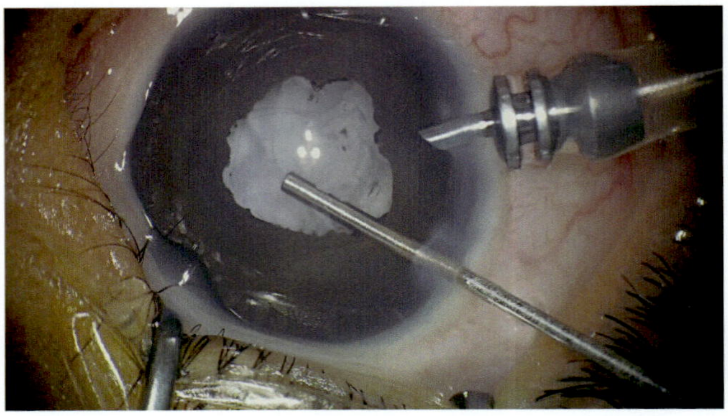

Fig. 14.2 Pupillary margin of the iris was dissected using a 25-gauge cutter

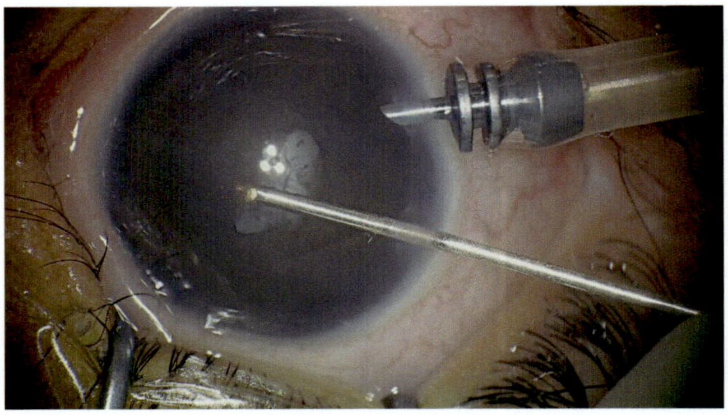

Fig. 14.3 Lensectomy was performed using a 25-gauge cutter

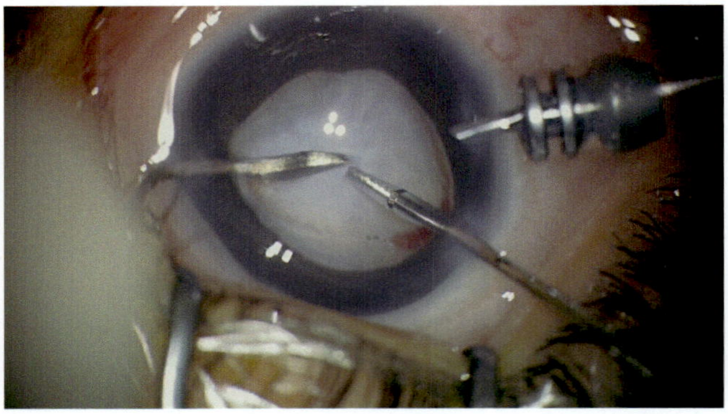

Fig. 14.4 Using a V-lance and forceps, the center of the retrolental fibrous membrane was dissected

After lens removal, dissection of the retrolental fibrous membranes is initiated from the center either using scissors or a sharp knife, such as the V-lance (Fig. 14.4). Separation of the membranes from the detached retina should be cautiously performed taking care to avoid any iatrogenic breaks. It is usually performed using forceps and scissors or a spatula with the bimanual technique (Fig. 14.5). Dissection can be extended peripherally in concentric and/or circumferential manners (Figs 14.6, 14.7, 14.8, 14.9, 14.10, and 14.11). To increase the chance of retinal reattachment (Fig. 14.12), the membranes should be removed as much as possible.

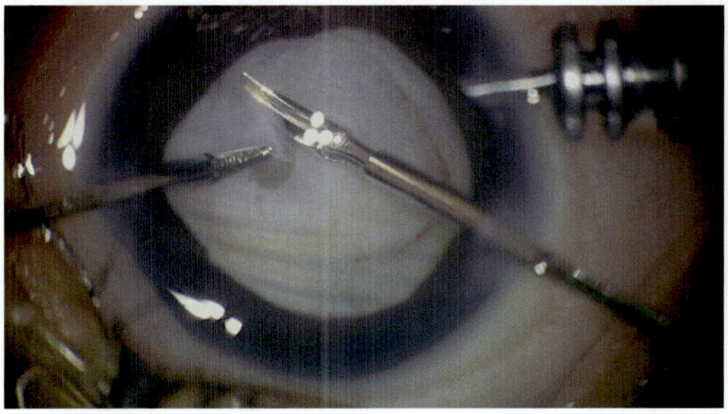

Fig. 14.5 Dissection of the membranes was extended peripherally using forceps and scissors

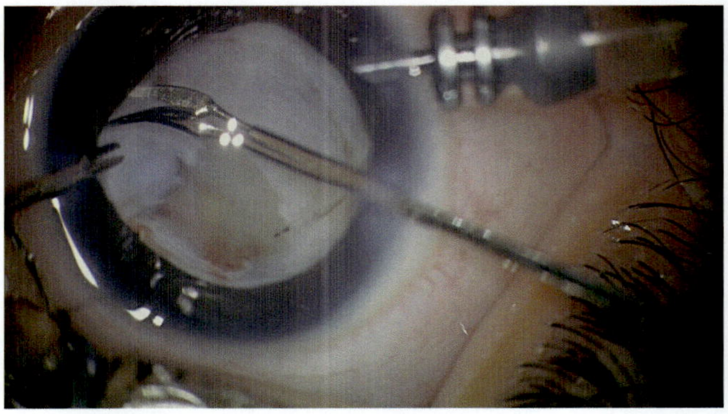

Fig. 14.6 Dissection of the membranes was extended in a circumferential manner

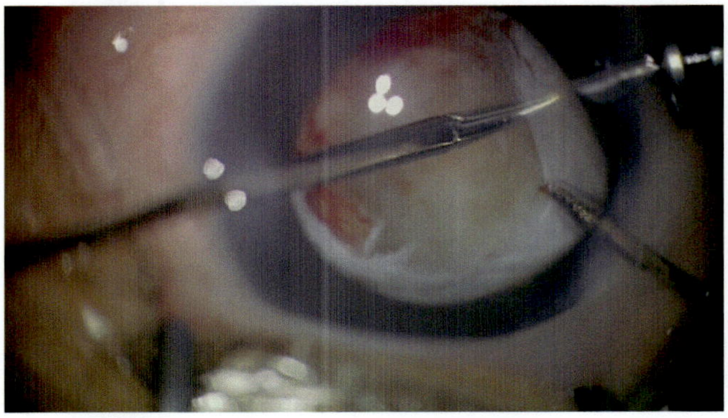

Fig. 14.7 Further dissection of the membranes

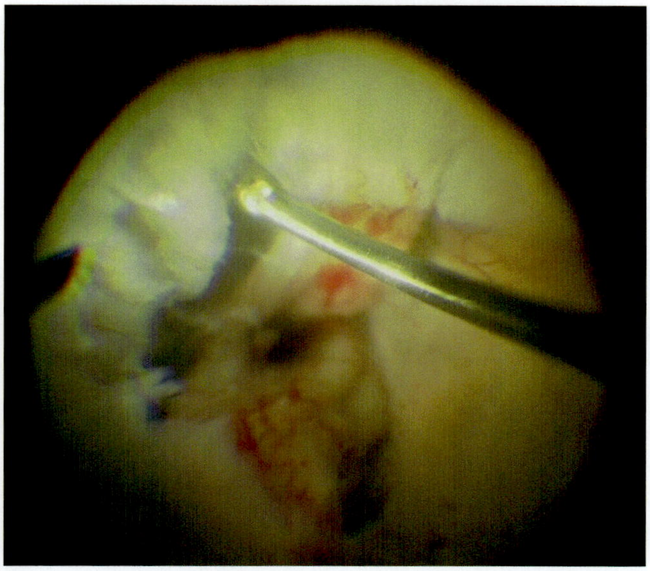

Fig. 14.8 After membrane dissection in the anterior part of the eye, further membrane dissection in the posterior part was conducted using a vitreous cutter under a wide-angle viewing system. Retinal detachment in complex figuration was observed

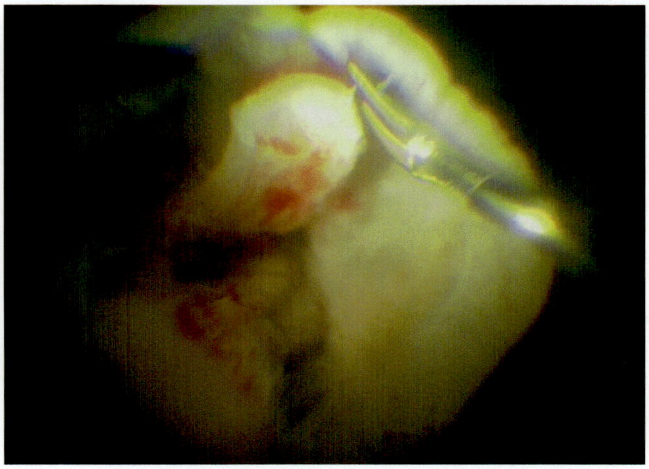

Fig. 14.9 Further membrane dissection in the posterior part was conducted using scissors under a wide-angle viewing system

Opening of the trough in the peripheral retina is critical; however, it is sometimes challenging and dangerous as a distinction between the thin membrane and avascular retina is often difficult. To avoid dialysis, caution must be taken to avoid pulling of the membranes too far in the peripheral region. The presence of a retinal break is highly associated with surgical failure in stage 5 ROP surgery. If most membranes can be removed, the retina is gradually reattached within several weeks. Otherwise, reoperation to remove residual membranes should be considered. Use of perfluoro-

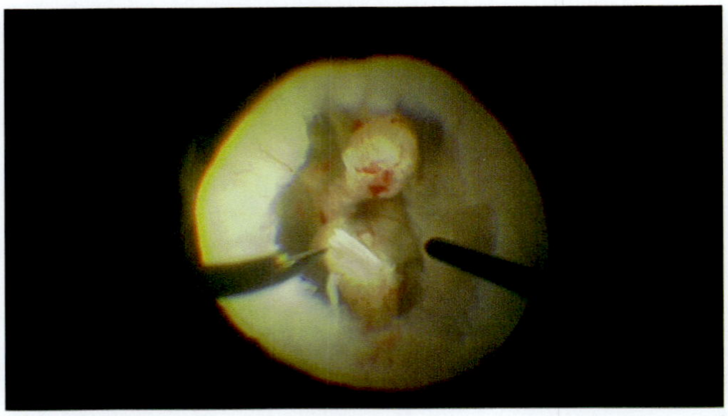

Fig. 14.10 After completion of membrane dissection. Some remaining membranes were observed. Complete removal of the membranes was not required for reattachment

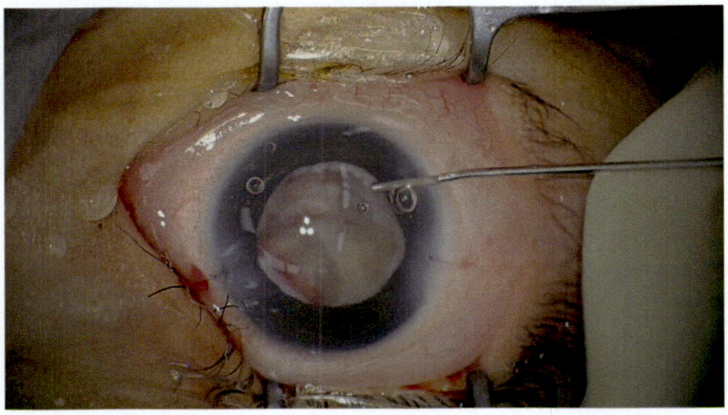

Fig. 14.11 Viscoelastic material is injected in the vitreous cavity to prevent adhesion of the retina. Postoperative high intraocular pressure will not occur in most cases. Every wound was securely sutured using 10-0 Vicryl in this case

carbon liquid as a short-term tamponade may be effective in such cases [9].

14.4 Surgical Results

Surgical results of vitrectomy for stage 5 ROP are generally unsatisfactory. In a clinical trial conducted in the USA [10], at least a portion of the retina was reattached in 11 (21%) of 52 eyes, and visual acuity was limited to light perception or no light perception in all but one eye after vitrectomy for stage 5 ROP at 5.5 years of age. Cusick et al. [11] have reported that at least partial retinal reattachment was achieved in 33% of 956 eyes from 601 infants, with a visual acuity better than 5/200 in 8 of 183 eyes. In a case series of 48 eyes with stage 5 ROPs evaluated 6 months postoperatively, 20 (42.6%) and 5 (10.6%) eyes exhibited total and partial reattachment of the retina, respectively (unpublished data). Similar results have been reported with retinal reattachment rates of approximately 40%–60% [12–19] and limited functional outcomes 12–16 [20–23], (Table 14.1). Regarding the factors related to anatomical success, the close shape of the funnel, presence of subretinal hemorrhage and vascularized membranes, and age at vitrectomy are associated with poor surgical outcomes [12, 13, 16].

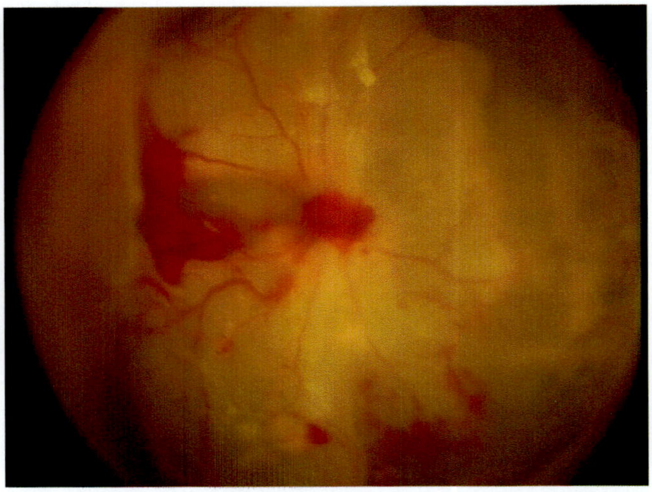

Fig. 14.12 Fundus view 1 week after surgery. The retina was partially reattached. Complete reattachment of the retina was achieved 2 weeks after surgery in this particular eye

14.5 Conclusions

Neonatologists should appropriately care for premature infants, and ophthalmologists must screen at appropriate timings and use proper techniques to reduce severe ROP that requires treatment. Interventions, such as laser ablation or anti-VEGF therapy, are critical in preventing the development of TRD. If tractional detachment occurs, vitrectomy should be performed at stage 4A before the macula is detached to achieve satisfactory outcomes.

Table 14.1 Summary of previous reports on vitrectomy for stage 5 ROP

Author(s)	Number of eyes	RA rate (%)	Functional results (%)	Birth weight (grams)	Gestational age at birth (weeks)	Publication
Cusick et al.	608	TRA: 25 PRA: 7	NLP:26, LP:59, HM:10, >20/2000: 4	871 (340 ~ 2750)	26 (20 ~ 35)	2006 [11]
Zilis et al.	121	TRA: 9 PRA: 31	F & F or greater: 11%, LP: 56% NLP: 25%	955 (560 ~ 1850)	26.3 (22 ~ 32)	1990 [19]
Trese	85	48	F & F:44, grasp object: 38, shape recognition: 15	640 ~ 1400	24 ~ 32	1986 [17]
Fuchino et al.	51	59	NLP:5, LP:19, HM:14, > 20/2000: 62	948 (515 ~ 1760)	27 (23 ~ 33)	1995 [13]
Tasman et al. (Open-sky Vtx)	23	35	NA	1038 (539 ~ 1950)	26 (24 ~ 32)	1987 [18]

RA retinal attachment, *g* gram, *TRA* total retinal attachment, *PRA* partial retinal attachment, *F&F* fix and follow, *LP* light perception, *NLP* no light perception, *HM* hand movement, *Vtx* vitrectomy, *NA* not available

References

1. Early Treatment for Retinopathy of Prematurity Cooperative Group. Revised indications for the treatment of retinopathy of prematurity: results of the early treatment for retinopathy of prematurity randomized trial. Arch Ophthalmol. 2003;121(12):1684–94.
2. Quiroz-Mercado H, Martinez-Castellanos MA, Hernandez-Rojas ML, Salazar-Teran N, Chan RV. Antiangiogenic therapy with intravitreal bevacizumab for retinopathy of prematurity. Retina. 2008;28(3 Suppl):S19–25.
3. Kusaka S, Shima C, Wada K, Arahori H, Shimojyo H, Sato T, Fujikado T. Efficacy of intravitreal injection of bevacizumab for severe retinopathy of prematurity: a pilot study. Br J Ophthalmol. 2008;92(11):1450–5.
4. Mintz-Hittner HA, Kennedy KA, Chuang AZ, BEAT-ROP Cooperative Group. Efficacy of intravitreal bevacizumab for stage3+ retinopathy of prematurity. N Engl J Med. 2011;364(7):603–15.
5. Sonmez K, Drenser KA, Capone A Jr, Trese MT. Vitreous levels of stromal cell-derived factor 1 and vascular endothelial growth factor in patients with retinopathy of prematurity. Ophthalmology. 2008;115(6):1065–70.
6. Sato T, Kusaka S, Shimojyo H, Fujikado T. Vitreous levels of erythropoietin and vascular endothelial growth factor in eyes with retinopathy of prematurity. Ophthalmology. 2009;116(9):1599–603.
7. Sato T, Kusaka S, Hashida N, Saishin Y, Fujikado T, Tano Y. Comprehensive gene-expression profile in murine oxygen-induced retinopathy. Br J Ophthalmol. 2009;93(1):96–103.
8. Greven C, Tasman W. Scleral buckling in stages 4B and 5 retinopathy of prematurity. Ophthalmology. 1990;97(6):817–20.
9. Imaizumi A, Kusaka S, Noguchi H, Shimomura Y, Sawaguchi S. Efficacy of short-term postoperative perfluoro-n-octane tamponade for pediatric complex retinal detachment. Am J Ophthalmol. 2014;157(2):384–9.
10. Quinn GE, Dobson V, Barr CC, Davis BR, Palmer EA, Robertson J, Summers CG, Trese MT, Tung B. Visual acuity of eyes after vitrectomy for retinopathy of prematurity: follow-up at 5 1/2 years. The Cryotherapy for Retinopathy of Prematurity Cooperative Group. Ophthalmology. 1996;103(4):595–600.
11. Cusick M, Charles MK, Agrón E, Sangiovanni JP, Ferris FL 3rd, Charles S. Anatomical and visual results of vitreoretinal surgery for stage 5 retinopathy of prematurity. Retina. 2006;26(7):729–35.
12. Hirose T, Katsumi O, Mehta MC, Schepens CL. Vision in stage 5 retinopathy of prematurity after retinal reattachment by open-sky vitrectomy. Arch Ophthalmol. 1993;111(3):345–9.
13. Fuchino Y, Hayashi H, Kono T, Ohshima K. Long-term follow up of visual acuity in eyes with stage 5 retinopathy of prematurity after closed vitrectomy. Am J Ophthalmol. 1995;120(3):308–16.
14. Trese MT, Droste PJ. Long-term postoperative results of a consecutive series of stages 4 and 5 retinopathy of prematurity. Ophthalmology. 1998;105(6):992–7.
15. Kono T, Oshima K, Fuchino Y. Surgical results and visual outcomes of vitreous surgery for advanced stages of retinopathy of prematurity. Jpn J Ophthalmol. 2000;44(6):661–7.
16. Jabbour NM, Eller AE, Hirose T, Schepens CL, Liberfarb R. Stage 5 retinopathy of prematurity. Prognostic value of morphologic findings. Ophthalmology. 1987;94(12):1640–6.
17. Trese MT. Visual results and prognostic factors for vision following surgery for stage V retinopathy of prematurity. Ophthalmology. 1986;93(5):574–9.
18. Tasman W, Borrone RN, Bolling J. Open sky vitrectomy for total retinal detachment in retinopathy of prematurity. Ophthalmology. 1987;94(4):449–52.
19. Zilis JD, de Juan E, Machemer R. Advanced retinopathy of prematurity. The anatomic and visual results of vitreous surgery. Ophthalmology. 1990;97(6):821–6.
20. Karacorlu M, Hocaoglu M, Sayman Muslubas I, Arf S. Long-term functional results following vitrectomy for advanced retinopathy of prematurity. Br J Ophthalmol. 2017;101(6):730–4.
21. Mintz-Hittner HA, O'Malley RE, Kretzer FL. Long-term form identification vision after early, closed, lensectomy-vitrectomy for stage 5 retinopathy of prematurity. Ophthalmology. 1997;104(3):454–9.
22. Hartnett ME, Rodier DW, McColm JR, Thompson HW. Long-term vision results measured with Teller Acuity Cards and a new Light Perception/Projection Scale after management of late stages of retinopathy of prematurity. Arch Ophthalmol. 2003;121(7):991–6.
23. Seaber JH, Machemer R, Eliott D, Buckley EG, deJuan E, Martin DF. Long-term visual results of children after initially successful vitrectomy for stage V retinopathy of prematurity. Ophthalmology. 1995;102(2):199–204.

15 Endoscopic Surgery in ROP

Gaurav Bhardwaj and Sui Chien Wong

In complex intraocular surgery, inadequate visualization can be a major limiting factor to surgical success. The inability to visualize the surgical field effectively prevents any possible surgical intervention. Endoscopy is a valuable tool in complex intraocular surgery [1–3], which provides the vitreoretinal surgeon with a unique perspective and surgical approach. It confers a particular advantage in procedures involving structures in the anterior retina, pars plana, and ciliary body, which conventional top-down viewing systems are unable to adequately visualize. Endoscopy also provides a useful adjunct to modern-day visualization with an operating microscope and wide-angle contact or non-contact viewing systems. Table 15.1 lists the indications where visualization with modern-day microscope viewing has limitations and an endoscopic approach has been studied.

Table 15.1 Indications for Endoscope-assisted vitrectomy (EAV)

Corneal opacities preventing fundal view [4–7] Severe ocular trauma [8, 9] Removal of intraocular foreign body [10] Endophthalmitis [5, 11–14]
ROP-RD [15]
RRD with anterior PVR [16–18]
Removal of cyclitic membranes [17, 19]
Cyclodialysis cleft repair [20]
Prognostication for advanced cases [21]
Haptic visualization for sutured IOLs [22–24]

ROP retinopathy of prematurity, *RRD* rhegmatogenous retinal detachment, *PVR* proliferative vitreoretinopathy, *IOL* intraocular lens

Apart from media opacities, where endoscopic viewing replaces modern-day microscope viewing systems, the endoscope is often a complementary tool to assist in parts of vitrectomy surgery. Therefore, the authors prefer the term endoscope-assisted vitrectomy (EAV) as opposed to endoscopic vitrectomy.

To many vitreoretinal surgeons, EAV remains a black-box and therefore a largely unutilized technique. Due to its learning curve and the fact that it is not commonly learned by training vitreoretinal surgeons in fellowship programs, its use is limited to a few specialized centers. It is most commonly utilized in tertiary centers that manage a large volume of pediatric vitreoretinal cases (such as ROP-RD) or ocular trauma. EAV however may be advantageous in a wide variety of surgical indications (Table 15.1). We hope that this chapter will be of equal value to surgeons who are just starting out in EAV or may only need to use EAV occasionally as opposed to more experienced EAV surgeons. We will cover a broad range of applications, and focus on its use in ROP-RD.

15.1 Advent of EAV

Endoscopes are commonly used in medicine for viewing internal cavities through small incisions. Their basic premise is the capturing of images and their transmission via a conduit to a proximal eyepiece or camera. Although the first endoscope for ophthalmic use was developed almost 90 years ago, [25] endoscopy has been a rarely utilized technique in most centers. This is likely due to numerous factors including advances in microscope viewing systems and microincision vitrectomy surgery, and lack of training and instrumentation for the endoscopic approach. The number of publications relating to EAV, however, has increased steadily over the last few decades, from just two papers in the 1980s to almost 40 in the current decade from 2010. This is due to technological advances in endoscopy and a recognition of its superiority over microscope-based viewing systems in certain situations. There are no randomized trials compar-

G. Bhardwaj (✉)
Sydney Children's Hospital Network, Sydney, Australia

Faculty of Medicine and Health, Discipline of Ophthalmology and Eye Health and Save Sight Institute, Sydney Medical School, Sydney, Australia

S. C. Wong
ROP Retinal Detachment Service, Great Ormond Street Hospital for Children, de facto UK National Centre, London, UK

Great Ormond Street Hospital for Children, Moorfields Eye Hospital, Royal Free Hospital, London, UK

W.-C. Wu, W.-C. Lam (eds.), *A Quick Guide to Pediatric Retina*, https://doi.org/10.1007/978-981-15-6552-6_15

ing EAV with microscope-based viewing; however, these are unlikely to occur due to case-mix, surgeon preference, and experience of one technique over the other.

The integration of the charge-coupled device (CCD) with endoscopy in 1983 [26] allowed electronic transmission of the image to a monitor, a key factor in improving the utility of the endoscope in ophthalmic surgery. Flexible fiber-optics, with its smaller diameter instruments and greater maneuverability has also largely replaced the gradient index lens system (GRIN).

Recently, a hybrid system was described [27] utilizing a combination of standard endoscopy with a 3D heads-up display (NGENUITY 3D® visualization system, Alcon Laboratories, Fort Worth, TX, USA). The purported advantage of this technique was that the images of the two modalities were side by side, and therefore, the surgeon did not need to alternate viewing through a microscope and a screen. A follow-up paper to this technique also reported using a 3D converter for the 2D endoscopic view along with the use of polarized glasses to improve the stereopsis of the image [28].

In the future, it is likely that a true 3D endoscopic view may be achievable, thus making the technique safer and more intuitive. At the present time, the endoscope image resolution is also limited to standard rather than high definition, due to the number and type of fibers the endoscope houses.

15.2 Advantages Over Modern-Day Microscope Viewing

There are two optical properties unique to the endoscope that confers advantages over modern-day microscope viewing in certain surgical scenarios.

Firstly, the unique surgeon's perspective (Fig. 15.1a) with the endoscope is advantageous in viewing structures anterior to the vitreous base, including the ora serrata, pars plicata, pars plana, ciliary body, and posterior iris, as the view is from where the endoscope tip is positioned in the posterior segment, rather than a top-down microscope-based view that relies on the optics of the patient's cornea and lens. This is particularly useful in ROP-RD, where the pars plicata can be visualized, enabling safer sclerotomy formation under direct guidance, avoiding iatrogenic retinal trauma and unnecessary lensectomy. Additionally, there is improved access to anterior PVR and retro-irideal pathology such as cyclitic membranes and intraocular foreign bodies around the ciliary body.

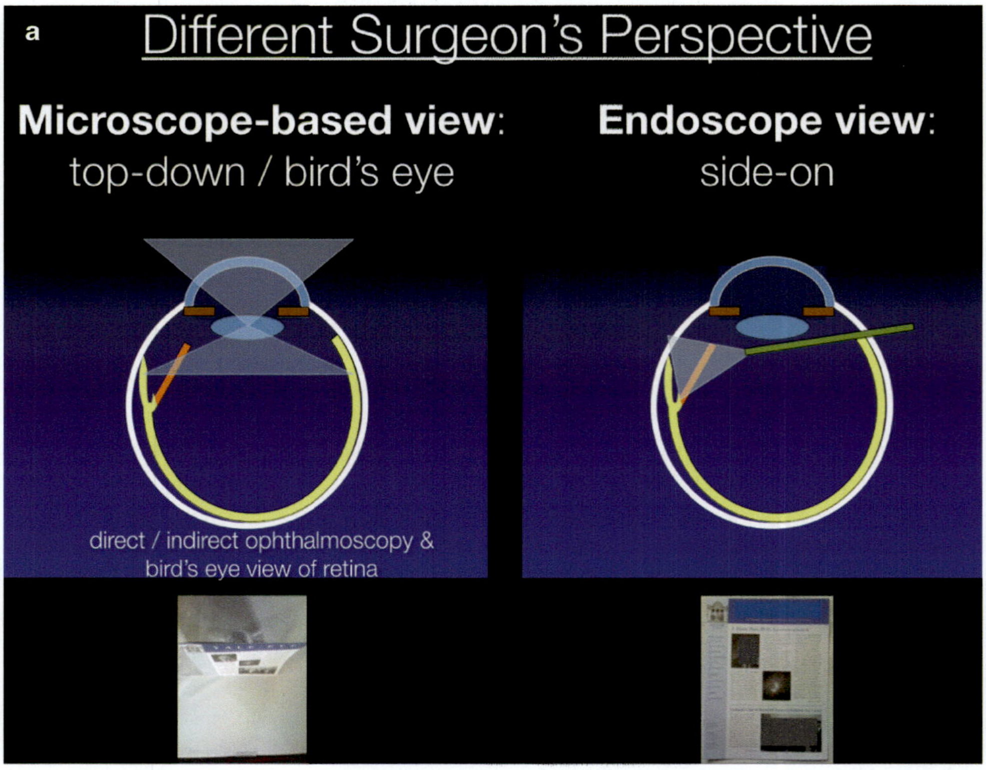

Fig. 15.1 (**a**). This figure illustrates the different perspective which is obtained with the endoscope compared with the microscope-based view. The side-on view of the endoscope allows better visualization of structures that appear almost end-on through the microscope. (**b**). These two photographs of text viewed through frosted tape to simulate vectors of vitreous traction illustrates the ease with which the semi-transparent tape is seen with the endoscopic view compared with the microscope-based view

Fig. 15.1 (continued)

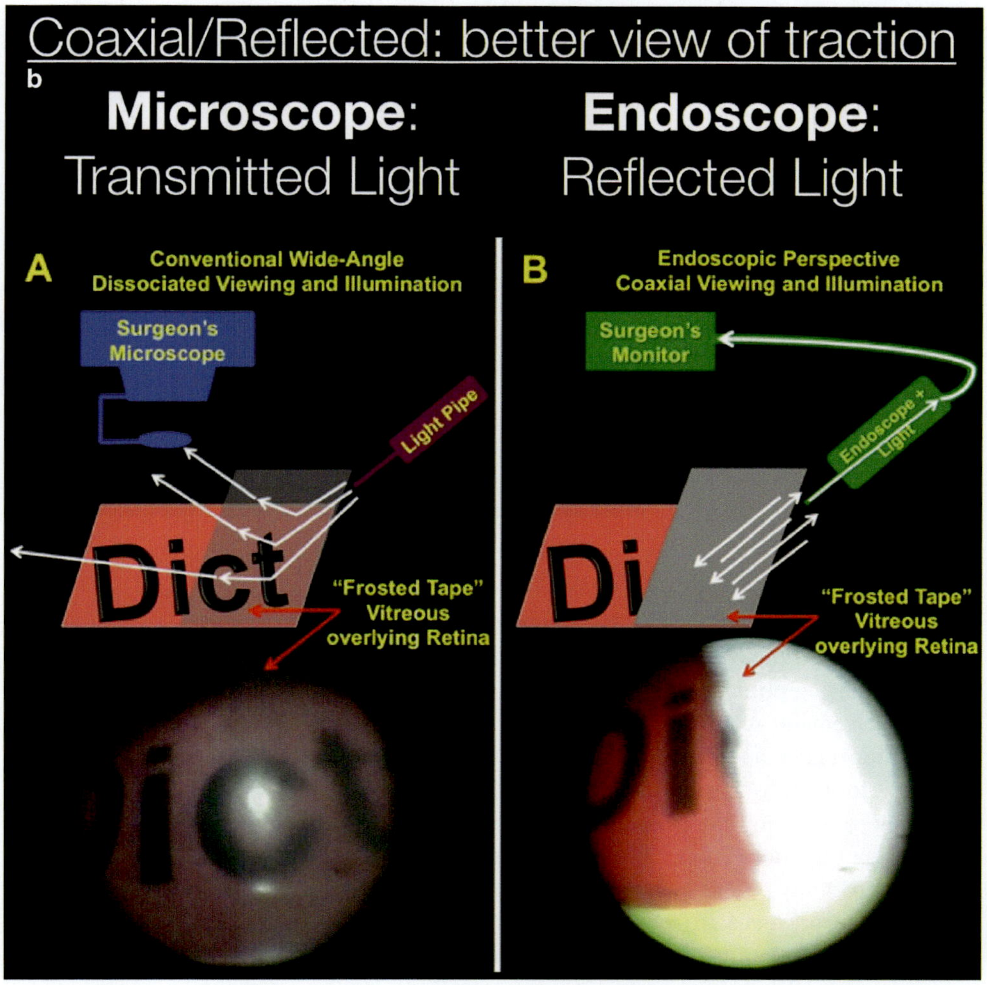

Secondly, visualization of structures that mostly appear transparent with the microscope, such as the anterior hyaloid face, vitreous cortex, and transvitreal traction, is superior with EAV. The reason for this is the effect of direct coaxial illumination, in which the illumination and viewing are performed in the same direction as light emanates from the endoscope tip and is reflected back into it. In traditional microscope viewing of the posterior segment, the endoillumination is directed from an angle, reflects off the retina away from its source, and is transmitted through the patient's anterior segment into the microscope to be viewed by the surgeon. Visualization of semi-transparent structures is superior with direct reflection of light off the structures than with transmission through the structures. This effect is illustrated in Fig. 15.1b. This is advantageous in various conditions such as retinopathy of prematurity associated retinal detachments (ROP-RD) where up to five different vectors of traction contribute to the pathology and surgical success relies on identifying and alleviating these.

EAV has also been utilized in the identification of undetected peripheral retinal breaks [29]. Subretinal surgery to remove fibrotic bands is also feasible without the need for an extensive relieving retinotomy.

15.3 ROP Traction Retinal Detachment

The advantages of EAV is seen particularly in ROP-RD due to the anterior nature of the traction RD that often extends toward the pars plicata and lens, as well as the multiple vectors of traction that are well recognized.

Port placement can be risky in ROP-RD due to a combination of traction RD that can be anteriorly positioned close to the pars plicata paired with a physiologically smaller vitreous compartment and a proportionately larger lens. This leaves a very small area for safe port placement that avoids iatrogenic retinal trauma. A study by El Rayes et al. [30] demonstrated that 57% of patients with Stage 4B ROP having conventional microscope-based vitrectomy required primary lensectomy. This has the downsides of increased amblyopia, visual rehabilitation needs including dependence on aphakic spectacles or contact lenses, and long-term risk

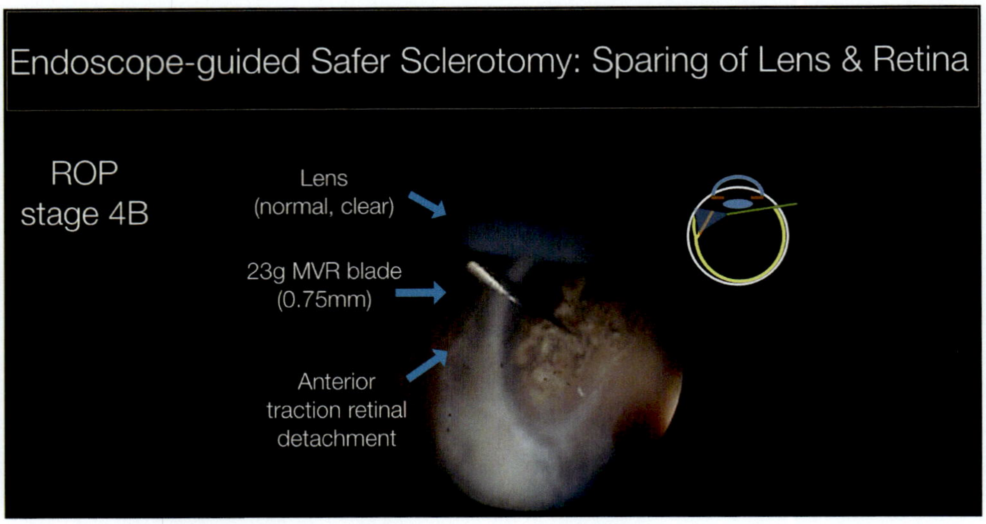

Fig. 15.2 Endoscopic visualization of port insertion allows for safe placement of trocars by avoiding anterior structures such as the lens or anterior tractional retinal detachments

of aphakic glaucoma [31]. A recent nationwide study [15] on endoscopic vitrectomy in the United Kingdom in 51 consecutive patients with Stage 4A and 4B ROP reported 0% of patients requiring primary lensectomy.

Port placement requires careful planning. Firstly, an examination under anesthetic (EUA) with scleral indentation is performed, to identify an area for placement of the endoscope sclerotomy port which is relatively safer, away from areas of traction. Once the endoscope is inserted, subsequent vitrectomy port placement can be directly visualized (Fig. 15.2) to prevent iatrogenic lens or retinal trauma. In cases of ROP-RD, iatrogenic retinal breaks have been found to lead to surgical failure in up to 100% of cases [32]. It is thus vital that all measures are taken to prevent such complications. The authors have found it safer and more controlled to use an MVR blade to make the pars plicata sclerotomy incision under direct endoscopic visualization, rather than a trocar as more force to get through the more elastic sclera is needed than the flatter MVR profile.

In stage 4A or 4B ROP-RD, up to five vectors of traction have been documented [33], ridge-to-ridge (transvitreal), ridge-to-optic disc, ridge-to-lens, ridge-to-vitreous base, and circumferential. Before the advent of EAV, a common approach in management of Stage 4A and 4B ROP was encirclement and more recently vitrectomy alone. Vitrectomy does not reliably relieve all vectors particularly anteroposterior traction from the ridge to the lens or ridge to vitreous base as it is more peripheral and more challenging to visualize. EAV, with the side-on surgeon's perspective as well as the use of coaxial lighting, optimizes visualization of these vectors. Persistent traction can prevent primary retinal reattachment, and increase the long-term risk of redetachment. It can also contribute to the development or worsening of macular dystopia and dragging which impacts vision.

Table 15.2 Advantages and disadvantages of EAV

Advantages	Disadvantages
Visualize pars plicata and pars plana, enabling direct guidance of sclerotomy formation	Resolution not as good as modern-day microscope-based view
Optimal visualization of transvitreal traction and identification of all vectors of traction, particularly anterior traction	Lack of stereopsis
Reduced possibility of lens trauma	Larger incision required
Allows for safe port placement with reduced iatrogenic breaks	Bimanual surgery not possible

Other tractional retinopathies where EAV has similar benefits include familial exudative vitreoretinopathy and posterior persistent fetal vasculature (PFV). The principles are similar to ROP-RD surgery. A detailed discussion of these conditions is outside the scope of this chapter.

Advantages and disadvantages of EAV compared with modern-day microscope-based vitrectomy are listed in Table 15.2.

15.4 Surgical Tips

15.4.1 Practical Guide to Setup and How to Perform Surgery

A widely utilized platform is the Endo Optiks Ophthalmic Laser Endoscopy system (Beaver Visitec, Waltham, MA). The Endo Optics 19G endoscope integrates high-resolution video imaging, wide-field illumination (175 or 300 watt xenon light source), and a diode laser (810 nm) for retinal or cyclo-photocoagulation. It has a resolution of 17,000 pixels and 140-degree field of view. The 23G probe has a resolution of 10,000 pixels and a field of view of 125 degrees.

Endoscopes are available in various gauges including 19G, 20G, 23G, and recently 25G [34]. The latter two fit through standard valved microcannulas and the two former require a limited peritomy and larger sclerotomy. The drawback of the larger gauges and the need for a larger incision is compensated for by the wider field of view and superior resolution. While a larger 19 g sclerotomy requires suturing, this is normally necessary in ROP surgery anyway even if 25 g or 27 g incisions are used due to the more elastic sclera. Thus, it is the authors' view that the larger incision is a small trade-off for the significant gains in visualization in complex cases, particularly ROP-RD surgery.

In the authors' experience, the 19G endoscope is superior for more complex cases and in cases where there is a greater reliance on the endoscopic view. There is also the choice between a straight tip and an angled tip and a straight probe and a curved probe. The curved probe, while reducing the risk of iatrogenic lens touch, adds an additional degree of complexity in the axis of rotation and therefore is more challenging to use.

Following a EUA and once the optimum position of the endoscope is determined, the surgical setup can be completed. To optimize endoscopic visualization of a particular pathological area of interest, it is best to place the endoscope port within 6 clock hours of it. In ROP-RD surgery, typically, the most relevant area of traction is temporal, causing macular dragging. Therefore, to optimize visualization of the temporal transvitreal traction bands, it is recommended that the surgeon sits temporally, placing the endoscope and vitrectomy ports at about the 11 and 7'o clock positions, respectively (in the scenario where the right eye was being operated on). Thus, the area of temporal traction would be sandwiched between the ports and be most accessible to surgical removal. Figure 15.3 demonstrates a setup where the surgeon is positioned temporally, while in Fig. 15.4 the surgeon is positioned superiorly. The aim is to have the endoscope screen as close to the surgeon's line of sight as possible to ease the alternation between the microscope and endoscope view.

Placement of the ports is carried out in the standard fashion. A peritomy is performed in the desired area and an incision made with a 20G microvitreoretinal (MVR) blade (Fig. 15.5). Depending on the extent and nature of the pathology, a second pars plana incision may occasionally be required on the other side.

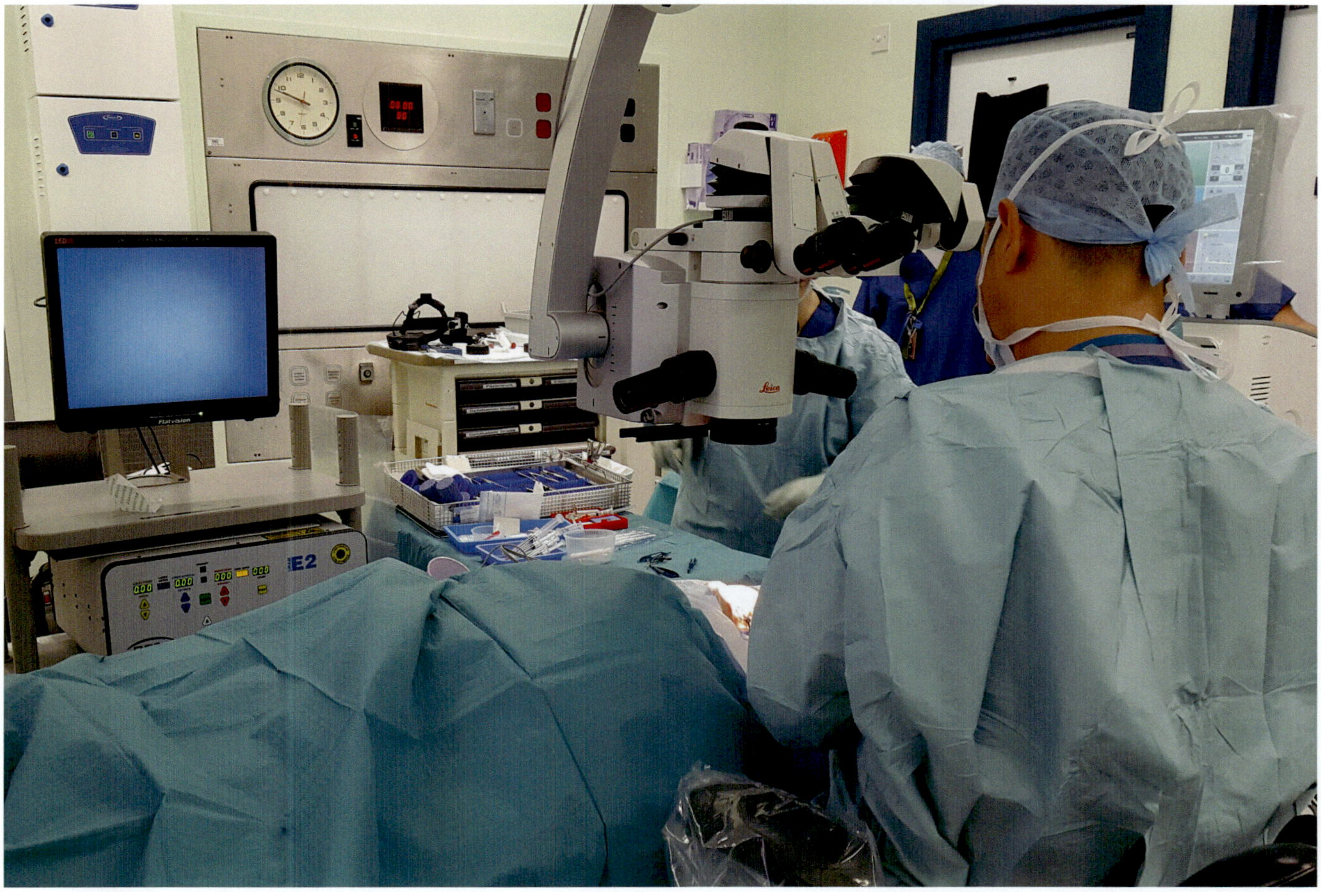

Fig. 15.3 Temporal approach EAV, with the scrub assistant at the head of the bed. This approach allows good access to the temporal retina, which is typically involved in ROP-RD. EAV-endoscope-assisted vitrectomy

If the operating microscope is also being utilized for parts of the surgery, illumination can either be provided by a regular endoilluminator or the endoscope. The advantage of using the endoscope as an illuminator is that the surgeon can always alternate between the endoscopic view and the microscope view. Alternating between the microscope and endoscope view is initially challenging and is one of the components of the learning curve. The hand–eye coordination learned during traditional surgical approaches must be modified and re-learned. The orientation is also different as structures are viewed from a side-on perspective as opposed to a top-down perspective.

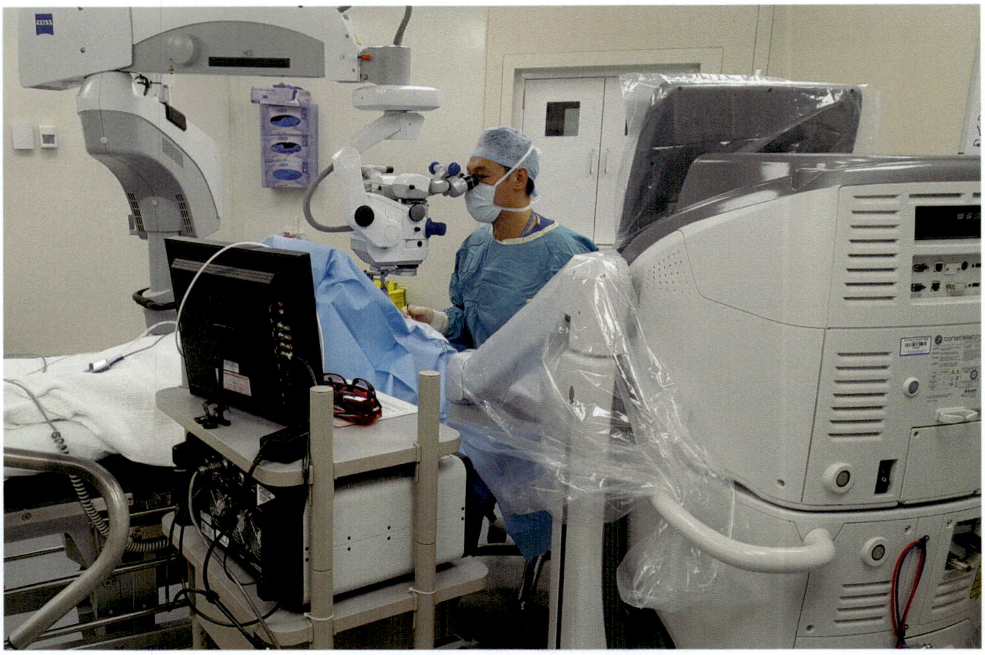

Fig. 15.4 Superior approach EAV, which is familiar to most vitreoretinal surgeons. The endoscope screen is positioned as close as possible to the line of light of the surgeon

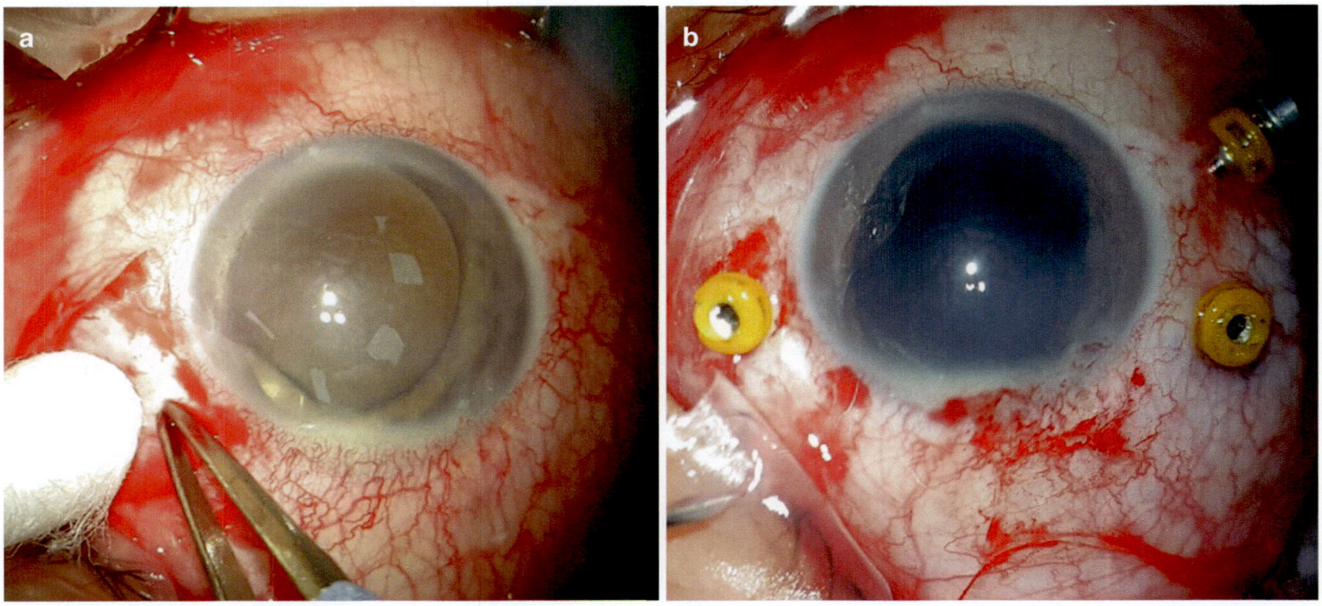

Fig. 15.5 (**a–d**) Steps involved in port placement in EAV (setup shown is 23G vitrectomy with a 19G endoscope in an adult patient). (**a**). A limited peritomy is made in preparation for the endoscope. Surface vessels are cauterised (**b**). Three ports are placed in the standard fashion (**c**). A 20G MVR blade is used to make the incision for endoscope insertion, the opening is slightly enlarged on removal of the blade. (**d**). The endoscope is inserted as shown. If endoscopic guidance is required for port placement, then the other ports are placed after endoscope insertion. MVR—microvitreoretinal

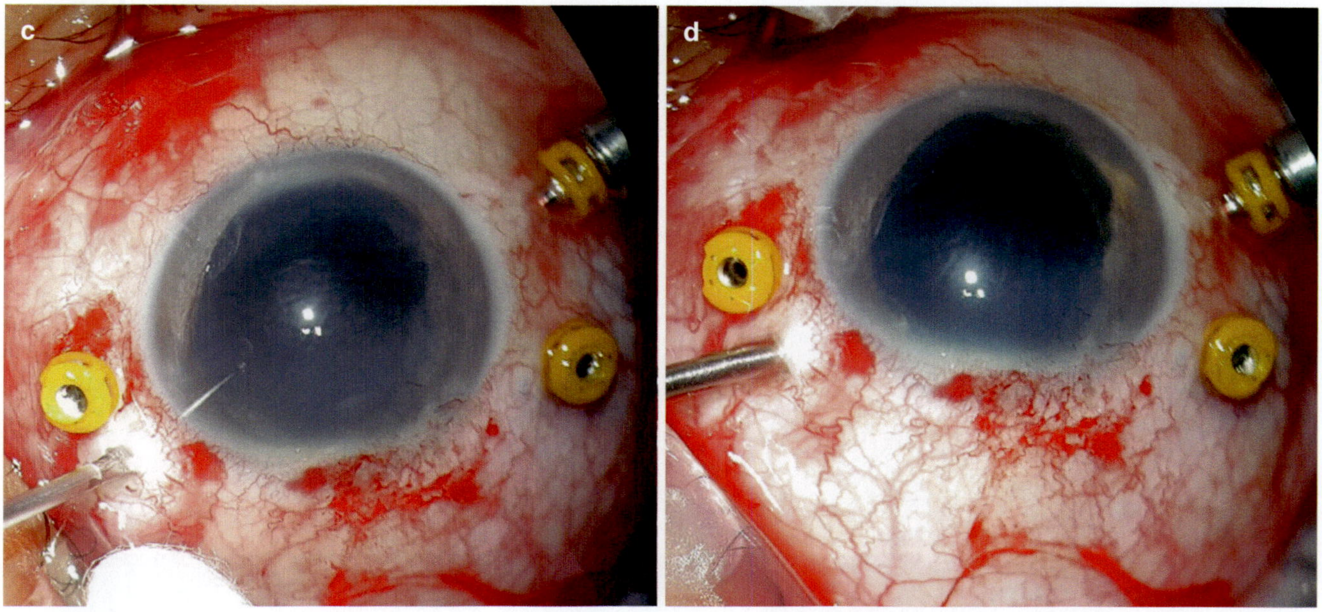

Fig. 15.5 (continued)

15.4.2 Staying Out of Trouble

The endoscopic view can be disorienting in the early stages, due to the extra axis of rotation, potentially narrower field of view, and higher magnification. To maintain orientation, image focusing, and orientation is initially performed with the endoscope outside the eye. Once in the eye, the endoscope should be rotated so that the lens always remains at the top of the image to help maintain orientation, while initially viewing at low magnification (and thus wider field of view). Gauging distance from the retina or other structures is also more difficult due to the lack of stereopsis. Other visual cues, such as shadows and relative size of structures compared with the known gauge of the instruments, need to be employed to maintain a safe working distance. A working distance of 3–4 mm is optimal when trying to view at high magnification, at which a 19 gauge endoscope can resolve detail down to 20 microns. Given that a first-order retinal arteriole is 125 microns, this level of detail is sufficient for fine surgical maneuvers, including the peeling of the internal limiting membrane [35] and fibrovascular membranes.

The narrow field of view necessitates care when moving instruments to avoid iatrogenic retinal or lens touch. The zoom of the image is changed by bringing the endoscope closer or further away. The light intensity also needs to be reduced the closer the endoscope is brought to the area of interest, otherwise a whiteout phenomenon will occur.

During initial insertion of the endoscope into an opaque vitreous cavity, such as in trauma cases or endophthalmitis, a whiteout or blackout view on the monitor may occur. If the anterior segment allows, a core vitrectomy can be performed with a top-down view prior to endoscope insertion to prevent this. If there is no view through the anterior segment, then the cutter needs to be brought into contact with the endoscope tip and a localized clearance performed in order to allow a sufficient view. While this has inherent risks of iatrogenic complications, the risk decreases with surgeon experience. In any case, there is no other way to be able to proceed with surgery and the risks must be balanced against the prospect of not operating.

Due to the significant differences between endoscopic surgery and microscope-based vitrectomy surgery, wet or dry-lab training is recommended to accelerate the process of familiarization and allow relearning of the hand–eye coordination.

15.5 Case Study Example

15.5.1 ROP

This is a case of a baby born at 26 weeks gestational age at 755 g. The child presented at 44 weeks postmenstrual age, with right eye stage 4B (macular involving) ROP and left inoperable stage 5 ROP. Figure 15.6a demonstrates the degree of traction in the right eye, with inferior macular heterotopia. Figure 15.6b demonstrates the first and second attempts at sclerotomy formation with an MVR blade. The first attempt, the tip of the MVR blade can be seen to be in contact with anterior traction RD. Not recognizing this, as would normally be the case with standard non-endoscope trocar insertion, could have led to an iatrogenic retinal break

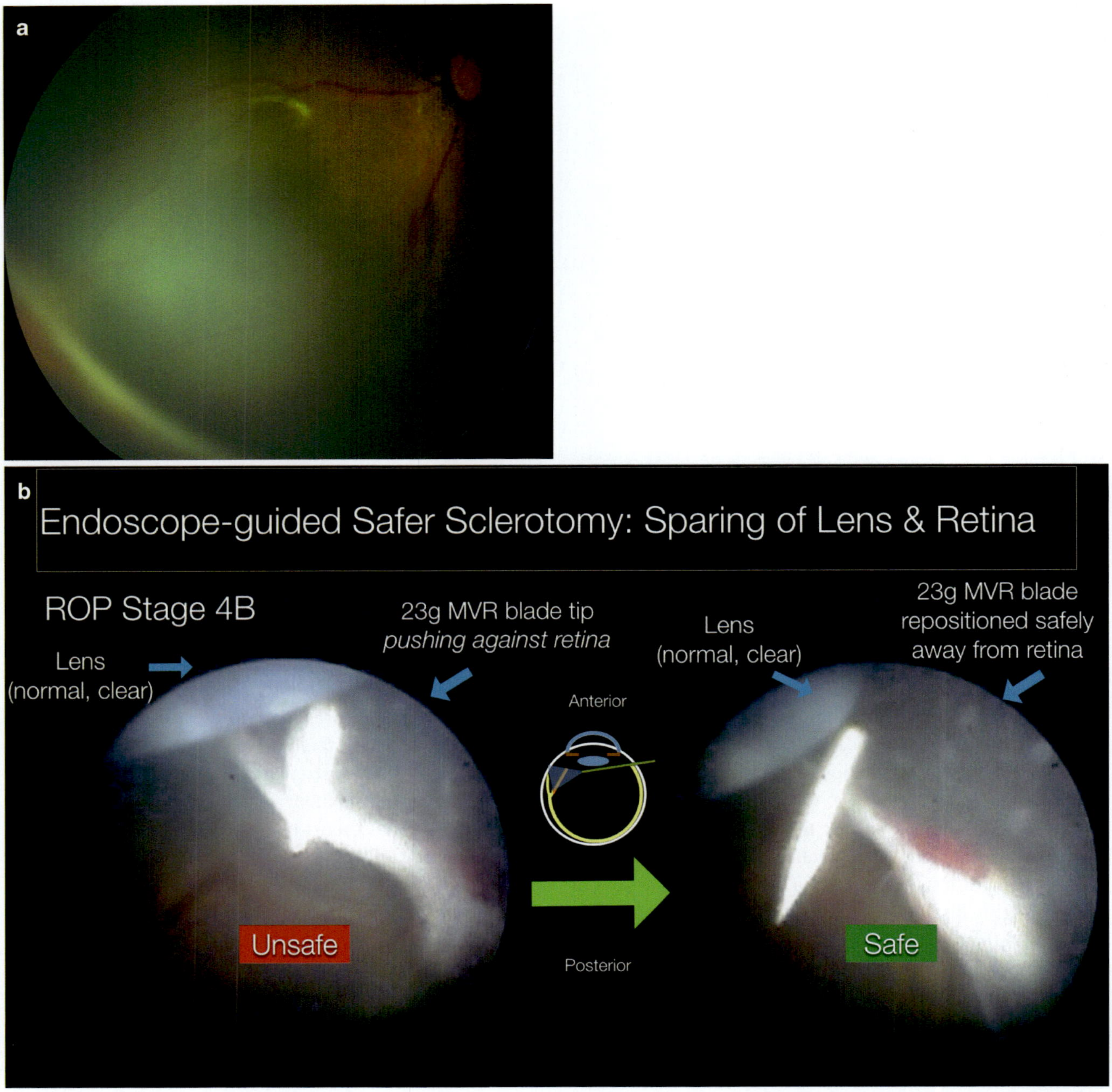

Fig. 15.6 (**a**). Right RetCam fundus photo of premature baby born at 26 weeks with 4B ROP. Note the macular heterotopia. (**b**). Endoscopic guidance of sclerotomy creation with 23G MVR blade, demonstrating the utility of EAV in ensuring safe sclerotomy formation

and surgical failure and blindness in this child's only seeing eye. The endoscope view highlighted this risk, and enabled repositioning of the MVR blade by 1 clock hour and is now seen to have safely entered the eye in a zone free of both lens and retina.

15.6 Conclusions

The endoscopic view during vitrectomy has a range of applications and is a useful adjunct to the modern-day microscope. It is particularly helpful in unique ROP-RD specific pathology, increasing the safety and efficacy of surgery by reducing the risk of iatrogenic lens and retinal trauma.

References

1. Wong SC, Lee TC, Heier JS. 23-Gauge endoscopic vitrectomy. Dev Ophthalmol. 2014;54:108–19.
2. Wong SC, Lee TC, Heier JS, Ho AC. Endoscopic vitrectomy. Curr Opin Ophthalmol. 2014;25(3):195–206.
3. Yeo DCM, Nagiel A, Yang U, Lee TC, Wong SC. Endoscopy for pediatric retinal disease. Asia Pac J Ophthalmol. 2018;7(3):200–7.
4. Huang YF, Chang CJ. Endoscope-assisted vitrectomy in the management of retinal detachment with corneal opacity. Taiwan J Ophthalmol. 2017;7(3):164–7.
5. Shen L, Zheng B, Zhao Z, Chen Y. Endoscopic Vitrectomy for severe posttraumatic Endophthamitis with visualization constraints. Ophthalmic Surg Lasers Imaging. 2010;9:1–4.
6. de Smet MD, Mura M. Minimally invasive surgery-endoscopic retinal detachment repair in patients with media opacities. Eye (Lond). 2008;22(5):662–5.
7. Ben-nun J. Cornea sparing by endoscopically guided vitreoretinal surgery. Ophthalmology. 2001;108(8):1465–70.
8. Yonekawa Y, Papakostas TD, Marra KV, Arroyo JG. Endoscopic pars plana vitrectomy for the management of severe ocular trauma. Int Ophthalmol Clin. 2013;53(4):139–48.
9. Sabti KA, Raizada S. Endoscope-assisted pars plana vitrectomy in severe ocular trauma. Br J Ophthalmol. 2012;96(11):1399–403.
10. Yang X, Li QY, Du S, Ren H, Jia CY, Tang XH. Extraction of intraocular foreign body at or near the ciliary body under endoscopic vitrectomy. Chin J Ophthalmol. 2013;49(8):691–6.
11. Pan Q, Liu Y, Wang R, Chen T, Yang Z, Deng Y, et al. Treatment of *Bacillus cereus* endophthalmitis with endoscopy-assisted vitrectomy. Medicine. 2017;96(50):e8701.
12. Martiano D, L'Helgoualc'h G, Cochener B. Endoscopy-guided 20-G vitrectomy in severe endophthalmitis: report of 18 cases and literature review. J Fr D'ophtalmol. 2015;38(10):941–9.
13. Ren H, Jiang R, Xu G, Chang Q, Lv J, Chen Q, et al. Endoscopy-assisted vitrectomy for treatment of severe endophthalmitis with retinal detachment. Graefes Arch Clin Exp Ophthalmol. 2013;251(7):1797–800.
14. De Smet MD, Carlborg EA. Managing severe endophthalmitis with the use of an endoscope. Retina (Philadelphia, PA). 2005;25(8):976–80.
15. Wong SC, Yeo D, et al. Acute retinal detachment in retinopathy of prematurity: UK national outcomes of endoscopic vitrectomy in 51 consecutive cases. Association for Research and Vision in Ophthalmology Annual Meeting; April 29 to May 2; Honolulu, HI2018.
16. Lee GD, Goldberg RA, Heier JS. Endoscopy-assisted vitrectomy and membrane dissection of anterior proliferative vitreoretinopathy for chronic hypotony after previous retinal detachment repair. Retina (Philadelphia, PA). 2016;36(6):1058–63.
17. Boscher C, Kuhn F. An endoscopic overview of the anterior vitreous base in retinal detachment and anterior proliferative vitreoretinopathy. Acta Ophthalmol. 2014;92(4):e298–304.
18. Boscher C, Kuhn F. Endoscopic evaluation and dissection of the anterior vitreous base. Ophthalmic Res. 2015;53(2):90–9.
19. Marra KV, Yonekawa Y, Papakostas TD, Arroyo JG. Indications and techniques of endoscope assisted vitrectomy. J Ophthal Vis Res. 2013;8(3):282–90.
20. Gnanaraj L, Lam WC, Rootman DR, Levin AV. Endoscopic closure of a cyclodialysis cleft. J AAPOS. 2005;9(6):592–4.
21. Reddy Pappuru RR, Tyagi M, Paulose RM, Dave VP, Das T, Chhablani J, et al. Role of diagnostic endoscopy in posterior segment evaluation for definitive prognostication in eyes with corneal opacification. Am J Ophthalmol. 2017;176:9–14.
22. Olsen TW, Pribila JT. Pars plana vitrectomy with endoscope-guided sutured posterior chamber intraocular lens implantation in children and adults. Am J Ophthalmol. 2011;151(2):287–96.e2.
23. Sasahara M, Kiryu J, Yoshimura N. Endoscope-assisted transscleral suture fixation to reduce the incidence of intraocular lens dislocation. J Cataract Refract Surg. 2005;31(9):1777–80.
24. Althaus C, Sundmacher R. Endoscopically controlled optimization of trans-scleral suture fixation of posterior chamber lenses in the ciliary sulcus. Der Ophthalmologe: Zeitschrift der Deutschen Ophthalmologischen Gesellschaft. 1993;90(4):317–24.
25. Thorpe HE. Ocular endoscope: an instrument for the removal of intravitreous nonmagnetic foreign bodies. Trans Am Acad Ophthalmol. 1934;34:422.
26. Eguchi S, Araie M. A new ophthalmic electronic videoendoscope system for intraocular surgery. Arch Ophthalmol (Chicago, Ill: 1960). 1990;108(12):1778–81.
27. Kita M, Mori Y, Hama S. Hybrid wide-angle viewing-endoscopic vitrectomy using a 3D visualization system. Clin Ophthalmol (Auckland, NZ). 2018;12:313–7.
28. Kita M, Kusaka M, Yamada H, Hama S. Three-dimensional ocular endoscope system for vitrectomy. Clin Ophthalmol (Auckland, NZ). 2019;13:1641–3.
29. Kita M, Yoshimura N. Endoscope-assisted vitrectomy in the management of pseudophakic and aphakic retinal detachments with undetected retinal breaks. Retina (Philadelphia, PA). 2011;31(7):1347–51.
30. El Rayes EN, Vinekar A, Capone A Jr. Three-year anatomic and visual outcomes after vitrectomy for stage 4B retinopathy of prematurity. Retina (Philadelphia, PA). 2008;28(4):568–72.
31. Iwahashi-Shima C, Miki A, Hamasaki T, Otori Y, Matsushita K, Kiuchi Y, et al. Intraocular pressure elevation is a delayed-onset complication after successful vitrectomy for stages 4 and 5 retinopathy of prematurity. Retina (Philadelphia, PA). 2012;32(8):1636–42.
32. Lakhanpal RR, Sun RL, Albini TA, Holz ER. Anatomical success rate after primary three-port lens-sparing vitrectomy in stage 5 retinopathy of prematurity. Retina (Philadelphia, PA). 2006;26:724–8.
33. Wu WC, Lai CC, Lin RI, Wang NK, Chao AN, Chen KJ, et al. Modified 23-gauge vitrectomy system for stage 4 retinopathy of prematurity. Arch Ophthalmol (Chicago, Ill: 1960). 2011;129(10):1326–31.
34. Kita M, Fujii Y, Hama S. Twenty five-gauge endoscopic vitrectomy for proliferative vitreoretinopathy with severe corneal opacity. Jpn J Ophthalmol. 2018;62(3):302–6.
35. Chen Y, Shen L, Zhao S, Wang L, Xu C. Internal limiting membrane peeling by 23-gauge endoscopy for macular hole retinal detachment in a pathological myopic eye. Ophthalmic Surg Lasers Imaging Retina. 2017;48(2):179–82.

Foveal Development in Retinopathy of Prematurity

16

William Raynor, Shwetha Mangalesh, Neeru Sarin, and Cynthia A. Toth

Abstract

Human foveal development is a complex process that can be altered by retinopathy of prematurity (ROP). Establishing a baseline of normal foveal development is paramount before understanding the impact caused by prematurity and ROP. It is important to recognize ROP as a *neurovascular* disease that impacts vascular development, neuronal development, and the complex interplay between them.

Keywords

Retinopathy of prematurity · Preterm infant · Premature infant · Foveal development · Inner retinal layers · Outer retinal layers · Photoreceptor layers · Retinal layer morphology · Retinal anatomy · Neurovascular development

Our understanding of the normal foveal development comes from histopathological studies conducted in detail in primate retinae [1–3]. Over the last decade, significant advancement in human infant retinal imaging, particularly in optical coherence tomography (OCT) and OCT angiography (OCTA), has allowed for bedside imaging of infants, thereby affording in vivo and longitudinal visualization of foveal development in both term and preterm infants [4, 5]. This chapter aims to highlight the process of normal foveal development and the influence of retinopathy of prematurity (ROP) on this process, using histopathology, OCT, and OCTA studies.

W. Raynor · S. Mangalesh · N. Sarin
Department of Ophthalmology, Duke University School of Medicine, Durham, NC, USA

C. A. Toth (✉)
Department of Ophthalmology, Duke University School of Medicine, Durham, NC, USA

Pratt School of Engineering, Duke University, Durham, NC, USA
e-mail: Cynthia.Toth@Duke.edu

16.1 Normal Foveal Development

All retinal layers are derived from the neuroectoderm, specifically a portion of the neural plate, during the first trimester [6]. Early in the first trimester (around 4 weeks postovulatory age), two distinct progenitor layers become identifiable: the neural retinal layer and the retinal pigment epithelial layer, separated by an intraretinal space. Thereafter, the intraretinal space vanishes as these layers collapse onto each other; a continuous membrane is formed containing all precursor retinal layers [6]. The fovea serves as the anatomical foundation for visual acuity and color vision; the development of which begins at 12 weeks of gestation (Fig. 16.1) [7].

16.1.1 Early Development

The primitive layers of the central retina are first established in the region of the developing macula. At around 10–12 weeks of gestation, the ganglion cell layer (GCL) and inner plexiform layer (IPL) are clearly defined and visualized in the central retina [8]. By 16 weeks, all the retinal laminae can be easily identified. A single layer of choriocapillaris develops at around 8 weeks gestation. It becomes more densely packed with medium and large-sized vessels in the outer stromal portion [9].

16.1.2 20–40 Weeks of Gestation

The first step in the formation of the foveal pit is the definition of the foveal avascular zone (FAZ) at the posterior pole, into which the blood vessels do not grow [10, 11]. At 24 weeks of gestation, more than half of the retina is still engaged in neurogenesis but not at the posterior pole [12]. The FAZ develops in the GCL between 25 and 27 weeks of gestation. At 28 weeks of gestation, the FAZ is defined by the innermost vascular plexus at the GCL/IPL interface; how-

W.-C. Wu, W.-C. Lam (eds.), *A Quick Guide to Pediatric Retina*, https://doi.org/10.1007/978-981-15-6552-6_16

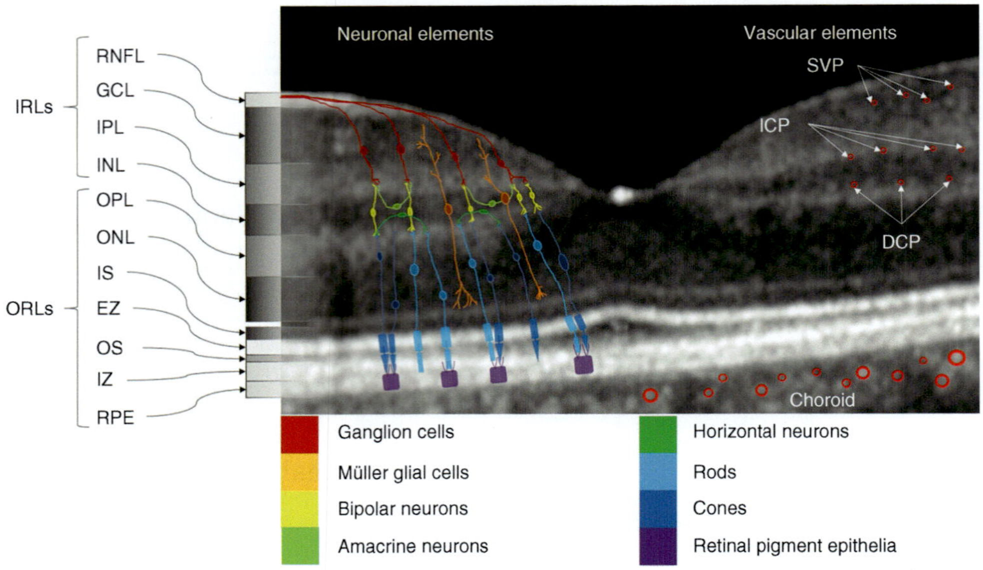

Fig. 16.1 Foveal microanatomy. Locations of neuronal elements (*left*) and vascular elements (*right*) superimposed on a spectral-domain optical coherence tomography (SDOCT) image of retinal layers. The inner retinal layers (IRLs) are divided into the retinal nerve fiber layer (RNFL), the ganglion cell layer (GCL), the inner plexiform layer (IPL), and the inner nuclear layer (INL). The outer retinal layers (ORLs) are divided into the outer plexiform layer (OPL), outer nuclear layer (ONL), the inner segments (IS) of photoreceptors, the ellipsoid zone (EZ), the outer segments (OS) of photoreceptors, the interdigitation zone (IZ), and the retinal pigment epithelium (RPE) with the choroid beneath. Cell bodies and nuclei are located in more hypo-reflective (darker) layers. Cellular projections are located in more hyper-reflective (lighter) layers. The vascular elements include the superficial vascular plexus (SVP), the deep capillary plexus (DCP), the intermediate capillary plexus (ICP) that bridges between the SVP and DCP, and the choroid. The SDOCT image is taken from a 10-year-old male born at term

ever, there are no vessels in the deeper foveal layers at this time [9]. These vessels (in the deeper plexuses) form by 32 weeks [9].

The formation of the structural layers below the pit occurs once the FAZ is fully enclosed by the perifoveal capillaries [10]. Between 25 and 27 weeks of gestation, the inner retinal layers are displaced peripherally to form the foveal pit, which is known as centrifugal migration [5]. During the formation of the pit, the GCL begins to thin in the fovea. Between 28 and 37 weeks of gestation, the foveal pit is distinct with the outward displacement of the GCL, IPL, and inner nuclear layer (INL) (Fig. 16.2). At the edges of the pit, the INL is divided by a layer of cytoplasm that separates the innermost cell bodies from the rest of the INL. This layer is known as the transient layer of Chievitz, which is constituted mainly by Muller cell processes that angle away from the foveal pit indicating the displacement of the neurons and the glia peripherally [2]. Between 37 and 39 weeks PMA, the layers are thinning at the foveal center (Fig. 16.3).

The foveal cones, although being the first cells to differentiate are the last to reach adult-like maturity [8, 13, 14]. The central foveal cones at 40 weeks gestation are only slightly more differentiated and taller than at 20 weeks. Retinal photoreceptors have a rudimentary inner segment and absent outer segments. The outer segments develop on the cones by 36 weeks gestation.

At birth, the fovea is still immature, as the outer nuclear layer (ONL) consists of morphologically immature cone photoreceptors and the foveal pit may still include the GCL and INL (Fig. 16.3). In the late prenatal and early postnatal periods, the choroid thickens due to an increased density of capillaries in the choriocapillaris and a large number of medium and large vessels in the inner and outer stroma also known as the Stattler's and Haller's layers, respectively [9].

16.1.3 After Birth

After birth, the overall layers at the foveal center continue to thicken, with the GCL, INL, and IPL becoming only 1–2 cells deep. Around 9–15 months, the GCL, IPL, and INL fuse into a single layer at the center of the foveal pit [4]. Between 28 months and 13 years, the pit becomes wider and shallower with only cone cell bodies at the center of the pit. The most striking changes after birth are in the outer plexiform layer (OPL) and the interdigitation zone (IZ) between the outer segments and RPE. The long cone axons are prominent across the central retina now making the OPL a much thicker layer. Central foveal cones develop elongated tapered inner segment and short outer segment when compared to the periphery [2, 5]. In general, IZ band is the last to mature and is not visualized before 46–47 weeks PMA [14–16]. By

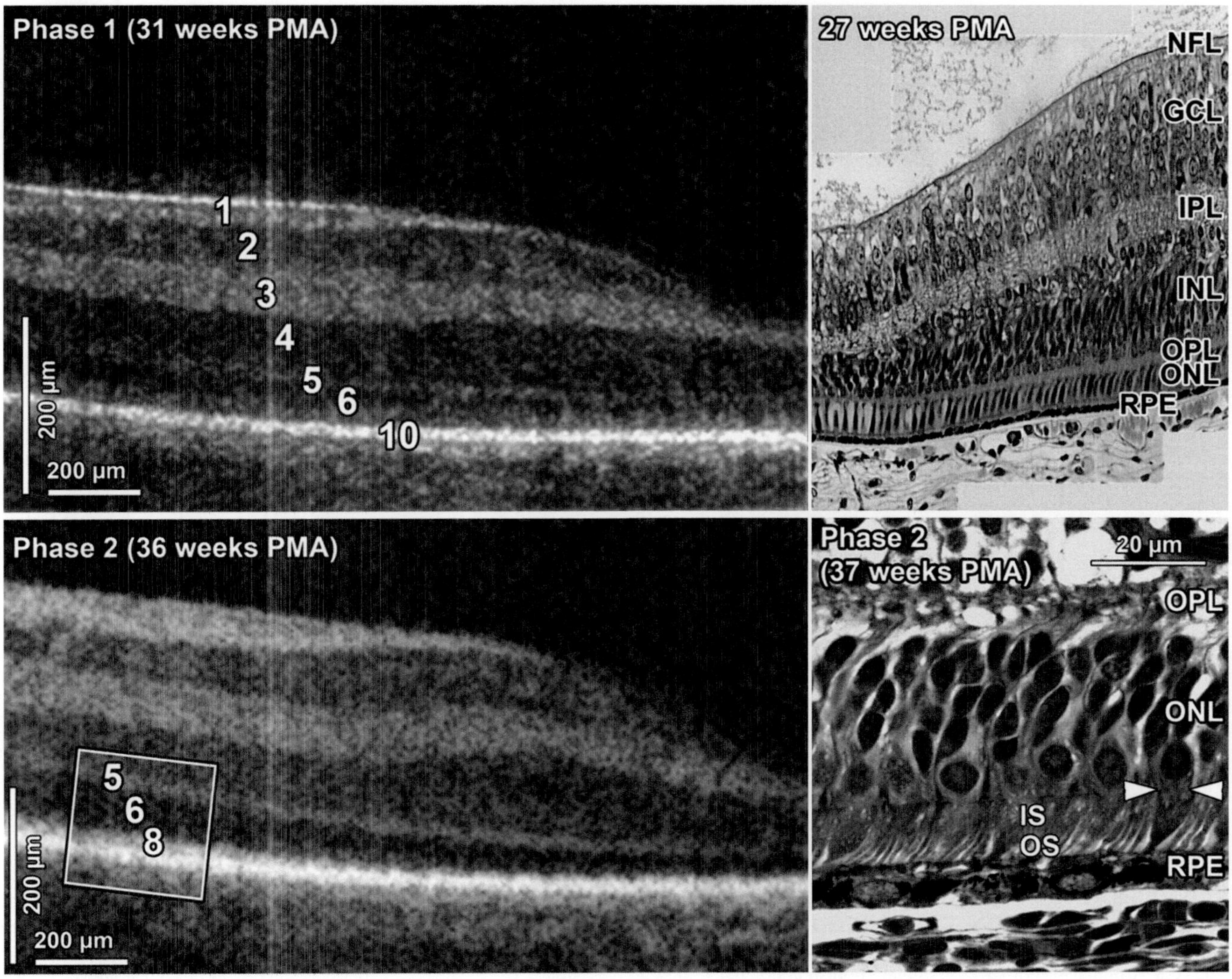

Fig. 16.2 Comparison of spectral-domain optical coherence tomography (SDOCT) to histology of foveal development in normal premature infant retinas early in the third trimester of development (top) and closer to term age (bottom). Inner layer development predominates here. SDOCT numeric bands are indicated on the OCT images (left) and can be compared to the light micrograph on the right (projected ~2:1 scale to match SDOCT). The GCL+IPL band at the fovea is primarily IPL. At 31 weeks the inner (IS) and outer (OS) segments are too short to separate band 8 from the RPE. By 36 weeks, the peripheral IS (bottom left, box) is now long enough to appear as a blurry band 8 in SDOCT. 1 = nerve fiber layer (NFL); 2 = ganglion cell layer (GCL); 3 = inner plexiform layer (IPL); 4 = inner nuclear layer (INL); 5 = outer plexiform layer on OCT and includes photoreceptor synapses (9 = OPL Photoreceptor synapses); however, Henle fibers (Ax) are hypo-reflective and included in 6 = outer nuclear layer (ONL/HFL) on OCT; 8 = immature ellipsoid zone (EZ); 10 = thin immature retinal pigment epithelium (RPE). (Adapted from Vajzovic L, Hendrickson AE, O'Connell RV, Clark LA, Tran-Viet D, Possin D, et al. Maturation of the human fovea: correlation of spectral-domain optical coherence tomography findings with histology. Am J Ophthalmol. 2012;154(5):779-82; with permission)

12–13 years, the fovea is mature in all aspects [5, 13, 14]. The choroidal pigmentation is first seen on the outer stroma after birth, which progressively increases within the stroma until adulthood [9].

16.1.4 OCT Imaging of Foveal Development

With the use of high-resolution, spectral-domain OCT (SDOCT) from 30 weeks PMA, the correlation of human foveal development on OCT with histopathology has been demonstrated (Fig. 16.4) [4, 17]. The retinal layer thicknesses change during foveal development. On SDOCT, the layers of the retina are displayed as alternating bands of hyper- and hypo-reflectivity that correspond to the layers defined by histology. These SDOCT bands are labeled from inner to outer: nerve fiber layer (NFL); GCL; IPL; INL; OPL; ONL, which includes Henle fiber layer (ONL+HFL); external limiting membrane (ELM); ellipsoid zone (EZ); outer segments (OS); and retinal pigment epithelium (RPE) [18, 19]. On SDOCT, axons are typically hyper-reflective. However, the photoreceptor axons in Henle's fiber layer are

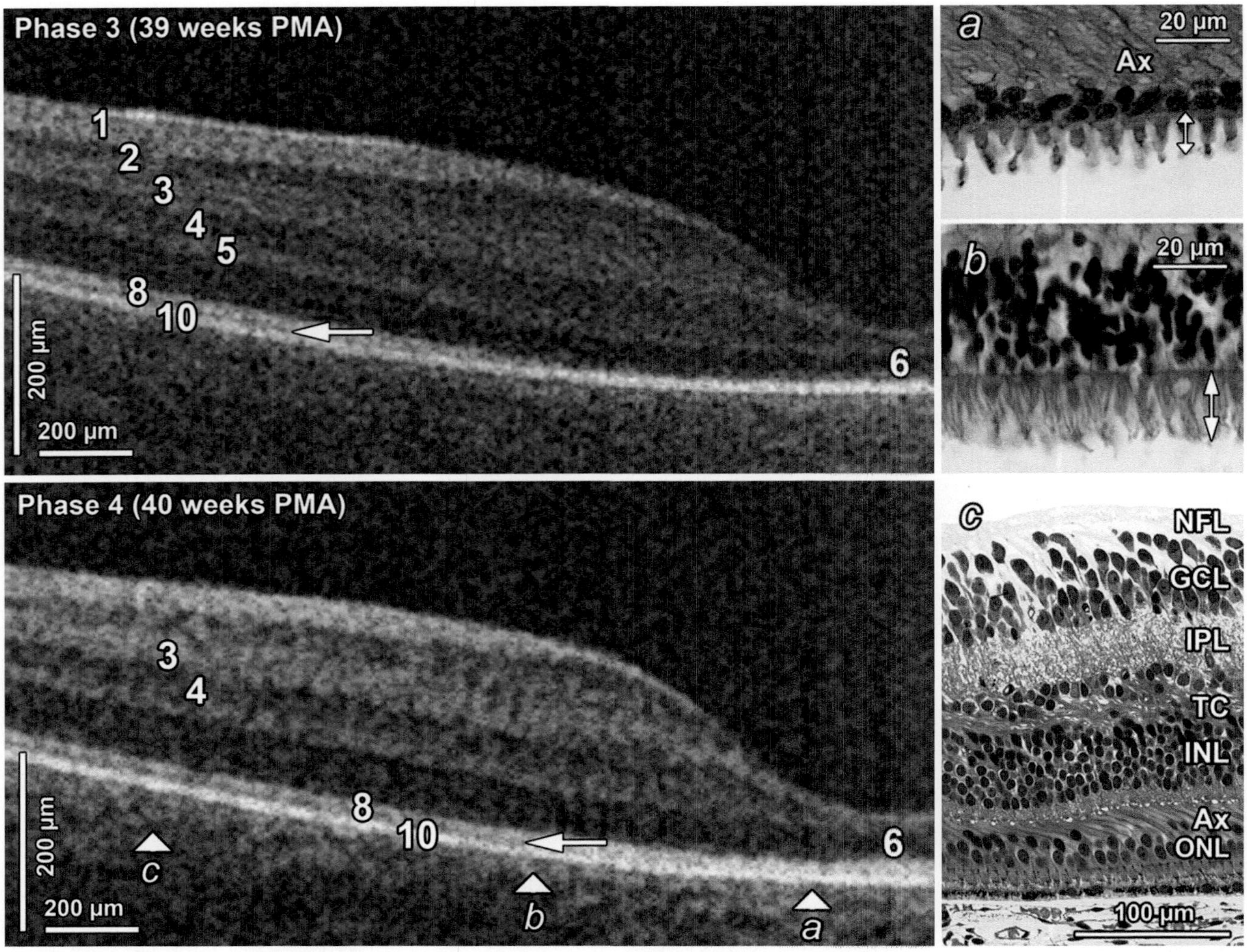

Fig. 16.3 Comparison of spectral domain optical coherence tomography (SDOCT) to histology of foveal development of the photoreceptor layers in normal term infants. Infants with retinopathy of prematurity may have delay. Inner retinal layers have collapsed together at the fovea, more so at 40 weeks PMA. Photoreceptors at the fovea begin their rapid growth in these phases. In phase 3 (Top left) the IS band was generally not discernable at the foveal center, while in phase 4 (Bottom left) this band is visible. The equivalent location of regions a, b, and c on the light micrographs (Right) are indicated on the SDOCT scan (Bottom left). On histology, lengths of IS+OS are notably shorter at the fovea than in the periphery (region a vs c, Right, white double-headed arrows). The elongation of OS in the periphery results in hypo-reflective band 9 (horizontal white arrow in SDOCT Top and Bottom left) that separates EZ from RPE. Henle axons (Ax, in regions a and c) would appear hypo-reflective and contribute to the thickness of band 6 outside the foveal center in SDOCT (Bottom left). 1 = nerve fiber layer (NFL); 2 = ganglion cell layer (GCL); 3 = inner plexiform layer (IPL); 4 = inner nuclear layer (INL); 5 = outer plexiform layer on OCT and includes photoreceptor synapses (OPL/PSL); however, Henle fibers (Ax) are included in 6 = outer nuclear layer (ONL/HFL) on OCT; 8 = photoreceptor inner segments ellipsoid (EZ); 10 = retinal pigment epithelium (RPE). (Adapted from Vajzovic L, Hendrickson AE, O'Connell RV, Clark LA, Tran-Viet D, Possin D, et al. Maturation of the human fovea: correlation of spectral-domain optical coherence tomography findings with histology. Am J Ophthalmol. 2012;154(5):779-89 e2; with permission)

hypo-reflective because of their alignment and distribution from the fovea. They are generally not distinguished from the photoreceptor nuclei. Thus, the hypo-reflective band, labeled ONL+HFL, includes the axons and nuclei and has been conventionally termed ONL [18].

Several groups have demonstrated a progressive increase in neurosensory retinal thickness across the macula from 30 weeks PMA (Fig. 16.5) [4, 14, 16]. The total neurosensory retinal thickness is found to be the thinnest in the fovea and the thickest in the periphery. As the age advances, the pit deepens, and the pit shoulders increase in height to create the greatest thickness difference in the foveal center and the parafoveal region (foveal/parafoveal ratio). The NFL is consistently thin in the fovea and changes very little here with age. The GCL+IPL layers are found to be thinner at the fovea than at the periphery. The INL shows pronounced thinning at

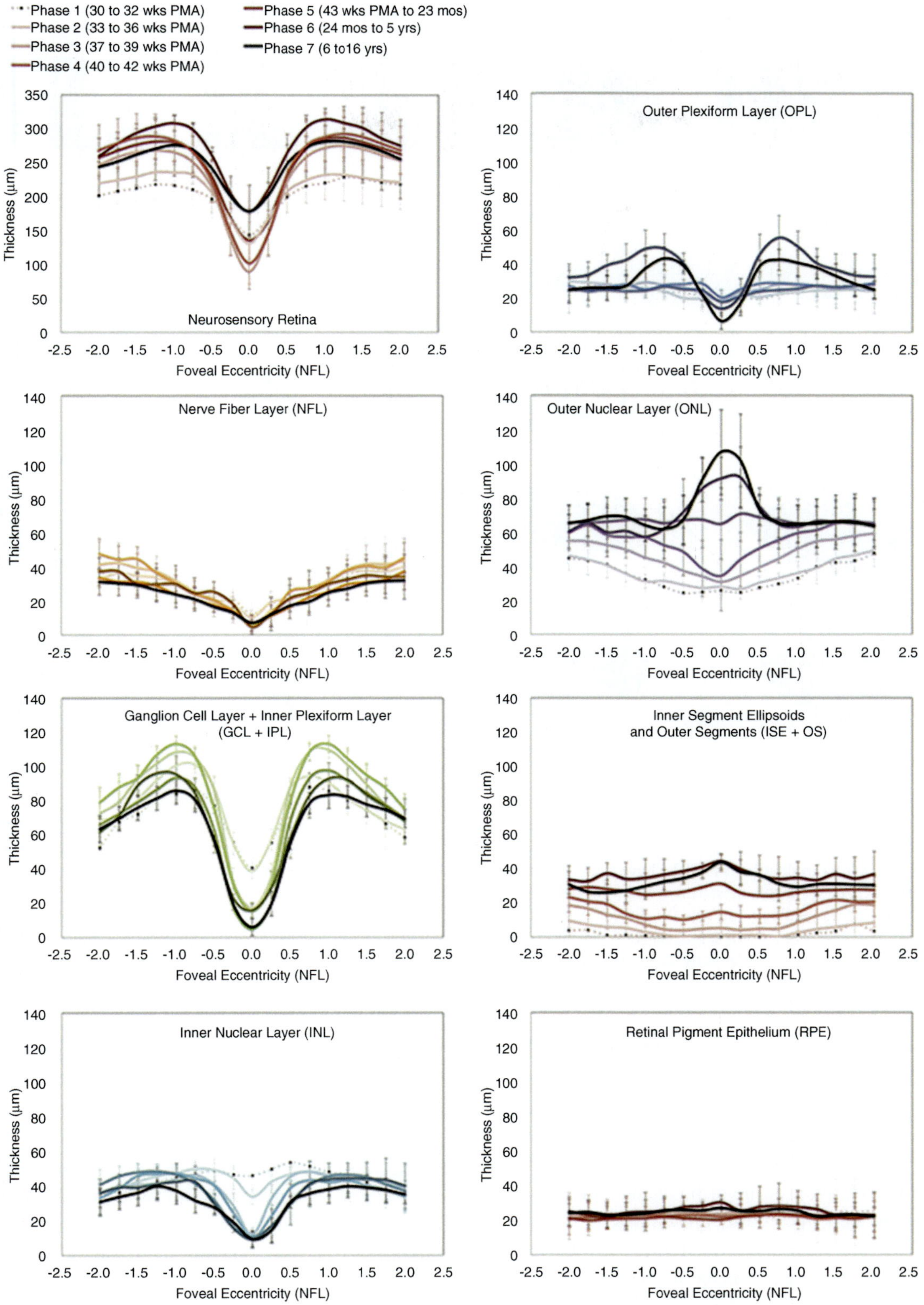

Fig. 16.4 Changes in Thickness of Foveal Layers from Preterm Period to Teenage Years. Mean retinal layer thicknesses are shown relative to their eccentricity from the foveal center at 0.0 mm. Measurements were from groups of infants and children (5–9 per subgroup in Phases 1–7) from 30 weeks postmenstrual age (PMA) to 16 years of age. The total retina is upper left. Inner retinal layers are in the left column and most of the change occurs in Phases 1–3 (the thickness lines are palest for the youngest phase (imaged from 30–32 weeks PMA) and darkest for the oldest phase (imaged at ages 6–16 years). Outer retinal layers are in the right column and the majority of the change is after Phase 2–3. Infants with macular edema of prematurity were excluded. (Adapted from Vajzovic L, Hendrickson AE, O'Connell RV, Clark LA, Tran-Viet D, Possin D, et al. Maturation of the human fovea: correlation of spectral-domain optical coherence tomography findings with histology. Am J Ophthalmol. 2012;154(5):779-89 e2; with permission)

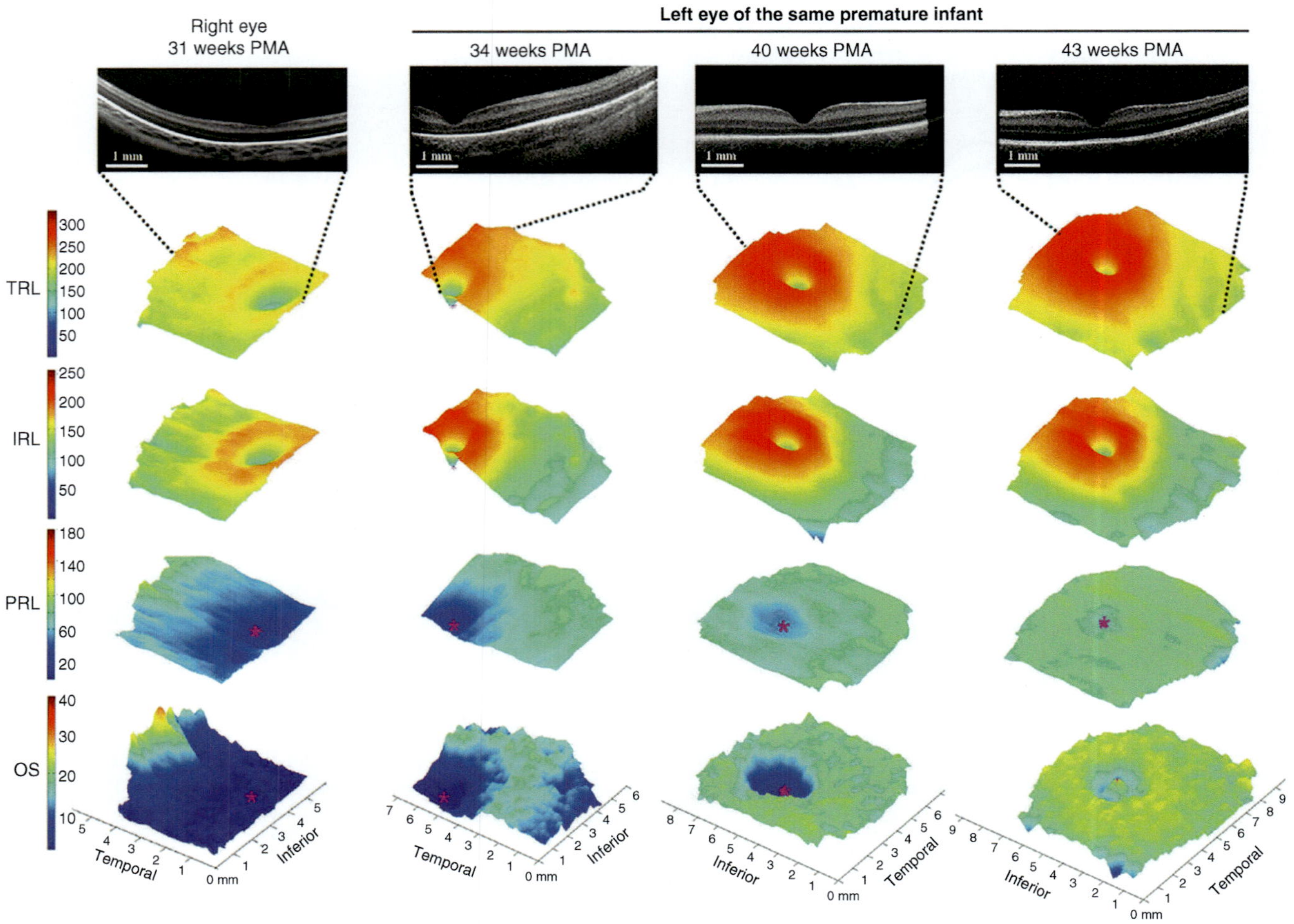

Fig. 16.5 A three-dimensional view of retinal layer development from 31 to 43 weeks postmenstrual age (PMA) in a preterm infant with zone II, stage 2 ROP. The total retinal layers (TRL) have the greatest contribution from the IRL (second thickness row), while the photoreceptor layer (PRL) remains exceedingly thin at the foveal center until 43 weeks PMA. The photoreceptor outer segments (OS) develop in a parafoveal annulus at 34 weeks and gradually develop toward the foveal center. Thickness quantities at a given region are represented by a color scale (on left). Foveal centers are marked by magenta asterisks. The central foveal B-scan (cross-sectional view) is shown at the top of each column. (Adapted from Maldonado RS, O'Connell RV, Sarin N, Freedman SF, Wallace DK, Cotten CM, et al. Dynamics of human foveal development after premature birth. Ophthalmology. 2011;118(12):2315-25; with permission)

the foveal center around 37–42 weeks PMA, while the hyperreflective OPL attains a flat contour around term age [4]. With cone packing and development, the ONL shows a profound increase at the fovea from 40 weeks PMA onwards, creating a bulge. The ELM is first seen at around 40 weeks PMA and the RPE shows little or no change throughout the development process [4]. Putting this all together, the immature preterm fovea from approximately 30–39 weeks actually thins at the foveal center as the inner retinal centrifugal migration occurs, then from 40 weeks PMA onward, the foveal thickness increases as photoreceptor development progresses [4]. By 12 years, the foveal thickness is comparable to the adult retina [14].

16.2 Effect of Prematurity and Retinopathy of Prematurity on Foveal Development

Retinopathy of prematurity (ROP) is a leading cause of blindness in preterm infants and varies from country to country depending on their socioeconomic development [20]. It is influenced by both genetic and environmental factors. Several genetic variants in EPAS1, VEGF, SOD, the WNT family and intron of BDNF have been found to be associated with ROP [21]. Prior to 30 weeks PMA, a major consequence of preterm birth is reduced expression of vascular endothelial growth factor (VEGF) in the retina, due to exposure to higher oxygen levels than in utero, resulting in slowed growth of retinal vessels [22]. The resulting hypoxia then drives elevated VEGF levels and other factors to result in ROP which is often perceived as only avascular disease. The neurosensory retina is also immature and affected by these growth factors. Thus, the effect of ROP on foveal development is influenced by both environmental and genetic factors associated with ROP that modulate active developmental processes, at multiple stages of gestation [7].

16.2.1 Formation of the Foveal Pit

Various imaging tools such as color fundus photos, fluorescein angiography (FA), OCT, and OCTA can be used to detect and understand macular neurovascular abnormalities in ROP [23–25]. Prior to the imaging era, data on foveal microanatomy in ROP, besides histopathology was gathered by clinical examination of the sequential appearance of three macular features: pigmentation, annular ring, and foveolar pit [26]. Preterm infants were noted to have a decrease in prominent foveal pigmentation, lack of annular reflex, and a poorly visualized foveal pit [26].

In infants born very preterm, the foveal pit formation may have barely begun; therefore, the infants born at this age are more likely to experience a range of structural variations that may result in visual impairments [27, 28]. Two main abnormal morphological findings in the inner and outer retinal layers in ROP are: persistent inner retinal layers (IRL), and immature photoreceptor layers resulting in a fovea plana which may be indistinguishable from foveal maldevelopment of albinism [29]. This has become apparent with OCT exams of infants and children with a history of preterm birth [16]. The persistence of IRL is characterized by the presence of GCL, IPL, and INL as distinct measurable layers at the foveal center [16, 30]. The persistence of GCL and INL in the central fovea suggests reduced outward migration of inner retinal neurons. It is important to note that the mechanism that mediates centrifugal (or radially outward) migration of inner retinal cells leading to the formation of the pit is independent of that of the outer retina and the photoreceptor layer, which mediate centripetal (or radially inward) displacement of the cones [4, 16]. The only identified structural abnormality thus far in the outer retina is a delay in the development of the EZ in preterm infants when compared to term infants [28]. Within the macula, choroidal vascular filling defects are common in aggressive posterior ROP [23]. Choroidal thickness development also continues after preterm birth and OCT studies have shown a delay in development in preterm infants relative to that of term infants [31]. This may be due to the oxidative stress or VEGF impacting this vascular plexus.

16.2.2 Neurovascular Development in the Fovea

Small or absent FAZ, observed on FA, is a hallmark of prematurity observed on FA [23, 32]. The smaller FAZ in prematurely born people [33, 34] may be explained by the delayed retinal vascular growth due to the exposure to oxygen-rich environment and the halted process of apoptosis that leads to the regression of vessels forming the FAZ [2, 32, 35]. Therefore, environmental factors could modify the expression of antiangiogenic factors that define FAZ and/or the timing of plexus formation may result in the delayed formation of FAZ in preterm infants [7].

Children with a history of ROP have been found to have a smaller FAZ when compared to age-matched controls [24], and further, children with a history of Type I ROP have shown a smaller FAZ when compared to normal children [25]. The persistence of a spider-web like central foveal capillary network on OCTA has been associated with the absence of the foveal pit on the structural OCT [24, 36]. The reason for this may be that a small FAZ with the presence of capillaries and astrocytes close to the foveola retards the centrifugal migration of the inner retinal layers during development [37]. Chen and colleagues imaged the central macular region of a premature infant from 33 weeks to 35 weeks PMA and highlighted that the vascularized retina (adjacent to the FAZ-to-be) is thicker than the non-vascular retina and the deep vascular plexus is not visible at this age, consistent with historical histopathological findings [38, 39].

Retinal vascular filling defects, seen as hypoflouresence on FA, are known to occur in aggressive posterior ROP [23]. Macular microvascular anomalies have also been reported after treatment of type 1 ROP, and these show violation of vascular stratification, with large superficial vessels diving from the IPL into INL, and deeper superficial vascular complex vessels located closer to the IPL associated with incomplete perifoveal deep vascular complex development (Figs. 16.6 and 16.7) [40]. These findings demonstrate how the retinal perifoveal microvasculature undergoes an active developmental and remodeling process during the critical postnatal period of ROP pathogenesis [40].

16.2.3 Other Foveal Findings Associated with ROP

Macular edema of prematurity (MEOP) has been detected incidentally during SDOCT imaging of infants with ROP by various research groups across the world (Fig. 16.8) [41–44]. MEOP is bilateral, symmetric, isolated in the INL, and typically causes foveal bulging hypo-reflective cystoid spaces separated by hyper-reflective septae. This has generally not

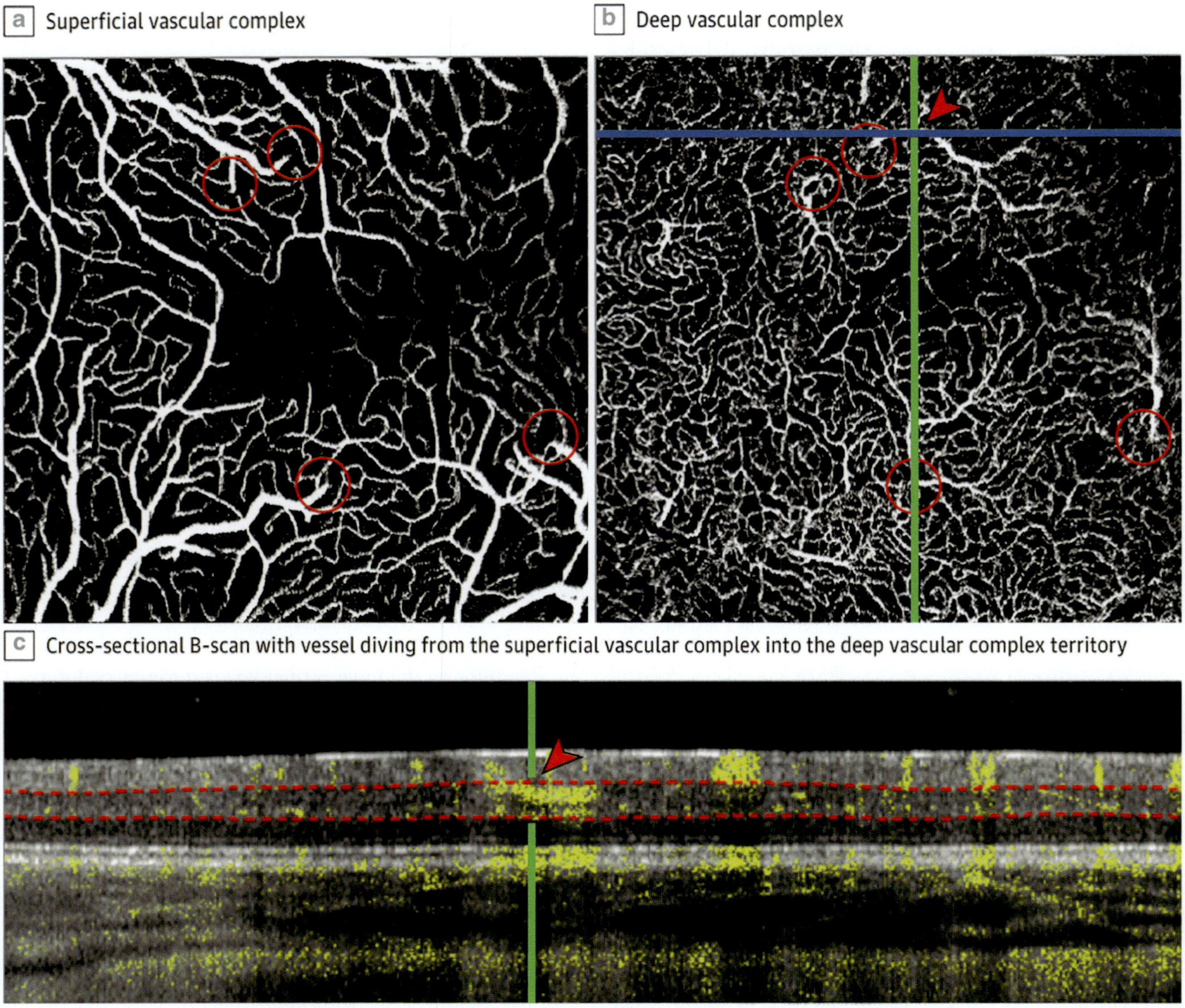

Fig. 16.6 Vascular anomalies on optical coherence tomography angiography (OCTA) in the macula of a 17-month-old child. The child was born at 24 weeks and 410 g and received intravitreal anti-VEGF and laser of avascular retina for retinopathy of prematurity. Large vessels from the superficial vascular complex (SVC) do not remain within the SVC as expected; they dive into the deep vascular complex (red circles in panel A and panel B; red arrow in panel C). (Adapted from Hsu ST, Chen X, House RJ, Kelly MP, Toth CA, Vajzovic L. Visualizing Macular Microvasculature Anomalies in 2 Infants With Treated Retinopathy of Prematurity. JAMA Ophthalmol. 2018;136(12):1422-4; with permission)

persisted beyond 42 weeks PMA [43, 45]; however, when it has persisted it has been associated with poor neurodevelopmental and visual outcomes [46, 47]. Whether this is intra- or extra-cellular fluid and due to oxygen or VEGF imbalance or other transient structural or fluid events or even inflammation is not yet known. Infants with MEOP have also demonstrated a delay in the development of photoreceptors [28]. The role of ROP in MEOP remains unclear, as the presence or absence of MEOP was not associated with ROP outcomes [42]. While the etiology of MEOP remains unclear, a number of studies have identified neurodevelopmental and functional outcomes suggesting that this is a pathological phenomenon rather than a phenotypic variant of development [45–48].

16.2.4 Retinal Schisis and Detachment in ROP

Schisis and detachment may affect the foveal center in ROP. Tractional retinal schisis in contrast to MEOP is often flat and associated with epiretinal membrane rather than bulging at the foveal center. The foveal involvement may be difficult to determine in advanced stages of ROP on clinical

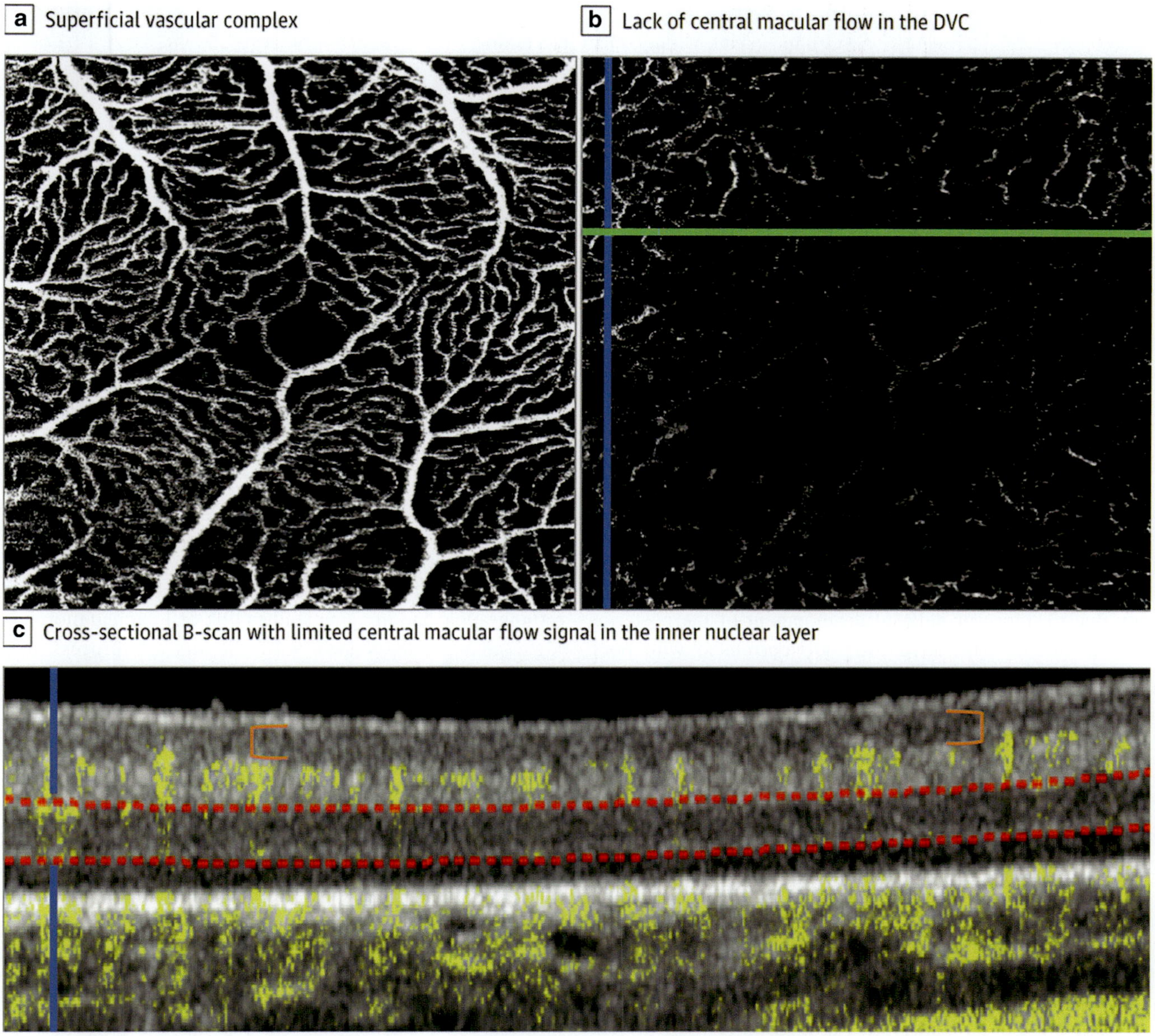

Fig. 16.7 A very small foveal avascular zone (FAZ) and abnormal location of vascular complexes within the retina observed on optical coherence tomography angiography (OCTA) of the macula of an infant with 4A retinopathy of prematurity (ROP). The infant was born at 24 weeks and had prior laser treatment for ROP OU. Panel A shows the small FAZ. Panel B shows the lack of vascular flow toward the center in the deep vascular complex (DVC) and the DVC segmentation is between the red dotted lines in panel C. Panel C shows the unusually deep location of the presumed SVC, below the orange brackets. (Adapted from Hsu ST, Chen X, House RJ, Kelly MP, Toth CA, Vajzovic L. Visualizing Macular Microvasculature Anomalies in 2 Infants With Treated Retinopathy of Prematurity. JAMA Ophthalmol. 2018;136(12):1422-4; with permission)

examination (Ex: Stage 4, whether 4A or 4B). These findings are readily visualized with macular SDOCT imaging which is especially helpful in advanced stages of ROP. For example, clinically undetected retinoschisis has been identified in multiple infants with Type I ROP [49] and OCT has been used to detect subclinical detachment at the fovea that was unrecognized on ophthalmoscopic examination, thus, revealing Stage 4B ROP [41, 50, 51]. OCT imaging of these findings, although transient during development, may be used to determine the response to novel clinical treatments for ROP [51].

Foveal development may be assessed by tests of function which currently involve preferential looking using Teller acuity cards [52], contrast sensitivity, and optotype visual acuity. The association between macular structure and visual function from the Early Treatment for Retinopathy of Prematurity study showed that while unfavorable morphol-

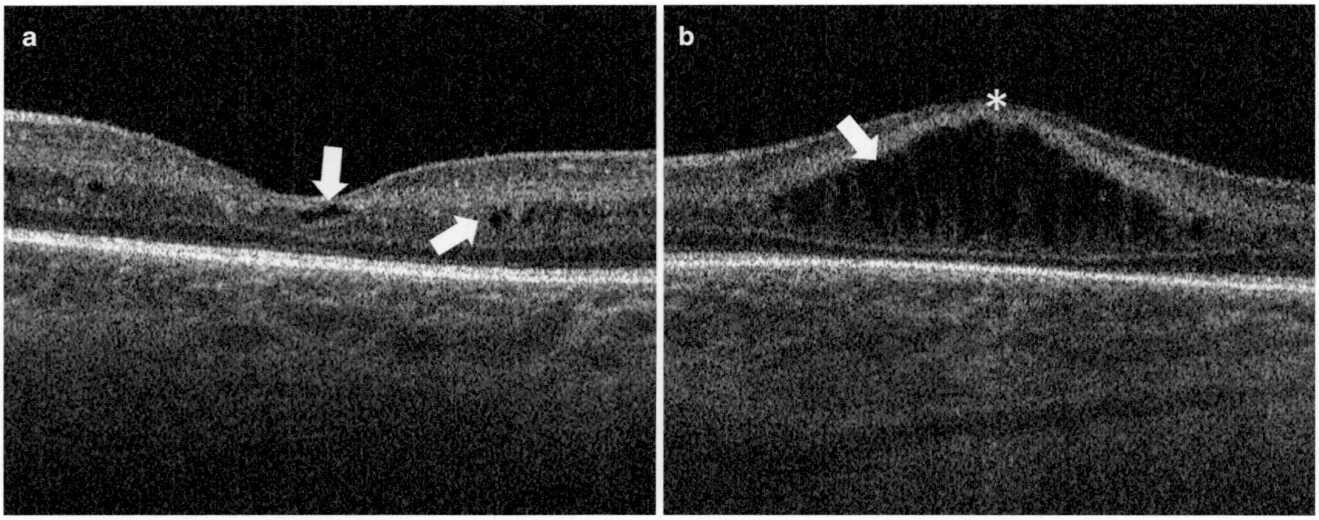

Fig. 16.8 Mild and severe cases of macular edema of prematurity (MEOP) in infants with retinopathy of prematurity. MEOP is located exclusively within the inner nuclear layer. (**a**) At 39 weeks PMA, the infant has mild MEOP with concave fovea and compact cystoid spaces (two white arrows). (**b**) At approximately 42 weeks, this infant still has severe MEOP with a bulging fovea and elongated cystoid spaces (white arrow). The white asterisk marks an approximation of the foveal center

ogy due to injury or delayed development of the posterior pole in infants with advanced ROP correlated with poor visual acuity, many of these infants had a normal-appearing macula and yet had subnormal visual acuity [53]. Thus, transient ROP effects on the fovea may have a lasting impact on vision. Additional more sensitive measures of distinct cone and rod function have been used to further investigate this impact. Maturation of normal rod photoreceptor and rod-driven post-receptor retinal processes can be demonstrated by analysis of the electroretinogram (ERG) a- and b-wave responses to full-field, brief flashes that span a several log unit range of stimulus intensities [54]. The multifocal ERG (mfERG) provides topographical information about the central retina. While cone-driven bipolar cells (post-receptor retina) are the main contributors to mfERG responses, both cones and rods are found in this region, ROP zone 1 [55]. Infants with mild ROP have delayed maturation of rod-mediated retinal sensitivity and also have deficits in cone-driven post-receptor activity [55].

16.3 Summary

The advent of OCT and OCTA imaging in preterm infant development and injury has significantly contributed to our understanding of the retinal and foveal microanatomy in the preterm infants, including those with ROP. These newer imaging modalities have provided useful new perspectives on macular neurovascular development and in in-vivo documentation of age-appropriate maturation associated with preterm birth and ROP. Information derived from electroretinographic and imaging studies link cellular and morphologic changes associated with the disease process and function. These point to the importance of recognizing ROP as a *neuro*vascular disease that not only affects vascular development, but it also has an impact on the development of neural tissue and their complex partnership in development.

References

1. Mann I. The development of the human eye. London: Cambridge University Press; 1928.
2. Hendrickson AE, Yuodelis C. The morphological development of the human fovea. Ophthalmology. 1984;91(6):603–12.
3. Hendrickson A. A morphological comparison of foveal development in man and monkey. Eye (Lond). 1992;6(Pt 2):136–44.
4. Vajzovic L, Hendrickson AE, O'Connell RV, Clark LA, Tran-Viet D, Possin D, et al. Maturation of the human fovea: correlation of spectral-domain optical coherence tomography findings with histology. Am J Ophthalmol. 2012;154(5):779–89 e2.
5. Hendrickson A, Possin D, Vajzovic L, Toth CA. Histologic development of the human fovea from midgestation to maturity. Am J Ophthalmol. 2012;154(5):767–78.e2.
6. Edward DP, Kaufman LM. Anatomy, development, and physiology of the visual system. Pediatr Clin N Am. 2003;50(1):1–23.
7. Provis JM, Madigan MC. Foveal development and photoreceptor development. In: Hartnett ME, editor. Pediatric retina. 2nd ed. Philadelphia, PA: Lippincott Williams & Wilkins; 2013.
8. Provis JM, van Driel D, Billson FA, Russell P. Development of the human retina: patterns of cell distribution and redistribution in the ganglion cell layer. J Comp Neurol. 1985;233(4):429–51.
9. Gariano RF, Iruela-Arispe ML, Hendrickson AE. Vascular development in primate retina: comparison of laminar plexus formation in monkey and human. Invest Ophthalmol Vis Sci. 1994;35(9):3442–55.

10. Provis JM, Sandercoe T, Hendrickson AE. Astrocytes and blood vessels define the foveal rim during primate retinal development. Invest Ophthalmol Vis Sci. 2000;41(10):2827–36.
11. Hendrickson A, Troilo D, Possin D, Springer A. Development of the neural retina and its vasculature in the marmoset Callithrix jacchus. J Comp Neurol. 2006;497(2):270–86.
12. Sandercoe TM, Madigan MC, Billson FA, Penfold PL, Provis JM. Astrocyte proliferation during development of the human retinal vasculature. Exp Eye Res. 1999;69(5):511–23.
13. Yuodelis C, Hendrickson A. A qualitative and quantitative analysis of the human fovea during development. Vis Res. 1986;26(6):847–55.
14. Lee H, Purohit R, Patel A, Papageorgiou E, Sheth V, Maconachie G, et al. In vivo foveal development using optical coherence tomography. Invest Ophthalmol Vis Sci. 2015;56(8):4537–45.
15. Lee H, Proudlock FA, Gottlob I. Pediatric optical coherence tomography in clinical practice—Recent progress in pediatric OCT in clinical practice. Invest Ophthalmol Vis Sci. 2016;57(9):OCT69–79.
16. Maldonado RS, O'Connell RV, Sarin N, Freedman SF, Wallace DK, Cotten CM, et al. Dynamics of human foveal development after premature birth. Ophthalmology. 2011;118(12):2315–25.
17. Dubis AM, Costakos DM, Subramaniam CD, Godara P, Wirostko WJ, Carroll J, et al. Evaluation of normal human foveal development using optical coherence tomography and histologic examination. Arch Ophthalmol. 2012;130(10):1291–300.
18. Spaide RF, Curcio CA. Anatomical correlates to the bands seen in the outer retina by optical coherence tomography: literature review and model. Retina. 2011;31(8):1609–19.
19. Lujan BJ, Roorda A, Knighton RW, Carroll J. Revealing Henle's fiber layer using spectral domain optical coherence tomography. Invest Ophthalmol Vis Sci. 2011;52(3):1486–92.
20. Gilbert C. Retinopathy of prematurity: a global perspective of the epidemics, population of babies at risk and implications for control. Early Hum Dev. 2008;84(2):77–82.
21. Hartnett ME, Cotten CM. Genomics in the neonatal nursery: focus on ROP. Semin Perinatol. 2015;39(8):604–10.
22. Hellstrom A, Smith LE, Dammann O. Retinopathy of prematurity. Lancet. 2013;382(9902):1445–57.
23. Lepore D, Molle F, Pagliara MM, Baldascino A, Angora C, Sammartino M, et al. Atlas of fluorescein angiographic findings in eyes undergoing laser for retinopathy of prematurity. Ophthalmology. 2011;118(1):168–75.
24. Falavarjani KG, Iafe NA, Velez FG, Schwartz SD, Sadda SR, Sarraf D, et al. Optical coherence tomography angiography of the fovea in children born preterm. Retina. 2017;37(12):2289–94.
25. Nonobe N, Kaneko H, Ito Y, Takayama K, Kataoka K, Tsunekawa T, et al. Optical coherence tomography angiography of the foveal avascular zone in children with a history of treatment-requiring retinopathy of prematurity. Retina. 2017;39:1.
26. Isenberg SJ. Macular development in the premature infant. Am J Ophthalmol. 1986;101(1):74–80.
27. O'Connor AR, Wilson CM, Fielder AR. Ophthalmological problems associated with preterm birth. Eye (Lond). 2007;21(10):1254–60.
28. Vajzovic L, Rothman AL, Tran-Viet D, Cabrera MT, Freedman SF, Toth CA. Delay in retinal photoreceptor development in very preterm compared to term infants. Invest Ophthalmol Vis Sci. 2015;56(2):908–13.
29. Lee H, Purohit R, Sheth V, Papageorgiou E, Maconachie G, McLean RJ, et al. Retinal development in albinism: a prospective study using optical coherence tomography in infants and young children. Lancet. 2015;385(Suppl 1):S14.
30. Vinekar A, Mangalesh S, Jayadev C, Maldonado RS, Bauer N, Toth CA. Retinal imaging of infants on spectral domain optical coherence tomography. Biomed Res Int. 2015;2015:782420.
31. Moreno TA, O'Connell RV, Chiu SJ, Farsiu S, Cabrera MT, Maldonado RS, et al. Choroid development and feasibility of choroidal imaging in the preterm and term infants utilizing SD-OCT. Invest Ophthalmol Vis Sci. 2013;54(6):4140–7.
32. Mintz-Hittner HA, Knight-Nanan DM, Satriano DR, Kretzer FL. A small foveal avascular zone may be an historic mark of prematurity. Ophthalmology. 1999;106(7):1409–13.
33. Yanni SE, Wang J, Chan M, Carroll J, Farsiu S, Leffler JN, et al. Foveal avascular zone and foveal pit formation after preterm birth. Br J Ophthalmol. 2012;96(7):961–6.
34. Mintz-Hittner HA, Kretzer FL. Postnatal retinal vascularization in former preterm infants with retinopathy of prematurity. Ophthalmology. 1994;101(3):548–58.
35. Balasubramanian S, Borrelli E, Lonngi M, Velez F, Sarraf D R. Sadda S, et al. Visual function and optical coherence tomography angiography features in children born preterm. Retina 2018, 39(11):2233-2239
36. Takagi M, Maruko I, Yamaguchi A, Kakehashi M, Hasegawa T, Iida T. Foveal abnormalities determined by optical coherence tomography angiography in children with history of retinopathy of prematurity. Eye. 2019;
37. Chui TY, Zhong Z, Song H, Burns SA. Foveal avascular zone and its relationship to foveal pit shape. Optom Vis Sci. 2012;89(5):602–10.
38. Chen X, Viehland C, Tran-Viet D, Prakalapakorn SG, Freedman SF, Izatt JA, et al. Capturing macular vascular development in an infant with retinopathy of prematurity. JAMA Ophthalmol. 2019;137(9):1083–6.
39. Provis JM. Development of the primate retinal vasculature. Prog Retin Eye Res. 2001;20(6):799–821.
40. Hsu ST, Chen X, House RJ, Kelly MP, Toth CA, Vajzovic L. Visualizing macular microvasculature anomalies in 2 infants with treated retinopathy of prematurity. JAMA Ophthalmol. 2018;136(12):1422–4.
41. Lee AC, Maldonado RS, Sarin N, O'Connell RV, Wallace DK, Freedman SF, et al. Macular features from spectral-domain optical coherence tomography as an adjunct to indirect ophthalmoscopy in retinopathy of prematurity. Retina. 2011;31(8):1470–82.
42. Maldonado RS, O'Connell R, Ascher SB, Sarin N, Freedman SF, Wallace DK, et al. Spectral-domain optical coherence tomographic assessment of severity of cystoid macular edema in retinopathy of prematurity. Arch Ophthalmol. 2012;130(5):569–78.
43. Vinekar A, Avadhani K, Sivakumar M, Mahendradas P, Kurian M, Braganza S, et al. Understanding clinically undetected macular changes in early retinopathy of prematurity on spectral domain optical coherence tomography. Invest Ophthalmol Vis Sci. 2011;52(8):5183–8.
44. Dubis AM, Subramaniam CD, Godara P, Carroll J, Costakos DM. Subclinical macular findings in infants screened for retinopathy of prematurity with spectral-domain optical coherence tomography. Ophthalmology. 2013;120(8):1665–71.
45. Vinekar A, Mangalesh S, Jayadev C, Bauer N, Munusamy S, Kemmanu V, et al. Macular edema in Asian Indian premature infants with retinopathy of prematurity: Impact on visual acuity and refractive status after 1-year. Indian J Ophthalmol. 2015;63(5):432–7.
46. Rothman AL, Tran-Viet D, Gustafson KE, Goldstein RF, Maguire MG, Tai V, et al. Poorer neurodevelopmental outcomes associated with cystoid macular edema identified in preterm infants in the intensive care nursery. Ophthalmology. 2015;122(3):610–9.
47. Rothman AL, Tran-Viet D, Vajzovic L, Tai V, Sarin N, Holgado S, et al. Functional outcomes of young infants with and without macular edema. Retina. 2015;35(10):2018–27.
48. Rothman AL, Mangalesh S, Chen X, Toth CA. Optical coherence tomography of the preterm eye: from retinopathy of prematurity to brain development. Eye Brain. 2016;8:123–33.

49. Muni RH, Kohly RP, Charonis AC, Lee TC. Retinoschisis detected with handheld spectral-domain optical coherence tomography in neonates with advanced retinopathy of prematurity. Arch Ophthalmol. 2010;128(1):57–62.
50. Chavala SH, Farsiu S, Maldonado R, Wallace DK, Freedman SF, Toth CA. Insights into advanced retinopathy of prematurity using handheld spectral domain optical coherence tomography imaging. Ophthalmology. 2009;116(12):2448–56.
51. Smith LEH, Hellstrom A, Stahl A, Fielder A, Chambers W, Moseley J, et al. Development of a retinopathy of prematurity activity scale and clinical outcome measures for use in clinical trials. JAMA Ophthalmol. 2018;137(3):305–11.
52. Mayer DL, Beiser AS, Warner AF, Pratt EM, Raye KN, Lang JM. Monocular acuity norms for the teller acuity cards between ages one month and four years. Invest Ophthalmol Vis Sci. 1995;36(3):671–85.
53. Wallace DK, Bremer DL, Good WV, Fellows R, Summers CG, Tung B, et al. Correlation of recognition visual acuity with posterior retinal structure in advanced retinopathy of prematurity-recognition visual acuity and retinal structure. JAMA Ophthalmol. 2012;130(12):1512–6.
54. Fulton AB, Hansen RM, Moskowitz A, Akula JD. The neurovascular retina in retinopathy of prematurity. Prog Retin Eye Res. 2009;28(6):452–82.
55. Moskowitz A, Hansen RM, Fulton AB. Retinal, visual, and refractive development in retinopathy of prematurity. Eye Brain. 2016;8:103–11.

Neurodevelopmental Outcomes Following Anti-VEGF Treatment for ROP

17

Yuan-Yao Fan and Wei-Chi Wu

Abstract

Although BEAT-ROP study has demonstrated no increased rates of death or severe ocular adverse events in ROP infants receiving IVB compared to those receiving conventional laser, concerns about the safety of IVB in newborns are still being raised. Pharmacokinetic studies have shown suppression of serum VEGF levels after IVB in ROP infants, and laboratory studies have shown that VEGF plays a role in neurogenesis in embryo and newborn. Investigation of the impact of IVB in newborns on neurodevelopment have been addressed in only a few studies. However, those studies have shown inconsistent conclusion, also all of them had certain bias and were limited by their small case number. Currently, there is no consensus on how to use IVB properly in ROP patients in regard to both its safety and effectivity. Further studies are needed to provide stronger evidence regarding the impact of IVB on neurodevelopment.

Keywords

ROP · IVI · Anti-VEGF · Bevacizumab · BEAT-ROP
Safety · Pharmacokinetics · Neurodevelopment
Bayley-II · Bayley-III

Y.-Y. Fan (✉)
Department of Ophthalmology, Chang Gung Memorial Hospital, Taoyuan, Taiwan

W.-C. Wu
Department of Ophthalmology, Chang Gung Memorial Hospital, Taoyuan, Taiwan

College of Medicine, Chang Gung University, Taoyuan, Taiwan

Abbreviations

BEAT-ROP	Bevacizumab eliminates the angiogenic threat of ROP
BW	Birth weight
ETROP	Early treatment for ROP
GA	Gestational age
IVB	Intravitreal injection of bevacizumab
IVI	Intravitreal injection
IVR	Intravitreal injection of ranibizumab
NICU	Neonatal intensive care unit
ROP	Retinopathy of prematurity
VEGF	Vascular endothelial growth factor

The treatment of retinopathy of prematurity (ROP) aims at halting the pathological neovascularization propelled by an elevation in intraocular vascular endothelial growth factor (VEGF) [1]. Although laser photoablation of the peripheral avascular retina remains the standard ROP treatment, VEGF inhibition treatment by intraocular delivery of anti-vascular endothelial growth factor (anti-VEGF) has gradually increased after Bevacizumab Eliminates the Angiogenic Threat of ROP (BEAT-ROP) study showed a significant benefit of intravitreal injections of bevacizumab (IVB) over laser treatment for zone I stage 3+ (i.e., stage 3 with plus disease) ROP cases [2]. However, safety issues were too difficult to address in the BEAT-ROP study owing to the small sample size and relatively low rates of severe adverse events recorded in the study (i.e., cornea opacity requiring corneal transplant, lens opacity requiring cataract removal, and death). Power analysis has determined that a patient population as large as 2800 infants, which is difficult to achieve, would be needed to demonstrate whether IVB is associated with a significantly higher mortality rate compared to laser treatment [2, 3]. Therefore, although currently no data have been reported regarding increased rates of death or severe adverse events in ROP infants receiving IVB [2, 4], ongoing concerns about the safety of IVB in those newborns have still been raised

W.-C. Wu, W.-C. Lam (eds.), *A Quick Guide to Pediatric Retina*, https://doi.org/10.1007/978-981-15-6552-6_17

[5–7], and there are currently no definite conclusions regarding how to properly use IVB for ROP treatment.

Studies of the pharmacokinetics of IVB in ROP infants have shown that bevacizumab molecules enter systemic circulation and affect serum VEGF levels. A study by Sato et al. demonstrated a suppression of systemic VEGF levels for at least 2 weeks after intravitreal injection (IVI) of either 0.25 mg or 0.5 mg bevacizumab in infants with stages 3, 4, and 5 ROP [8]. Kong et al. showed that serum VEGF levels dropped 2 days after either laser treatment or IVB at different doses (0.25 mg or 0.625 mg) was given to ROP infants and that the reductions were more significant in IVB-treated patients [9]. They also found a detectable level of serum bevacizumab in those infants 60 days after IVB [9]. A series of studies by Wu et al. [10–12] further showed that serum VEGF levels in type 1 ROP infants were suppressed for as long as 12 weeks after 0.625 mg IVB was given [10–12].

Laboratory studies have shown a role of VEGF in neurogenesis in embryos as well as in newborn infants. Breier et al. [13] found abundant VEGF mRNA levels in the ventricular neuroectoderm of embryonic and neonatal murine brains when endothelial cells rapidly proliferate, while adult murine brains had reduced levels of VEGF transcripts when endothelial cell proliferation ceased [13]. Bagnard et al. [14] found that VEGF165 promotes the migration, survival, and proliferation of a neural progenitor cell line [14]. Jin et al. [15] found that VEGF treatment enhances embryonic cortical neural progenitor cell proliferation in vitro and that intracerebroventricular administration of VEGF stimulates neurogenesis, astrocyte production, and endothelial cell growth in the hippocampus and the lateral subventricular zone in adult rats [15]. Zhang et al. [16] found that neural progenitors derived from the newborn rat rostral subventricular zone expressed VEGF receptors after fibroblast growth factor 2 (FGF2) stimulation, and VEGF guided the directed migration of those undifferentiated neural progenitors [16]. In a study by Malik et al. [17], VEGF expression was found to be lower in preterm rabbit newborns than in term newborns [17]. Additionally, treatment with hypoxia-mimetics after preterm delivery not only significantly increased VEGF levels but also restored neurogenesis in these preterm rabbit pups [17]. Furthermore, by studying human samples from spontaneous abortus and dead premature infants, Malik et al. also found that significant neurogenesis continued in human preterm infants born at a gestational age (GA) of less than or equal to 28 weeks [17]. Therefore, deprivation of serum VEGF may lead to neurodevelopmental delay and reduced growth of the cerebral cortex in preterm newborns.

Since VEGF plays a role in neurogenesis in embryos and preterm infants, the impact of IVI anti-VEGF, when performed on premature newborns, on neurodevelopment is of interest for a better understanding of the safety issues (Fig. 17.1). However, neurodevelopmental outcomes after IVB for ROP have been addressed in only a few studies. In a prospective noncomparative case series by Martínez-Castellanos et al. [18], infants who received IVB for ROP were evaluated annually by the pediatricians using the standardized Denver Developmental Screening Test II. The majority of patients showed normal neurodevelopmental scores 5 years after the use of IVB, while one patient experienced developmental delay in personal social skills (25th percentile), language skills (25th percentile), and fine motor adaptive skills (50th percentile) [18]. However, the study was limited by its relatively small number of patients (18 eyes of 13 patients) as well as its noncomparative design, making it difficult to determine whether there were actual neurodevelopmental differences between IVB-treated preterm infants and untreated infants.

Morin et al. [6] first compared the neurodevelopmental outcomes of 125 preterm infants treated with IVB ($n = 27$) and laser ablation ($n = 98$) using the Bayley Scales of Infant and Toddler Development (Bayley-III) for assessment. In this retrospective study, they found a significantly lower motor composite score in patients receiving IVB than in those receiving laser ablation (median: 81 vs. 88, respectively; $p = 0.02$), while no differences were noted in the cognitive and language composite scores. They further investigated the risks of neurodevelopmental impairment and found higher odds of motor composite score <85, neurodevelopmental impairment (defined as cerebral palsy, sensorineural/mixed hearing loss, visual impairment, or Bayley-III composite scores <85), and severe neurodevelopmental disability (defined as cerebral palsy with Gross Motor Function Classification Scale of 3,4, or 5, requirements for hearing

Fig. 17.1 Concerns about the effects of IVB on neurodevelopment in newborns have been raised

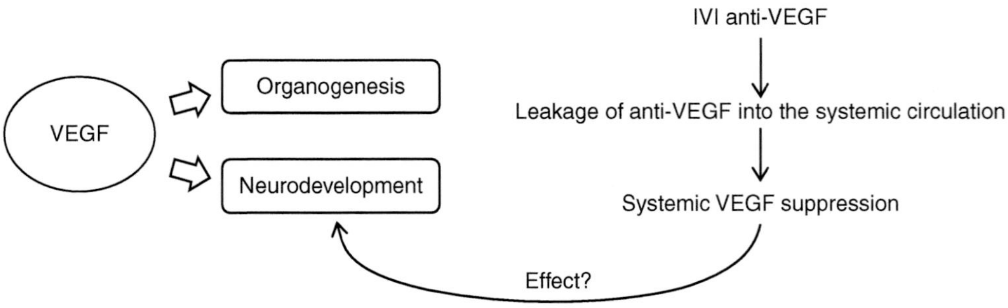

aids or cochlear implants, bilateral visual impairment, visual acuity poorer than 20/70, or Bayley-III composite scores <70) in patients receiving IVB than in those receiving laser ablation [6]. However, it is worth noting that the neurodevelopmental disabilities in that study may not be reliable indicators of neurodevelopmental outcomes, since some of the included items were questionable. First, cerebral palsy is not a postnatal neurodevelopmental disorder. In contrast, it is a movement disorder that is present and diagnosed at birth. Infants born with cerebral palsy would have cerebral palsy before any treatments, and treatments would not change it. Second, visual outcomes are highly related to the severity and treatment outcome of ROP itself. Therefore, including visual impairment as a criterion for neurodevelopmental impairment related to the ROP treatments would be highly confounded by those patients' ROP consequences. Blair et al. [19] also commented that the treatment indications were not mentioned in this study and that the IVB group in this study included sicker infants with worse ROP statuses compared to the laser group, which may be related to differences in treatment indications [19]. In addition, more patients were excluded from the laser group due to an inability to undergo Bayley-III assessment, which may have been related to poorer neurodevelopment [19].

Lien et al. [20] retrospectively compared the neurodevelopment of 61 preterm infants with type 1 ROP treated with IVB only ($n = 12$), laser only ($n = 33$), and a combination of laser and IVB treatment ($n = 16$), with assessments performed at the corrected ages of 6, 12, 18, and 24 months with the Bayley-II as the assessment tool. They found that patients treated with laser treatment alone and IVB alone did not significantly differ in mental or psychomotor development and that the worst neurodevelopmental outcomes were noted in the combined IVB and laser group. Patients in the combined IVB and laser group had significantly lower mental developmental index ($p = 0.028$) and psychomotor developmental index ($p = 0.002$) values as well as a higher risk of severe psychomotor impairment at 24 months ($p = 0.042$) than patients in the laser group [20]. However, as commented by Blair et al. [19], patients in the combined IVB and laser group in this study were younger, had a lower birth weight (BW), and were also significantly more likely to have zone I disease, which would have certain impact on neurodevelopmental outcomes [19].

Kennedy et al. [21] analyzed the medical and neurodevelopmental outcomes of a subgroup of 18 inborn infants at one study site of the BEAT-ROP study. In the study, infants with stage 3+ ROP were randomized to either IVB or laser treatment, as in the BEAT-ROP study, and neurodevelopmental outcomes were evaluated at the corrected age of 18–22 months using the Bayley-III for assessment. The results showed that there were no significant differences between the IVB group and laser group in all three composite scores (cognitive, language, and motor), but there seemed to be a trend toward higher scores in the IVB group. However, this study was limited by its small number of patients (7 and 9 patients in the IVB and laser groups, respectively), which might not be sufficiently powered to demonstrate small but important differences. Additionally, it must be noted that the treatment criteria in this study, as in the BEAT-ROP study, were stage 3+ ROP in zone I or zone II posterior, which differs from the currently more widely accepted criteria, i.e., type 1 ROP defined by the ETROP study.

More recently, Fan et al. [22] conducted the first prospective comparative study regarding neurodevelopmental outcomes after IVB. In the study, three groups of premature infants were enrolled, including premature infants without ROP ($n = 79$), premature infants with ROP without requirements of treatment ($n = 31$), and premature infants with type 1 ROP treated with one dose of IVB ($n = 38$). Based on the study by Morin et al. [6], a prestudy power analysis was performed to determine the sample size needed to identify a significant difference in odds ratios of severe neurodevelopmental disability. Neurodevelopmental assessment was conducted at a corrected age of 1–3 years using the Bayley-III assessment tool. The results showed that the patients with ROP without treatment and the patients with ROP with IVB treatment had no significant differences in any aspects of the Bayley-III or in their risks of severe neurodevelopmental disability after adjustment for confounding factors. However, although satisfying the prestudy power analysis, the patient number in this study was still relatively small. Furthermore, the three groups, who had different ROP severities, were not comparable in their baseline conditions, such as GA, BW, and comorbidities. Although the comparisons of neurodevelopmental outcomes were adjusted for some of these factors, it is still difficult to weigh the potential impacts of these and other factors (that were not recorded) on neurodevelopment.

The patient number, assessment tools, and main findings of the abovementioned comparative studies are summarized in Table 17.1. While interpreting those studies comparing the effects of IVB and laser treatment on neurodevelopmental outcomes, one should notice that the laser groups in those studies should not be viewed as "negative controls." Although laser treatment is currently the standard treatment for ROP, lasers may also have certain effects on neurodevelopment. First, the need for general anesthesia or sedation while applying the laser is an issue, since general anesthesia and sedative drugs in children less than 3 years of age may affect neurodevelopment, as indicated by the warning from the US Food and Drug Administration (https://www.fda.gov/drugs/drug-safety-and-availability/fda-drug-safety-communication-fda-approves-label-changes-use-general-anesthetic-and-sedation-drugs accessed July 22, 2020). Second, as demonstrated by Kong et al. [9], serum VEGF

Table 17.1 Comparison of comparative studies regarding neurodevelopmental outcomes following IVB and laser treatment in ROP patients.

	Design	Grouping and patient number	Treatment indication	Assessment tool	Main findings	Potential source of bias
Morin et al. Pediatrics. (2016)	Retrospective	• IVB (27) • Laser (98)	Not mentioned	Bayley-III	• Significantly lower motor composite scores in IVB group. • Significantly higher risk of motor composite score <85, neurodevelopmental impairment, and severe neurodevelopmental disability in IVB group.	• Including patients with cerebral palsy and including them in the severe neurodevelopmental disability category. • More severe systemic illnesses and more severe ROP statuses in IVB group patients. • More excluded patients from the laser group due to an inability to undergo Bayley-III assessment, which may be related to poorer neurodevelopment.
Lien et al. PLoS One. (2016)	Retrospective	• IVB (12) • Laser (33) • IVB + laser (16)	Type 1 ROP	Bayley-II	• Significantly lower mental developmental index and psychomotor developmental index values in the IVB + laser group than in the laser group. • Significantly higher risk of severe psychomotor impairment in the IVB + laser group than in the laser group. • No significant differences in neurodevelopmental outcomes between the IVB group and laser group.	• Lower GA and BW in IVB + laser group.
Kennedy et al.J AAPOS. (2018)	Retrospective analysis of patients in one study site of a randomized trial (BEAT-ROP study)	• IVB (7) • Laser (9)	Stage 3+ ROP in zone I or zone II posterior	Bayley-III	• No significant differences in neurodevelopmental outcomes between the IVB group and laser group, but there seemed to be a trend toward better neurodevelopmental outcomes in the IVB group.	• Relatively small number of patients.
Fan et al. Ophthalmology. (2019)	Prospective	• Prematurity without ROP (79) • ROP without treatment (31) • IVB (38)	Type 1 ROP	Bayley-III	• No significant differences in neurodevelopmental outcomes and risk of severe neurodevelopmental disability between ROP without treatment group and IVB group.	• Lower GA and BW and higher prevalence of comorbidities in IVB group.

levels decreased not only following IVB but also following laser treatment, although the reductions were more significant and occurred more rapidly after IVB [9]. It cannot be excluded that the suppression of serum VEGF following laser treatment may also have a certain effect on neurodevelopment.

Hwang et al. [23] also conducted an animal study that investigated the systemic impact of IVB in rabbits. In the study, newborn rabbits received either one or two IVB or sham injections and were sacrificed 2 months later. Histology and immunohistochemistry examinations of the central nervous system as well as major organs did not show significant differences among groups with different injection regimens [23]. As the first animal study designed to mimic IVB in newborns and to investigate its effect on organ development, this study provided important information regarding the systemic safety of intravitreal anti-VEGF injection in newborn individuals, although anatomic similarity may not guarantee similarity of function in those organs, especially the central nervous system.

In conclusion, previously published studies all had certain biases and were limited by their small patient number. Furthermore, those studies showed inconsistent results. Currently, there remains no consensus on how to use IVB properly in ROP patients in regard to both its safety and efficacy. Further larger-scale randomized controlled trials are needed to better address the impact of IVB on the neurodevelopment of ROP infants.

References

1. Alon T, Hemo I, Itin A, Pe'er J, Stone J, Keshet E. Vascular endothelial growth factor acts as a survival factor for newly formed retinal vessels and has implications for retinopathy of prematurity. Nat Med. 1995;1:1024–8.
2. Mintz-Hittner HA, Kennedy KA, Chuang AZ, Group B-RC. Efficacy of intravitreal bevacizumab for stage 3+ retinopathy of prematurity. N Engl J Med. 2011;364:603–15.
3. Micieli JA, Surkont M, Smith AF. A systematic analysis of the off-label use of bevacizumab for severe retinopathy of prematurity. Am J Ophthalmol. 2009;148:536–43 e2.
4. Wu WC, Kuo HK, Yeh PT, Yang CM, Lai CC, Chen SN. An updated study of the use of bevacizumab in the treatment of patients with prethreshold retinopathy of prematurity in Taiwan. Am J Ophthalmol. 2013;155:150–8 e1.
5. Hård AL, Hellström A. On safety, pharmacokinetics and dosage of bevacizumab in ROP treatment – a review. Acta Paediatr. 2011;100:1523–7.
6. Morin J, Luu TM, Superstein R, et al. Neurodevelopmental outcomes following bevacizumab injections for retinopathy of prematurity. Pediatrics. 2016;137:e20153218.
7. Quinn GE, Darlow BA. Concerns for development after bevacizumab treatment of ROP. Pediatrics. 2016;137:e20160057.
8. Sato T, Wada K, Arahori H, et al. Serum concentrations of bevacizumab (avastin) and vascular endothelial growth factor in infants with retinopathy of prematurity. Am J Ophthalmol. 2012;153:327–33 e1.
9. Kong L, Bhatt AR, Demny AB, et al. Pharmacokinetics of bevacizumab and its effects on serum VEGF and IGF-1 in infants with retinopathy of prematurity. Invest Ophthalmol Vis Sci. 2015;56:956–61.
10. Wu WC, Lien R, Liao PJ, et al. Serum levels of vascular endothelial growth factor and related factors after intravitreous bevacizumab injection for retinopathy of prematurity. JAMA Ophthalmol. 2015;133:391–7.
11. Wu WC, Shih CP, Lien R, et al. Serum vascular endothelial growth factor after bevacizumab or ranibizumab treatment for retinopathy of prematurity. Retina. 2017;37:694–01.
12. Huang CY, Lien R, Wang NK, et al. Changes in systemic vascular endothelial growth factor levels after intravitreal injection of aflibercept in infants with retinopathy of prematurity. Graefes Arch Clin Exp Ophthalmol. 2018;256:479–87.
13. Breier G, Albrecht U, Sterrer S, Risau W. Expression of vascular endothelial growth factor during embryonic angiogenesis and endothelial cell differentiation. Development. 1992;114:521–32.
14. Bagnard D, Vaillant C, Khuth ST, et al. Semaphorin 3A-vascular endothelial growth factor-165 balance mediates migration and apoptosis of neural progenitor cells by the recruitment of shared receptor. J Neurosci. 2001;21:3332–41.
15. Jin K, Zhu Y, Sun Y, Mao XO, Xie L, Greenberg DA. Vascular endothelial growth factor (VEGF) stimulates neurogenesis in vitro and in vivo. Proc Natl Acad Sci U S A. 2002;99:11946–50.
16. Zhang H, Vutskits L, Pepper MS, Kiss JZ. VEGF is a chemoattractant for FGF-2-stimulated neural progenitors. J Cell Biol. 2003;163:1375–84.
17. Malik S, Vinukonda G, Vose LR, et al. Neurogenesis continues in the third trimester of pregnancy and is suppressed by premature birth. J Neurosci. 2013;33:411–23.
18. Martinez-Castellanos MA, Schwartz S, Hernandez-Rojas ML, et al. Long-term effect of antiangiogenic therapy for retinopathy of prematurity up to 5 years of follow-up. Retina. 2013;33:329–38.
19. Blair MP, Shapiro MJ. Re: Good: Bevacizumab for retinopathy of prematurity: treatment when pathology is embedded in a normally developing vascular system (Ophthalmology. 2016;123:1843-1844). Ophthalmology. 2017;124:e74–5.
20. Lien R, Yu MH, Hsu KH, et al. Neurodevelopmental outcomes in infants with retinopathy of prematurity and bevacizumab treatment. PLoS One. 2016;11:e0148019.
21. Kennedy KA, Mintz-Hittner HA. Medical and developmental outcomes of bevacizumab versus laser for retinopathy of prematurity. J AAPOS. 2018;22:61–5.e1.
22. Fan YY, Huang YS, Huang CY, et al. Neurodevelopmental outcomes after intravitreal bevacizumab therapy for retinopathy of prematurity: a prospective case-control study. Ophthalmology. 2019;126:1567–77.
23. Hwang YS, Liu CH, Huang YC, et al. Systemic effects after intravitreal injection of bevacizumab in new born rabbit eyes. Cutan Ocul Toxicol. 2018;37:41–51.

Artificial Intelligence for Retinopathy of Prematurity Diagnosis

18

J. Peter Campbell, Susan R. Ostmo, and Michael F. Chiang

Abstract

Retinopathy of prematurity is a leading cause of childhood blindness. There are several challenges to care delivery in the real-world including inter-observer diagnostic error due to subjective diagnosis, human resource limitations for trained examiners, and a growing incidence of disease in low- and middle-income countries. Digital fundus imaging has facilitated the development of telemedicine programs with central grading, and the application of artificial intelligence to improve the objectivity of diagnosis. In this chapter, we review the background, early advances, and potential future applications of artificial intelligence to improve care for patients with ROP.

Keywords

Artificial intelligence · Machine learning · Deep learning Retinopathy of prematurity

Retinopathy of prematurity (ROP) is a leading cause of childhood blindness throughout the world [1]. ROP did not exist before the mid-twentieth century because the survival of premature infants was limited before that time. In the mid-twentieth century, with the development of modern neonatal care, and the use of supplemental oxygenation to support immature pulmonary development, neonatal survival rates began to increase. Unfortunately, this led to an epidemic of blindness from this new disease, initially called retrolental fibroplasia (RLF) reflecting the end-stage of the disease. It was soon determined that the incidence of RLF declined with more careful oxygen monitoring, and clinicians began to observe the earlier stages of the disease using ophthalmoscopy.

The International Classification for ROP (ICROP) first formalized the disease characteristics of ROP in 1984, and again in 2005, dividing the spectrum of disease into three characteristics: zone, stage, and plus disease [2, 3]. The zone of the disease refers to the posterior border of avascular retina—it is generally recognized that the more posterior the disease the worse the prognosis (zone "I" is worse than zone "II"). The stage of disease refers to the degree of vascular abnormality at the vascular–avascular border, from 0 (no disease) to 5 (total retinal detachment). Plus disease refers to the degree of vascular dilation and tortuosity in the posterior retina in severe ROP. Technically, per ICROP, the definition of plus disease is "arteriolar tortuosity and venous dilation in the posterior retina" more than depicted in a standard published photograph. The National Institutes of Health (NIH) funded Cryotherapy for ROP (CRYO-ROP) and Early Treatment for ROP (ETROP) studies have defined the criteria for evidence-based intervention with pan-retinal photocoagulation to reduce the risk of retinal detachment [4, 5]. Post-ETROP, treatment is initiated for type 1 ROP, defined as any zone I, any stage ROP with plus disease; zone II, stage 2 or 3 ROP with plus disease; or zone I, stage 3 (even if plus disease is absent). Thus, plus disease is the critical disease feature defining the need for treatment in ROP (Fig. 18.1).

18.1 Real-World Problems

In practice, are several challenges in plus disease diagnosis: (1) Qualitative analysis of diagnostic processes suggest that clinicians develop a gestalt of disease severity and rely on clinical factors that are not part of the technical definition of plus disease [6, 7]. (2) It is challenging to compare the level

J. P. Campbell · S. R. Ostmo
Department of Ophthalmology, Casey Eye Institute, Oregon Health and Science University, Portland, OR, USA

M. F. Chiang (✉)
Department of Ophthalmology, Casey Eye Institute, Oregon Health and Science University, Portland, OR, USA

Department of Medical Informatics and Clinical Epidemiology, Oregon Health and Science University, Portland, OR, USA
e-mail: chiangm@ohsu.edu

W.-C. Wu, W.-C. Lam (eds.), *A Quick Guide to Pediatric Retina*, https://doi.org/10.1007/978-981-15-6552-6_18

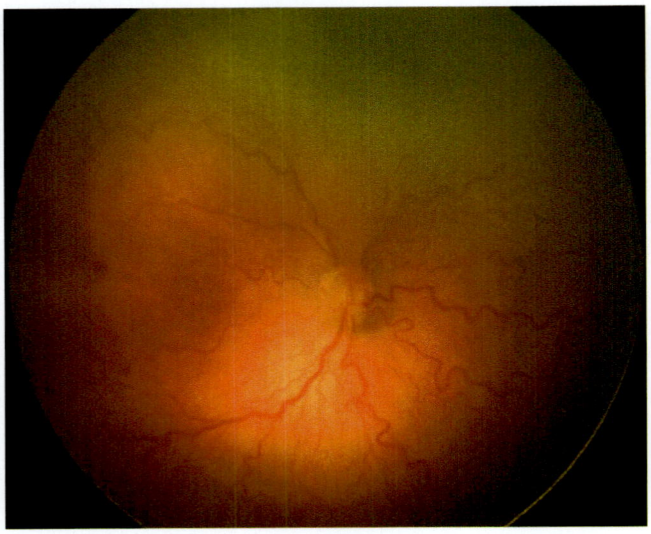

Fig. 18.1 Representative image of an eye with plus disease

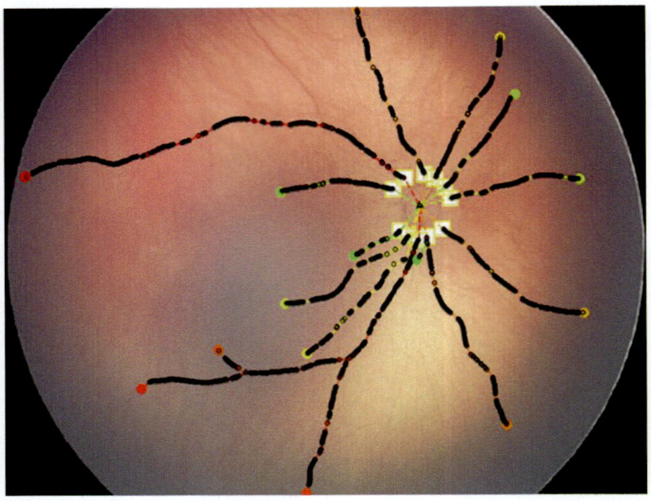

Fig. 18.2 Example of node-based vascular tracing. Starting from the optic nerve, a vascular tree of nodes and segment is developed. Both segments, and individual points along a segment can then be used to extract quantitative features of dilation and tortuosity (Credit to Esra Ataer-Cansizoglu, PhD)

of disease to the standard photograph, which had a narrow field of view and high magnification [7, 8]. (3) There is some evidence that the classification of plus disease has changed over time toward less severe disease [9]. (4) Vascular abnormalities in ROP range from mild to severe, yet plus disease is classified into categories. Evidence suggests that different experts are systematically biased as to his/her cut-points between categories along the spectrum of severity [10, 11]. (5) These and other factors contribute to significant variability in plus disease classification even among world experts. This has been shown in research studies [10, 12, 13], NIH funded clinical trials [14], and international randomized trials [15].

There are also severe human resources limitations to meet the need for ROP screening worldwide. Even in the USA, due to medicolegal concerns, and limited training, fewer ophthalmologists feel comfortable and/or willing to manage ROP. This problem is compounded in low- and middle-income countries (LMIC) where the disease is epidemic for two reasons: (1) improving neonatal mortality leading to higher at-risk population and (2) heterogeneous oxygen monitoring practices leading to higher incidence of any and severe ROP [16]. For both of these reasons (problems with plus disease diagnosis and limited workforce), several groups have explored quantitative computer-based analysis of vascular disease in ROP.

18.2 Feature Extraction and Machine Learning

This avenue of research was enabled by the development of wide-angle digital fundus photography, notably the Retcam (Natus Medical Incorporated, Pleasanton, CA). Early attempts used specific measurements of dilation and tortuosity as a surrogate for the clinical entity of plus disease [17]. While several of these systems were developed, none of the feature extraction-based systems were routinely incorporated into ROP screening outside of research purposes primarily due to poor correlation with the clinical diagnosis of plus disease. Feature extraction methods begin with vessel segmentation (Fig. 18.2) and then utilize various measurements of dilation and tortuosity to quantify plus disease. A machine-learning-based system developed by the Imaging and Informatics in ROP (i-ROP) consortium was able to meet or exceed classification performance of ROP experts on three-level (plus, pre-plus, no plus) classification, but required manually processed (hand-traced) vessel maps as inputs, severely limiting real-world usefulness (Fig. 18.3) [7, 18].

18.3 Deep Learning

Deep learning was first applied to plus disease in ROP by Worrall et al. in 2016 with some success, though notably limited by variable ground truth labels for plus disease [19]. In 2018, Brown et al. published the results of the "i-ROP DL" system that was trained on more than 5000 images with a robust reference standard diagnosis (RSD) consisting of four independent classifications (three based on images and one based on ophthalmoscopy) [20]. The i-ROP DL system reported an area under the receiver operating characteristic curve (AUC) of 0.98 for the detection of plus disease, and 0.94 for the detection of "worse than normal" disease against the RSD. On an independent test set of 100 images with 15

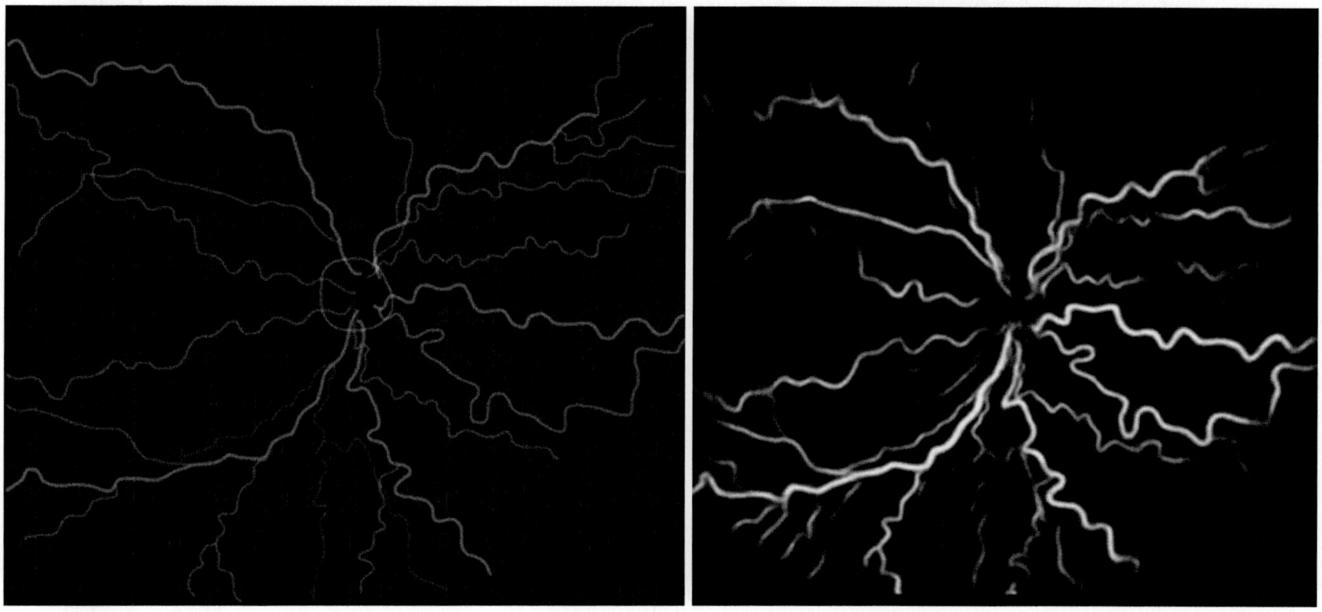

Fig. 18.3 Manual (left) and automated (right) segmentation of image from Fig. 18.1. Feature extraction-based methods require manual or automated segmentation of the optic nerve and blood vessels

plus images and 32 pre-plus images, the system outperformed 7/8 international ROP experts with a kappa of 0.92 on three level plus disease classification. The i-ROP DL network consists of two serial networks: the first network takes a raw wide-angle digital fundus image and creates a vessel map, and the second classifies plus disease from the vessel map (as shown in Fig. 18.3) [20].

18.4 Translating to Clinical Practice: Development of a Severity Scale for ROP Screening

In theory, the diagnosis of zone and stage could also be performed using montaged images, and thus a parallel network could diagnose not only plus, but the full ICROP classification of zone, stage and plus. One practical challenge for direct implementation of an AI-based plus disease classification system in ROP is that physicians may not accept a computer-based diagnostic system that has medicolegal implications for treatment. Under current treatment paradigms, a diagnosis of plus disease requires treatment; therefore, it may be problematic to have that as the output of the system, if it is in conflict with clinical judgment. Given the fact that the vascular changes in ROP run a continuum, and that agreement on relative disease severity is better than agreement on classification, the i-ROP team developed a continuous severity score for ROP, based on the plus disease classification probability. The rationale behind a continuous score for vascular severity is that: (1) it could be used in screening to identify patients at a point in time or over time with clinically significant disease; (2) it would provide an objective metric of disease severity; and (3) it would not have the same therapeutic implication as a diagnosis of "plus disease." In 2018, Redd et al. reported the results of a vascular severity score applied to the database of more than 5000 eye exams each classified with image grading and ophthalmoscopy with an RSD [21]. The 1–9 score demonstrated an AUC of 0.95 for the detection of type 1 (treatment-requiring) ROP, and 0.91 for the detection of type 2 (or pre-plus) or worse disease. Separately applied to the independent test set of 100 images, a cut-off of 3 demonstrated 100% sensitivity, 94% specificity for detection of pre-plus or worse disease. This reflects the fact that though ROP is classified as zone, stage and plus independent, these sub-classifications are physiologically related. Eyes with more posterior disease (zone 1), and more severe stage (stage 3) tend to have more severe dilation and tortuosity. Figure 18.4 demonstrates the mean severity score for eyes with zone 1 vs. zone 2, and stage I–III disease. This suggests that in a telemedicine model, this automated score could add objectivity to the detection of clinically significant disease.

18.5 Disease Monitoring Using an AI-Based Severity Score

Recent work has applied this concept to track disease severity over time. Using a small cohort of patients in each of five groups categories (no progression, progression to mild ROP, progression to pre-plus disease, progression to plus disease, and progression to APROP), Brown et al. demonstrated that

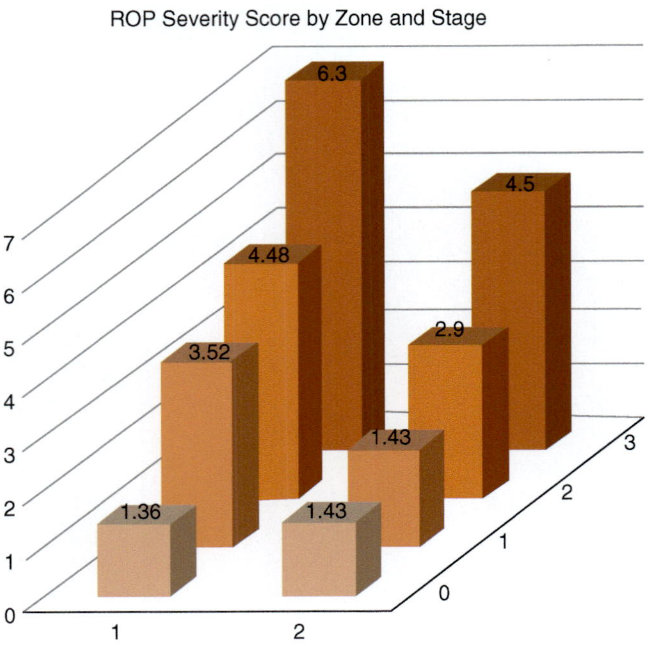

Fig. 18.4 Mean severity score by zone and stage. This figure represents the mean vascular severity score (vertical axis) by zone and stage in 5511 examinations from the Imaging and Informatics in the ROP study. Eyes with more posterior disease (zone 1) and higher stage have higher vascular severity scores

each cohort has both rates of change, and peak severity levels, that reflect the relative level of disease severity [22]. Taylor et al. expanded this to the entire i-ROP database, demonstrating that eyes that progression to treatment demonstrate a rapid and separable pace of disease, and suggest that eyes may be identified as high risk as early as a month prior to treatment [23]. This suggests that incorporated into an ROP screening program, a continuous score may correlate with clinical disease severity at a point in time, and change in score may have prognostic implications and identify eyes progressing to more severe ROP enabling early referral, diagnosis, and treatment.

Though NIH-funded clinical trials have defined the level of disease severity at which treatment is recommended, the regression of severe ROP after treatment has not been as well defined. Gupta et al. evaluated the ability of the ROP severity score to monitor disease regression in eyes with treatment-requiring ROP [24]. They found: (1) the vascular severity score dramatically increased in the month before treatment, and decreased after treatment; (2) eyes treated with anti-VEGF tended to have more aggressive disease and responded more rapidly than laser; and (3) eyes that required additional treatment tended to have higher severity scores at baseline. These results need to be further evaluated in larger prospective trials, but further suggest that the vascular severity score may help optimize the timing of treatment, and identify eyes that are responding suboptimally to treatment.

18.6 Future Applications

Artificial intelligence has demonstrated the ability to perform image recognition for numerous medical applications [25]. With enough quality data, it seems this technology can be trained to do many of the image-recognition tasks that humans can do, and perhaps better and more efficiently than humans. However, with the exception of IDx-DR™, the autonomous artificial intelligence (AI) system developed by Abramoff and colleagues for diabetes, no AI systems have been implemented into clinical practice in ophthalmology (at the time of this writing) [25]. There are several reasons for this that are beyond the scope of this chapter, but it is important to compare and contrast how these systems are developed with how they would be used in the real world. In the case of diabetes, this is being implemented using an autonomous DR screening camera in primary care offices. In every other application, there is a persistent implementation gap that needs to be overcome. Part of the resistance to the incorporation of artificial intelligence in medicine has been the "black box" nature of the algorithms—it is not clear how they work in all cases. Thus, there have been movements toward "explainability" methods to try to illuminate the low-level features that are utilized in the networks (as in Fig. 18.5), as well as develop networks a priori that are interpretable [25]. In ROP, we foresee increasing use of telemedicine networks with digital fundus photography and with appropriate

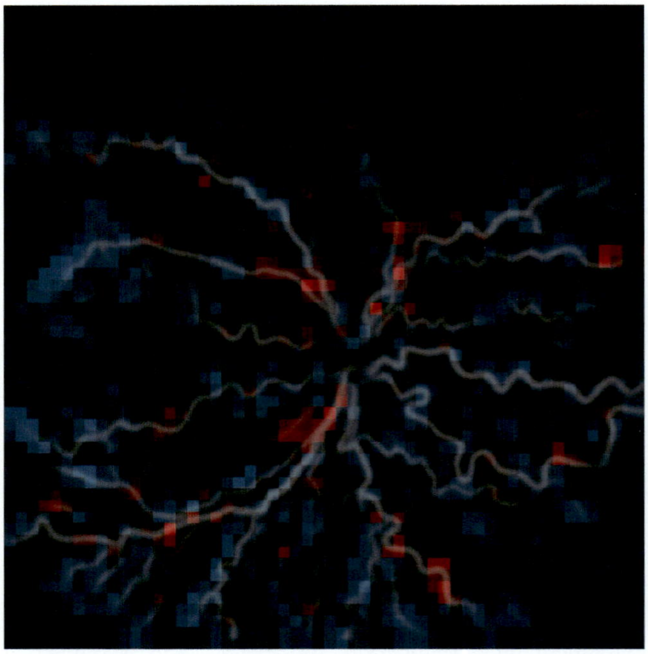

Fig. 18.5 Representative image of a heatmap. There have been multiple attempts to explain the inner workings of a convolutional neural network, which operates as a black box. Heatmaps work by identifying patches that seem to contribute more (red) to the overall diagnostic classification than other patches (Credit to James M. Brown, PhD)

validation, the use of a vascular severity score to monitor clinical disease progression in the future [26]. The challenge will be for physicians to learn to incorporate this technology into clinical practice in a way that is safe, effective, and improves our ability to take care of patients.

Financial Disclosure JPC, SO, and MFC are supported by grants R01EY19474, K12EY027720, and P30EY10572 from the National Institutes of Health (Bethesda, MD), by grant SCH-1622679 from the National Science Foundation (Arlington, VA), by grant funding from Genentech (South San Francisco, CA), and by unrestricted departmental funding from Research to Prevent Blindness (New York, NY). MFC is an unpaid member of the Scientific Advisory Board for Clarity Medical Systems (Pleasanton, CA), a Consultant for Novartis (Basel, Switzerland), and an initial member of Inteleretina (Honolulu, HI).

References

1. Gilbert C, Foster A. Childhood blindness in the context of VISION 2020: the right to sight. Bull World Health Organ. 2001;79:227–32.
2. The Committee for the Classification of Retinopathy of Prematurity. An international classification of retinopathy of prematurity. Arch Ophthalmol. 1984;102:1130–4.
3. International Committee for the Classification of Retinopathy of Prematurity. The International Classification of Retinopathy of Prematurity revisited. In: Archives of ophthalmology: American Medical Association; 2005. p. 991–9.
4. Cryotherapy for Retinopathy of Prematurity Cooperative Group. Multicenter trial of cryotherapy for retinopathy of prematurity. Preliminary results. Arch Ophthalmol. 1988;106:471–9.
5. Early Treatment for Retinopathy of Prematurity Cooperative Group. Revised indications for the treatment of retinopathy of prematurity: results of the early treatment for retinopathy of prematurity randomized trial. Arch Ophthalmol. 2003;121:1684–94.
6. Hewing NJ, Kaufman DR, Chan RVP, Chiang MF. Plus disease in retinopathy of prematurity. JAMA Ophthalmol. 2013;131:1026–7.
7. Campbell JP, Ataer-Cansizoglu E, Bolon-Canedo V, et al. Expert diagnosis of plus disease in retinopathy of prematurity from computer-based image analysis. JAMA Ophthalmol. 2016;134:651–7.
8. Rao R, Jonsson NJ, Ventura C, Gelman R, Lindquist MA, Casper DS, Chiang MF. Plus disease in retinopathy of prematurity: diagnostic impact of field of view. Retina (Philadelphia, PA). 2012;32:1148–55.
9. Moleta C, Campbell JP, Kalpathy-Cramer J, Chan RP, Ostmo S, Jonas K, Chiang MF, Imaging & Informatics in ROP Research Consortium. Plus disease in retinopathy of prematurity: diagnostic trends in 2016 vs. 2007. Am J Ophthalmol. 2007; https://doi.org/10.1016/j.ajo.2016.12.025.
10. Campbell JP, Kalpathy-Cramer J, Erdogmus D, et al. Plus disease in retinopathy of prematurity: a continuous spectrum of vascular abnormality as a basis of diagnostic variability. Ophthalmology. 2016;123:2338–44.
11. Kalpathy-Cramer J, Campbell JP, Erdogmus D, et al. Plus disease in retinopathy of prematurity: improving diagnosis by ranking disease severity and using quantitative image analysis. Ophthalmology. 2016;0:2345–51.
12. Chiang MF, Jiang L, Gelman R, Du YE, Flynn JT. Interexpert agreement of plus disease diagnosis in retinopathy of prematurity. Arch Ophthalmol. 2007;125:875–80.
13. Kalpathy-Cramer J, Campbell JP, Erdogmus D, et al. Plus disease in retinopathy of prematurity: improving diagnosis by ranking disease severity and using quantitative image analysis. Ophthalmology. 2016;123:2345–51.
14. Reynolds JD, Dobson V, Quinn GE, et al. Evidence-based screening criteria for retinopathy of prematurity: natural history data from the CRYO-ROP and LIGHT-ROP studies. Arch Ophthalmol. 2002;120:1470–6.
15. Fleck BW, Williams C, Juszczak E, et al. An international comparison of retinopathy of prematurity grading performance within the Benefits of Oxygen Saturation Targeting II trials. Eye (Lond). 2017;123:1–7.
16. Gilbert C, Rahi J, Eckstein M, O'Sullivan J, Foster A. Retinopathy of prematurity in middle-income countries. The Lancet. 1997;350:12–4.
17. Wittenberg LA, Jonsson NJ, Paul Chan RV, Chiang MF. Computer-based image analysis for plus disease diagnosis in retinopathy of prematurity. J Pediatr Ophthalmol Strabismus. 2011;49:11–9.
18. Ataer-Cansizoglu E, Bolon-Canedo V, Campbell JP, et al. Computer-based image analysis for plus disease diagnosis in retinopathy of prematurity: performance of the "i-ROP" system and image features associated with expert diagnosis. Transl Vis Sci Technol. 2015;4:5.
19. Worrall DE, Wilson CM, Brostow GJ. Automated retinopathy of prematurity case detection with convolutional neural networks. In: Deep learning and data labeling for medical applications. Cham: Springer; 2016. p. 68–76.
20. Brown JM, Campbell JP, Beers A, et al. Automated diagnosis of plus disease in retinopathy of prematurity using deep convolutional neural networks. JAMA Ophthalmol. 2018; https://doi.org/10.1001/jamaophthalmol.2018.1934.
21. Redd TK, Campbell JP, Brown JM, et al. Evaluation of a deep learning image assessment system for detecting severe retinopathy of prematurity. Br J Ophthalmol. 2018;bjophthalmol–2018–313156.
22. Brown JM, Kalpathy-Cramer J, Campbell JP, et al. Fully automated disease severity assessment and treatment monitoring in retinopathy of prematurity using deep learning. In: Zhang J, Chen P-H, editors. Imaging informatics for healthcare, research, and applications: SPIE; 2018. p. 22–8.
23. Taylor S, Campbell JP, Gupta K, et al. A quantitative severity scale for retinopathy of prematurity using deep learning: monitoring disease progression. JAMA Ophthalmol. 2019. In Press.
24. Gupta K, Campbell JP, Taylor S, et al. A quantitative severity scale for retinopathy of prematurity using deep learning: monitoring disease regression after treatment. JAMA Ophthalmol. 2019. In Press.
25. Ting DSW, Pasquale LR, Peng L, Campbell JP, Lee AY, Raman R, Tan GSW, Schmetterer L, Keane PA, Wong TY. Artificial intelligence and deep learning in ophthalmology. Br J Ophthalmol. 2018;bjophthalmol–2018–313173.
26. Ting DSW, Wu W-C, Toth C. Deep learning for retinopathy of prematurity screening. Br J Ophthalmol. 2018;bjophthalmol–2018–313290.

E-Education in ROP

19

Emily D. Cole, Nita Valikodath, Tala Al-Khaled,
Samir N. Patel, Michael F. Chiang, J. Peter Campbell,
and R. V. Paul Chan

Abstract

Web-based educational resources are available for providers managing patients with retinopathy of prematurity (ROP). These tools include web-based tutorials and training modules, integrated software tools, online toolkits with standardized patient education, consents, and reference materials.

Keywords

Retinopathy of prematurity · Web-based education
Online resources · Retinopathy of prematurity toolkit
ROP tutorial

In both developed and developing countries, there is a shortage of specialists who are able to provide adequate care for infants with retinopathy of prematurity (ROP). This is due to a multitude of factors, including a lack of adequate training in residency and fellowship programs [1]. In ophthalmology residency programs, as well as in pediatric ophthalmology and retina fellowship training, there is variability in the number of ROP exams performed with direct supervision by an attending, no standardization in the number of cases required to attain competency, and limited use of formal evaluation to assess fellow competency in ROP management [2–6].

Web-based, self-directed educational tools are becoming increasingly prevalent in residency, fellowship, and for use in continuing medical education. These tools are important resources for increasing the knowledge and skills of providers who provide ROP care in all contexts, as well as standardizing screening, consent, and follow-up protocols. It is important that the proper resources provided by the appropriate stakeholders are utilized. This chapter will provide a review of ROP web-based training modules and resources provided by the American Academy of Ophthalmology (AAO), Ophthalmic Mutual Insurance Company (OMIC), and others.

Telemedicine for ROP is frequently described in the context of using images acquired at one location to make a diagnosis by a provider at a different location. The definition of telemedicine in this setting is the use of information technology to support healthcare between entities geographically separated from each other [7]. With this definition, it can also encompass tele-education programs which can be used for local resource-building, increasing the number of trained clinicians in middle-income and low-income countries. This tele-mentoring approach has also been demonstrated in other surgical subspecialties including urology and gynecology and can be applied to ROP treatment and surgical approaches to increase treatment capacity, particularly in low- and middle-income countries [8–10]. Tele-education systems can enable access to high-quality ROP education and alleviate the strain on local ROP experts who may be otherwise unavailable to devote time to education.

The Global Education Network for ROP (GEN-ROP) and the Imaging and Informatics for ROP (i-ROP) groups developed a web-based platform that allows users around the world to access an ROP training module, and given the increasing access to Internet in low- and middle-income countries, web-based learning is now more highly accessible [11]. The program consists of pretest, posttest, and case-based training chapters in which trainees work through cases consisting of retinal images from infants with varying degrees of ROP. Trainees are also provided with feedback during the training in order to reinforce their learning [11].

The GEN-ROP/i-ROP training module has previously shown to improve ophthalmology trainees' ability to diagnose ROP in the United States, Mexico, the Philippines, and Brazil

E. D. Cole · N. Valikodath · R. V. P. Chan (✉) · T. Al-Khaled
Department of Ophthalmology and Visual Sciences,
Illinois Eye and Ear Infirmary, University of Illinois at Chicago,
Chicago, IL, USA

S. N. Patel
Wills Eye Hospital, Philadelphia, PA, USA

M. F. Chiang · J. P. Campbell
Department of Ophthalmology, Casey Eye Institute,
Oregon Health and Science University, Portland, OR, USA

W.-C. Wu, W.-C. Lam (eds.), *A Quick Guide to Pediatric Retina*, https://doi.org/10.1007/978-981-15-6552-6_19

[10, 12, 13]. Resident and fellow trainees demonstrated improvement in the sensitivity for diagnosis of plus disease, ROP zone/stage/category as well as the presence of aggressive posterior-ROP. A comparison of the two groups found no significant differences between trainees in higher income countries compared to lower income countries in the sensitivity or specificity of diagnosing clinically significant disease. A post-module assessment showed that both groups felt their understanding of ROP improved after participating in the web-based training. Participants in the tele-education program also demonstrated improvement in intra-grader reliability when provided with the same case, improving from fair/moderate agreement to substantial agreement for all subtypes of ROP. This is notable considering that the literature reports poor intra- and inter-grader reliability amongst experts diagnosing ROP [13, 14].

The WISE-ROP (Widefield Imaging for Screening and Education for ROP) is another example of an online training module that was used in the KID-ROP (Karnataka Internet Assisted Diagnosis of Retinopathy of Prematurity) program. KID-ROP is one of the largest telemedicine networks for screening ROP in India. The 90-day training module used in this program is now available as an online training module, which consists of image grading, self-assessment, and scheduled video sessions with an assigned mentor for individualized feedback and assessment. This program grades participants prior to awarding them with certification [15].

Online resources are a valuable tool for the standardization of ROP care around the world. The Ophthalmic Mutual Insurance Company provides a comprehensive set of resources entitled the OMIC ROP Safety Net Toolkit, which was first developed in 2006 and recently revised in 2018 and reviewed by ophthalmologists. These toolkits include procedures for screening, discharge, and coordination of care for ophthalmologists who are involved in the screening and treatment of ROP. The toolkit outlines specific protocols for the following procedures in order to ensure standardization of care and optimize outcomes. These procedures include tracking of hospitalized infants, the ROP examination in the hospital-based setting, transfer to a treating hospital, discharge, and transfer for non-ROP care. OMIC also provides a comprehensive risk analysis of ROP-related claims with root cause analysis to address preventable breakdowns in the process of care. Additionally, there are three in-depth case analyses of claims in which there was failure to coordinate follow-up care, delayed referral for progressive ROP, and a case that outlines the challenges of navigating the legal system in ROP cases. The hospital and office toolkits provide standardized consent forms, educational tools, and letters to parents about ROP in English and Spanish. Finally, OMIC provides an overview of anti-vascular endothelial growth factor (VEGF) treatment in ROP with a comprehensive review of safety and liability risks [16].

Software tools that integrate documentation and telemedicine systems represent platforms that can be utilized in the hospital and clinic settings. FocusROP is one such HIPAA and FDA compliant image handling and storage platform which was developed in collaboration with pediatric vitreoretinal specialists. It includes tools for user-driven image analysis such as identification of zone I, the optic nerve, macula, and vessel tracing tools. This system can be integrated into telemedicine systems which allow for electronic expert opinions when needed. It also includes manuscripts for patient and family education. The software provides reminders for exam scheduling based on current evidence-based guidelines for screening.

The AAO also provides specific resources for ROP. In collaboration with GEN-ROP and i-ROP, the AAO offers case-based training for ROP which consists of 20 virtual patients for participants to evaluate and determine zone, stage, and category of ROP and whether or not the patient needs treatment (Fig. 19.1) [17]. The vitreoretinal section of the Knights Templar Eye Foundation Pediatric Ophthalmology and Strabismus Resource Center is an AAO resource which provides regularly updated articles and videos regarding current treatment and screening options for ROP. This resource includes specific articles and discussions on the topics of anti-VEGF and laser treatment, telemedicine, and management of retinal detachments [18].

Providers working in low-resource settings can utilize resources provided by Every Preemie—SCALE (Scaling, Catalyzing, Advocating, Learning, and Evidence-Driven), which is a 5-year USAID cooperative agreement which is designed to provide scalable approaches to preterm birth and low birthweight interventions. The Do No Harm technical briefs highlight the safe and effective use of specific inpatient newborn care interventions and include topics such as oxygen use, infection prevention, thermal protection, and ROP prevention and screening. The ROP technical brief highlights the importance of ROP screening, risk factors, current World Health Organization recommendations, and a summary of evidence-based practices for primary, secondary, and tertiary prevention of ROP-related blindness. Importantly, the technical briefs address actions that can be taken by policymakers, program planners, facility managers, as well as clinicians and nurses to advocate for an agenda that prioritizes ROP. These resources are available in English, Spanish, and French. Current ROP screening programs supported by USAID include those in India, Mongolia, and Nepal [19].

While there is yet to be a standardization of certification for healthcare professionals providing ROP care, a multitude of online resources have been developed to build knowledge, standardize treatment and screening protocols, decrease preventable blindness, and mitigate risk. These

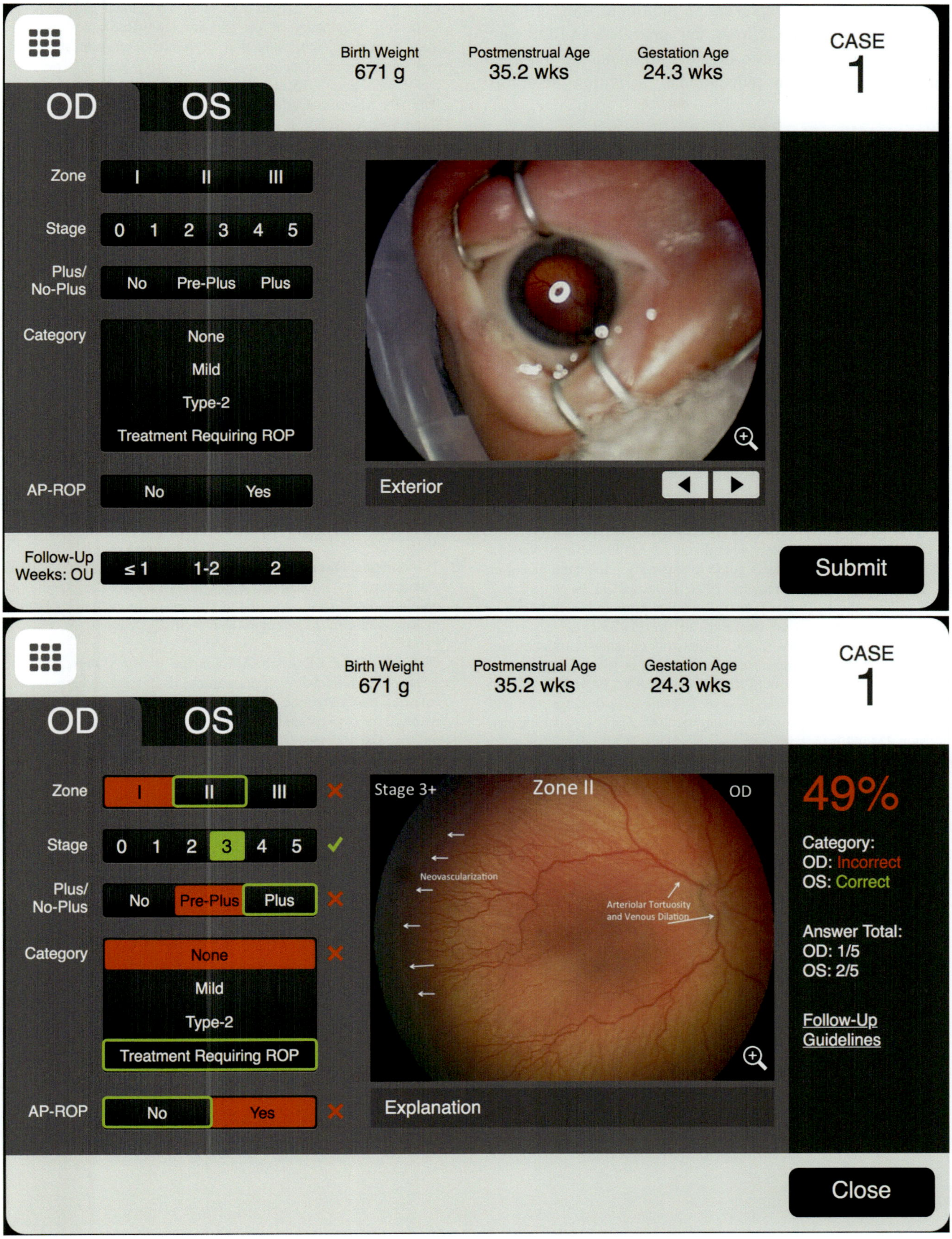

Fig. 19.1 Example of online case-based retinopathy of prematurity (ROP) tutorials available through the American Academy of Ophthalmology. These cases include standardized views and background information including birth weight, gestational age, and postmenstrual age. The second image shows the individualized feedback with visual explanations of the correct stage

web-based resources represent an important starting point for training residents, fellows, and providers of ROP care and are complementary to mentorship, hands-on training, and participation in educational activities such as conferences.

References

1. Chiang MF, Jiang L, Gelman R, Du YE, Flynn JT. Interexpert agreement of plus disease diagnosis in retinopathy of prematurity. Arch Ophthalmol. 2007;125(7):875–80.
2. Chan RVP, Williams SL, Yonekawa Y, et al. Accuracy of retinopathy of prematurity diagnosis by retinal fellows. Retina. 2010;30(6):958–65.
3. Myung JS, Chan RVP, Espiritu MJ, et al. Accuracy of retinopathy of prematurity image-based diagnosis by pediatric ophthalmology fellows: implications for training. J AAPOS. 2011;15(6):573–8.
4. Nagiel A, Espiritu MJ, Wong RK, et al. Retinopathy of prematurity residency training. Ophthalmology. 2012;119(12):2644–2645. e1–e2.
5. Wong RK, Ventura CV, Espiritu MJ, et al. Training fellows for retinopathy of prematurity care: a web-based survey. J AAPOS. 2012;16(2):177–1781.
6. Swamy L, Patel S, Jonas KE, Ostmo S, Chiang MF, Chan RVP. Characterization of errors in retinopathy of prematurity (ROP) diagnosis by ophthalmology residents. J AAPOS. 2016;20(4):e44.
7. Field MJ. Telemedicine: a guide to assessing telecommunications in healthcare. J Digit Imaging. 1997;10(3 Suppl 1):28.
8. Challacombe B, Wheatstone S. Telementoring and telerobotics in urological surgery. Curr Urol Rep. 2010;11(1):22–8.
9. Gambadauro P, Magos A. NEST (network enhanced surgical training): a PC-based system for telementoring in gynaecological surgery. Eur J Obstet Gynecol Reprod Biol. 2008;139(2):222–5.
10. Mendez I, Hill R, Clarke D, et al. Robotic long-distance telementoring in neurosurgery. Neurosurgery. 2005;56(3):434–40; discussion 434–440.
11. Chan RVP, Patel SN, Ryan MC, et al. The global education network for retinopathy of prematurity (Gen-Rop): development, implementation, and evaluation of a novel tele-education system (an American Ophthalmological Society Thesis). Trans Am Ophthalmol Soc. 2015;113:T2.
12. Patel SN, Martinez-Castellanos MA, Berrones-Medina D, Swan R, Ryan MC, Jonas KE, et al. Assessment of a tele-education system to enhance retinopathy of prematurity (ROP) training by international ophthalmologists-in-training in Mexico. Ophthalmology. 2017;124(7):953–61.
13. Campbell JP, Swan R, Jonas K, Ostmo S, Ventura CV, Martinez-Castellanos MA, Chan RP. Implementation and evaluation of a tele-education system for the diagnosis of ophthalmic disease by international trainees. In: AMIA Annual Symposium Proceedings, vol. 2015: American Medical Informatics Association; 2015. p. 366.
14. Al-Khaled T, Mikhail M, Jonas KE, Wu W, Anzures R, Amphonphruet A, Campbell P, Chan RVP. Training of residents and fellows in retinopathy of prematurity (ROP) around the world: an international web-based survey. J AAPOS. 2018;22(4):e57.
15. Vinekar A, Bhende P. Innovations in technology and service delivery to improve Retinopathy of Prematurity care. Community Eye Health. 2018;31(101):S20–2.
16. "OMIC's ROP Resources." https://www.omic.com/rop-resources/. Accessed 3 Feb 2019.
17. Chan RV, Chiang M, Jonas K. Retinopathy of prematurity: case-based training. 2015. https://www.aao.org/interactive-tool/retinopathy-of-prematurity-case-based-training. Accessed 3 Feb 2019.
18. "Vitreoretinal Disease." Knights Templar Eye Foundation Pediatric Ophthalmology Education Center. https://www.aao.org/pediatric-ophthalmology-strabismus-listing?subspecialty=pediatric-ophthalmology-strabismus&subtopic=Vitreoretinal_Diseases. Accessed 3 Feb 2019.
19. Chan RVP, Jonas KE, Litch JA, Campbell JP, Yap V. Prevention and screening of retinopathy of prematurity (ROP), do no harm technical brief. Every Preemie—SCALE. April 2018. https://www.everypreemie.org/wp-content/uploads/2018/04/ROP_4.20.18-FINAL.pdf. Accessed 25 Oct 2018.

Ultra-widefield Imaging in Pediatric Retinal Diseases

20

Igor Kozak, Syed M. Ali, and Maram E. A. Abdalla-Elsayed

Abstract

High-resolution imaging is an indispensable part of pediatric retina practice. It provides necessary diagnostic information and monitoring of disease or follow-up of treatment. Imaging of the peripheral retina has revolutionized the science of retinal diseases and the care of pediatric patients. Reliable (ultra)wide-angle cameras and systems are available for health care professionals as the popularity of this type of imaging has been growing in spite of some challenges. Alternative approaches and techniques have appeared to facilitate imaging in order to overcome the barriers. Ultra-widefield imaging technology will be *sine qua non* for the routine pediatric retina practice.

Keywords

Pediatric retina · Imaging · Ultra-widefield · Retina camera · Retinal diseases

20.1 Introduction

Careful clinical examination of patient's ocular fundus and, especially, peripheral retina with scleral indentation is crucial for clinical decision making. However, there is a need for an objective and reproducible documentation of encountered findings. The peripheral retina is the site of pathology in many ocular diseases. In uncooperative children, a detailed examination of the retinal periphery may pose a unique challenge. Technological advances in diagnostic imaging techniques have played an important role in improved assessment of the retina and its periphery. Ultra-widefield (UWF) imaging is one of the new technologies available to pediatric and adult retinal specialists. Current UWF imaging modalities can provide documentation and evaluation, including options for color images, red-free and fluorescein angiography, and fundus autofluorescence [1, 2]. Data from these modern imaging devices has led to more understanding of the role of the peripheral pathology in both adult and pediatric retinal diseases.

20.2 Imaging Technology

Few commercially available systems have been used in clinical practice. The Retcam (Natus Medical Inc., Pleasanton, CA, USA) is a portable wide-angle camera system available since 1997. It is a contact-based, coaxial illumination system, which obtains 130° field of view [3]. The system is particularly well-suited for imaging pediatric patients because it is portable and can be placed directly on patients unable to position themselves, such as neonates and infants (Fig. 20.1a, b). Specifically, this device has been well studied in patients with retinopathy of prematurity. A major limitation in this technology, however, was its inability to image through lens opacities [3].

The Optos camera (Optos, Dunfermline, UK) is a UWF imaging system which produces a 200° view of the retina (about 82% of the surface area). The Optos technology utilizes a combined scanning laser ophthalmoscope with an ellipsoidal mirror to obtain images of the retinal periphery with one capture without the need for bright illumination lighting or a contact lens, and in some patients, pupillary dilation (Figs. 20.2a, b and 20.3). The system provides the ability to capture red and green reflectance imaging, as well as fundus autofluorescence and fluorescein angiography (Fig. 20.4a, b) [4].

The 3nethra/Neo system (Forus Health Ltd, Bangalore, India) is a portable hand-held unit for imaging of retina with

I. Kozak (✉) · S. M. Ali
Moorfields Eye Hospital UAE, Abu Dhabi, United Arab Emirates
e-mail: igor.kozak@moorfields.ae

M. E. A. Abdalla-Elsayed
Jeddah Eye Hospital, Jeddah, Saudi Arabia

W.-C. Wu, W.-C. Lam (eds.), *A Quick Guide to Pediatric Retina*, https://doi.org/10.1007/978-981-15-6552-6_20

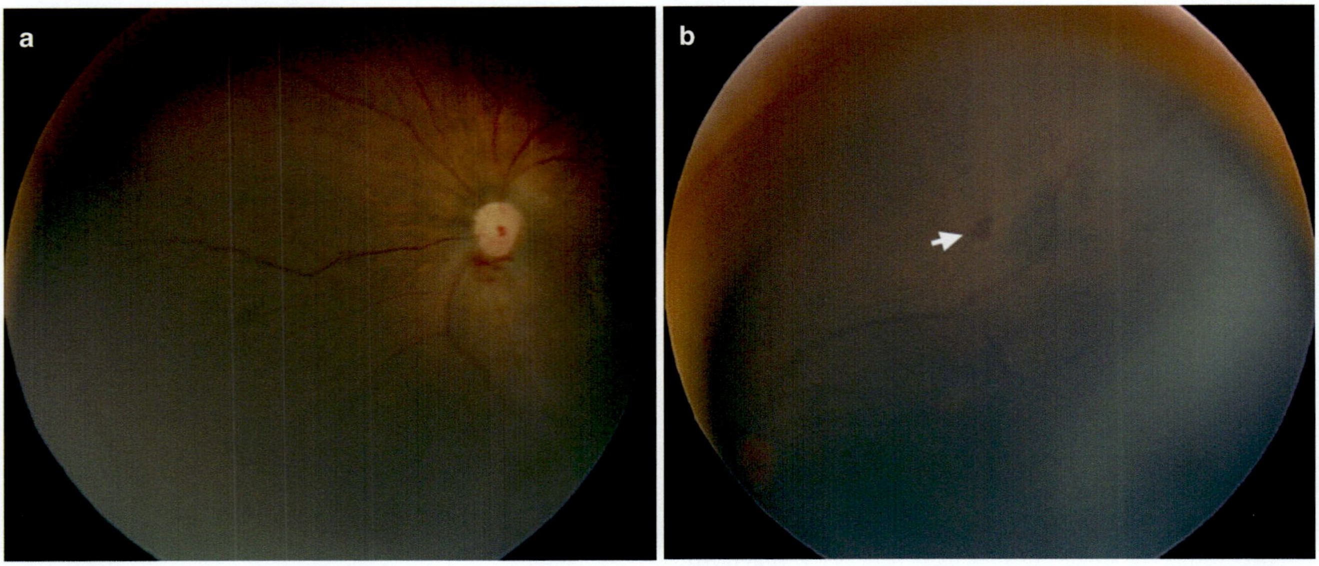

Fig. 20.1 (**a**) Birth trauma. Retcam image of left eye of newborn baby following spontaneous delivery demonstrates peripapillary and optic disc hemorrhage. (**b**) Birth trauma. Retcam image of the same eye demonstrates intraretinal hemorrhages superior to the arcade (white arrow)

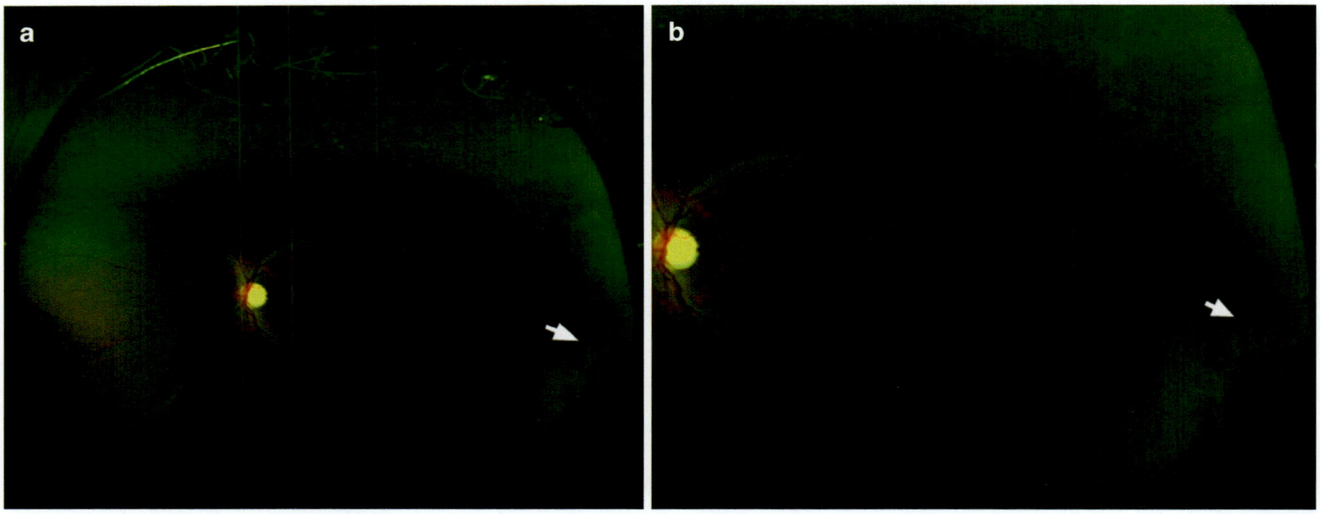

Fig. 20.2 (**a**) Peripheral retinal hole. Optos color fundus image of the left eye of a 9-year-old myopic girl demonstrates inferotemporal lattice degeneration with atrophic hole inside lattice lesion (white arrow). (**b**) Peripheral retinal hole. Optos color fundus blow-up image of the same eye demonstrates a small atrophic hole inside the lattice lesion (white arrow)

120° field of view. It is capable of capturing both still and video images and commonly used in pediatric retina (Figs. 20.5 and 20.6).

Wide-field imaging of the retina and vitreous using biomicroscopic system utilizing 3 CCD video camera and a personal computer was described in 2000 [5]. The advantage of the system is its ease of use, practicality, and ability to capture dynamic images. It is suitable for older and younger cooperative children (Figs. 20.7 and 20.8).

20.3 Challenges and New Techniques

20.3.1 Patient Cooperation

Obtaining discernible and reproducible images in pediatric patients can be challenging as times. Uncooperative children require a great amount of patience on part of physician and parents. A good relation and rapport are crucial in gaining a chance to perform retinal imaging. In children too small to be seated for camera chin rest a technique of flying baby imaging has been successful in selected cases (Fig. 20.9a, b).

20.3.1.1 Artifacts

Another challenge in pediatric imaging even in cooperative children or adult patients is the presence of imaging artifacts. A major cause of artifact with any fundus imaging arises from the reflection of light from interfaces in the ocular media. Elimination of these reflections is achieved using confocal scanning laser ophthalmoscopy (cSLO), which separates the illuminating and imaging beam within the eye [6]. Even after the elimination of central reflections, some peripheral artifacts may appear. The presence of eyelashes at the margin of the captured image has been a frequent artifact with Optos system.

20.3.1.2 Mercator Projection

An inevitable discrepancy in ultra-widefield imaging is to map a three-dimensional image onto a two-dimensional map, so-called Mercator projection known from cartography [7]. Peripheral retina is non-linear with image distortions. Hence, the dimensions are changed which may not necessarily reflect the true distances of the structures.

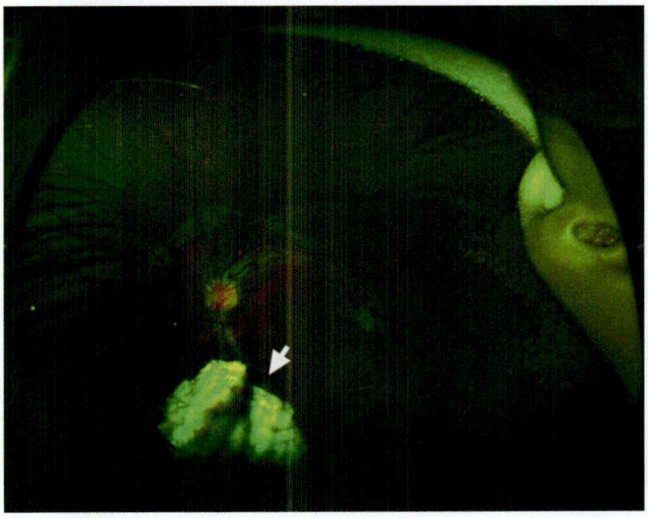

Fig. 20.3 Intraocular retinoblastoma following intraarterial chemotherapy. Optos color fundus image of the eye of a 2-year-old girl demonstrates retinoblastoma tumor after intraarterial chemotherapy (white arrow)

20.3.2 Oral FFA

Another challenge in the pediatric population is associated with invasive procedures such as injecting contrast dyes in fundus fluorescein angiography (FFA). The inability to find and safely enter small or fragile veins in children or fear of needles can prevent from performing this important diagnostic study. Ultra-widefield fundus fluorescein angiography (FFA), in particular, has contributed significantly to the detection of peripheral fundus disease in pediatric retinal conditions [8]. An alternative to intravenous injection of fluorescein is oral fluorescein angiography. Oral FFA has been successfully used with standard and wide-field camera systems [9]. The technique of oral ultra-widefield fluorescein angiography in children using noncontact high-resolution Optos 200Tx imaging system (Dunfermline, UK) has been described by Ali et al. [10]. The peripheral retinal anatomy, vascular network, and necessary clinical information can be obtained by this technique (Figs. 20.10a, b and 20.11).

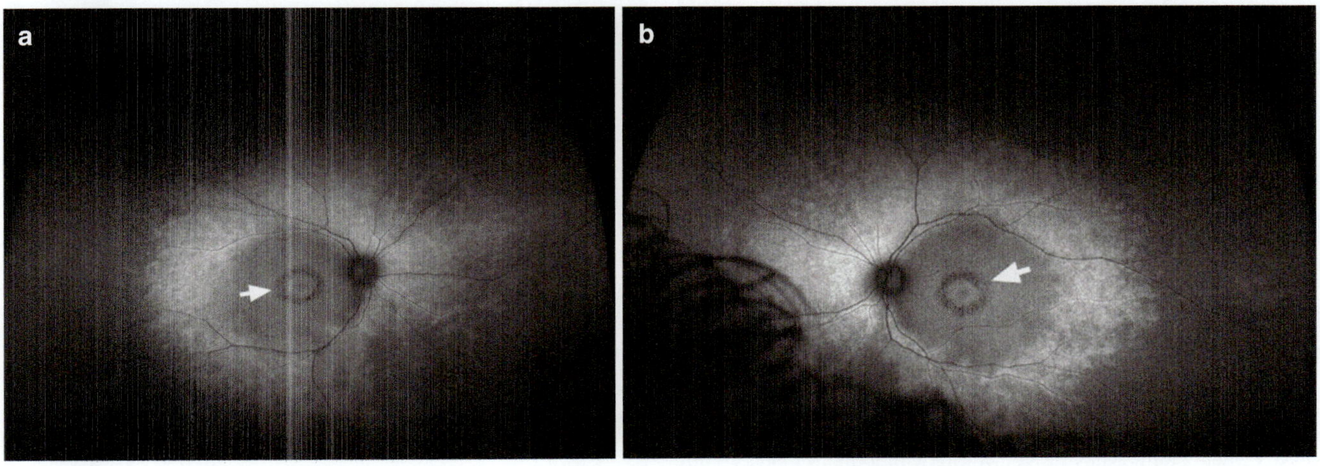

Fig. 20.4 (**a**) Bull's eye maculopathy. Optos fundus autofluorescence image of the right eye of a 9-year-old patient with decreased central vision (20/80) demonstrates hypoautofluorescence ring of bull's eye maculopathy (white arrow). (**b**) Bull's eye maculopathy. Optos fundus autofluorescence image of the left eye of the same patient with decreased central vision (20/70) demonstrates hypoautofluorescence ring of bull's eye maculopathy (white arrow)

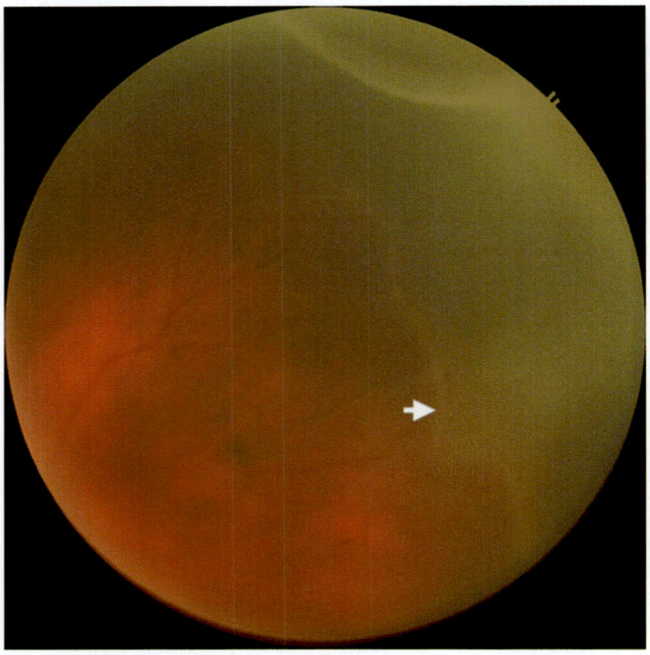

Fig. 20.5 Retinopathy of prematurity—stage 3. 3nethra/Neo system color fundus image of the left eye of a 4-week-old baby demonstrates stage 3, zone 2 retinopathy of prematurity (white arrow) with peripheral retinal image under scleral indentation superiorly

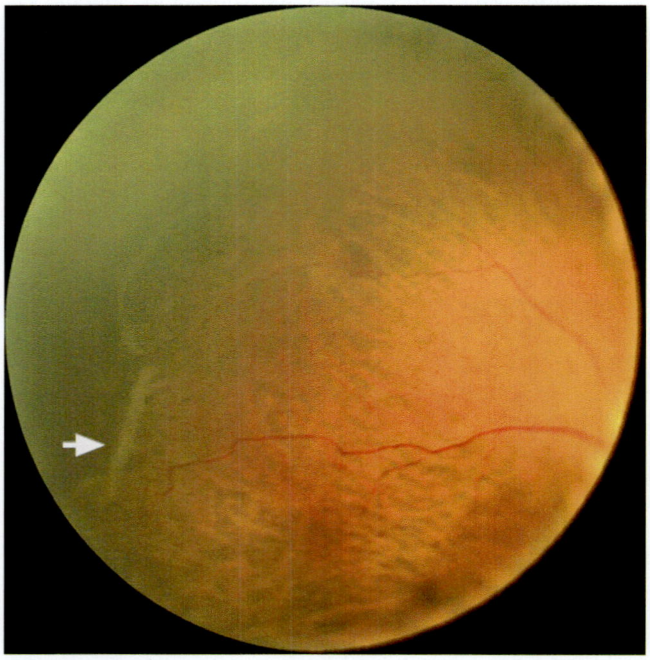

Fig. 20.6 Retinopathy of prematurity—stage 3. 3nethra/Neo system color fundus image of the left eye of a 6-week-old baby demonstrates stage 3, zone 2 retinopathy of prematurity with tortuous blood vessels anterior to the ridge (white arrow)

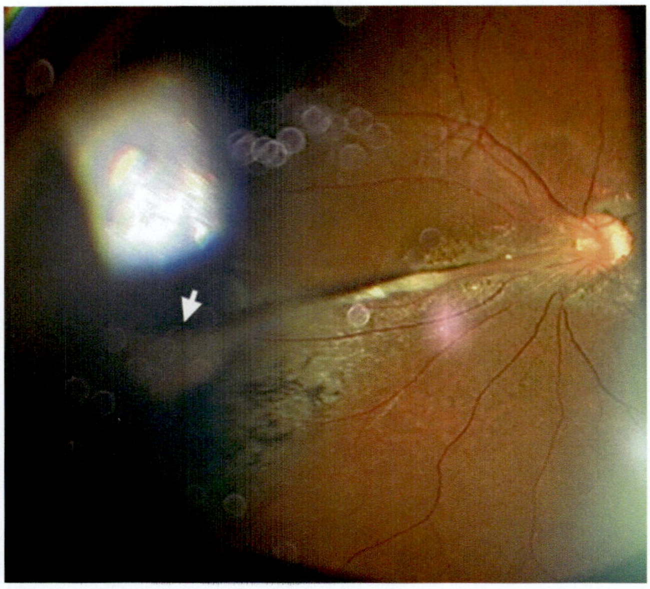

Fig. 20.7 Granuloma of toxocariasis. Wide-angle biomicroscopic color fundus image of the right eye of a 15-year-old patient demonstrates peripheral granuloma (white arrow) due to intraocular toxocariasis with connecting stalk reaching up to the optic disc. Reflex artifact is present above the lesion (image by Prof. ByungRo Lee, Seoul, Korea)

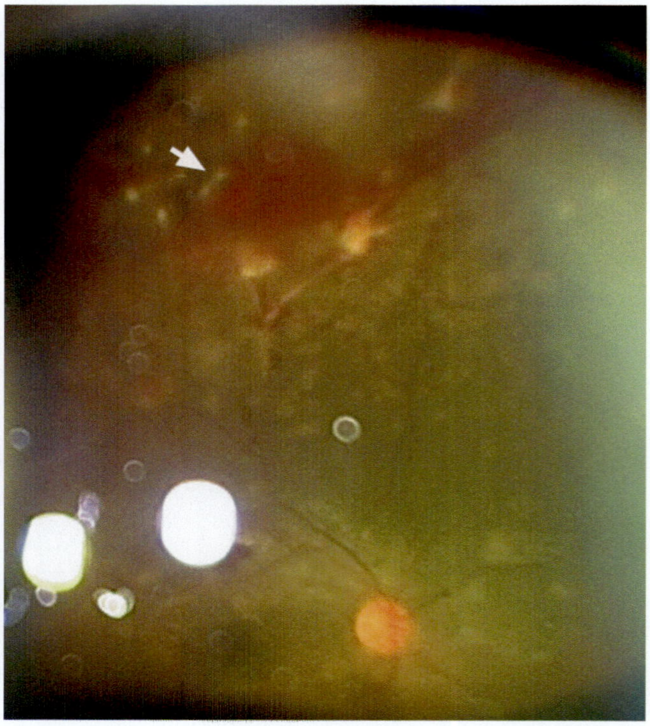

Fig. 20.8 Retinal vasculitis of Eales disease. Wide-angle biomicroscopic color fundus image of the right eye of an 18-year-old patient demonstrates retinal vasculitis (white arrow) with both pre- and intraretinal hemorrhages. Image captures both the central and far peripheral retinal areas. Reflex artifacts are present along the superior arcade (image by Prof. ByungRo Lee, Seoul, Korea)

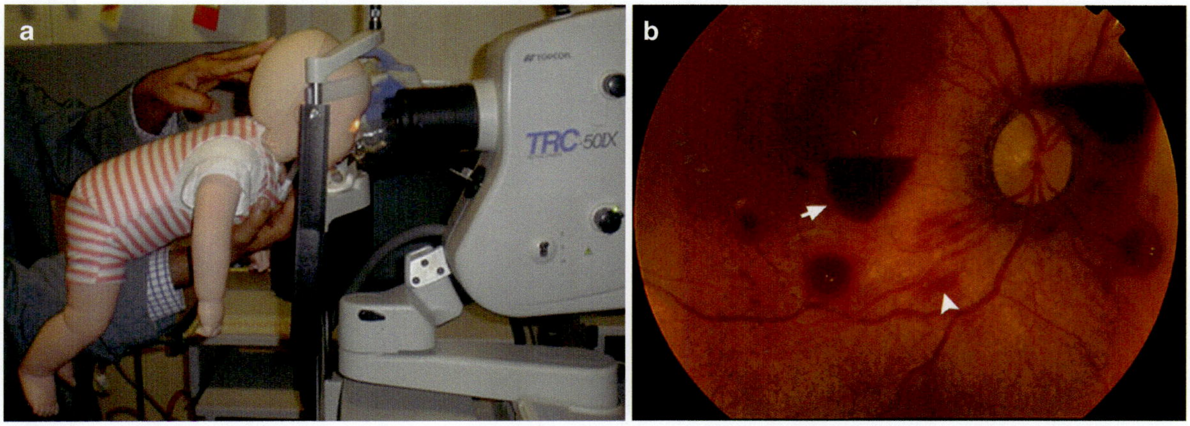

Fig. 20.9 (**a**) Flying baby photography technique. Demonstration of positioning infants for fundus photography. (**b**) Shaken baby syndrome. Color fundus photography acquired by flying baby technique on a 3-month-old baby brought in with reduced consciousness and fracture ribs. It shows subhyaloid (white arrow) and intraretinal (white arrowhead) hemorrhages at different stages of resolution confirming diagnosis of shaken baby syndrome

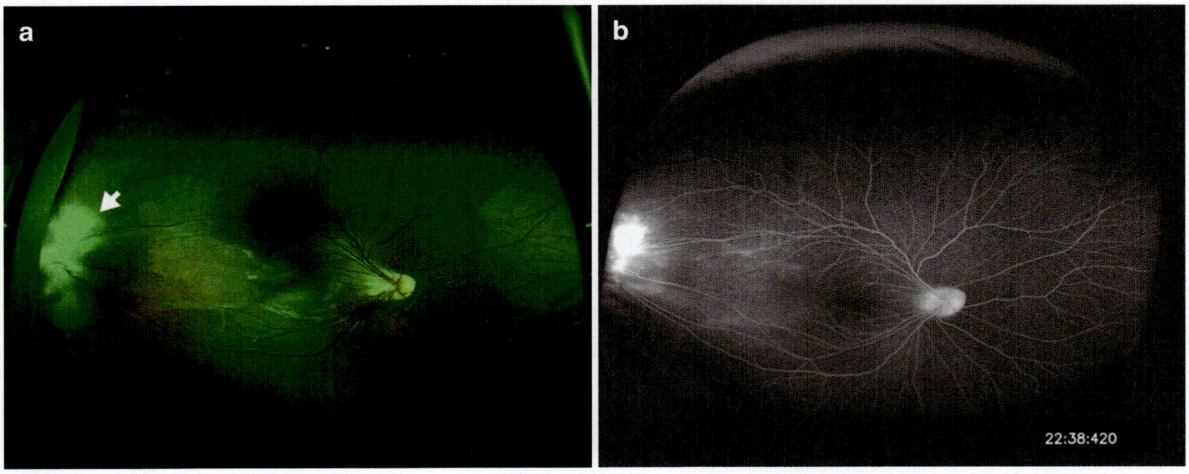

Fig. 20.10 (**a**) Familial exudative vitreoretinopathy. Optos color fundus image of right eye of a 7-year-old patient with mild peripheral retinal elevation, vascular tortuosity and retinal dragging (white arrow). (**b**) Familial exudative vitreoretinopathy. Optos fundus fluorescein image of the same eye following ingestion of oral fluorescein demonstrates dye leakage from peripheral retinal vessels

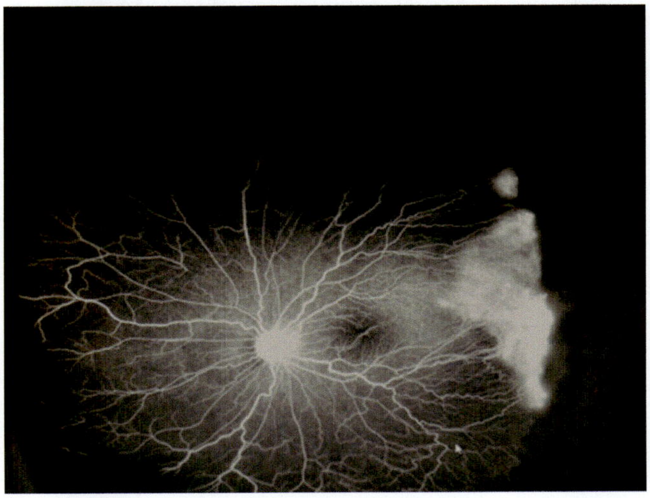

Fig. 20.11 Coat's disease. Optos fundus fluorescein image of the left eye of an 11-year-old boy with Coat's disease following ingestion of oral fluorescein. It shows dye leakage from temporal peripheral telangiectatic retinal vessels

References

1. Tan CS, Sadda SR, Hariprasad SM. Ultra-widefield retinal imaging in the management of diabetic eye diseases. Ophthalmic Surg Lasers Imaging Retina. 2014 Sep 1;45(5):363–6.
2. Shoughy SS, Arevalo JF, Kozak I. Update on wide- and ultra-widefield retinal imaging. Ind J Ophthalmol. 2015;63:575–81.
3. Roth DB, Morales D, Feuer WJ, Hess D, Johnson RA, Flynn JT. Screening for retinopathy of prematurity employing the retcam 120: sensitivity and specificity. Arch Ophthalmol. 2001;119:268–72.
4. Witmer MT, Parlitsis G, Patel S, Kiss S. Comparison of ultra-widefield fluoresceuin angiography with the Heidelberg Spectralis noncontact ultra-widefield module versus the Optos Optomap. Clin Ophthalmol. 2013;7:389–94.
5. Lee BR, Chang HR. Biomicroscopic vitreous observation using a 3 CCD video camera and a personal computer for image capture and archiving. Korean J Ophthalmol. 2000;14:74–9.
6. Kaines A, Oliver S, Reddy S, Schwartz SD. Ultrawide angle angiography for the detection and management of diabetic retinopathy. Int Ophthalmol Clin. 2009;49(2):53–9.
7. Van Cader TC. History of ophthalmic photography. J Ophthalmic Photogr. 1978;1:7–9.

8. Tsui I, Franco-Cardenas V, Hubschman JP, Schwartz SD. Pediatric retinal conditions imaged by ultra wide field fluorescein angiography. Ophthalmic Surg Lasers Imaging Retina. 2013;44(1):59–67.
9. Kelley JS, Kincaid M. Retinal fluorography using oral fluorescein. Arch Ophthalmol. 1979;97:2331–2.
10. Ali SMA, Khan I, Khurram D, Kozak I. Ultra-widefield angiography with oral fluorescein in pediatric patients with retinal diseases. JAMA Ophthalmol. 2018;136(5):593–4.

Part II

Non-ROP Pediatric Retina

21 Retinoblastoma

Sameh E. Soliman, Brenda Gallie, and Wai-Ching Lam

Abstract

Retinoblastoma management is a success story of a genetic cancer. Nowadays, advances in diagnostic and therapeutic approaches have provided approximately 99% survival in developed countries. Later diagnosis lowers survival in developing countries. In this chapter, we present the concepts of pathogenesis, diagnosis, treatment, and long-term surveillance for retinoblastoma patients and their families.

Keywords

Retinoblastoma · Genetics · Cancer · Heritability Enucleation · Chemoreduction · Vitreous seeds · RB1 pathogenic allele · Leukocorea

Retinoblastoma is the most common pediatric intraocular malignancy that arises from the developing retinal cells. It can affect one or both eyes with around 8000 new cases annually worldwide. The survival is high when it is timely diagnosed and managed through a multidisciplinary team of ophthalmologists, oncologists, geneticists, radiologists, pediatricians, anesthesiologists, and social workers [1].

21.1 Epidemiology

Retinoblastoma affects 1 in 18,000 live births. The live-birth rate is the main factor-affecting incidence where India followed by China has the largest number of annual cases. Multiple factors such as parental age and occupation, method of conception, and exposure to mutagens as X-rays, viral agents, or sunlight exposure were studied but never proven [2].

Retinoblastoma affects children under 5 years of age with a mean age of 12 and 24 months for bilateral versus unilateral disease respectively. The mean age is higher in developing than developed countries [3] due to later diagnosis with more advanced disease. Retinoblastoma affects males and females equally [4].

21.2 Genetics

Retinoblastoma develops secondary to loss of both copies of *RB1* gene (13q14). The *RB1* gene is a tumor suppressor gene encoding for a protein that regulates normal cell cycle and prevents uncontrolled proliferation. A pathogenic allele affecting the *RB1* gene causes absent/dysfunctional (null pathogenic alleles) or a poorly functional *RB1* protein (low-penetrance pathogenic alleles) [5].

There are two distinct genetic forms of retinoblastoma according to the timing of the first *RB1* gene pathogenic allele (M1) [4]. Heritable (germline) form when prezygotic/zygotic or early post-zygotic pathogenic allele leads to a mutated copy of *RB1* gene involving the whole body cells or a subset of cells (mosaicism). Retinoblastoma develops after the second pathogenic allele (M2) occurs (two-hit hypothesis) [6]. Individuals with heritable retinoblastoma usually

S. E. Soliman
Department of Ophthalmology and Vision Science, Hospital for Sick Children, Toronto, Canada

Department of Ophthalmology, Faculty of Medicine, University of Alexandria, Alexandria, Egypt

B. Gallie
Department of Ophthalmology and Vision Science, Hospital for Sick Children, Toronto, Canada

Department of Ophthalmology and Vision Science, University of Toronto, Toronto, Canada
e-mail: brenda.gallie@sickkids.ca

W.-C. Lam (✉)
Department of Ophthalmology and Vision Science, Hospital for Sick Children, Toronto, Canada

Department of Ophthalmology, University of Hong Kong, Hong Kong, Hong Kong
e-mail: waichlam@hku.hk

W.-C. Wu, W.-C. Lam (eds.), *A Quick Guide to Pediatric Retina*, https://doi.org/10.1007/978-981-15-6552-6_21

develop multiple (multifocal) retinoblastoma tumors usually affecting both eyes (bilateral) and diagnosed earlier. Their other body cells have the same pathogenic allele and are prone to second primary neoplasms with a 50% chance of transmission of the pathogenic allele to each offspring [7]. Patients with the *RB1* can be associated with a midline intracranial tumor most probably pinealoblastoma in 3–5% of cases [8]. Heritable cases have a higher risk of developing second primary malignancies later in life. Moreover, avoidance of irradiation whether therapeutic (external beam irradiation) or unnecessary diagnostic procedures (computed tomography and X-rays) is recommended [9].

In contrast, non-heritable (non-germline) *RB1* pathogenic alleles that occur later in a single retinal cell are associated with a single (unifocal) unilateral retinoblastoma tumor that is diagnosed later with no risk of second primary neoplasms, pinealoblastoma, or vertical transmission [2, 5, 7, 10]. A rare form of non-heritable retinoblastoma (2%) develops due to the amplification of N-MYC oncogene rather than *RB1* pathogenic alleles (normal *RB1* gene) characterized by early unilateral aggressive presentation within the first few months after birth [11].

In 94% of germline retinoblastoma, the *RB1* allele arises de novo, with no family history; 6% inherit the pathogenic allele from an affected parent (familial). The first affected child in the family is called the proband and the exact pathogenic allele can be detected with full molecular diagnostic techniques. In rare instances, an unaffected parent may carry the pathogenic allele and pass it to his offspring and can be detected by molecular analysis of the parent's serum for the proband's pathologic allele or simply predicted if more than one sibling have retinoblastoma (Fig. 21.1) [5].

Retinoblastoma is the first cancer to include heritability in its initial staging (tumor, node, metastasis and heritability staging, American Joint Committee of Cancer 8th edition). H1 designates heritable retinoblastoma and assigned if bilateral/trilateral retinoblastoma, positive family history in a first-degree relative or positive molecular diagnosis. H0 designates non-heritable retinoblastoma and assigned in unilateral cases with negative genetic testing. If genetic testing is unavailable, unilateral cases are assigned Hx [12].

Rigorous postnatal screening of retinoblastoma survivors' offspring, each of which has a 60% chance of having tumors in at least one eye, helps to diagnose the tumors earlier with less treatment burden and better visual and ocular outcomes [13]. Prenatal screening includes molecular diagnosis of the fetal amniocytes obtained via amniocentesis during the second trimester of pregnancy to determine if the fetus carries the proband's pathogenic allele. If positive, the option of late preterm/early term delivery reduces the incidence of tumors at birth to 20% [14]. Nowadays, detection and even the management of invisible tumors is reviving the concept of secondary prevention in retinoblastoma [15]. Proper genetic counseling is essential in the management of every patient to

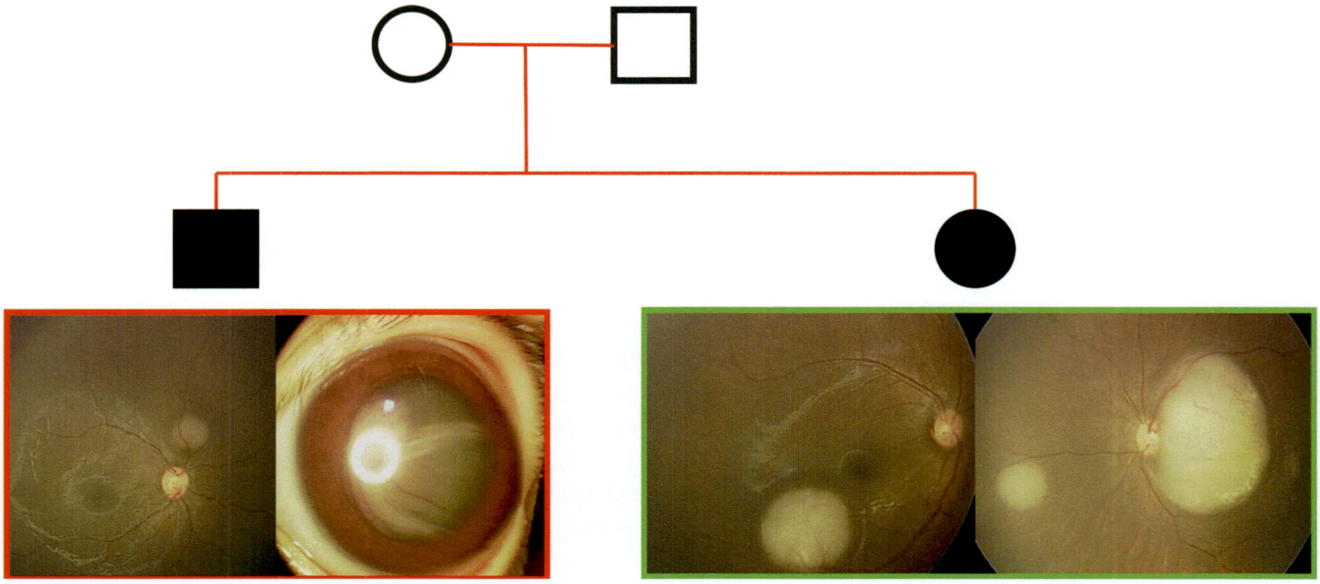

Fig. 21.1 Showing a family pedigree of a non-consanguineous couple. No known family history of retinoblastoma. The family presented because of left leukocorea in the left eye of their elder son (Red box—age: 2 years). On examination, the left eye harbored a large tumor with total retinal detachment without vitreous seeds and was staged as (IIRC group D eye/cT2a). The right eye had one small tumor that lied within 1.5 mm from the optic disc and was staged as (IIRC group B eye/cT1b). Due to bilateral disease, the child was designated as H1. No genetic testing was available, so the sibling (green box—2 months old) was examined at the same session and revealed bilateral multifocal retinoblastoma (both eyes classified as IIRC group B/cT1b H1). The parents declined to be examined but one of them has to be a carrier of the RB1 pathogenic allele

communicate the knowledge for the importance of screening and life-long surveillance for second cancers [16].

21.3 Natural History of Retinoblastoma (Fig. 21.2)

Retinoblastoma arises from a developing retinal cell within the inner nuclear layer. At first, a small round tumor is clinically invisible and detected only by optical coherence tomography (OCT) in screened eyes of patients with positive family history [17, 18]. Uniform growth elevates the developing tumor above the retinal surface to become clinically visible as a rounded white single mass. A visible separate blood supply can be observed with increase in size and tortuosity with the enlarging tumor. Different growth rates of the tumor cell clones make the tumor lose its rounded appearance into a mass with lobules or nipples. When the tumor overgrows its blood supply, areas of necrosis with dystrophic calcification appear that are highly diagnostic on clinical or sonographic examination [19].

The tumor breaks through the inner limiting membrane and the serous effusion from the actively growing tumor causes the retina to detach [19]. Tumor cells lose cohesiveness and tumor seeds separate from the main mass into the vitreous cavity or the subretinal space. Seeds can be in the form of fine dust, spheres, or clouds [20]. They can be localized within 3 mm from the main tumor or diffuse (>3 mm). Large greasy seeds or subretinal tumor plaques are dangerous and difficult to be treated [21]. Landed seeds on the retinal surface or the pars plana of the ciliary body can grow into new tumors especially at the inferior periphery.

The enlarging tumor involves most of the posterior segment and may involve the ciliary body and back of the iris. It might push the iris lens diaphragm forward causing pupillary block or angle-closure glaucoma. Furthermore, iris and anterior chamber angle neovascularization can cause neovascular glaucoma [22]. Glaucoma may present as buphthalmos at such young age. Tumor involvement of the anterior chamber can appear in the form of tumor seeds or can produce an irregular pseudohypopyon in advanced cases [20]. The tumor may bleed causing either vitreous hemorrhage or hyphema. If massive necrosis in the tumor occurs secondary to vascular occlusion and tumor autoinfarction, the release of inflammatory mediators can produce an aseptic inflammatory response involving the whole orbit (aseptic orbital cellulitis) or can cause ciliary body shut down with atrophic or phthisic ocular changes [22].

Tumor can spread outside the eye posteriorly through the optic nerve (ON) into the central nervous system and involves the cerebrospinal fluid (CSF) or through the choroid and sclera into the orbital cavity. Anteriorly the tumor can spread through the anterior chamber angle and trabecular meshwork into the episclera and the conjunctiva and might involve the draining preauricular and cervical lymph nodes [23]. Hematogenous spread mainly to the bone marrow and liver occurs secondary to massive uveal (choroid, ciliary body, or iris) invasion.

After enucleation of an eye for advanced retinoblastoma, meticulous histopathologic assessment can point to high-risk

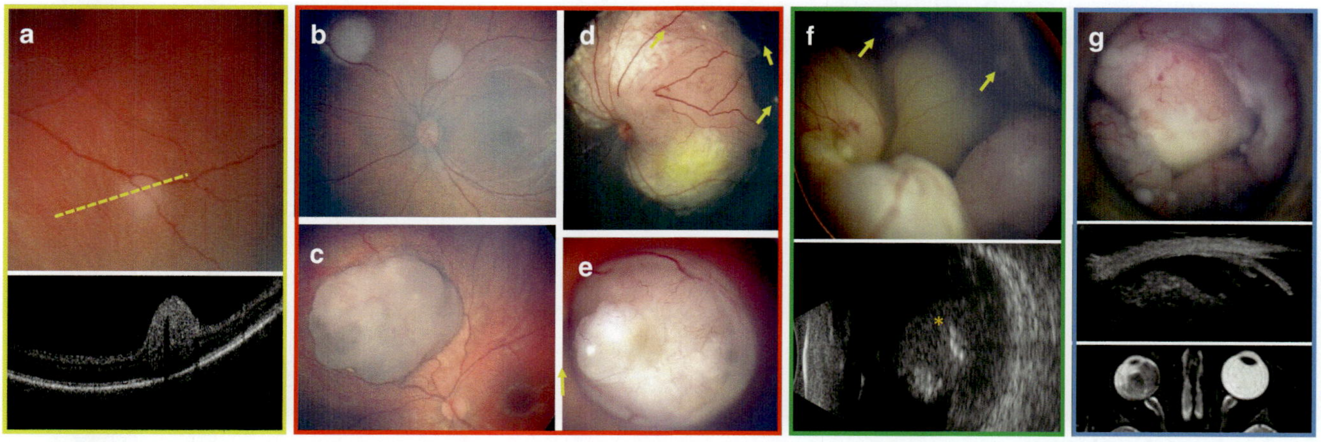

Fig. 21.2 Natural history of intraocular retinoblastoma at different stages of growth. Yellow Box: (**a**) small rounded white retinoblastoma staged as group A (<3 mm in size and >1.5 mm away from optic nerve and >3 mm from foveal center) by the international intraocular retinoblastoma classification (IIRC, note the retinal vessels passing on top). OCT scan showing a homogenous elevated dome-shaped intra-retinal lesion. Red Box: (**b**) multifocal small retinoblastomas (IIRC group A). (**c**) Large lobulated retinoblastoma staged as IIRC group B (>3 mm in size or <1.5 mm away from optic nerve and <3 mm from foveal center, no retinal detachment or vitreous seeding). (**d**, **e**) Large retinoblastoma with subtle surrounding retinal detachment and localized fine tumor seeding (arrows) staged as IIRC group C. Green Box: (**f**) diffuse tumor >1 quadrant retinal detachment and greasy distant tumor seeds (arrows) staged as IIRC group D. B-scan ultrasonography shows the mass with classic calcifications (*). Blue Box: (**g**) A diffuse tumor occupying most of the posterior segment of the eye with elevated intraocular pressure and rubeosis irides staged as IIRC group E. Ultrasound biomicroscopy identifies the anterior extent of the tumor and magnetic resonance imaging assesses the optic nerve and scleral intactness to exclude extraocular spread

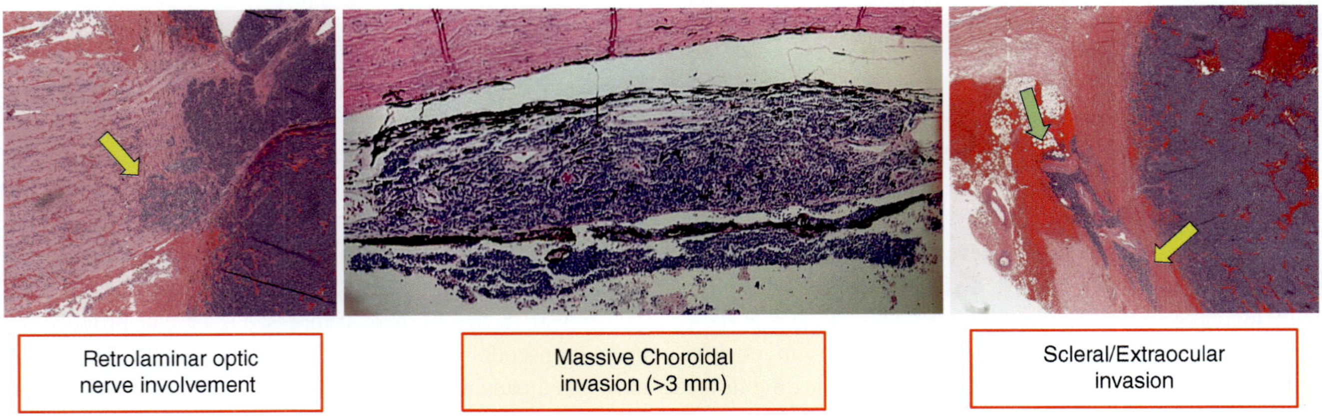

Fig. 21.3 High-risk histopathologic features assessed after enucleation

features suggestive of risk of extraocular or metastatic spread (Fig. 21.3) namely ON involvement beyond the lamina cribrosa (retrolaminar ON invasion) especially if extending up to the cut end of the ON. Massive choroidal invasion >3 mm in any dimension or total involvement of the choroidal thickness is the risk of hematogenous spread. Scleral invasion (partial or complete) and definitive extraocular disease are at higher risk metastasis. Anterior segment involvement is debatable as a high-risk feature [24].

21.4 Clinical Presentation

Leukocorea (white pupil) is the most common presentation in both forms of retinoblastoma. Parents usually notice the white glow caused by light reflection from the white tumor occupying the posterior pole. Parents often describe it similar to a cat's eye. Retinoblastoma can also be first recognized in non-modified photographs (photoleukocorea) [1]. Strabismus can occur earlier if the tumor involves the fovea. Glaucoma and/or buphthalmos occur in advanced cases with large tumors elevating the intraocular pressure through the forward push of the lens-iris diaphragm or iris and anterior chamber neovascularization. Proptosis is considered a later presentation secondary to extraocular spread. Rare presentations include hypopyon, hyphema, vitreous hemorrhage, phthisis bulbi, or aseptic orbital cellulitis [22].

21.5 Investigations

B-scan ultrasonography identifies the mass and its measurements and highlights tumor relation to the nerve and detects associated retinal detachment. The presence of echogenic calcifications is suggestive but not pathognomonic [25]. Ultrasound biomicroscopy (UBM) shows the anterior extent of the tumor in relation to the ciliary body and the crystalline lens [26]. Optical coherence tomography (OCT) can highlight small and clinically invisible tumors and show tumor relation to the fovea [15, 17]. Fluorescein angiography has a minimal role in diagnosing retinoblastoma. Magnetic resonance angiography (MRI) is essential to determine the risk of optic nerve or extrascleral invasion and exclude pinealoblastoma or suprasellar masses. Computed tomography is best avoided because of its high radiation dose.

21.6 Differential Diagnosis

Unilateral advanced retinoblastoma may be confused with Coats' disease [25] (telangiectatic vessels, yellowish-red reflex and absence of perpendicular vascular dipping into an underlying mass), persistent fetal vasculature (prominent ciliary processes and vascular stalk on ultrasonography), and ocular toxocariasis (pets, inflammatory signs, and serology). Small tumors may be mistaken for astrocytomas (moth-eaten appearance on OCT, other manifestations of tuberous sclerosis).

21.7 Intraocular Classification (Staging)

Eyes harboring retinoblastoma are classified according to the tumor size, tumor location within the eye, presence and characters (size, location, and shape) of tumor seeds, presence and extent of serous retinal detachment and any associated signs of elevated intraocular pressure, neovascularization (iris or anterior chamber angle), or hemorrhage [1]. Multiple classifications have been used over years, mainly related to the available treatment modalities. Reese–Ellsworth classification [6] was developed to predict the outcome of external beam irradiation (EBRT). This was replaced by the international intraocular retinoblastoma classification (IIRC) [19] when systemic chemotherapy prevailed. Three versions of IIRC were described that have significant differences in classifying advanced eyes [1]. The American joint classifica-

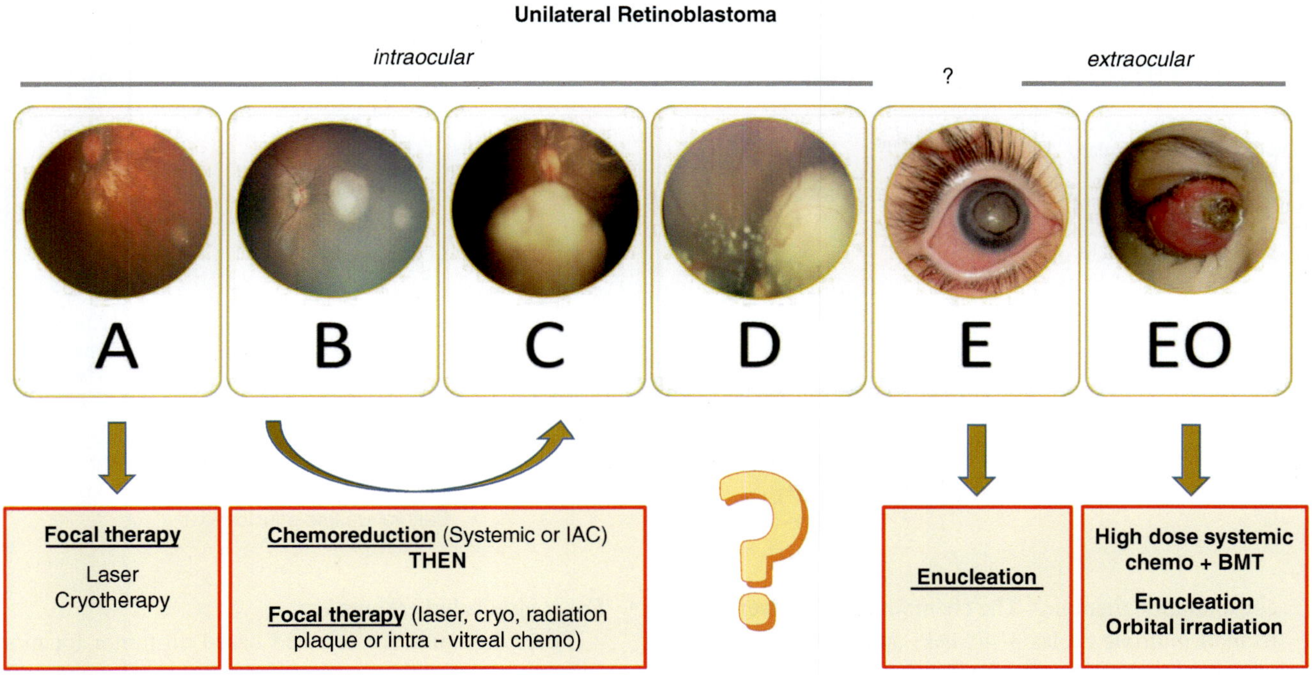

Fig. 21.4 Schematic representation of the management of unilateral retinoblastoma. Group D is debatable

tion of cancer (AJCC, 8th ed.) is the current consensus classification [12]. It depends on the tumor, lymph nodes, and metastatic involvement assessment (TNM). Furthermore, heritability (H) was added to highlight its importance in decision-making in retinoblastoma management and lifelong surveillance.

21.8 Management

Goals: Saving the child's life is the main goal of management plans to prevent local or metastatic tumor spread. Saving any visual potential follows. Saving a blind eye for cosmetic purposes is controversial.

21.9 General Principles

- Treatment is carried by a multidisciplinary team lead by the ophthalmologist.
- Rationale, expectations, and available modalities of therapy are discussed with parents/guardians (informed consent).
- The importance of compliance with the treatment plan is emphasized.
- Lifelong follow-up includes ocular and systemic surveillance.
- Genetic counseling is key including genetic testing if available [4, 16].
- Recurrence or poor response to therapy can happen even after an initial favorable response.
- Unilateral retinoblastoma has special considerations during management planning, as the other eye is normal [27–29] (Figs. 21.4 and 21.5).

21.10 Treatment Modalities

- ***Enucleation***:

  Primary enucleation with an 8–12 mm optic nerve stump is recommended in cT3/E eyes regardless of laterality to reduce the chance of tumor spread [12]. Primary enucleation allows accurate histopathologic assessment for high-risk features without being masked by chemotherapy [30]. Some centers recommend primary enucleation for unilateral cT2/D eyes unless they have predictive clinical signs of low-risk histopathology namely visible optic disc, foveal sparing, and <1 quadrant of retinal detachment [31]. Enucleation with primary implant using the myoconjunctival technique (vertical and horizontal recti sutured to their respective conjunctival fornices) improves cosmesis and motility and reduces the implant extrusion rate [32, 33]. Secondary enucleation is recommended for refractory retinoblastoma (progressive, recurrent, or nonresponsive) after failure of primary trial salvage [10].
- ***Chemoreduction:***

  The goal of chemotherapy is to reduce the size of the tumor into a size appropriate for the application of focal

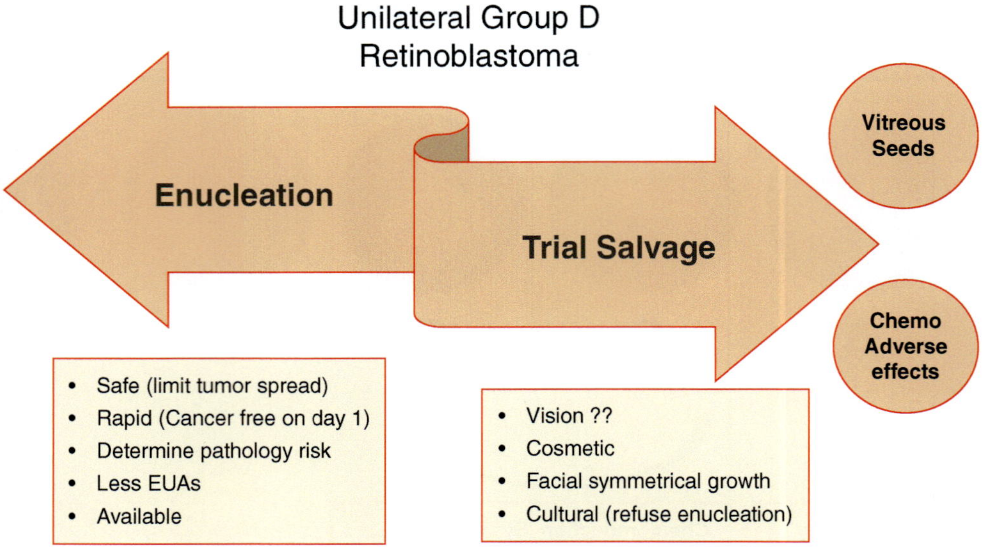

Fig. 21.5 Schematic representation of the management of unilateral retinoblastoma (IIRC group D) showing the pros of each modality. The trial ocular salvage failure is highly related to the resistance of vitreous seeds and the chemotherapy adverse effects

consolidation therapies. The chemotherapy is given in the form of multiple cycles 3–4 weeks apart [34]. Two routes of delivery for chemotherapy are currently available, depending on laterality, staging, and informed discussion with parents regarding the pros and cons of each procedure [35].

– **Systemic chemotherapy**

  Intravenous chemotherapy using multiple drugs (to reduce incidence of cancer cell resistance) is given on 2 or 3 days for 4–6 cycles by a pediatric oncologist. Multiple regimens are reported but vincristine, etoposide, and carboplatin (VEC) are the most commonly utilized worldwide. Myelosuppression, susceptibility to infection, peripheral neurotoxicity (Vincristine), and gastrointestinal disturbances are the most significant short-term side effects. Ototoxicity (Carboplatin, 25%, more in children less than 6 months) [36] and Leukemia (1%, etoposide) are significant long-term adverse effects.

– **Intra-arterial chemotherapy**

  Direct delivery of chemotherapeutic drugs (melphalan, topotecan, and/or carboplatin) via catheterization of the ophthalmic artery can be used for the treatment of one or both eyes. It involves an intracranial procedure that requires high technical preparation and is performed by an experienced interventional radiologist [37]. It has less systemic side effects than systemic chemotherapy. Locally, there is risk of vascular occlusion (ophthalmic, central retinal artery, or sectorial choroidal vessels), transient nerve palsies (ptosis, optic neuritis, or third nerve palsy), localized forehead erythema, and temporary loss of eyebrow hair. As an intracranial procedure, there is a risk of cerebrovascular stroke which is extremely rare but very serious [28].

• ***Focal ophthalmic therapies:***

  Focal therapies are selected based on tumor location and size. Posterior tumors are better consolidated with Lasers, while cryotherapy is more appropriate for anterior non-calcified tumors. Brachytherapy is reserved for tumors that cannot be consolidated with laser or cryotherapy and can be covered completely. Focal chemotherapy can be used to treat tumor seeds [38].

– **Laser therapy:**

  Tumors can be treated by photocoagulation or thermotherapy using transpupillary and rarely transscleral approach. Indirect ophthalmoscopy or operating microscope-mount laser delivery systems can be used. OCT can be used to ensure complete laser treatment and to identify skipped areas [39]. Treated tumors appear swollen, hyper-reflective with shadowing, and interrupted retinal pigment epithelial line on ultrasound. Misplaced laser burns can destroy normal retina and laser treatment scars can show expansion, migration, or traction [38].

– **Cryotherapy:**

  Transconjunctival cryotherapy is used to treat anteriorly located tumors. Triple freeze–thaw cryotherapy cycles (a complete ice ball covers the tumor followed by complete thawing of the ice ball before the next freeze). Tumor cells die during thawing. Cryotherapy near calcified tumors can induce iatrogenic retinal tears; cryotherapy covering >2 retinal quadrants risks anterior segment ischemia [40].

– **Plaque radiotherapy:**

  A radiation physicist plans the radioactive plaque (Ruthenium, Iodine, Strontium, or palladium) based on the prescribed radiation dose, tumor location, and height. The plaque is sutured to the sclera overlying the tumor (corresponding muscle might be disinserted to ensure proper tumor coverage) and left for a planned number of days. A dose of 40 Gy is sufficient in retinoblastoma. Common complications include radiation-induced cataract in anteriorly treated tumors and radiation-induced optic neuropathy and maculopathy in posteriorly treated tumors [41].

- ***Focal chemotherapy***
  - **Intravitreal chemotherapy (IvitC):**

    Munier et al. [42, 43] developed an anti-reflux injection technique to reduce the potential for extraocular tumor spread. The injection site is 3.5 mm behind the limbus in an area free of tumor, retinal detachment, or massive seeding. Anterior chamber paracentesis (30G needle) of 0.1 ml aqueous humor precedes intravitreal injection (32/33G needle) of chemotherapy. The injection tract is sterilized using three brief freeze–thaw cryotherapy applications.

    Multiple chemotherapeutic agents can be injected including melphalan (most common, 20–30 μg/0.1 ml), topotecan or carboplatin. Multiple injections are required 1–2 weeks apart. IvitC is usually effective against all types of vitreous seeds (dust, spheres, and clouds). No extraocular spread has been reported after this procedure [21]. Complications include infection, vitreous or preretinal hemorrhage, and phthisis bulbi (associated with improper high dose) [44].
  - **Periocular chemotherapy**

    Periocular injection of carboplatin was utilized in refractory cases with limited success regarding tumor control and significant local adverse effects including inflammation and extensive fibrosis [45]. Topotecan has milder local side effects with proven efficacy in localized small subretinal, or preretinal seeds. Systemic absorption of the drug occurs reducing the eye dose and fibrin sealant was used to limit this possibility [46]. Presently, a local episcleral implant (FDA approved) is being studied for safety and effectiveness as sustained release chemotherapy over 6–9 weeks [47].
- ***Tumor Endoresection:***

  Report of planned pars-plana vitrectomy (PPV) under melphalan infusion with tumor endoresection for eyes with refractory tumor opens a new approach [48]. The risk of extraocular tumor spread is very low with a carefully planned approach and tight collaboration between experienced vitreoretinal surgeon and retinoblastoma expert and meticulous follow-up.
- ***External beam irradiation therapy (EBRT):***

  External beam radiotherapy is a last desperate option for eyes with refractory tumors. EBRT increases the risk of second primary malignancy especially if combined with alkylating chemotherapy in H1 patients [49]. Proton beam and stereotactic radiation may carry similar risks despite the intent of reducing radiation dose to normal tissue [50]. Other local long-term EBRT complications include facial asymmetry, keratoconjunctivitis, and cataract [51].
- ***Metastatic retinoblastoma:***

  Multimodal approach is required including high-dose systemic chemotherapy, enucleation, and orbital irradiation followed by bone marrow transplantation. Mortality is >50% in these situations mainly due to central nervous system metastasis [52].

References

1. Dimaras H, Corson TW, Cobrinik D, et al. Retinoblastoma. Nat Rev Dis Primers. 2015;1:15021.
2. Dimaras H, Kimani K, Dimba EA, et al. Retinoblastoma. Lancet. 2012;379(9824):1436–46.
3. Soliman SE, Eldomiaty W, Goweida MB, Dowidar A. Clinical presentation of retinoblastoma in Alexandria: a step toward earlier diagnosis. Saudi J Ophthalmol. 2017;31(2):80–5.
4. Soliman SE, Racher H, Zhang C, MacDonald H, Gallie BL. Genetics and molecular diagnostics in retinoblastoma–an update. Asia Pac J Ophthalmol (Phila). 2017;6(2):197–207.
5. Corson TW, Gallie BL. One hit, two hits, three hits, more? Genomic changes in the development of retinoblastoma. Genes Chromosomes Cancer. 2007;46(7):617–34.
6. Knudson AG. Mutation and cancer: statistical study of retinoblastoma. Proc Natl Acad Sci U S A. 1971;68(4):820–3.
7. Canadian RS. National Retinoblastoma Strategy Canadian Guidelines for Care: Strategie therapeutique du retinoblastome guide clinique canadien. Can J Ophthalmol. 2009;44(Suppl 2):S1–88.
8. de Jong MC, Kors WA, de Graaf P, Castelijns JA, Kivela T, Moll AC. Trilateral retinoblastoma: a systematic review and meta-analysis. Lancet Oncol. 2014;15(10):1157–67.
9. Kletke S, Soliman SE, Gallie BL. Radiation compromised survival of patients with heritable retinoblastoma (H1): what will be the long-term consequences of current eye salvage therapies? Ann Eye Sci. 2017;2(5).
10. Gallie BL, Soliman S. Retinoblastoma. In: Lambert B, Lyons C, editors. Taylor and Hoyt's paediatric ophthalmology and strabismus. 5th ed. Oxford: Elsevier; 2017. p. 424–42.
11. Squire J, Goddard AD, Canton M, Becker A, Phillips RA, Gallie BL. Tumour induction by the retinoblastoma mutation is independent of N-myc expression. Nature. 1986;322(6079):555–7.
12. Mallipatna A, Gallie BL, Chévez-Barrios P, et al. Retinoblastoma. In: Amin MB, Edge SB, Greene FL, editors. AJCC Cancer staging manual. 8th ed. New York, NY: Springer; 2017. p. 819–31.
13. Imhof SM, Moll AC, Schouten-van Meeteren AY. Stage of presentation and visual outcome of patients screened for familial retinoblastoma: nationwide registration in the Netherlands. Br J Ophthalmol. 2006;90(7):875–8.
14. Soliman SE, Dimaras H, Khetan V, et al. Prenatal versus postnatal screening for familial retinoblastoma. Ophthalmology. 2016;123(12):2610–7.
15. Soliman SE, VandenHoven C, MacKeen LD, Gallie BL. Secondary prevention of retinoblastoma revisited: laser photocoagulation of invisible new retinoblastoma. Ophthalmology. 2020;127(1):122–27.
16. Soliman SE, ElManhaly M, Dimaras H. Knowledge of genetics in familial retinoblastoma. Ophthalmic Genet. 2017;38(3):226–32.

17. Soliman SE, VandenHoven C, MacKeen LD, Heon E, Gallie BL. Optical coherence tomography-guided decisions in retinoblastoma management. Ophthalmology. 2017;124(6):859–72.
18. Rootman DB, Gonzalez E, Mallipatna A, et al. Hand-held high-resolution spectral domain optical coherence tomography in retinoblastoma: clinical and morphologic considerations. Br J Ophthalmol. 2013;97(1):59–65.
19. Murphree AL. Intraocular retinoblastoma: the case for a new group classification. Ophthalmol Clin N Am. 2005;18:41–53.
20. Munier FL. Classification and management of seeds in retinoblastoma. Ellsworth Lecture Ghent August 24th 2013. Ophthalmic Genet. 2014;35(4):193–207.
21. Francis JH, Abramson DH, Gaillard MC, Marr BP, Beck-Popovic M, Munier FL. The classification of vitreous seeds in retinoblastoma and response to intravitreal melphalan. Ophthalmology. 2015;122(6):1173–9.
22. Balmer A, Zografos L, Munier F. Diagnosis and current management of retinoblastoma. Oncogene. 2006;25(38):5341–9.
23. Ali MJ, Honavar SG, Reddy VA. Orbital retinoblastoma: present status and future challenges – a review. Saudi J Ophthalmol. 2011;25(2):159–67.
24. Sastre X, Chantada GL, Doz F, et al. Proceedings of the consensus meetings from the International Retinoblastoma Staging Working Group on the pathology guidelines for the examination of enucleated eyes and evaluation of prognostic risk factors in retinoblastoma. Arch Pathol Lab Med. 2009;133(8):1199–202.
25. Soliman SE, Wan MJ, Heon E, Hazrati LN, Gallie B. Retinoblastoma versus advanced Coats' disease: is enucleation the answer? Ophthalmic Genet. 2017;38(3):291–93.
26. Moulin AP, Gaillard MC, Balmer A, Munier FL. Ultrasound biomicroscopy evaluation of anterior extension in retinoblastoma: a clinicopathological study. Br J Ophthalmol. 2012;96(3):337–40.
27. Soliman SE, Dimaras H, Souka AA, Ashry MH, Gallie BL. Socioeconomic and psychological impact of treatment for unilateral intraocular retinoblastoma. J Francais D Ophtalmologie. 2015;38:550–8.
28. Yousef YA, Soliman SE, Astudillo PP, et al. Intra-arterial chemotherapy for retinoblastoma: a systematic review. JAMA Ophthalmol. 2016;134(6):584–91.
29. Kletke SN, Feng ZX, Hazrati LN, Gallie BL, Soliman SE. Clinical predictors at diagnosis of low-risk histopathology in unilateral advanced retinoblastoma. Ophthalmology. 2019;126(9):1306–14.
30. Zhao J, Dimaras H, Massey C, et al. Pre-enucleation chemotherapy for eyes severely affected by retinoblastoma masks risk of tumor extension and increases death from metastasis. J Clin Oncol. 2011;29(7):845–51.
31. Kletke SN, Feng ZX, Hazrati LN, Gallie BL, Soliman SE. Clinical predictors at diagnosis of low-risk histopathology in unilateral advanced retinoblastoma. Ophthalmology. 2019.
32. Shome D, Honavar SG, Raizada K, Raizada D. Implant and prosthesis movement after enucleation: a randomized controlled trial. Ophthalmology. 2010;117(8):1638–44.
33. Milne M, Soliman SE. Prosthetic fabrication in identical triplets with bilateral retinoblastoma and a single enucleated globe using a myoconjuntival enucleation procedure. J Ophthalmic Prosthetics. 2015;20(1):5–11.
34. Shields CL, De Potter P, Himelstein BP, Shields JA, Meadows AT, Maris JM. Chemoreduction in the initial management of intraocular retinoblastoma. Arch Ophthalmol. 1996;114(11):1330–8.
35. Kaliki S, Shields CL. Retinoblastoma: achieving new standards with methods of chemotherapy. Indian J Ophthalmol. 2015;63(2):103–9.
36. Soliman SE, D'Silva CN, Dimaras H, Dzneladze I, Chan H, Gallie BL. Clinical and genetic associations for carboplatin-related ototoxicity in children treated for retinoblastoma: a retrospective noncomparative single-institute experience. Pediatr Blood Cancer. 2018;65(5):e26931.
37. Gobin YP, Dunkel IJ, Marr BP, Brodie SE, Abramson DH. Intra-arterial chemotherapy for the management of retinoblastoma: four-year experience. Arch Ophthalmol. 2011;129(6):732–7.
38. Soliman S, Kletke S, Roelofs K, VandenHoven C, McKeen L, Gallie B. Precision laser therapy for retinoblastoma. Expert Rev Ophthalmol. 2018;13(3):149–59.
39. Soliman SE, VandenHoven C, MacKeen LD, Gallie BL. Vision and visual potential for perifoveal retinoblastoma after optical coherence tomographic guided sequential laser photocoagulation. Br J Opthalmol. 2019;103(6):753–60.
40. Shields JA, Shields CL, De-Potter P. Cryotherapy for retinoblastoma. Int Ophthalmol Clin. 1993;33(3):101–5.
41. Shields CL, Shields JA, Cater J, Othmane I, Singh AD, Micaily B. Plaque radiotherapy for retinoblastoma: long-term tumor control and treatment complications in 208 tumors. Ophthalmology. 2001;108(11):2116–21.
42. Munier FL, Gaillard MC, Balmer A, et al. Intravitreal chemotherapy for vitreous disease in retinoblastoma revisited: from prohibition to conditional indications. Br J Ophthalmol. 2012;96(8):1078–83.
43. Munier FL, Soliman S, Moulin AP, Gaillard MC, Balmer A, Beck-Popovic M. Profiling safety of intravitreal injections for retinoblastoma using an anti-reflux procedure and sterilisation of the needle track. Br J Ophthalmol. 2012;96(8):1084–7.
44. Smith SJ, Smith BD, Mohney BG. Ocular side effects following intravitreal injection therapy for retinoblastoma: a systematic review. Br J Ophthalmol. 2014;98(3):292–7.
45. Kim JW, Yau JW, Moshfeghi D, Fishman M. Orbital fibrosis and intraocular recurrence of retinoblastoma following periocular carboplatin. J Pediatr Ophthalmol Strabismus. 2010;47 Online:e1–4.
46. Mallipatna AC, Dimaras H, Chan HS, Heon E, Gallie BL. Periocular topotecan for intraocular retinoblastoma. Arch Ophthalmol. 2011;129(6):738–45.
47. Carcaboso AM, Chiappetta DA, Opezzo JA, et al. Episcleral implants for topotecan delivery to the posterior segment of the eye. Invest Ophthalmol Vis Sci. 2010;51(4):2126–34.
48. Zhao J, Li Q, Wu S, et al. Pars plana vitrectomy and endoresection of refractory intraocular retinoblastoma. Ophthalmology. 2018;125(2):320–2.
49. Wong JR, Morton LM, Tucker MA, et al. Risk of subsequent malignant neoplasms in long-term hereditary retinoblastoma survivors after chemotherapy and radiotherapy. J Clin Oncol. 2014;32(29):3284–90.
50. Sethi RV, Shih HA, Yeap BY, et al. Second nonocular tumors among survivors of retinoblastoma treated with contemporary photon and proton radiotherapy. Cancer. 2014;120(1):126–33.
51. Blach LE, McCormick B, Abramson DH. External beam radiation therapy and retinoblastoma: long-term results in the comparison of two techniques. Int J Radiat Oncol Biol Phys. 1996;35(1):45–51.
52. Palma J, Sasso DF, Dufort G, et al. Successful treatment of metastatic retinoblastoma with high-dose chemotherapy and autologous stem cell rescue in South America. Bone Marrow Transpl. 2012;47(4):522–27.

22 Paediatric Intra-ocular Tumours (Non-RB)

Harshit Vaidya and Vikas Khetan

Abstract

Tumours of the eye are broadly classified as extra-ocular and intra-ocular. Among intra-ocular tumours of the eye in the paediatric age group, a majority of the tumours comprise of retinoblastoma. In this chapter, we are focussed primarily on three intra-ocular tumours other than retinoblastoma. The reason it is essential to learn about these tumours is because these tumours can vary significantly in presentation, management as well as prognosis. Timely identification and management can significantly alter the prognosis of these patients.

Keywords

Medulloepithelioma · Retinal astrocytoma

22.1 Retinal Astrocytoma (Astrocytic Hamartoma)

22.1.1 History

In 1880, Bournville described a group of hereditary disorders known as Tuberous sclerosis (TSC) or Morbus Bourneville–Pringle disease characterised by disseminated hamartomas involving the central nervous system, skin and kidney. Van der Hoeve (1921) described the ocular involvement as a part of the same entity [1].

22.1.2 Etiopathogenesis

It is a rare benign tumour arising from the astrocytes of the sensory retina, typically forming early in life and diagnosed during childhood or adolescence. No racial or gender differences have been noted [2]. They can be acquired or congenital. Unilateral unifocal patterns are seen in the sporadic non-syndromic disorders, whereas bilateral multifocal disease is often associated with tuberous sclerosis [2]. It is the most common ophthalmic finding in tuberous sclerosis (50% are bilateral tumours) [3].

Histology—it comprises of a mass of intertwined spindle-shaped fibrous astrocytes containing small elongated oval nuclei having indistinct wavy cytoplasmic borders. Undifferentiated glioneurocytes during the embryonal development of the retina and giant astrocytes (plump polygonal cells with eosinophilic cytoplasm) are seen in syndromic astrocytomas [2, 4].

22.1.3 Clinical Features

Unless the tumour involves the macula, these patients can often be asymptomatic. On examination, the acquired form can be associated with retinal traction, retinal and vitreous haemorrhage, cystoid macular oedema, feeder vessels and exudation in absence of calcification [5, 6]. Congenital form seen in younger patients can intrinsically develop calcification and may be associated with TSC complex [7]. The tumour appears as a white superficial retinal mass (tumour basal dimension: 0.3–12 mm) which can range from translucent intra-retinal patches to opaque white nodular lesions to partly calcified mulberry like tumours (Table 22.1) [2, 4]. Figure 22.1 shows vascularization of the tumour arising from the retinal vessels, although these vessels are neither dilated nor tortuous. Syndromic disease can often have multiple and peripheral tumours as opposed to

H. Vaidya · V. Khetan (✉)
Department of Ocular Oncology and Vitreoretina Services, Medical Research Foundation, Sankara Nethralaya, Chennai, India

W.-C. Wu, W.-C. Lam (eds.), *A Quick Guide to Pediatric Retina*, https://doi.org/10.1007/978-981-15-6552-6_22

Table 22.1 Morphological features of reinal astrocytoma

Morphological features of retinal astrocytoma	
Type 1 (most common)	Circular or oval solitary lesion (0.5 mm disc diameter) Relatively flat, light grey, semi-transparent glistening mass in NFL No calcification
Type 2	Multiple calcific nodular areas, mulberry-like appearance
Type 3	Contains features of both type 1 and 2 Peripheral semitranslucent and irregular rim Whitish-grey glistening central calcification

Incorporated from Mennel S, Meyer CH, Eggarter F, Peter S. Autofluorescence and angiographic findings of retinal astrocytic hamartomas in tuberous sclerosis. Ophthalmologica. 2005;219(6):350–6

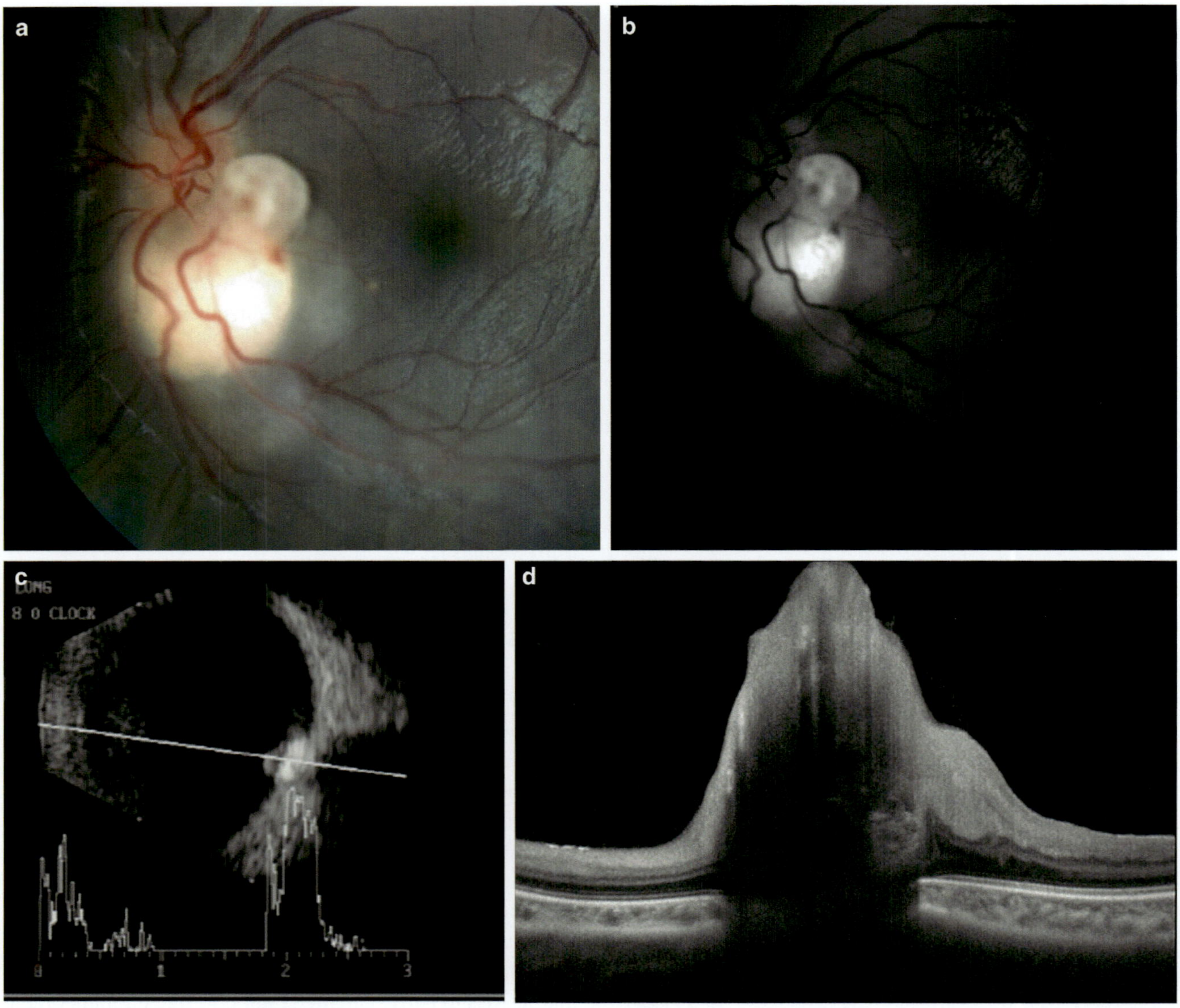

Fig. 22.1 (**a**) Colour fundus photograph of the left eye of a 3 year old male child with a retinal astrocytoma presenting as a whitish raised retinal lesion with normal overlying vessels. (**b**) Red free image of the same patient. (**c**) Ultrasound (**a**) and (**b**) scan through the astrocytoma showing a high reflective structure with backshadowing due to calcification. (**d**) Swept source Optical coherence tomography (DRI OCT-1 Atlantis by Topcon, USA) through the lesion showing a elevated retinal lesion with areas of intralesional calcifications and backshadowing

Table 22.2 Autofluorescence and angiographic findings of retinal astrocytic hamartomas

	Lesion type		
	1	2	3
AF	No lesion-specific AF, blockade of physiologic background AF	Lesion-specific AF	Central part: lesion-specific AF Peripheral part: no lesion-specific AF, partial blockade of physiologic background AF
Early FA	Partial blockade	Total blockade	Central part: total blockade Peripheral part: partial blockade
Late FA	Hyperfluorescence, leakage	Hyperfluorescence, leakage	Hyperfluorescence, leakage
Early ICG A	Subtly visible due to partial blockade	Total blockade	Central part: total blockade Peripheral part: partial blockade
Late ICGA	Partial blockade with good visibility due to high contrast to surrounding background fluorescence	Total blockade	Central part: total blockade Peripheral part: partial blockade, high contrast to surrounding background fluorescence

Table reprinted with permission from Mennel S, Meyer CH, Eggarter F, Peter S. Autofluorescence and angiographic findings of retinal astrocytic hamartomas in tuberous sclerosis. Ophthalmologica. 2005;219(6):350–6

the non-syndromic disease [8]. Unilateral, isolated non-syndromic tumour in an otherwise healthy patient is often considered an atypical variant of the tumour [2]. These tumours can cause severe vision loss due to large size, macular location and associated subretinal fluid [5, 6]. These tumours can often be misdiagnosed as amelanotic choroidal melanoma, which can lead to enucleation [2]. On rare occasions, a non-foveal tumour can result in a non-rhegmatogenous retinal detachment involving the macula and causing a drop in vision [2].

22.1.4 Diagnosis

Fundus autofluorescence (AF), Fundus fluorescein angiography (FFA) and Indocyanine green angiography (ICGA)—Angiographic findings tpyically show relatively slow filling of the undilated and normal calibre intralesional vasculature with limited late staining of the tumour. Prominent surface vascularity of the isolated retinal astrocytomas helps differentiate these lesions from amelanotic choroidal melanomas with retinal invasion [2, 8]. ICG angiography allowed the diagnosis and localisation of type 1 tumours due to blockade of choroid especially in the late phases of angiogram [9]. FFA and ICGA are useful in detection of tumours, especially the morphological type 1, which can be missed on clinical examination. FFA helps in the differentiation between type 2 and type 3 lesions [9] (Table 22.2).

B-scan Ultrasonography (USG)—Small noncalcified tumours appear as ill-defined lesions having reflectivity similar to that of normal retina. The larger calcific tumours have focal strong intralesional reflections and orbital shadowing by the mass. USG is helpful in measuring the dimensions of peripheral tumours whereas OCT which is useful in paramacular or peripapillary tumours [3, 8].

Optical Coherence Tomography (OCT)—The tumour was localised to the inner retina based on Time Domain OCT (TD-OCT), while Spectral Domain OCT (SD-OCT) localised it to the nerve fibre layer (Table 22.3). Moth eaten appearance was identified on TD-OCT, but the features were further explored on SD-OCT [3]. The moth-eaten optically empty spaces (OES) are hypothesised to represent intralesional calcifications in the calcific astrocytomas, whereas they represent intralesional cavitation in non-calcific tumours. The numbers of OES is believed to be significantly more in macular tumours compared to extramacular tumours. The size of OES was larger in calcified tumours and had a positive correlation with increasing tumour size and a drop in vision [4]. OCT has helped identify vitreous seeds, which are cells spreading from the tumour surface into the vitreous [8]. Caution must be exerted as vitreous seeding is associated with other amelanotic retinal lesions. A striking feature noted recently was the presence of hyperreflective dots which are similar to those observed in occult choroidal neovascular membrane in eyes with AMD and proposed to represent fibrovascular activity [10] (Table 22.3).

OCT-angiography- features show a dense vascular network within the tumour which could represent dilated anastomotic and dilated superficial and deep capillary plexuses. Feeder vessels have been documented in some reports [11].

Table 22.3 SD-OCT features to predict systemic features in retinal astrocytomas

SD-OCT features to predict systemic features in retinal astrocytomas		
Type 1	Flat without traction	No systemic features
Type 2	Thickness <500 μ with traction	Cutaneous fibrous plaques
Type 3	Thickness >500 μ with calcification	Subependymal astrocytoma
Type 4	Thickness >500 μ with cavitation	Pulmonary lymphangiomyomatosis

Incorporated from Pichi F, Massaro D, Serafino M, Carrai P, Giuliari GP, Shields CL, Veronese C, Ciardella AP, Nucci P. Retinal astrocytic hamartoma. Retina. 2016 Jun 1;36(6):1199-208

Computed Tomography and Magnetic Resonance Imaging—do not help in differentiating ocular condition but can reveal characteristic central nervous system lesions of tuberous sclerosis. Occasionally, fine-needle aspiration biopsy can help to establish the diagnosis of an atypical retinal astrocytoma [2].

22.1.5 Differential Diagnosis

Amelanotic choroidal melanoma, retinoblastoma, toxocara granuloma, isolated myelinated retinal nerve fibre, massive gliosis of retina.

22.1.6 Treatment

- Observation—most cases.
- Enucleation—painful blind eye (in cases of neovascular glaucoma) in progressively large tumours.
- Radiotherapy or charged particle beam—ineffective.
- Other treatment modalities—
  1. Photodynamic therapy and transpupillary thermotherapy have been used in symptomatic tumours.
  2. Intravitreal anti-VEGF agents have been used to treat choroidal neovascular membrane and macular oedema associated with the tumour.
  3. Recently systemic Everolimus (mTOR inhibitor) has shown efficacy in the management of aggressive retinal astrocytomas in a dose-dependent manner. Sirolimus has also been used with moderate success and has lesser bioavailability compared to everolimus [2, 12, 13].

22.1.7 Outcomes

Limited progression has been noted in childhood. They have extremely low malignant potential and do not metastasize. Progressive visual loss can be noticed in tumours around the fovea, but most patients retain normal vision [2, 13, 14]. Reports of spontaneous regression of the tumour have been documented [15].

22.2 Combined Hamartoma of Retina and Retinal Pigment Epithelium

22.2.1 History

The term combined hamartoma was first used by Gass in 1973 to describe the findings in a series of seven patients with similar features.

22.2.2 Origin

Hamartoma is an abnormal growth of tissue that normally occur at the affected site. It has been proposed that this tumour could actually be a hamartoma of the retina, retinal pigment epithelium and the vitreous [16].

22.2.3 Clinical Features

CHRRPE is believed to be a congenital tumour often observed in young children with symptoms of visual loss or strabismus [17, 18]. Floaters, leukocoria and ocular pain are other occasionally observed complaints. Visual acuity can range from 20/20 to light perception. Common clinical features noted are intra-retinal corkscrew vessels/vascular tortuosity, pigmentation, retinal traction/elevation, epiretinal membrane/vitreo-retinal interface disturbances and lipid exudation [17] (Fig. 22.2). Choroidal neovascular membrane, tractional or rhegmatogenous retinal detachment are known complications of this tumour. It is a unilateral pathology, but bilateral cases can be observed in certain systemic conditions [16, 18].

Based on predominant tissue type, the tumour has been classified as melanocytic, vascular or glial [17]. A recent classification system was proposed by Dedania et al. [18]. Based on the location the, tumour was classified into three zones: Zone 1—macular/peripapillary, Zone 2—mid-periphery, Zone 3—far periphery. Second component of the classification was anatomical status of the retina: Stage 1—no traction, stage 2—retinal traction or schisis, stage 3—retinal detachment. The third component was tumour anatomy on the OCT: A—epiretinal membrane only, B—partial retinal involvement, C—retinal and RPE involvement. Peripheral lesions may not cause macular distortion and may be asymptomatic.

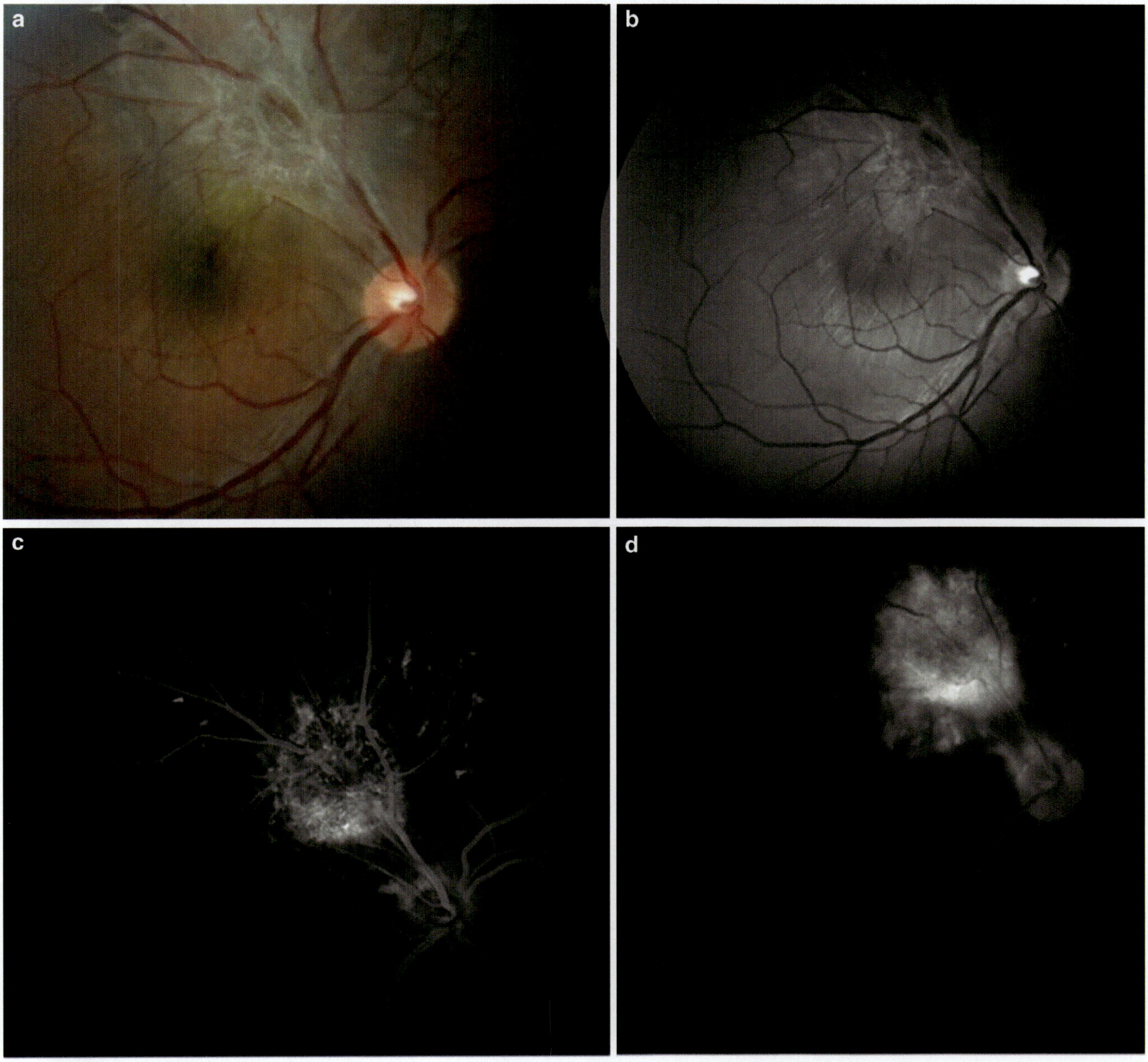

Fig. 22.2 (**a**) Colour fundus photo of the right eye of a 10-year-old male child (patient 1) with combined hamartoma of the retina and retinal pigment epithelium at the supero-temporal arcade with epiretinal membrane extending over the macular area. (**b**) Red-free image of the same patient showing epiretinal membrane. (**c**) Fundus fluorescein angiogram (1.04 min)—showing mild hyperfluorescence corresponding to the area of CHRRPE. (**d**) Late phase fundus fluorescein angiogram (7.48 min)—showing staining of the tissue

22.2.4 Systemic Associations

Neurofibromatosis type II (less commonly type I), tuberous sclerosis, Gorlin–Goltz syndrome, Poland anomaly, branchio-oculo-facial syndrome, juvenile nasopharyngeal angiofibroma [16].

22.2.5 Diagnosis

Optical Coherence Tomography (OCT)—On imaging with optical coherence tomography, CHRRPE appears to be a thickened retinal mass with hyperreflective surface, epiretinal membrane with retinal folds and full-thickness retinal disorganisation (Figs. 22.3 and 22.4). The vitreoretinal traction can lead to "mini peak" (saw tooth pattern) of the inner retina or "maxi-peaks" (retina folded pattern) involving the full thickness of the retina [19]. Distinction between macular CHRRPE and idiopathic ERMs can be made by identification of "omega sign" in the former [20]. It is an omega-shaped disorganisation of the inner retinal layers bounded posteriorly by the outer plexiform layer. "Shark teeth sign" is seen as small hyperreflective triangles at the edge of the hamartoma without any back-shadowing [21]. This sign seems to persist even post surgery despite normalisation of other structural abnormalities. A recent OCT-based study stated that these lesions originate and primarily involve the inner retinal layers up to the outer plexiform layer and that outer retinal layers and

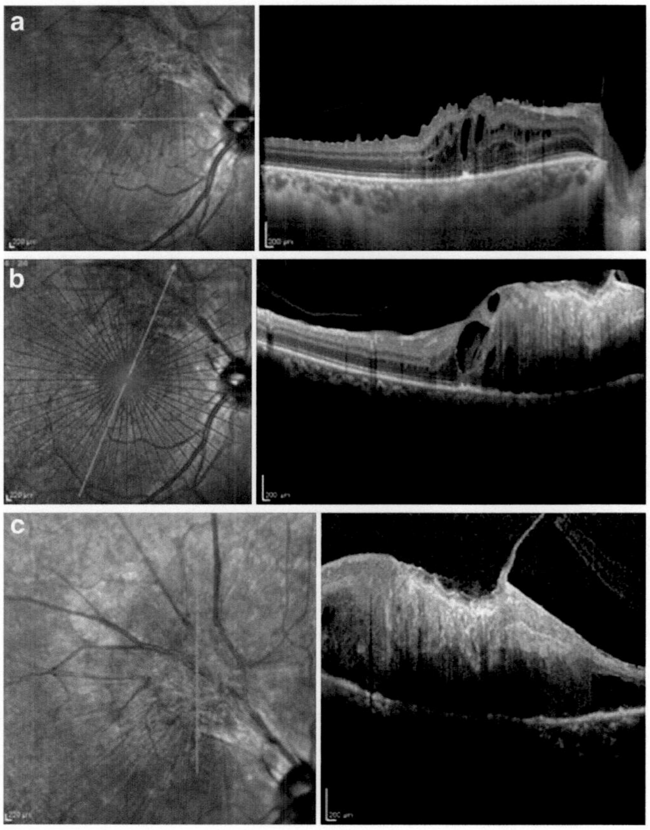

Fig. 22.3 (**a**) Spectral domain Optical coherence tomography (Heidelberg engineering, Germany) of patient 1. Horizontal line scan through the fovea showing "mini-peaks" along with cystoid spaces. (**b**) Radial line scan through the fovea showing cystoid spaces along with disorganized retinal structures, superonasal to the fovea along with epiretinal membrane. (**c**) Vertical line scan through the CHRRPE lesion, superonasal to the fovea showing an epiretinal membrane along with disorganized retinal structure occupied by the lesion with some amount of back-shadowing over the RPE

RPE under the hamartoma are intact in most of the cases [22]. The epiretinal membrane associated with CHRRPE, which was once considered intrinsic to the tumour, is now believed to be extrinsic and the cleavage plane between the two can be identified on SD-OCT [23].

Fundus fluorescein angiography (FFA)—reveal dilated, telangiectatic capillaries in the early phase with leakage in the late phase of the angiogram [17, 24] (Fig. 22.5).

Optical Coherence Tomography—Angiography (OCT-A)—increased tortuosity of the superficial vessels, plexa rarefactions, and reduced detection or disappearance of the FAZ are features prominent of OCT-A [21]. Another hypothesis states that flow signals in deep capillary plexus in the absence of any vascular network corresponding to the normal retinal vasculature can be attributed only to intra-retinal vascularity of CHRRPE (filigree pattern) [25].

B-scan Ultrasonography (USG)—scan reveals a solid mildly elevated lesion often involving the optic nerve head. A scan reveals an irregular pattern of medium to high reflective lesion.

Multicolour imaging—multicolour imaging along with near infra-red reflectance help in delineating the tumour boundaries and defining the macular extent thereby aiding in prognostication of the tumour when planning any surgical intervention. Green reflectance helps in assessing the epiretinal gliosis and inner retinal involvement [26].

22.2.6 Differential Diagnosis

Epiretinal membrane is the most common differential diagnosis but the presence of retinal folds, hyperpigmentation, vessel tortuosity on FFA and OCTA features in CHRRPE helps in distinction from epiretinal membrane. Choroidal melanoma, congenital hypertrophy of retinal pigment epithelium, retinoblastoma, chorio-retinal scar and vascular anomaly are other differential diagnoses.

22.2.7 Treatment

Surgical removal of the epiretinal membrane in CHRRPE is believed to damage the NFL and muller cells, making it difficult to strip the membrane and does not result in any visual improvement [23, 24]. However, certain studies have found the membrane to be extrinsic to the tumour and thereby proposing a role of ERM removal in CHRRPE for visual recovery [23]. Macular CHRRPEs having progressive visual loss are often due to the vitreous traction and epiretinal gliosis [27]. Surgical removal of membranes in these cases can be attempted, although the visual outcomes are guarded. Continuous glial proliferation is known

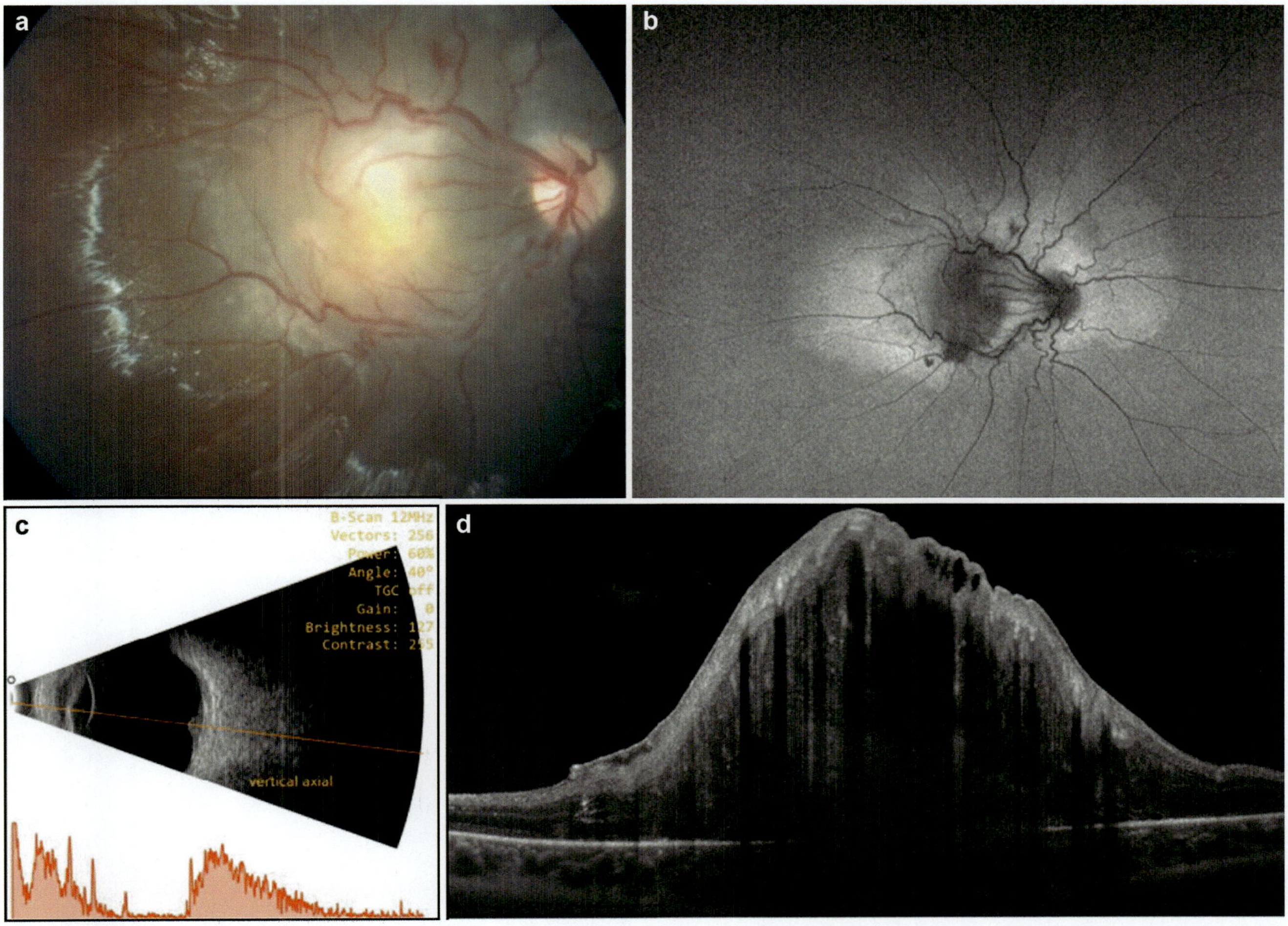

Fig. 22.4 (**a**) Colour fundus photograph of the right eye of a 11 year old girl (Patient 2) who came for consultation after noticing drop in vision after trivial trauma to her head. Shows a whitish retinal lesion over the posterior pole measuring about 1.5 disc diameters in size with slightly dilated retinal vessels overlying the lesion. (**b**) Widefield (Optos) fundus autofluorescence of the lesion showing area of hypoautofluorescence corresponding to the retinal lesion and areas of hyperautofluorescence surrounding the lesion. (**c**) Ultrasound (**b**) and (**a**) scan showing an area of retinal elevation with moderate surface reflectivity and low internal reflectivity. (**d**) Swept source optical coherence tomography, showing a retinal lesion over the macular area with disorganization of the retinal structures and few cystoid spaces

to occur in CHRRPE and a tendency for recurrent ERM even after surgery [23, 27]. Surgical option is generally deferred in cases of long-standing visual loss or in presence of marked cystoid macular oedema [28].

22.2.8 Prognosis

The factors resulting in poor visual outcome include macular location, clock hour meridian of the tumour, clinically visible epimacular membrane and male gender [17].

22.3 Medulloepithelioma

22.3.1 History

Badel and Lagrange in 1892 were the first to identify the condition as "carcinoma primitive". Vaerhoff in 1904 coined the term "neuroteratoma". In 1908, Fuchs used the term "diktyoma" to describe a net-like pattern of poorly differentiated ribbon cells. The term medulloepithelioma was coined by Grinker in 1931 [29–31].

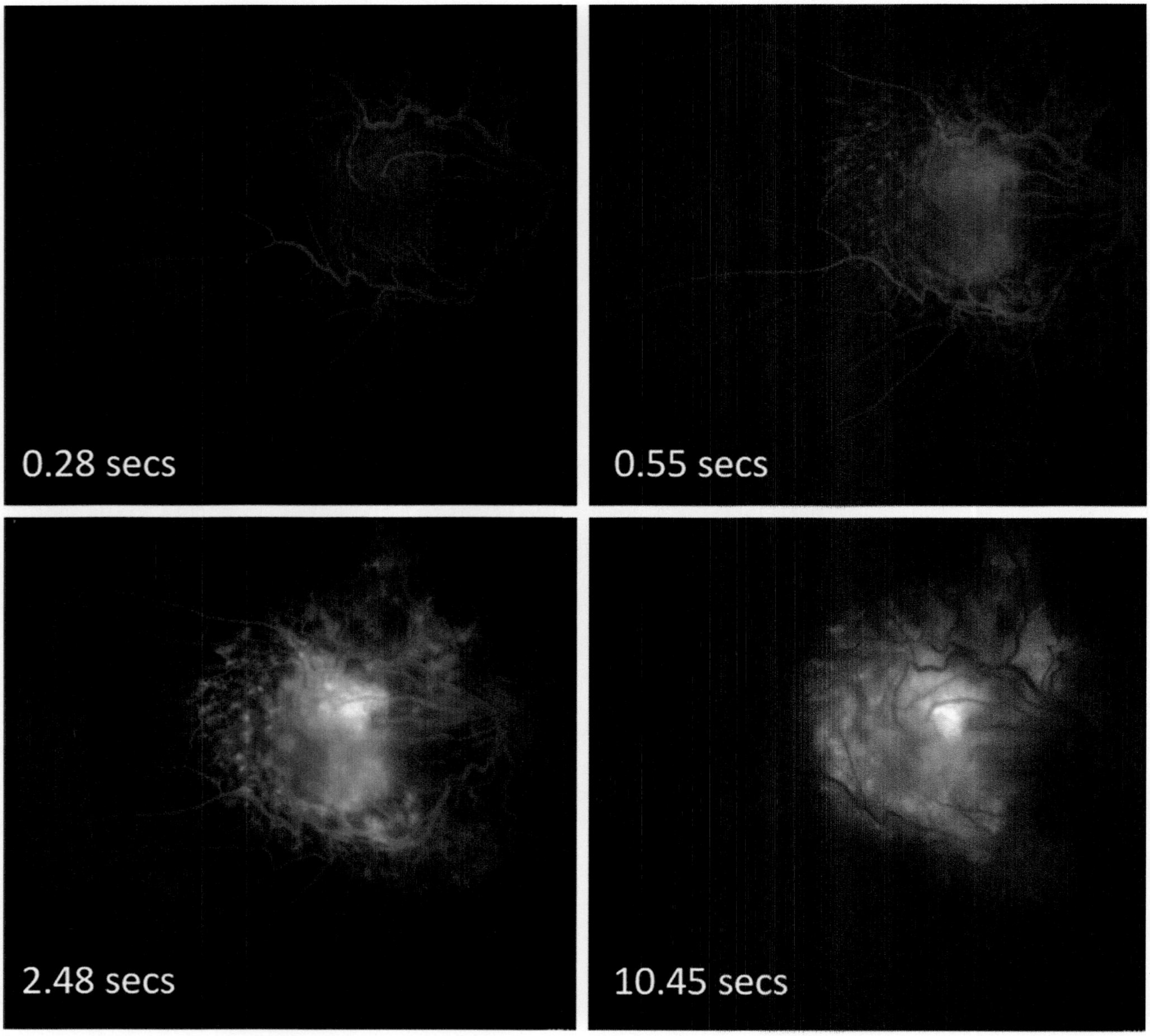

Fig. 22.5 Fundus fluorescein angiogram of the right eye (Patient 2) showing a hypofluorescent lesion which shows leakage in later phases

22.3.2 Origin

Retina arises from the optic cup as an outgrowth of the medullary epithelium of the medullary tube. At 6 weeks of gestation, the embryonal retina appears similar to the medullary epithelium of the brain. Anterior portion of the optic cup forms the epithelium of the iris and ciliary body (CB) [31, 32].

Medulloepithelioma is a congenital tumour of non-pigmented ciliary epithelium of the eye. It is an embryonal tumour arising from the primitive medullary epithelium along the inner layer of the optic cup [31]. These tumours can be benign or malignant and teratoid (heteroplastic elements like hyaline cartilage, neuroglial tissue, rhabdomyoblasts) or non-teratoid (purely primitive medullary epithelium). Rarely, they can arise from the iris, optic disc and retinal stalk [33, 34].

Most often seen in children, it is hypothesised to derive from incompletely differentiated embryonic ciliary epithelium [31, 32]. When observed in adults, it is believed to arise from completely differentiated ciliary epithelium undergoing hyperplasia [35].

22.3.3 Clinical Presentation

Medulloepithelioma typically presents as unilateral tumours between 2 and 6 years of age, with more than 75% of cases presenting in the first decade of life [32]. Adult manifestation of the disease has been well documented [35]. There is no known gender or racial predilection. These tumours are often asymptomatic. Until tumours are large enough to be seen through the pupil or cause symptoms due to secondary effects, the smaller tumours are often unnoticeable. Patients often receive treatment for the secondary effects even before the mass is identified [32] (Table 22.4).

Tumour description—often present as irregular grey-white to pink mass (rarely pigmented) located in the ciliary body region [36, 37] (Fig. 22.6). Multiple intra-tumoural cysts are found in more than 50% of cases [36]. These cysts can also be found in the anterior chamber, angle or vitreous cavity [32, 38]. It may contain chalky grey-white areas of cartilage or it may have vessels running over the surface or feeder episcleral vessels [39].

Secondary effects—Zonular loss adjacent to the tumour leads to a notch/coloboma of the lens. This could in turn cause lens subluxation with occasional cataract. Ciliary body adjacent to the tumour has long ciliary zonules covered with neoplastic cyclitic membranes. The tumour tends to grow along the posterior lens capsule and anterior hyaloid forming a vascular retrolental membrane. Child presenting with a normal fundus and unilateral neovascular glaucoma must be suspected to have medulloepithelioma. Rarely, retina can be involved ("retro-invasive medulloepithelioma"). Retinal involvement is believed to be associated with old age, chronicity and glaucoma [32, 36, 37, 39].

Table 22.4 Signs and symptoms of medulloepithelioma

Symptoms	Signs
• Loss of vision • Leucocoria • Painful red eye • Strabismus	• Grey-white CB mass with cysts • Iris (NVI/localised bowing/ectropion uveae/ correctopia) • Lens (cataract—sectoral or total/loss of zonules or subluxation/notch or coloboma) • Retrolental neoplastic cyclitic membrane • Secondary glaucoma (neovascular or angle closure) • Vitreous haemorrhage

Systemic association: DICER-1 gene (member of ribonuclease III family) is a dominant trait located on chromosome 14q. It results in a familial cancer syndrome called Pleuropulmonary Blastoma Family Tumour and Dysplasia Syndrome (PPB-FTDS). Less than 1% of patients with PPB manifest CB medulloepithelioma and 5% cases with medulloepithelioma have a history of PPB. Recently somatic mutations of KMT2D have also been recognised [32, 40].

22.3.4 Diagnosis

B-scan Ultrasonography (USG)—displays a heterogeneous, highly echogenic mass in the CB region with irregular intratumoural cystic areas. Occasional calcification seen due to presence of cartilage can give a picture similar to that of a retinoblastoma [41].

Ultrasound Biomicroscopy (UBM)—helps in delineating the radial and circumferential extent of the tumour along with co-existing pathologies (intra-tumoural cysts, anterior chamber (AC) cysts, neoplastic cyclitic membranes, lens subluxation) [42].

Fundus fluoresecein angiogram (FFA)—reveals vessels arising from the ciliary body tumour and form a haphazard network within the retrolental membrane. Vascular stalk from the detached retina to the CB tumour has been noted as well [32].

Magnetic Resonance Imaging (MRI)—reveals a heterogeneous mass of both cystic and solid tumour arising from the CB region. The tumour is isointense to mildly hypertense on T1 imaging, with contrast enhancement [32, 43].

22.3.5 Histopathology

It is composed of pseudostratified primitive neuroepithelial cells surrounded by hyaluronic acid-rich hypocellular stroma. It resembles medullary epithelium of the developing neurosensory retina or embryonic neural tube before the fourth month of gestation. Rosettes are often larger and more cellular. Neuroepithelial tubules and absence of calcification are features specific to medulloepithelioma. Although it is primarily a tumour arising from the region of non-pigmented ciliary body epithelium, foci of pigmented tumour cells are relatively common [30, 32].

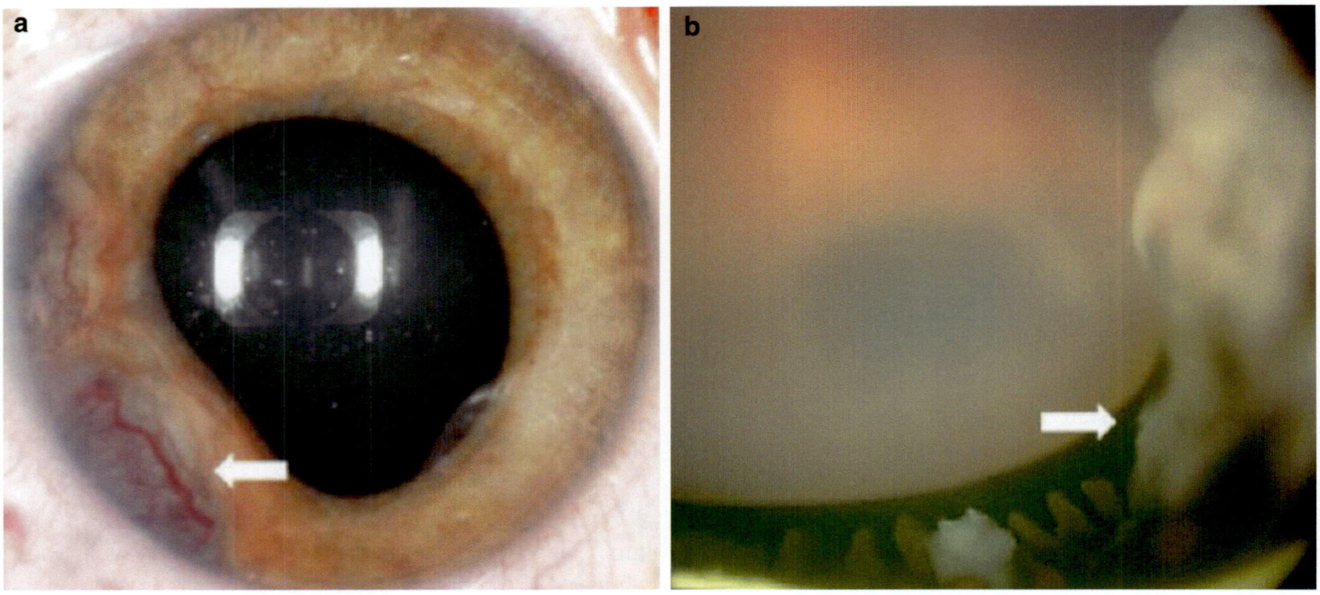

Fig. 22.6 Clinical features of medulloepithelioma in (**a**) 2-year-old girl who presented with translucent white mass (arrow) with intrinsic vascularity and iris neovascularisation. (**b**) In the ciliary body was a beige-white mass with loss of zonule, representing medulloepithelioma (Image courtesy Dr Santosh Honavar. Incorporated from Tadepalli SH, Shields CL, Shields JA, Honavar SG. Intraocular medulloepithelioma–A review of clinical features, DICER 1 mutation, and management. Indian journal of ophthalmology. 2019 Jun;67(6):755)

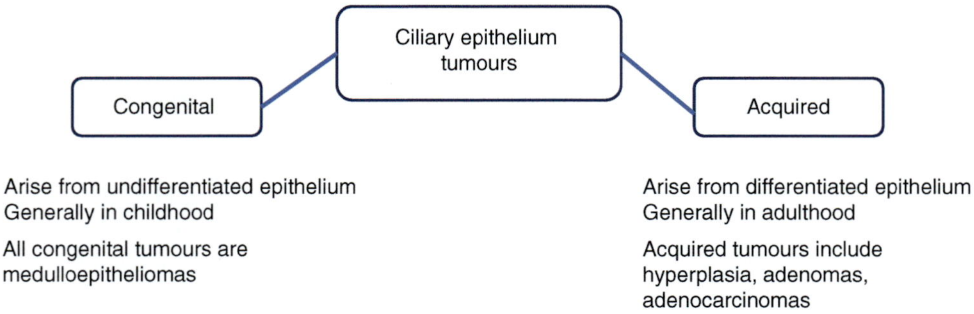

Malignant medulloepithelioma is diagnosed based on [31]:

1. Retinoblastoma-like elements (sheets of neuroblastic cells among the cords) with or without rosettes
2. Sarcoma-like elements
3. Pleomorphism and high mitotic index
4. Invasion into adjacent uvea, lens, sclera, cornea, optic nerve or orbit

Immunohistochemistry: Vimentin and neuron-specific enolase are positive in nonteratoid tumours. Immunohistochemistry for pancytokeratins and cytokeratin (CK) 18, with no reactivity for CK7, CK20, and epithelial membrane antigen has been described [32, 44].

Most common malignant features are high mitotic activity (60%) and retinoblastoma-like differentiation (37%). Intra-ocular medulloepithelioma has features similar to that of medulloepithelioma of the central nervous system, but survival rates are significantly better [32, 36].

22.3.6 Differential Diagnosis

1. Retinoblastoma—Neovascular glaucoma (NVG), CB invasion, AC seeds, total cataract can lead to misdiagnosis.
    - Presence of calcification is characteristic of retinoblastoma but intra-tumoural cartilage in medulloepithelioma may show a similar picture.
2. Coats disease—Present as unilateral retinal vascular telangiectasia with exudative retinal detachment
    - Lack of CB involvement helps in differentiation

- Retrolental neoplastic cyclitic membrane—serves to distinguish medulloepithelioma from retinoblastoma and Coats
- FFA: rapid filling of haphazard large vessels originating from the CB across the anterior hyaloid in medulloepithelioma. Total RD in coats and Rb, regular organised vessels emanate from the centre to the CB region.

3. PHPV—cells comprising of neoplastic membrane in medulloepithelioma multiply and produce collagen. This could lead to opacification of the membrane which resembles PHPV. Vessels arise from the periphery and there is no vascular stalk attaching to the disc as in PHPV.
4. Juvenile xanthogranuloma—they present as sudden hyphema with diffuse iris involvement and occasional skin involvement
5. Toxocariasis—patients are generally older than 5 years with a history of contact with dogs.
6. In adults
   - Adenoma
   - Hyperplasia
   - Carcinoma
   - Metastasis
   - CB melanoma

22.3.7 Management

Small tumours (<3–4 clock hours)

1. Cryotherapy—triple freeze–thaw technique for small or recurrent tumours [32, 39].
2. Local resection (partial lamellar sclerouvectomy—PLSU)—technically demanding with a high recurrence rate (up to 50%). The recurrence may be attributed to subclinical tumour not included in the excision [39].
3. Radiotherapy—successful treatment has been noted with plaque brachytherapy with I-125 and Ru-106 (apex dose: 40–50 Gy). EBRT (45–50 Gy) mainly used as adjuvant therapy for orbital and metastatic tumours [32, 45].

Large tumours

1. Enucleation—standard of treatment for advanced cases with large tumours and neovascular glaucoma. Spillage must be prevented while performing enucleation [36, 39].
2. Exenteration/extended enucleation—for cases with orbital extension [32].

22.3.8 Outcomes

Patients often present months after the onset of symptoms, with the secondary manifestations of the disease like cataract, glaucoma and uveitis and managed for the same for months. Unless extraocular or CNS involvement is noted, tumour- or metastasis-related death is uncommon [30, 36, 39]. Five-year survival post enucleation in ocular tumours is 90–95%. Prognosis in tumours with metastasis and recurrence is guarded [32, 46].

References

1. Van der Hoeve JV. Augengeschwülstebei der tuberösenHirnsklerose (Bourneville). Graefes Arch Clin Exp Ophthalmol. 1921 Jun 1;105(1):880–98.
2. Augsburger JJ, Cruess AF. Astrocytoma of retina. In: Ophthalmology. 3rd ed. St Louis, MO: Mosby Elsevier; 2009. p. 928.
3. Shields CL, Say EA, Fuller T, Arora S, Samara WA, Shields JA. Retinal astrocytic hamartoma arises in nerve fiber layer and shows "moth-eaten" optically empty spaces on optical coherence tomography. Ophthalmology. 2016 Aug 1;123(8): 1809–16.
4. Shields JA, Eagle RC, Shields CL, Marr BP. Aggressive retinal astrocytomas in 4 patients with tuberous sclerosis complex. Arch Ophthalmol. 2005 Jun 1;123(6):856–63.
5. Nyboer JH, Robertson DM, Gomez MR. Retinallesions in tuberous sclerosis. Arch Ophthalmol. 1976;94:1277–80.
6. Rowley SA, O'Callaghan FJ, Osborne JP. Ophthalmicmanifestations of tuberous sclerosis: a population-based study. Br J Ophthalmol. 2001;85:420–3.
7. Say EA, Shah SU, Ferenczy S, Shields CL. Optical coherence tomography of retinal and choroidal tumors. J Ophthalmol 2011;2011.
8. Semenova E, Veronese C, Ciardella A, Marcheggiani EB, Shah S, De-Pablo-Gomez-de-Liaño L, Finger PT. Multimodality imaging of retinal astrocytoma. Eur J Ophthalmol. 2015 Dec;25(6):559–64.
9. Mennel S, Meyer CH, Eggarter F, Peter S. Autofluorescence and angiographic findings of retinal astrocytic hamartomas in tuberous sclerosis. Ophthalmologica. 2005;219(6):350–6.
10. Xu L, Burke TR, Greenberg JP, Mahajan VB, Tsang SH. Infrared imaging and optical coherence tomography reveal early-stage astrocytic hamartomas not detectable by fundoscopy. Am J Ophthalmol. 2012 May 1;153(5):883–9.
11. Yung M, Iafe N, Sarraf D. Optical coherence tomography angiography of a retinal astrocytic hamartoma. Can J Ophthalmol. 2016 Apr 1;51(2):e62–4.
12. Nallasamy N, Seider MI, Gururangan S, Mruthyunjaya P. Everolimus to treat aggressive retinal astrocytic hamartoma in tuberous sclerosis complex. J Am Assoc Pediat Ophthalmol Strabismus. 2017 Aug 1;21(4):328–31.
13. Querques G, Kerrate H, Leveziel N, Coscas G, Soubrane G, Souied EH. Intravitreal ranibizumab for choroidal neovascularization associated with retinal astrocytic hamartoma.
14. Mennel S, Meyer CH, Peter S, Schmidt JC, Kroll P. Current treatment modalities for exudative retinal hamartomas secondary to tuberous sclerosis: review of the literature. Acta Ophthalmologica Scandinavica. 2007 Mar;85(2):127–32.
15. Kiratli H, Bilgic S. Spontaneous regression of retinal astrocytic hamartoma in a patient with tuberous sclerosis. Am J Ophthalmol. 2002;133:715–6.
16. Stallman JB. Visual improvement after pars plana vitrectomy and membrane peeling for vitreoretinal traction associated with combined hamartoma of the retina and retinal pigment epithelium. Retina. 2002 Feb 1;22(1):101–4.

17. Shields CL, Thangappan A, Hartzell K, Valente P, Pirondini C, Shields JA. Combined hamartoma of the retina and retinal pigment epithelium in 77 consecutive patients: visual outcome based on macular versus extramacular tumor location. Ophthalmology. 2008 Dec 1;115(12):2246–52.
18. Dedania VS, Ozgonul C, Zacks DN, Besirli CG. Novel classification system for combined hamartoma of the retina and retinal pigment epithelium. Retina. 2018 Jan 1;38(1):12–9.
19. Arepalli S, Pellegrini M, Ferenczy SR, Shields CL. Combined hamartoma of the retina and retinal pigment epithelium: findings on enhanced depth imaging optical coherence tomography in eight eyes. Retina. 2014 Nov 1;34(11):2202–7.
20. Kumar V, Chawla R, Tripathy K. Omega sign: a distinct optical coherence tomography finding in macular combined hamartoma of retina and retinal pigment epithelium. Ophthal Surg Lasers Imaging Retina. 2017 Feb 14;48(2):122–5.
21. Arrigo A, Corbelli E, Aragona E, Manitto MP, Martina E, Bandello F, Parodi MB. Optical coherence tomography and optical coherence tomography angiography evaluation of combined hamartoma of the retina and retinal pigment epithelium. Retina. 2019 May 1;39(5):1009–15.
22. Chawla R, Kumar V, Tripathy K, Kumar A, Venkatesh P, Shaikh F, Vohra R, Molla K, Verma S. Combined hamartoma of the retina and retinal pigment epithelium: an optical coherence tomography-based reappraisal. Am J Ophthalmol. 2017 Sep 1;181:88–96.
23. Bruè C, Saitta A, Nicolai M, Mariotti C, Giovannini A. Epiretinal membrane surgery for combined hamartoma of the retina and retinal pigment epithelium: role of multimodal analysis. Clin Ophthalmol (Auckland, NZ). 2013;7:179.
24. Schachat AP, Shields JA, Fine SL, Sanborn GE, Weingeist TA, Valenzuela RE, Brucker AJ. Combined hamartomas of the retina and retinal pigment epithelium. Ophthalmology. 1984 Dec 1;91(12):1609–15.
25. Gupta R, Pappuru RR, Fung KA, Lupidi M, Kaliki S, Yannuzzi L, Freund KB, Reid K, Zur D, Iglicki M, Chhablani J. Filigree vascular pattern in combined hamartoma of retina and retinal pigment epithelium on optical coherence tomography angiography. Ophthalmol Retina. 2019.
26. Cohn AD, Quiram PA, Drenser KA, Trese MT, Capone A Jr. Surgical outcomes of epiretinal membranes associated with combined hamartoma of the retina and retinal pigment epithelium. Retina. 2009 Jun 1;29(6):825–30.
27. Kaprinis K, Bobat H, De Salvo G. MultiColor TM imaging in combined hamartoma of the retina and retinal pigment epithelium. Eye. 2018 Sep;32(9):1478.
28. McDonald HR, Abrams GW, Burke JM, Neuwirth J. Clinicopathologic results of vitreous surgery for epiretinal membranes in patients with combined retinal and retinal pigment epithelial hamartomas. Am J Ophthalmol. 1985 Dec 1;100(6):806–13.
29. Canning CR, McCartney AC, Hungerford J. Medulloepithelioma (diktyoma). Br J Ophthalmol. 1988 Oct 1;72(10):764–7.
30. Saunders T, Margo CE. Intraocular medulloepithelioma. Arch Pathol Lab Med. 2012 Feb;136(2):212–6.
31. Zimmerman LE. Verhoeff's "terato-neuroma" a critical reappraisal in light of new observations and current concepts of embryonic tumors. Trans Am Ophthalmol Soc. 1971;69:210.
32. Tadepalli SH, Shields CL, Shields JA, Honavar SG. Intraocular medulloepithelioma–A review of clinical features, DICER 1 mutation, and management. Indian J Ophthalmol. 2019 Jun;67(6):755.
33. Takei H, Florez L, Moroz K, Bhattacharjee MB. Medulloepithelioma: two unusual locations. Pathol Int. 2007;57:91–5.
34. Morris AT, Garner A. Medulloepithelioma involving the iris. Br J Ophthalmol. 1975;59:276–8.
35. Ali MJ, Honavar SG, Vemuganti GK. Ciliary body medulloepithelioma in an adult. Surv Ophthalmol. 2013 May 1;58(3):266–72.
36. Kaliki S, Shields CL, Eagle RC Jr, Vemuganti GK, Almeida A, Manjandavida FP, Mulay K, Honavar SG, Shields JA. Ciliary body medulloepithelioma: analysis of 41 cases. Ophthalmology. 2013 Dec 1;120(12):2552–9.
37. Shields JA, Eagle RC, Shields CL, Singh AD, Robitaille J. Pigmented medulloepithelioma of the ciliary body. Arch Ophthalmol. 2002 Feb 1;120(2):207–10.
38. Zhou M, Xu G, Bojanowski CM, Song Y, Chen R, Sun X, Wang W, Chan CC. Differential diagnosis of anterior chamber cysts with ultrasound biomicroscopy: ciliary body medulloepithelioma. Acta Ophthalmologica Scandinavica. 2006 Feb;84(1):137–9.
39. Shields JA, Eagle RC Jr, Shields CL, De Potter P. Congenital neoplasms of the nonpigmented ciliary epithelium (medulloepithelioma). Ophthalmology. 1996;103:1998–2006.
40. Ramasubramanian A, Correa ZM, Augsburger JJ, Sisk RA, Plager DA. Medulloepithelioma in DICER1 syndrome treated with resection. Eye. 2013 Jul;27(7):896.
41. Sansgiri RK, Wilson M, McCarville MB, Helton KJ. Imaging features of medulloepithelioma: report of four cases and review of the literature. Pediatr Radiol. 2013;43:1344–56.
42. Ayres B, Brasil OM, Klejnberg C, Moura LR, Fernandes BF, Burnier MN Jr. Ciliary body medulloepithelioma: clinical, ultrasound biomicroscopic and histopathologic correlation. Clin Exp Ophthalmol. 2006 Sep;34(7):695–8.
43. Potter PD, Shields CL, Shields JA, Flanders AE. The role of magnetic resonance imaging in children with intraocular tumors and simulating lesions. Ophthalmology. 1996;103:1774–83.
44. Kivelä T, Tarkkanen A. Recurrent medulloepithelioma of the ciliary body: immunohistochemical characteristics. Ophthalmology. 1988;95:1566–75.
45. Davidorf FH, Craig E, Birnbaum L, Wakely P Jr. Management of medulloepithelioma of the ciliary body with brachytherapy. Am J Ophthalmol. 2002 Jun 1;133(6):841–3.
46. Vajaranant TS, Mafee MF, Kapur R, Rapoport M, Edward DP. Medulloepithelioma of the ciliary body and optic nerve: clinicopathologic, CT, and MR imaging features. Neuroimag Clin. 2005 Feb 1;15(1):69–83.

Congenital X-Linked Retinoschisis

23

Kimberly Drenser

Abstract

Congenital X-linked Retinoschisis (CXRS) is a vitreoretinopathy that is primarily inherited in an X-linked recessive pattern. It is typically bilateral and is the most common cause of juvenile macular degeneration in males. The primary defect is in the *RS1* gene, with a high correlation between clinical diagnosis and alterations within the gene. While this makes CXRS an excellent target for gene therapy, the current management remains predominantly surgical.

Keywords

Congenital X-linked retinoschisis · CXRS · OCT · RS1
Retinoschisin · X-linked · Inner wall · Foveal schisis
Flat schisis · Lamellar schisis

23.1 Introduction

Clinical Presentation Congenital X-linked Retinoschisis (CXRS) affects 1 in 5000–25,000 live births worldwide and occurs in a broad population, without demonstrating ethnic predisposition [1]. It is bilateral, although it may be asymmetric, and is the most common cause of juvenile macular degeneration in males. Typical of X-linked inheritance, mothers are asymptomatic obligate carriers, with normal retinal findings on examination. Generally, children present between the ages of 5 and 10 years after failing an eye exam or having difficulty with scholastic tasks, but severe cases may present in infancy with nystagmus or strabismus. The clinical course is variable with severity ranging from mild/moderate effect on visual acuity (20/50 to the 20/100 range), to very severe affectation with no light perception [2].

The vitreoretinopathy is due to the expression of an aberrant retinoschisin, caused by an alteration in the *RS1* gene [3–5]. The retinoschisin protein plays an important role in both the structural and functional integrity of the retina. Clinically, patients present with a wide array of retinal pathology but universally manifest a loss of intraretinal integrity. The hallmark for the disease is splitting, or schisis, of the retinal layers [2]. Optical coherence tomography (OCT) demonstrates that retinal splitting occurs in all layers of the retina, but appears to most commonly occur in the outer plexiform layer [6, 7]. Schisis in the fovea (Fig. 23.1), the area of the retina responsible for detailed visual acuity, is seen in nearly all cases to varying degrees and is responsible for the loss of fine visual acuity. Although foveal schisis may be the earliest change detected, retinal splitting can be seen in the mid-periphery and periphery, and present as a bullous (Fig. 23.2) or flat schisis (Fig. 23.3) cavity. Until the development of OCT, this flat, or lamellar schisis, was often missed, and it is now understood that this finding may be responsible for vision significantly worse than initial examination may reveal. The advent of OCT analysis, in combination with ophthalmoscopic exam, aids in the accurate diagnosis of CXRS and determining the extent of affected retina [6, 8, 9]. Based on these OCT findings a new classification system (Table 23.1) has been developed which better represents the spectrum of this disease [7].

The advent of the OCT has also aided in understanding how structure affects function. The electroretinogram (ERG) typically shows a normal a-wave amplitude and a reduced b-wave amplitude, and that both focal ERG and full-field ERG yield similar results. This has been attributed to the schisis cavity within the retina causing a delay in electrical impulse conductance [10, 11]. OCT findings demonstrating lamellar schisis explain the finding that ERG dysfunction is found

K. Drenser (✉)
Royal Oak, MI, USA

Eye Research Institute, Oakland University, Rochester, MI, USA
e-mail: kdrenser@arcpc.net

W.-C. Wu, W.-C. Lam (eds.), *A Quick Guide to Pediatric Retina*, https://doi.org/10.1007/978-981-15-6552-6_23

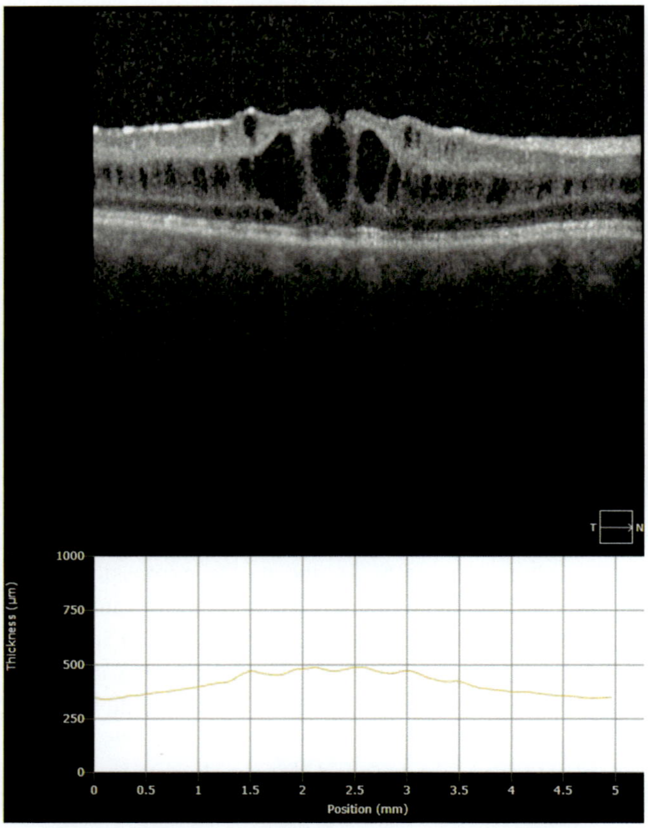

Fig. 23.1 OCT example of foveal schisis. The OCT shows spaces within the retina which are typical

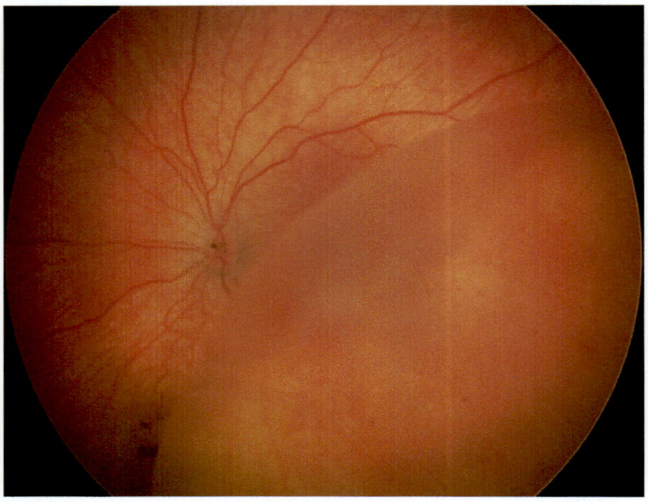

Fig. 23.2 Fundus photo example of a bullous schisis cavity. The outer retina remains attached but the inner wall is detached

Table 23.1 Classification of Congenital X-linked Retinoschisis

Type	Foveal schisis	Lamellar schisis	Peripheral schisis
Foveal	+	–	–
Foveal-lamellar	+	+	–
Complex	+	+	+
Foveal-peripheral	+	–	+

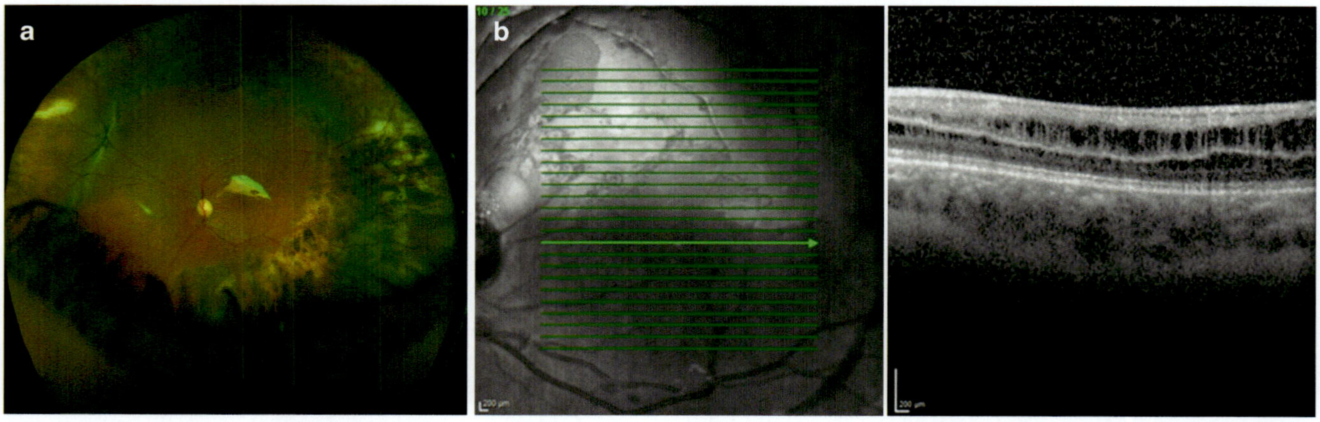

Fig. 23.3 Example of lamellar (or flat) schisis. (**a**) The color fundus photo shows an attached retinal following surgery for a combined tractional schisis and full-thickness rhegmatogenous retinal detachment. The retinal layers are tamponaded by silicone oil. (**b**) The OCT shows the persistent intraretinal structural schisis that persists despite repair

throughout the retina even when clinical evaluation reveals foveal pathology only. Foveal CXRS, with foveal schisis only, explains the occasional eye which has a normal ERG.

References

1. Tanatri A, Vrabec TR, Cu-Unjieng A, Frost A, Annesley WH, Donoso LA. X-linked retinoschisis: a clinical and molecular genetic review. Surv Ophthalmol. 2004;49:214–30.
2. Sieving PA, MacDonald IM, Trese MT. Congenital X-linked retinoschisis. In: Hartnett ME, Trese MT, Capone A, et al., editors. Pediatric retinal diseases: medical and surgical approaches. Philadelphia: Lippincott, Williams & Wilkins; In Press.
3. Hiriyanna KT, Bingham EL, Yashar BM, Ayyagari R, Fishman G, Small KW, Weinberg DV, Weleber RG, Lewis RA, Andreasson S, Richards JE, Sieving PA. Novel mutations in XLRS1 causing retinoschisis, including first evidence of a putative leader sequence change. Hum Mutat. 1999;14:423–7.
4. Zeng Y, Takada Y, Kjellstrom S, Hiriyanna K, Tanikawa A, Wawrousek E, Smaoui N, Caruso R, Bush RA, Sieving PA. RS-1 gene delivery to an adult Rs1h knockout mouse model restores ERG b-wave with reversal of the electronegative waveform of X-linked retinoschisis. Invest Ophthalmol Vis Sci. 2004;45:3279–85.
5. The Retinoschisis Consortium. Functional implications of the spectrum of mutations found in 234 cases with X-linked juvenile retinoschisis (XLRS). Hum Mol Genet. 1998;7:1185–92.
6. Chan WM, Choy KW, Wang J, Lam DS, Yip WW, Fu W, Pang CP. Two cases of X-linked juvenile retinoschisis with different optical coherence tomography findings and RS1 gene mutations. Clin Exp Ophthalmol. 2004;32:429–32.
7. Prenner JL, Capone A, Ciaccia S, Takada Y, Sieving PA, Trese MT. Congenital X-linked retinoschisis classification system. Arch Ophthalmol. 2004; accepted.
8. Azzolini C, Pierro L, Codenotti M, Brancato R. OCT images and surgery of juvenile macular retinoschisis. Eur J Ophthalmol. 1997;7:196–200.
9. Eriksson U, Larsson E, Holmstrom G. Optical coherence tomography in the diagnosis of juvenile X-linked retinoschisis. Acta Ophthalmol Scand. 2004;82:218–23.
10. Kahn NW, Jamison JA, Kemp JA, Sieving PA. Analysis of photoreceptor function and inner retinal activity in juvenile X-linked retinoschisis. Vis Res. 2001;41:3931–42.
11. Huang S, Wu D, Jiang F, Luo G, Liang J, Wen F, Yu M, Long S, Wu L. The multifocal electroretinogram in X-linked juvenile retinoschisis. Doc Ophthalmol. 2003;106:251–5.

Inherited Retinal Degenerations in the Pediatric Population

24

Birgit Lorenz and Markus N. Preising

Abstract

Inherited retinal degenerations (IRDs) are usually progressive disorders that may be difficult to diagnose in early childhood and look different from more advanced stages. This chapter focusses on early phenotypes visible with currently available imaging techniques and describes the clinical course during the first two decades. It also emphasizes the importance of recognizing carrier signs in X-linked disease.

Keywords

Inherited retinal degenerations · IRDs · Childhood manifestation · Phenotype · Genotype · Carrier status

24.1 Introduction and Short Overview on Inherited Retinal Degenerations (IRDs)

IRDs are genetically and phenotypically extremely heterogeneous. Figure 24.1 and Table 24.1 summarize the actually known genes. The data are constantly updated in the referenced electronic databases. The European Reference Network on Rare Eye Diseases (ERN-EYE) recently developed an ontological foundation for ocular phenotypes and rare eye diseases [1]. It is important to remember that most IRDs are progressive in nature, and the expressivity may be variable. Especially in infants and young children, the funduscopic features may be relatively unremarkable or show only subtle signs. In particular, they may be difficult to detect in the presence of nystagmus, usually noticed around the age of 6–10 weeks. Infantile nystagmus can be a sign of very different diseases but hereditary retinopathies are a frequent cause of sensory defect nystagmus [2, 3]. With disease progression, the funduscopic findings and visual functions will change over time. To familiarize the clinician dealing with hereditary retinal disease, we provide ample information of the findings of fundus photography, fundus autofluorescence (FAF), and optical coherence tomography (OCT) of various genotypes. This illustrates phenotypic variations with different degrees of severity due to genetic and allelic heterogeneity, intrafamilial variability, and disease progression from childhood into young adulthood.

24.2 Examination Techniques with Special Focus on the Pediatric Age Group

Adequate diagnosis and follow-up of inherited retinal degenerations require a whole set of examination methods. Because of emerging therapies, natural history studies are becoming increasingly important to provide insight if the therapies are slowing or stopping the disease course. Multimodal investigations including electrophysiology as well as common and advanced imaging techniques can identify specific phenotypes but nystagmus may limit the image quality. Table 24.2 lists the most important tests that are in clinical use, at least in centers focusing on IRDs [4]. Age adapted tests are highlighted as they are important to get reliable and meaningful results. Early in childhood, retinal changes visible by biomicroscopy may be subtle. Poor compliance at a young age hampers the feasibility of functional tests. These tests need special skills and experience of the examiner when applied in young children. Holder and Robson [5] have published a practical approach to pediatric ophthalmology. Handheld and portable imaging devices allow their use starting from infancy; therefore, examination under general anesthesia is only done exceptionally.

B. Lorenz (✉) · M. N. Preising
Department of Ophthalmology, Justus-Liebig-University Giessen, Universitaetsklinikum Giessen and Marburg, campus Giessen, Giessen, Germany
e-mail: birgit.lorenz@augen.med.uni-giessen.de; markus.preising@augen.med.uni-giessen.de

W.-C. Wu, W.-C. Lam (eds.), *A Quick Guide to Pediatric Retina*, https://doi.org/10.1007/978-981-15-6552-6_24

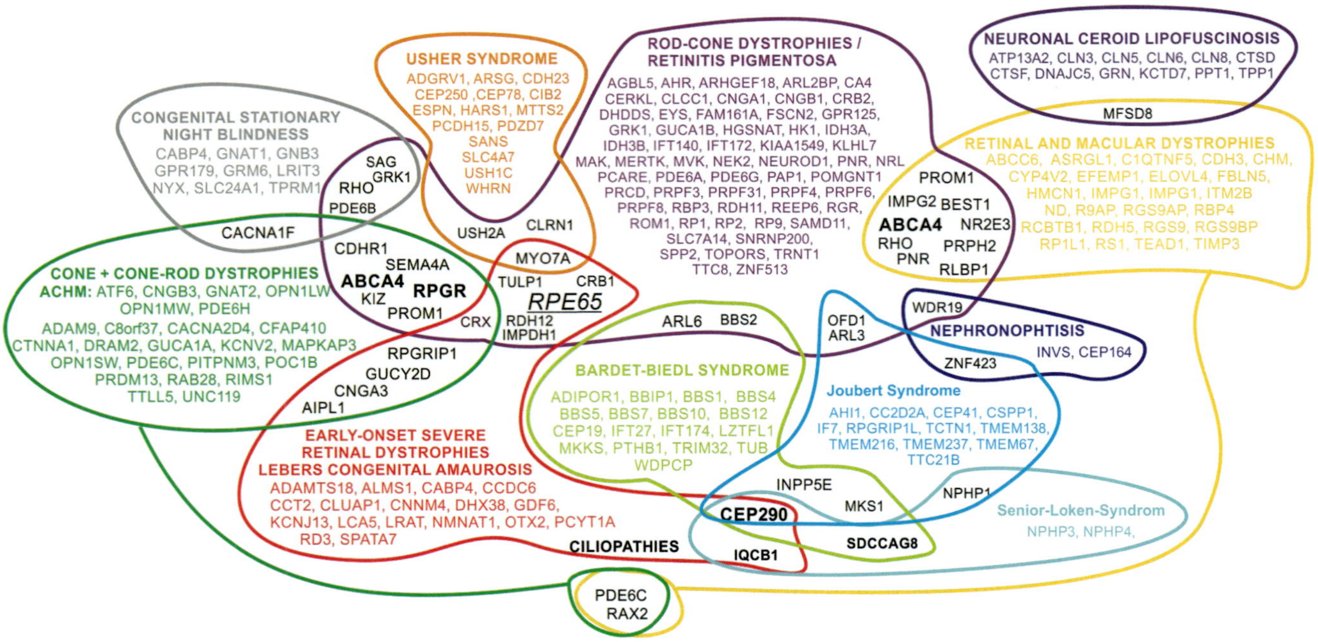

Fig. 24.1 Genes: Compilation of genes with sequence variations causing inherited retinal degenerations (IRDs). Genes written in black are involved in at least two disease entities. Genes involved in multiple disease entities are highlighted in bold. *RPE65* in italic font and underlined is currently the only gene with a clinically approved gene therapy. Diseases are in the order according to age of onset and pathophysiology

Table 24.1 The spectrum of inherited retinal disorders (IRD) (updated 02/2020) (according to OMIM (http://omim.org/), RetNet (https://sph.uth.edu/retnet/) and GeneBank (https://www.ncbi.nlm.nih.gov/gene/)

Function	Disease entities	Genes
Unknown	Rod-Cone Dystrophy (RCD)	*ABCC6, GPR125, ITM2B, KIAA1549, SPP2*
	Congenital Stationary night blindness (CSNB)	*NYX*
Ocular development, organogenesis	Cone-Rod-Dystrophy (CRD)	*ADAM9, ADAMTS18, C1QTNF5, CERKL, CRB1, CRB2, CTNNA1, DRAM2, MAPKAP3*
	Retinitis pigmentosa (RP)/RCD	*EYS, FAM161A, IMPG1, IMPG2, KLHL7, ND, NEK2, TEAD1, TIMP3, ZNF513*
	Early-onset severe retinal dystrophies (EOSRD) Ciliopathies	*CCDC6, GDF6, INVS, OTX2, PCYT1*
Transcriptional control DNA damage repair	Aniridia (AN2)	*PAX6*
	Achromatopsia (ACHM)	*ATF6*
	RP/RCD/CRD	*AHR, C21orf2, CRX, NEUROD1, NR2E3, NRL, PRDM13, RAX2, RCBTB1, REEP6, SAMD11, TRNT1*
	BBS	*TUB*
	USH	*HARS1*
Visual cascade	ACHM	*CNGA3*, ***CNGB3***, *GNAT2, PDE6C, PDE6H*
	Blue Cone Monochromacy (BCM)	*OPN1LW, OPN1MW*
	CRD	*GUCA1A*, ***GUCY2D***[a], *PDE6A, RD3*[a], *OPN1SW*
	RP/RCD	*CNGA1, CNGB1, GRK1, GUCA1B, PDE6B*[b], *PDE6G, PRKCG, R9AP, RGS9AP, RGS9, RGS9BP*, ***RHO***[b], *SAG*
	CSNB	*GNAT1, GNB3*
Retinol cycle	RP/RCD	*RDH11, RGR, RBP3, LRAT*, ***RPE65***[a], *RLBP1*[b], *RBP4*, ***ABCA4***[c]
	CRD	*RDH12*[a], *RDH5*[b]

Table 24.1 (continued)

Function	Disease entities	Genes
Neural function, Photoreceptor response, Impulse transmission Electrochemistry	CRD	*CACNA2D4, KCNV2, RS1, UNC119*
	Bestrophinopathies (VMD, ARB, ADVIRC)	***BEST1***[c]
	EOSRD	*KCNJ13*
	RP/RCD	*CA4, CLCC1*
	CSNB	*CABP4*[d], ***CACNA1F***, *GRM6, GRP179, SLC24A1, TPRM1*
	Usher Syndrome	*SLC4A7*
Ciliopathies and intraflagellar transport	EOSRD Joubert Syndrom Senior–Løken Syndrom Nephronophthisis	*AHI, ALMS1, C6orf152, CC2D2A, CEP41,* ***CEP290***[d], *CLUAP, CSPP1, INPP5E, IQCB1, KIF7, LCA5, MKS1, NPHP1, NPHP3, NPHP4,* ***RPGRIP1***, *RPGRIP1L SPATA7, TCTN1, TMEM67, TMEM138, TMEM216, TMEM237, TTC21B*
	CRD	*CDHR1, POC1B, RP1L1*
	RP/RCD	*AGBL5, ARL2BP, C8orf37, CDHR1, FSCN2, IFT140, IFT172, IMPDH1, KIZ, MAK, PCARE, PROM1,* ***PRPH2***, *ROM1, RP1, RP2,* ***RPGR***, *SEMA4A, TTC8, TTLL5*
	Bardet–Biedl Syndrome (BBS)	*ARL6*[c], *BBIP1, BBS1, BBS2,* ***BBS7***, *BBS4, BBS5, BBS7,* ***BBS10***, *BBS12, CEP19, IFT27, IFT174, INPP5E, LZTFL1, MKKS, MKS1, PTHB1, SDCCAG8, TRIM32, WDPCP*
	Usher Syndrome (USH)	*ADGRV1, CDH23, CDH3, CEP250, CIB2, CEP78, CLRN1, ESPN, FBLN5, GPR98, Harmonin, MTTS2,* ***MyoVIIa***, *PCDH15, PCDH21, PDZD7, SANS,* ***USH2A***[c], *USH2D, WHRN*
Intracellular transport	CSNB	*LRIT3*
	EOSRD	*AIPL1, CCT2*
	RP/RCD	*ARHGEF18, ARL3, MERTK, RAB28, TULP1*[d] *OCRL1, CHM*
	CRD	*RIMS1*
Metabolism and housekeeping functions	EOSRD	*CNNM4, NMNAT1, SRD5A3*
	RP/RCD	*ASRGL1, DHDDS, HGSNAT, HK1, IDH3A, IDH3B, MVK, PLA2G5, POMGNT1, PRCD, SLC7A14, TOPORS, TTPA*
	CRD	*CYP4V2, EFEMP1, ELOVL4, MFSD8*
	Syndromes	*MTP, PXMP3, TREX1, TTPA8, WDR19*
	BBS	*ADIPOR1*
	USH	*ARSG*
	Ceroid lipofuscinosis	*ATP13A2, CLN3, CLN5, CLN6, CLN8, CTSD, CTSF, DNAJC5, GRN, KCTD7, MFSD8, PPT1, TPP1*
Splicing	RP/RCD	*PAP1, PRPC8, PRPF3, PRPF4, PRPF6, PRPF8, PRPF31, SNRNP200*
	EOSRD	*DHX38*

Bold: frequent: sequence variations underlying overlapping phenotypes from allelic heterogeneity
[a]Predominant early-onset phenotypes, [b]With congenital stationary night blindness (CSNB), [c]With Retinitis pigmentosa (RP/RCD), [d]With early-onset severe retinal dystrophies (EOSRD)

24.3 Selected Examples of IRDs with Identified Genotypes

The high and still increasing number of genes correlated with inherited retinal degenerations precludes a comprehensive list of all currently known genes in the context of this book. It is important to note that complex disease phenotypes require an interdisciplinary approach, which has been demonstrated again recently by identifying the retinal phenotype in a new metabolic disorder, i.e., Taurin transporter SLC6A6 that might be amenable to therapy [6].

The selection includes genes associated with the following features: manifestation at birth or early childhood, relatively high frequency, involvement in complex pathways, importance in differential diagnosis and genetic counseling, or upcoming and already existing therapeutic approaches. Clinicians and researchers looking for more in-depth information should refer to the textbook by Traboulsi on Genetic

Table 24.2 Compilation of the most relevant clinical tests to diagnose IRDs in children

Imaging	Electrophysiology	Psychophysics
Fundus photography Infants: wide-field contact (e.g., RetCam) wide-field non contact (OPTOS) later on: wide-field, e.g.,OPTOS, Zeiss Clarus 700	Full-field ERG DTL electrodes Skin electrodes	Visual Acuity:Infants: Teller Acuity Cards TAC Toddlers: LEA, HOTV Thereafter: Snellen, ETDRS Visual Field Testing From about 6 years on
Fundus Autofluorescence FAF Spectralis (Heidelberg Eng.) OPTOS	mfERG (from about 6 years on)	Color vision: Matsubara plates, Waggoner plates Panel D 15
Optical coherence tomography SD-OCT, SD-OCT Hand-held, table-mounted		Dark adaptation Dark adapted VF testing Full-field stimulus threshold testing FST

Comment: Clinical diagnosis should precede molecular genetic diagnosis to describe the natural course of the disease. Molecular genetic analysis then confirms the clinical diagnosis. The best possible clinical diagnosis is important in order to preselect likely genes and to interpret the molecular genetic results for mutations of unknown significance. Segregation analysis of the mutations found is important in the case of compound heterozygous mutations to prove biallelic presence compatible with autosomal recessive inheritance. Gene directed therapies require a precise molecular genetic diagnosis

Diseases of the Eye (2nd edition 2012) [7]. We published a concise update on the basics of hereditary disease, genetic testing, phenotyping, and treatment in ocular disorders [8, 9]. Basic aspects and principles of genetic testing are described in Chap. 30 of this book.

24.3.1 Ocular Development and Metabolic Disease

In this section, three genes are discussed in more detail, i.e., *PAX6*, the master control gene for ocular development, Norrie Disease Protein (*NDP*) which was the first gene identified as part of the wnt signaling pathway, and Juvenile Ceroid Lipofuscinosis (CLN3) as an important differential diagnosis to juvenile Retinitis Pigmentosa (RP) because of its early fatal disease course.

24.3.1.1 *PAX6*

The most frequent cause of macular hypoplasia is albinism [10, 11] which is not included here because of its stationary course. Retinal diseases are a frequent cause of infantile nystagmus [2, 3]. *PAX* genes are a family of transcriptional regulators involved in the early development of organisms during embryogenesis. *PAX6* is the master control gene for ocular development in vertebrates and non-vertebrates. Heterozygous *PAX6* gene mutations are associated with a wide spectrum of phenotypes due to haploinsufficiency (For an overview, see [12]). The iris changes are most prominent, but the disease is panocular and includes also macular hypoplasia, retinal and choroidal colobomata. Cataract and corneal opacification are typically progressive and cause additional visual impairment later in life. Figure 24.2 shows representative examples. Recently, a nonsense suppression therapy in a *pax6* mouse model administered postnatally has reversed malformation defects [13].

24.3.1.2 Norrie Disease

Norrie disease is an X-linked disorder with typical congenital blindness, hearing problems, psychiatric features, and epilepsy. The gene (*NDP*) was identified in 1992 [14]. The disease may be limited to the eye. While non-attachment of the retina is the typical appearance, milder phenotypes with exudative vitreoretinopathy or falciform retinal fold may mimic retinopathy of prematurity although without prematurity. We reported this already in 1995 [15]. Figure 24.3 shows a collection of phenotypes. Norrie disease is part of diseases recognized as wnt-signaling pathway disorders manifesting as familial exudative vitreoretinopathy with autosomal dominant inheritance being the most frequent. Autosomal recessive inheritance may also occur (For an overview, see [16]). Knowledge of the pathophysiology of Norrie Disease may lead to effective therapeutic approaches. In milder phenotypes, early retinal photocoagulation may be effective to prevent disease progression (see Fig. 24.3a–c, unpublished data, courtesy Monika Andrassi-Darida, Dept. of Ophthalmology Giessen). Early vitrectomy has also been proposed [17].

24.3.1.3 Juvenile Ceroid lipofuscinosis (CLN3)

CLN3 is a rare autosomal recessive lysosomal storage disorder. The majority of patients suffer from neurological symptoms due to neuronal degeneration in the first decade of life leading to death in the second or third decade. One of the first symptoms usually preceding neurological symptoms is a rapid visual decline from severe retinal degeneration [18]. Children between 5 and 8 years present with rapidly progressing RP or bull's eye maculopathy. OCT is pathognomonic because, different from RP, not only photoreceptors, but also inner retinal layers are severely compromised early on (Fig. 24.4).

24.3.2 Ciliopathies

Motile and non-motile cilia are nearly ubiquitous cellular organelles. By 2017, 35 different ciliopathies have been described, with 187 established genes, and >240 candidate genes [19]. Sensory ciliopathies result specifically from defects in the sensory and/or signaling functions of non-

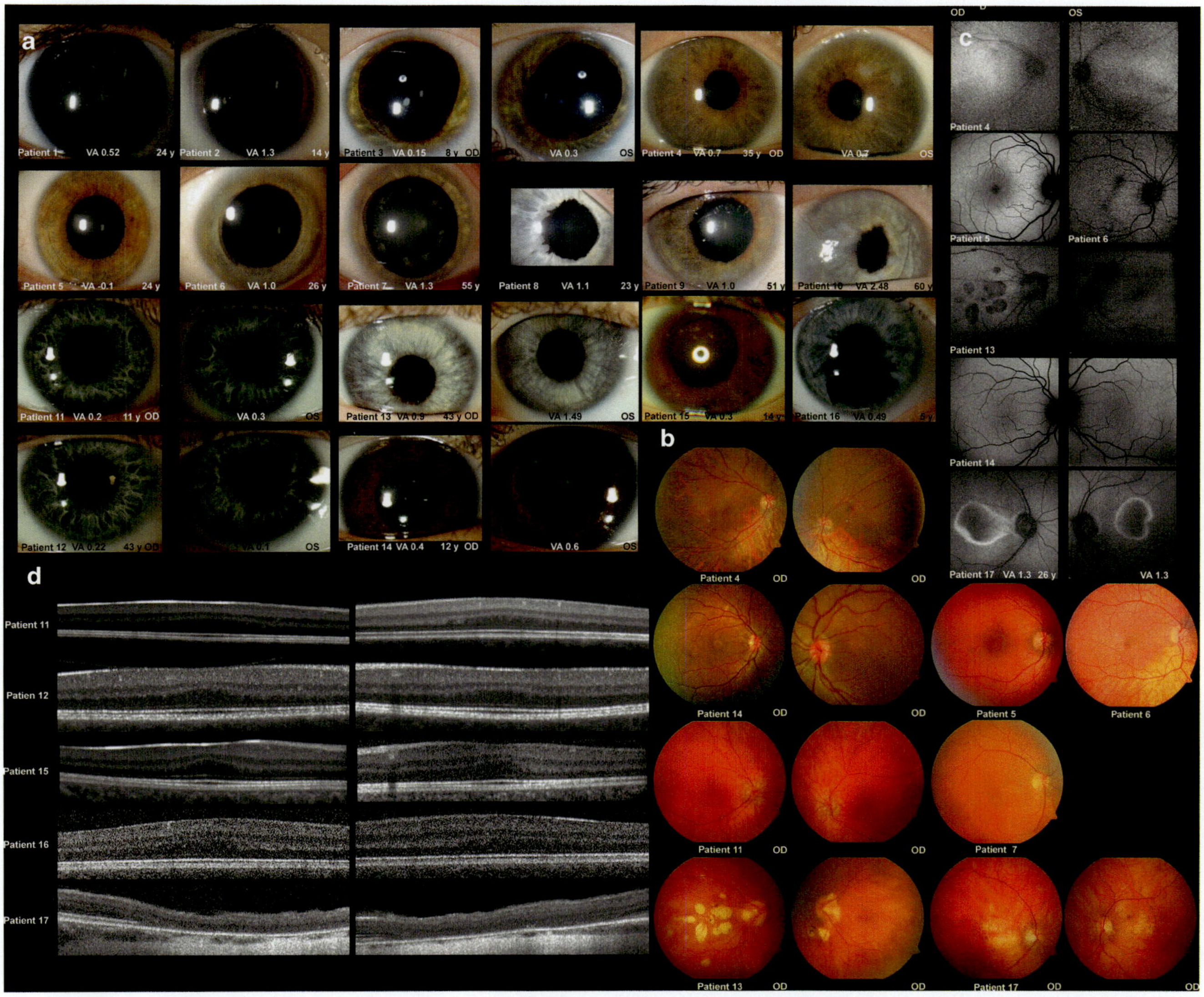

Fig. 24.2 *PAX6*: Compilation of phenotypic variations in patients with mutations in the prominent transcription factor PAX6 controlling major steps in eye development. Variations in disease severity are attributed to haploinsufficiency. (**a**) Iris hypoplasia including atypical coloboma as prime feature of PAX6 dysfunction presents with interpatient and intrafamilial variability shown for sequence variation p.*423Lfsext**180 in Patient 1–10. Patient 1 at 24 years presented with full aniridia, while Patient 2 at 14 years showed incomplete aniridia and Patient 3 at 8 years had partial aniridia while Patient 4 at 35 years had displaced pupil. Patient 5 at 24 years, patient 6 at 26 years, and their mother Patient 7 at 55 years, as well as Patient 8 at 23 years, her mother, patient 9 at 51 years, and aunt, Patient 10 at 60 years, all showed an appearance of intrafamilial variability including cataract formation. On the other hand, phenotypic expression can be unique and stable like in Patient 11 at 11 years (Sequence variation p.P249R (c.746C>G)) and her mother, patient 12 at 43 years. The expression in the iris can be very mild as in this family and patient 13 at 43 years (Sequence variation p.F217S (c.650T>C)), patient 14 at 12 years (Sequence variation p.E228K (c.682G>A)), Patient 15 at 14 years (Sequence variation p.L57P (c.170T>C)), Patient 16 at 5 years (Sequence variation p.G12R (c.34G>C)), and Patient 17 at 26 years (Sequence variation p.R128H (c.383G>A)). Assorted (**b**) Fundus photograph, (**c**) Fundus autofluorescence (FAF), and (**d**) SD-OCT images showed macular hypoplasia. Atypical chorioretinal hypoplasia is present in Patient 13 and 17, while Patient 5–7 are an example of intrafamilial variability of retinal affection. Visual acuity (VA) is reported in logMAR

motile cilia. Ciliopathies with retinal manifestation in early childhood are *CEP290*-associated IRDs (LCA, isolated or syndromic = Joubert Syndrome, JBTS), the Bardet–Biedl Syndromes (BBS), Senior–Løken Syndrome, and Alström Disease. The Usher Syndromes usually have a later retinal manifestation, although night blindness may be an early symptom. Inheritance is always autosomal recessive.

24.3.2.1 *CEP290*-Associated IRD

CEP290-associated IRD is a ciliopathy that may manifest as isolated LCA or as Joubert Syndrome (JBTS).

Biallelic *CEP290* mutations are one of the most frequent causes of IRDs with infancy onset. The interest in *CEP290*-associated LCA is high since recently a novel therapeutic approach, i.e., intravitreal injection of antisense

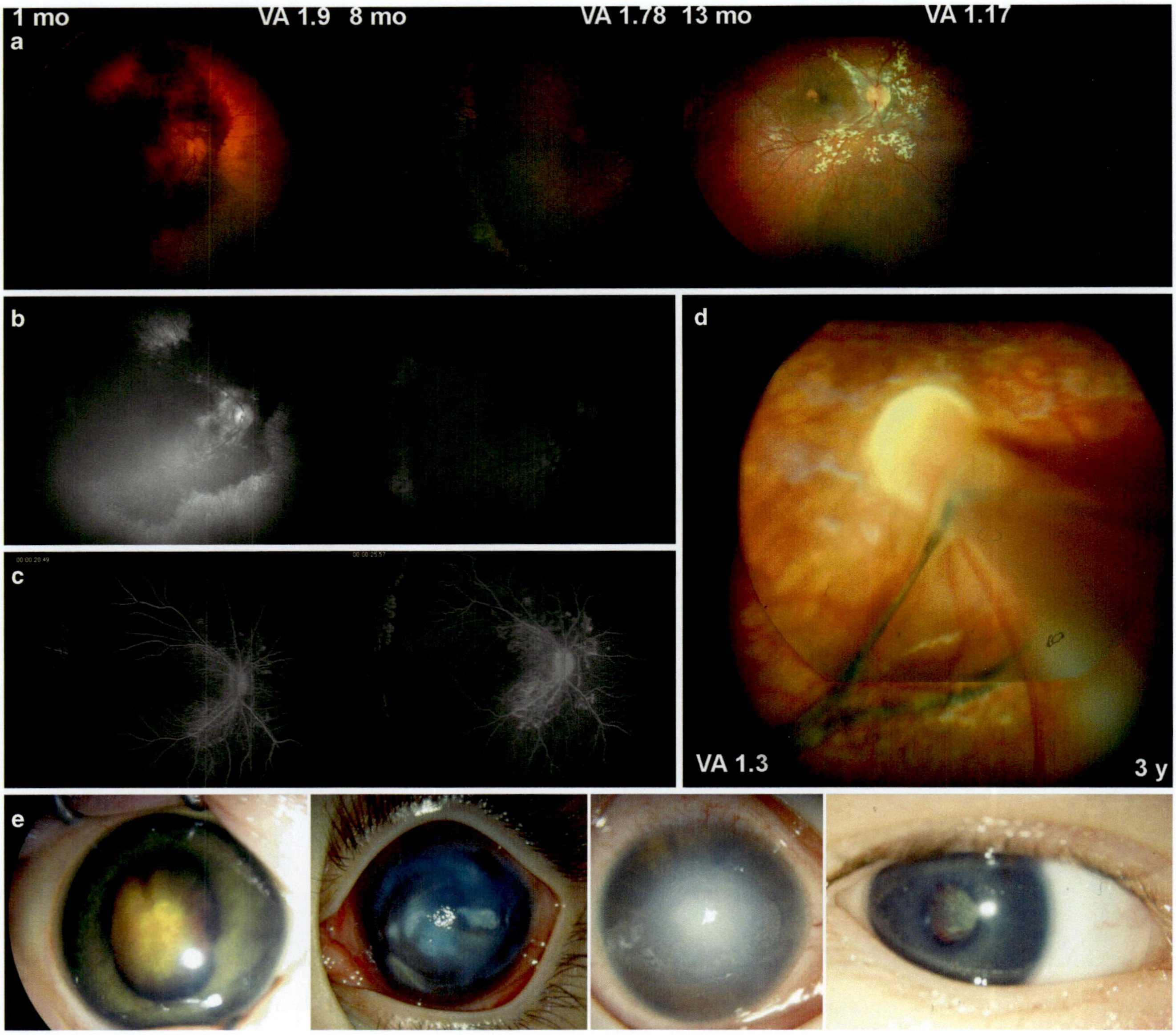

Fig. 24.3 NDG. (**a**) Fundus photograph with RetCam, Patient 1 with Norrie syndrome caused by sequence variant p.C95F (c.284G>T) at 1 month and 6 months, and with a Clarus 700 camera at 13 months. (**b**) Corresponding fundus autofluorescence images at 1 month and 6 months taken with Retcam. (**c**) Fluorescence angiogram taken by Retcam in Patient 1 at 20 min and 25 min post-injection at 6 months. Note the leaking vessels at the retinal arcades. (**d**) Retinal falciform fold in patient 2 at 3 years. (**e**) Examination challenge in Norrie disease in different patients. Visual acuity (VA) is reported in logMAR

oligonucleotide has shown promising results in a clinical trial [20]. Figure 24.5 is a compilation of typical phenotypes at a young age. A recent study on the natural phenotype included 66 patients carrying the most frequent *CEP290* mutation [c.2991+1655A>G (p.C998*)] either homozygous or heterozygous with another pathogenic sequence variant [21]. About 70% of patients had either light perception or no light perception. Among patients with measurable visual acuity, the range was 0.12–1.9 logMAR. Extra-ocular features were present in 18% of which delayed psychomotor development was most frequently encountered (42%). OCT data were available in 12 patients, 11 of whom had retained foveal outer nuclear layer and ellipsoid zone integrity, up until 48 years (median 23 years) of follow-up. Homozygous patients appeared less severely affected compared to their compound-heterozygous peers. Improvement of visual function may occur in the early years of life, possibly providing physicians with an optimal time window for therapeutic intervention. An intact foveal ONL and photoreceptor layer visible on OCT may extend this window, emphasizing the importance of thorough and regular patient phenotyping despite the presence of nystagmus that may complicate the examination procedures. Another study from our group [22], analyzed 30 patients with the full spectrum of pathogenic

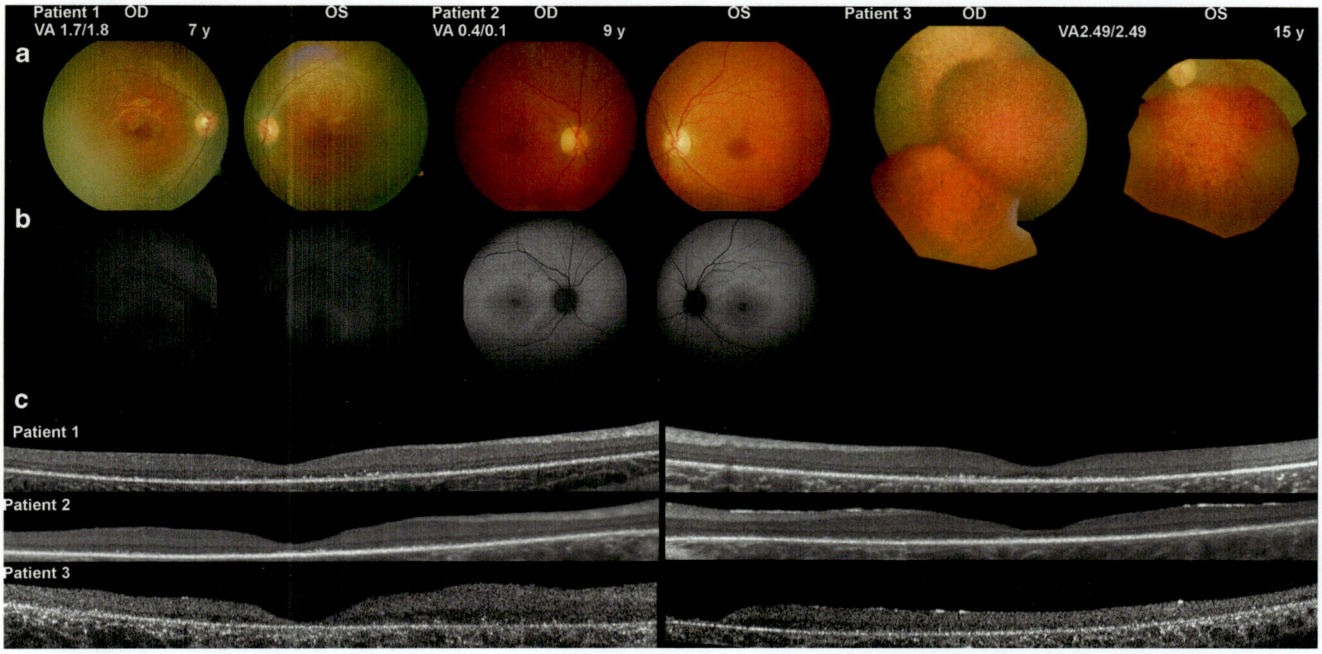

Fig. 24.4 *CLN3*. Three patients homozygous for the common 1.02 kb deletion covering the exons 7 and 8 in the *CLN3* gene causing juvenile ceroid lipofuscinosis. The patients were at the critical age range from onset to about 7 years (Patient 1), functional impairment at 9 years (Patient 2) to the advance stage at 15 years (Patient 3). (**a**) At onset (Patient 1) and in the period of severe and quick functional loss (Patient 2), the fundus may present with relatively mild changes with atypical foveal reflex and narrow retinal arteries (Patient 1) or bull's eye maculopathy (Patient 2) but develop pan-retinal photoreceptor degeneration that is typically very fast progression (Patient 3). (**b**) Fundus autofluorescence (FAF) with a rod-cone degeneration pattern with a paramacular ring of increased autofluorescence (Corresponding recordings to **a**). (**c**) SD-OCT explains the functional loss by a general reduction of retinal thickness with quickly progressing degeneration of photoreceptors including inner and outer segments together with severe involvement of the inner retina as well. Visual acuity (VA) is reported in logMAR

sequence variants including a 1-month-old infant. Only 33% of the 30 patients had no LP, 67% at least LP, and among these 26% had logMAR 2 to 0.7. Twenty-three of the 30 patients carried the c.2991+1655A>G mutation, 7 were homozygous. The homozygous patients are candidates for intravitreal antisense oligonucleotide therapy [20]. Full-field electroretinogram showed residual response in a few patients only who later deteriorated further. Fundus photography documented degenerative changes throughout the retina with macular degeneration and increased circular fundus autofluorescence signals in the perimacular ring, while the peripheral FAF appeared spotty in the rod ring. SD-OCT disclosed reduced photoreceptor layer thickness and preserved inner retinal thickness indicating anatomical potential for successful treatment.

24.3.2.2 Bardet–Biedl Syndromes

To date, biallelic mutations in as many as 25 different genes have been associated with the Bardet–Biedl Syndrome (BBS), a big surprise for such a rare syndrome. The cardinal features are rod-cone-dystrophy with early central involvement, polydactyly, truncal obesity, renal abnormalities, and mental retardation or learning disabilities but not all are present together. Polydactyly may have been corrected already at the time of the first presentation to the ophthalmologist. Therefore, clinicians should ask specifically for this feature. So far, no clear genotype–phenotype correlation arises for the different genes involved. A recent cross-sectional retrospective study demonstrates the early decline in visual acuity [23]. Figure 24.6 shows the early phenotypes of mutations in six BBS genes and demonstrates the macular involvement clearly visible on OCT and on FAF. An overview of the role of BBS genes on the eye has been published recently [24]. To date, no causal therapies are available. Therefore, supportive and rehabilitation therapies are important.

24.3.3 Early Onset Severe Retinal Dystrophies (EOSRD, EORD, SECORD)

Early-onset severe retinal dystrophies EOSRD (alternative terms Early Onset Retinal Dystrophies EORD, or Severe Early Onset Retinal Dystrophies SECORD) comprise a group of genetically and clinically heterogenous IRDs that are all characterized by onset in early infancy. The most severe phenotype is also called Leber Congenital Amaurosis (LCA) first described by Theodor Leber in 1869. For an overview, see the publication by Henderson, Lorenz, and Moore in 2006 [25]. The following sections present phenotypes for eight of the genes identified by February 2020.

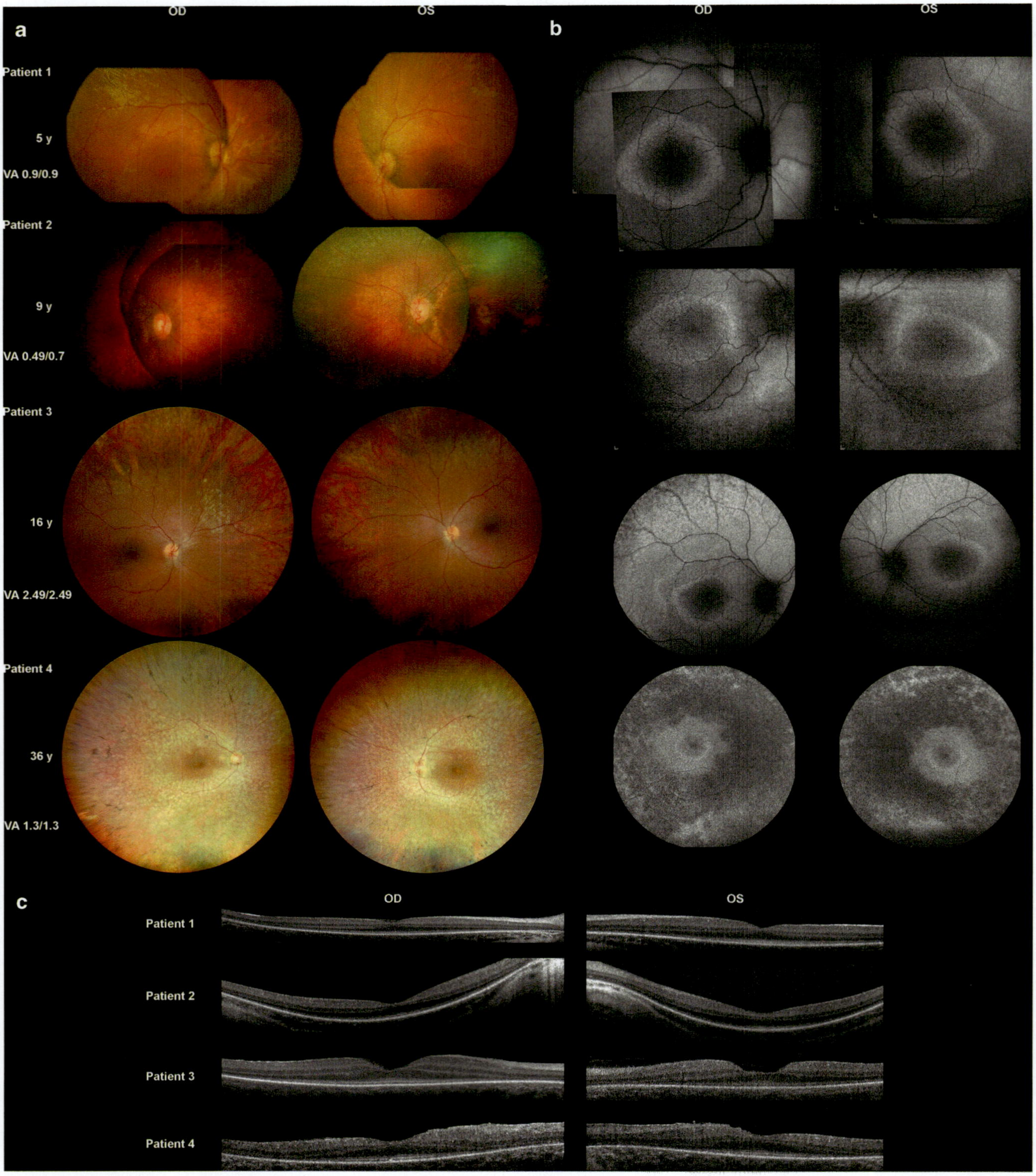

Fig. 24.5 *CEP290*. Course of retinal dystrophy in *CEP290*-associated early-onset retinal degeneration (EOSRD) and Leber congenital amaurosis (LCA). (**a**) Fundus photographs of four patients with different biallelic *CEP290* sequence variants. Patient 1 at 5 years (sequence variations p. G860* (c.2578G>T), [p.R1752W (c.5254C>T), p.R1253H (c.3758G>A)]) presented with a blunt fundus appearance in the center and yellowish spotty appearance in the periphery. A more obvious degenerative progression is visible in the retinal periphery of Patient 2 at 9 years (sequence variations c.2991+1655A>G (p.C998*) homozygous) and Patient 3 at 16 years (sequence variations c.2367+1G>A, c.2991+1655A>G (p.C998*)). In the latter, the peripheral RPE shows clear signs of degeneration, and the fovea looks abnormal as well. In Patient 4 at age of 36 years (sequence variations c.2991+1655A>G (p.C998*), c.6277delG (p.V2093fs*4)) the degeneration has progressed and shows pan-retinal involvement. (**b**) The corresponding fundus autofluorescence (FAF) images to (**a**) indicate major rod involvement by a ring of increased autofluorescence as commonly seen in rod-cone degeneration. (**c**) Spectral-domain Optical Coherence Tomography (SD-OCT) finding supports the advanced peripheral photoreceptor degeneration compared to the slower progression in the center with preserved layering of the outer and inner segments and the outer nuclear layer which gives hope to effective treatment approaches. Visual acuity (VA) is reported in logMAR

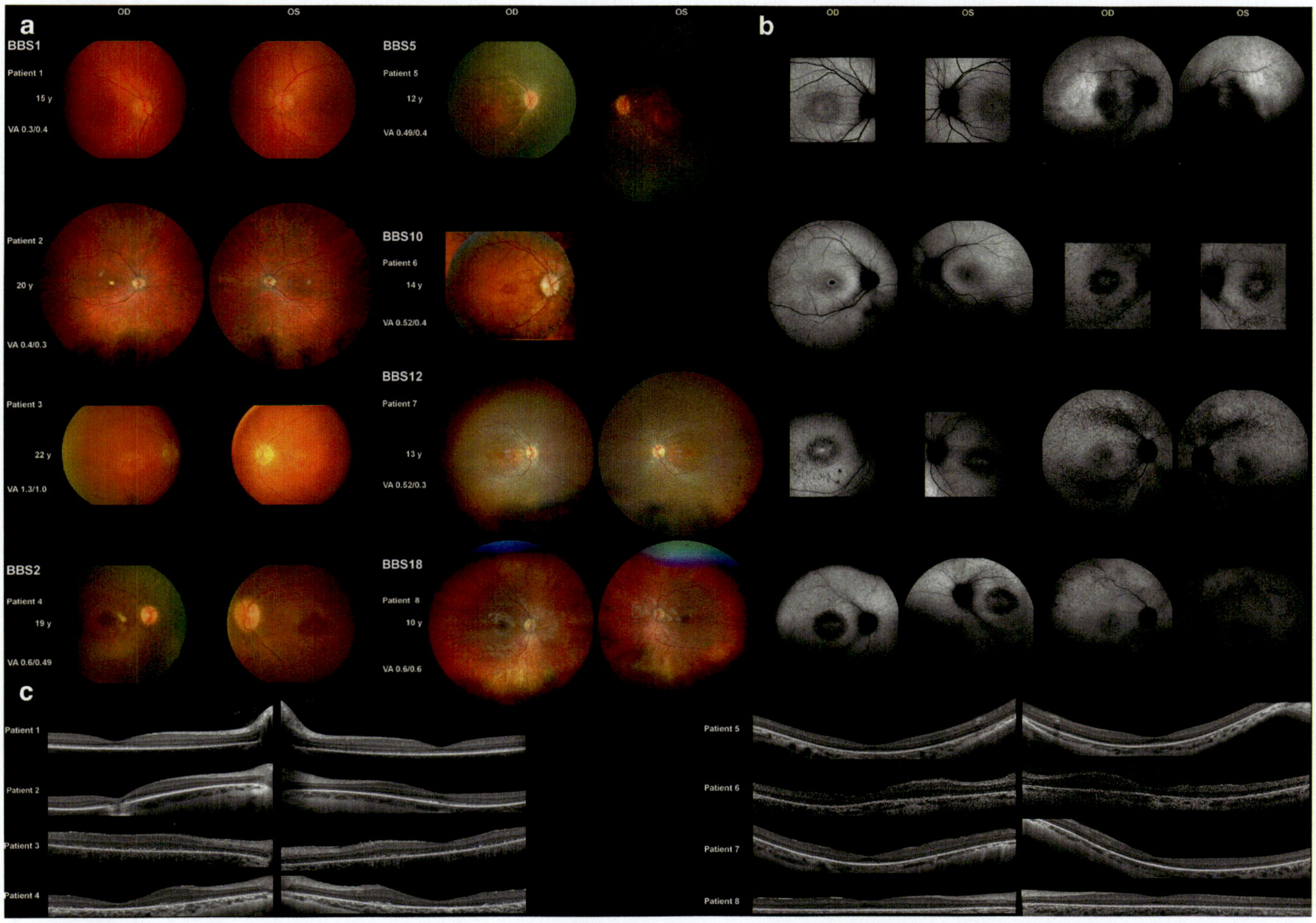

Fig. 24.6 BBS. Compilation of phenotypes of various Bardet–Biedl Syndrome (BBS) types. (**a**) Fundus photographs in three BBS1 patients with the most prevalent sequence variation p.M390R (c.1269T>G) in BBS1 in the homozygous state in Patient 1 at 15 years and Patient 2 at 20 years, as well as sequence variations c.479+4A>G, and a CNV deleting exons 14–17 in Patient 3 at 22 years. Patient 4 represents type *BBS2* at 19 years (sequence variations p.R23P (c.68C>G), p.R275* (c.823C>T)), followed by Patient 5 at 12 years with sequence variation c.412delCinsTTTAAATTAAGAA (p.R138delinsFKLRS) in *BBS5* in the homozygous state. The figure continues with Patient 6 at 14 years carrying the second most prevalent BBS sequence variation c.271insT (p.C91fs*95) in *BBS10* in the homozygous state and closes with Patient 7 at 14 years with sequence variation p.E254* (c.724GG>T) in *BBS12* in the homozygous state and Patient 8 at 10 years the homozygous sequence variation c.216+1G>T in *BBIP1* (BBS18). (**b**) Corresponding fundus autofluorescence (FAF) images, (**a**) shows pan-retinal involvement and advanced macular degeneration which is more prominent than postulated in a "typical pure ocular retinitis pigmentosa form" of inherited retinal degeneration, also in line with an early and severe reduction in visual acuity in patients with BBS. (**c**) SD-OCT recordings and FAF images as in (**b**). Visual acuity (VA) is reported in logMAR

Typically, inheritance mode is autosomal recessive due to biallelic mutations. In LCA, the full-field-ERG is usually non-recordable from infancy onward, and nystagmus or roving eye movements are also early signs.

24.3.3.1 Photoreceptor Guanylate Cyclase (*GUCY2D*) Phenotypes

Mutations in *GUCY2D* (the gene coding for photoreceptor guanylate cyclase GC-E) can give rise to either autosomal recessive LCA (LCA1, biallelic mutations), or to autosomal dominant cone-rod-degeneration (adCRD, CORD5, monoallelic mutations). LCA1 means that this was the first LCA gene attributed to a specific chromosomal location, CORD5 similarly means that this was the fifth CORD gene localized. The autosomal recessive form (LCA type) is associated with severe visual impairment to complete blindness usually from infancy onward but sometimes also better preserved visual function, due to the absence of an essential enzyme in the visual cascade. Interestingly, the retinal structure typically remains relatively well preserved into adulthood (Fig. 24.7a, d, g). In contrast, the autosomal CORD is typically associated with early and severe loss of macular function (Fig. 24.7b, e, h), although milder phenotypes also exist (Fig. 24.7c, f, i). A comprehensive overview of phenotype–genotype correlations has been published recently [26]. The preserved retinal structure in LCA 1 gives hope to future gene therapeutic approaches [27] and was recently confirmed in a natural history study in preparation of a clinical trial [28].

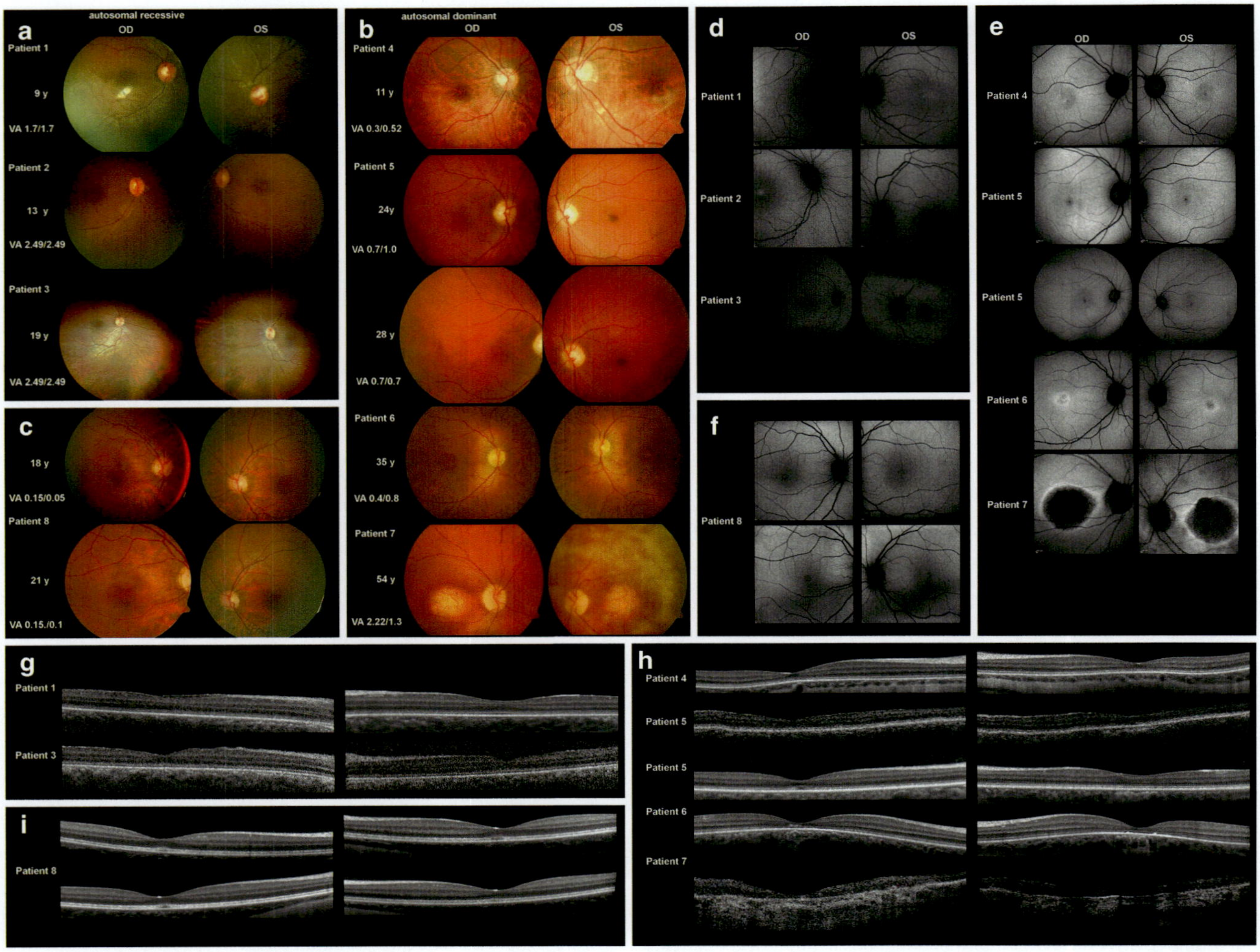

Fig. 24.7 *GUCY2D.* Autosomal recessive Leber Congenital Amaurosis (LCA) versus autosomal dominant cone-rod degeneration (CORD5) all caused by sequence variants in *GUCY2D.* (**a**) Three patients with autosomal recessive LCA from different biallelic sequence variations in *GUCY2D* at ages from late childhood to early adulthood. Patient 1 (9 years, sequence variations p.L176P (c.527T>C), p.Y351C (c.1052A>G)), Patient 2 (18 years, sequence change, p.Y922* (c.2766C>G) homozygous), Patient 3 (19 years, sequence variations c.3027delG (p.E1010Sfs*11) homozygous). Note the unremarkable fundus appearance throughout adolescence. (**b**) Four patients with autosomal dominant CORD15 from monoallelic sequence change p.R838C (c.2512C>T) in *GUCY2D* presenting disease development between late childhood and late adulthood. Note the increasing degeneration in the fovea. Patient 4 (11 years), Patient 5 (24 years, 28 years), Patient 6 (35 years), Patient 7 (54 years). (**c**) Patient 8 (18 years, 21 years) with autosomal dominant CORD15 from the minor frequent sequence change p.R838H (c.2513G>A) in *GUCY2D* at early adulthood. (**d**)–(**f**) Fundus autofluorescence (FAF) images corresponding to (**a**)–(**c**). (**d**) Minor changes with diminished blocking of FAF in the center. FAF signal appears relatively weak, possibly due to nystagmus typically present in a.r. *GUCY2* disease. (**g**)–(**i**) Optical coherence tomography (OCT) recordings corresponding to (**a**)–(**c**). Patients 1 and 3 with autosomal recessive inheritance showed subnormal to normal thickness in the layers of the outer and the inner retina. RPE is within normal limits. Patients with autosomal dominant inheritance present with obvious degenerative lesions in the macula in line with the FAF images. OCT of Patient 5 at 24 years and Patient 7 assessed by a time-domain device (*Stratus OCT3*, Zeiss Meditec). All others are spectral-domain OCT (Spectralis, Heidelberg Engineering). Visual acuity (VA) is reported in logMAR

24.3.3.2 *AIPL1* (Aryl Hydrocarbon Receptor Interacting Protein-Like 1)

Biallelic *AIPL1* mutations cause one of the most severe forms of inherited retinal degeneration (IRD). They are associated with rapid and extensive photoreceptor degeneration challenging the development of potential treatments [29]. Nevertheless, the same authors report that the preclinical studies of both gene augmentation and photoreceptor transplantation show regeneration and restoration of retinal function in animal models of *AIPL1*-associated LCA. Figure 24.8a–c confirm the presence of severe retinal degeneration in early childhood.

24.3.3.3 *TULP1* (Tubby-Like Protein 1)

An increasing number of genes are discussed as candidate genes for future therapeutic approaches, including *TULP1* [30]. TULP1 is part of the TULP family. Biallelic *TULP1* mutations are rarely causative of autosomal recessive LCA

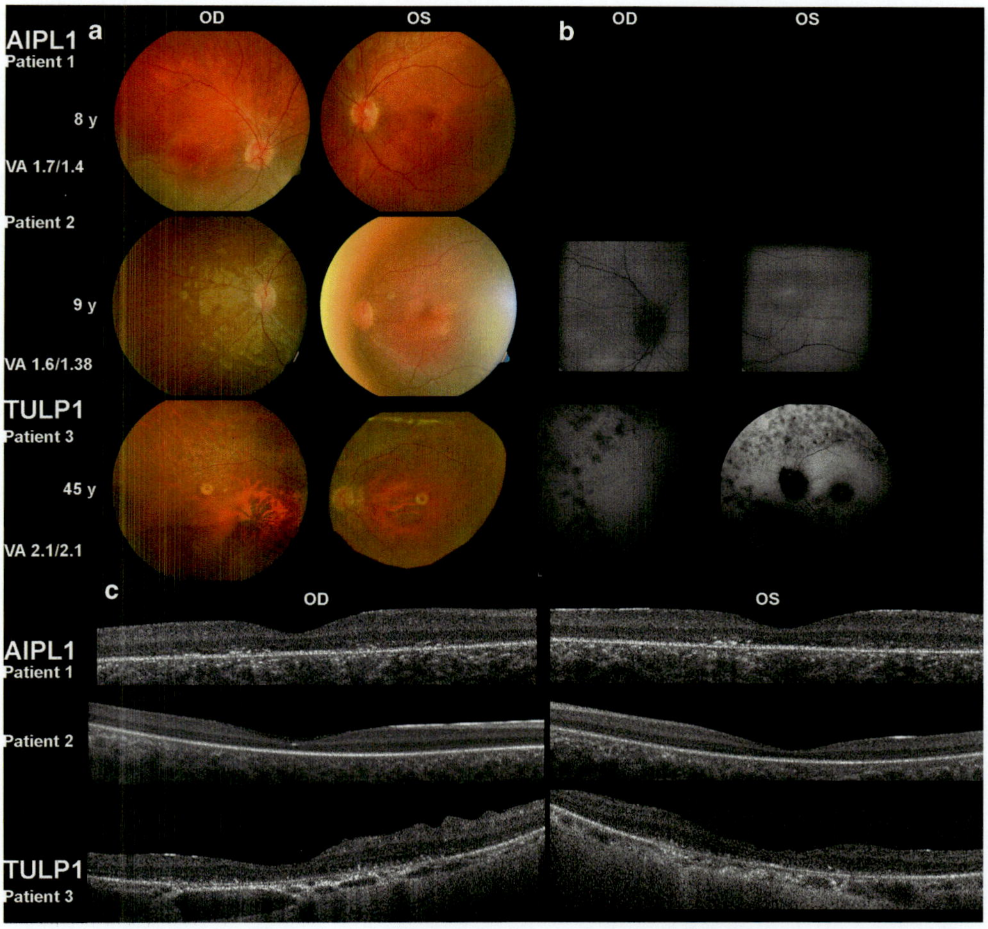

Fig. 24.8 Early-Onset Severe Retinal Dystrophy (EOSRD) *AIPL1* and *TULP1*. Compilation of very early-onset retinal dystrophies with severe course commonly summarized as Leber congenital amaurosis (LCA). The figure depicts phenotypes of patients with sequence changes in *AIPL1* and*TULP1*. Sequence changes in these two genes cause a generalized cone-rod dystrophy with severe degeneration of the photoreceptor layers from early infancy on. The visual impairment associated with nystagmus can also interfere with the photo documentation. (**a**) Fundus photograph in *AIPL1* (Patient 1 at 7 years (Sequence change p.W278* (c.834G>A) homozygous)) and Patient 2 at 9 years (Sequence change p.L17P (c.50T>C) homozygous)), and *TULP1* (Patient 3 at 45 years (Sequence change c.718+2T>C homozygous)). Abnormal features already present in childhood. (**b**) Corresponding fundus autofluorescence (FAF) images in (**a**). (**c**) Corresponding SD-OCTs to (**a**) and (**b**) documenting the severe degeneration of the photoreceptor layers down to the RPE in advanced stages. Visual acuity (VA) is reported in logMAR

[31], but rather a rare cause of autosomal recessive retinitis pigmentosa [32]. The protein is implicated in the maintenance and functioning of neuronal cells during development and post-differentiation [33] and affects intra-photoreceptor ciliary transport processes like in *CEP290* and *RPGRIP* associated retinopathies [31]. Patient 3 in Fig. 24.8 demonstrates a case of arRP with advanced pan-retinal degeneration.

24.3.3.4 *CRB1* (Crumbs Cell Polarity Complex Component 1)

Biallelic mutations in the *CRB1* gene are associated with variable phenotypes of severe retinal dystrophies, ranging from LCA to RP. Moreover, specific fundus features may be present such as preservation of the para-arteriolar retinal pigment epithelium (PPRPE) and retinal telangiectasia with exudation ("Coats-like vasculopathy"). Analysis of a large cohort of >240 patients with *CRB1* mutations did not find a clear genotype–phenotype correlation, though null mutations tended to be more frequent in the LCA phenotype [34]. We emphasized its early disease course [35]. During the first decade, we saw some improvement in visual acuity. Visual fields were severely reduced early on. Hypomorphic missense mutations with the predicted residual function of the gene product resulted in a more moderate disease. In the severe phenotypes, reduced retinal stratification indicated a general loss of structural integrity of the retinal layers. Figure 24.9 shows two patients, patient 1 with early-onset and severe phenotype, and patient 2 with a somewhat later onset. A recent study on 55 patients with RP associated with biallelic mutations in *CRB1* including 34 individuals from a Dutch genetic isolate indicated an eventual therapeutic window within the first 2–3 decades in the RP phenotype [36].

24.3.3.5 *MERTK* (MER Tyrosine Kinase) Phenotype

MER tyrosine kinase (*MERTK*) encodes a surface receptor localized at the apical membrane of the retinal pigment epithelium RPE. It plays a critical role in photoreceptor outer segment internalization prior to phagocytosis. Macular involvement occurs early, and OCT discloses debris-like changes in the outer retina compatible with the disturbed outer segment internalization [37]. SD-OCT findings in patients 3 and 4 in Fig. 24.9 are compatible with this description. A comprehensive review of all reported *MERTK* disease-causing variants with the associated phenotype was reported in 2018 [38]. Recently, rescue of the MERTK phagocytic defect has been shown in a human iPSC disease model using translational read-through inducing drugs [39], eventually leading to an effective therapeutic approach for specific *MERTK mutations*.

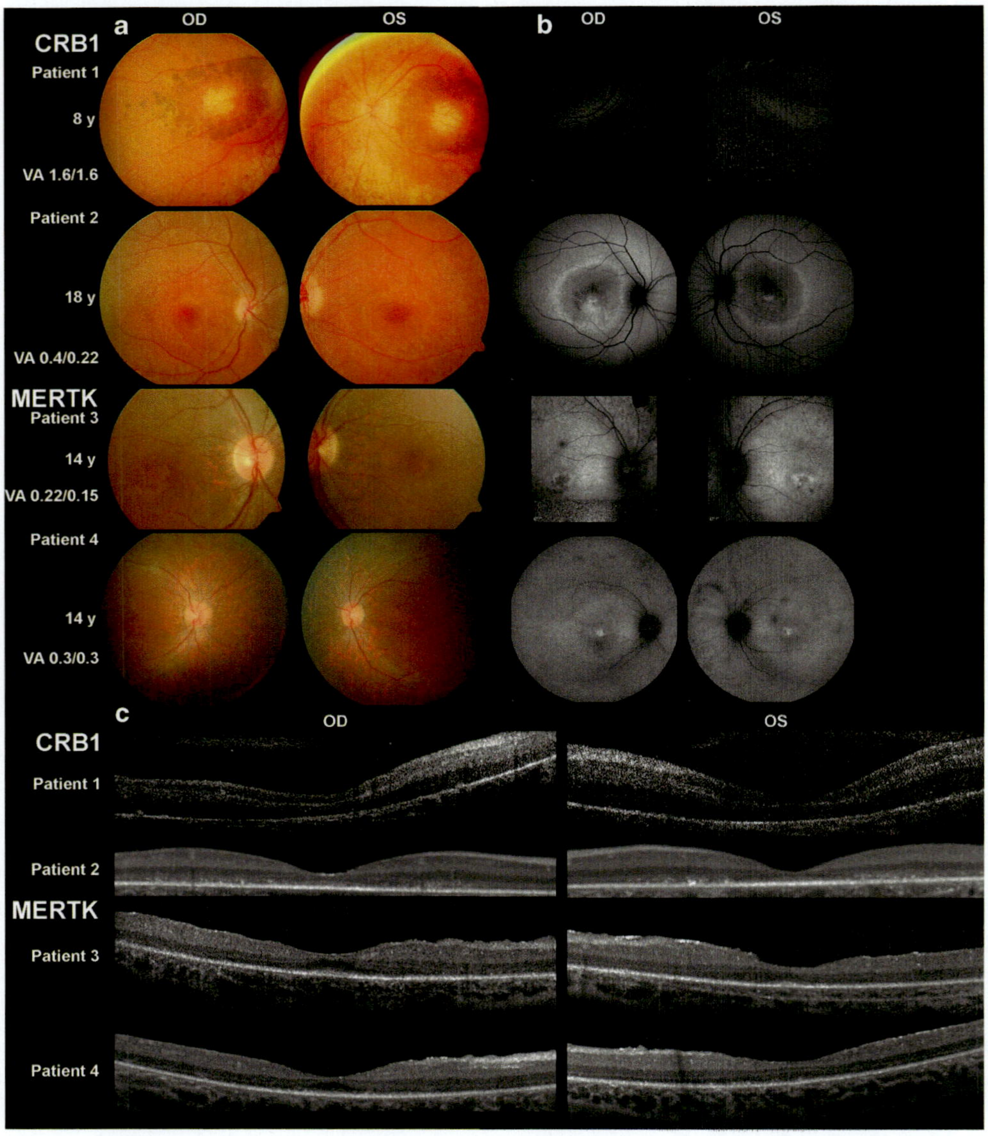

Fig. 24.9 Early-Onset Severe Retinal Dystrophy (EOSRD) *CRB1* and *MERTK*. The figure depicts phenotypes of patients with sequence changes in *CRB.1* and *MERTK*. *CRB1* is characterized by a broad individual spectrum from LCA to juvenile rod-cone dystrophy. *MERTK* causes a generalized cone-rod dystrophy with severe degeneration of the photoreceptor layers from early infancy. (**a**) Fundus photograph in *CRB1* (Patient 1 at 8 years (Sequence change p.C948Y (c.2843G>A); p.K801* (c.2401A>T))) and Patient 2 at 18 years (Sequence change c.498_506del (p.I167_G169del), p.H1035L (c.3104A>T))) and *MERTK* (Patient 3 at 14 years (Sequence change p. C115W (c.345C>G); c.1530delT (p.C510Wfs*5))) and Patient 4 at 14 years (Sequence change c.1744_1751del insT (p.I582*) homozygous)). (**b**) Corresponding fundus autofluorescence (FAF) images to (**a**). Patient 1 with early-onset disease presents with the pigmented paravenous chorioretinal atrophy with increased FAF, while patient 2, a case of rod-cone dystrophy shows the characteristic para-macular circle of increased FAF. (**c**) Corresponding SD-OCTs to (**a**) and (**b**) documenting the severe degeneration of the photoreceptor layers down to the RPE in advanced stages. Visual acuity (VA) is reported in logMAR

24.3.3.6 *RDH12* (Retinol Dehydrogenase 12) Associated Retinal Degeneration

RDH12 is expressed in the inner segments of the photoreceptors. It functions as part of the visual cycle. Mutations in *RDH12* have been linked to Leber congenital amaurosis (LCA) and autosomal dominant RP. A number of in-vitro studies have shown that mutations in *RDH12* result in little or no enzyme activity. Knockout mouse models however do not recapitulate the severe phenotype observed in patients, resulting in a limited understanding of the disease mechanisms [40]. A recent paper describes the natural history including some genotype–phenotype correlations in *RDH12*-Associated Retinal Degeneration [41]. Typical early macular involvement evident on funduscopy results in early severely reduced visual acuity. Some rare mutations may be associated with better visual functions throughout adulthood. Therapeutic intervention, which is not yet available, would best work in early childhood. Patients 1–3 in Fig. 24.10 illus-

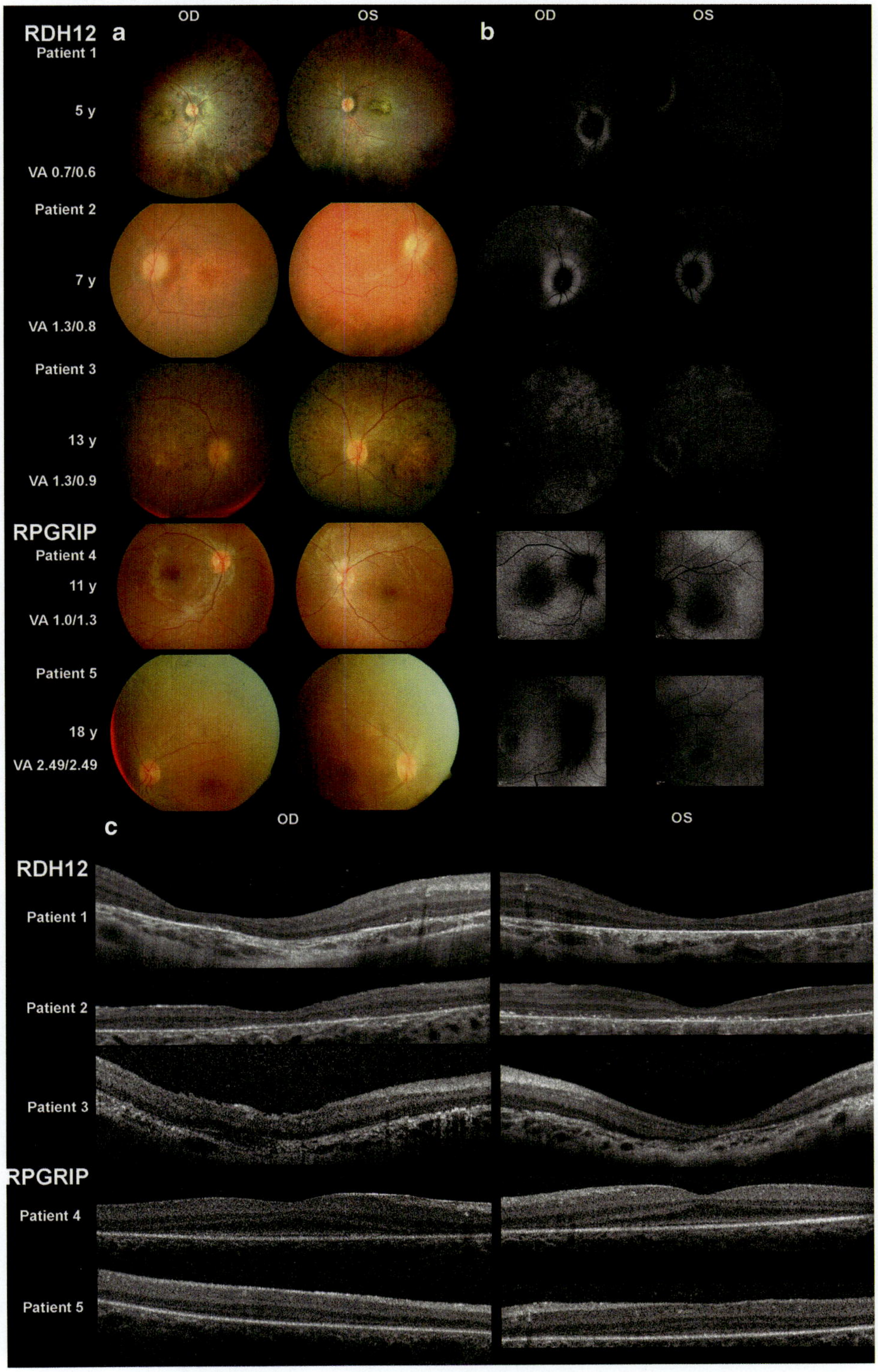

Fig. 24.10 Early-Onset Severe Retinal Dystrophy (EOSRD) *RDH12* and *RPGRIP*. The figure depicts phenotypes of patients with sequence changes in *RDH12* and *RPGRIP*. Mutations in both genes cause a generalized cone-rod dystrophy with severe degeneration of the photoreceptor layers from early infancy. (**a**) Fundus photographs in *RDH12* (Patient 1 at 5 years (Sequence change p.G127* (c.379G>T) homozygous)), Patient 2 at 7 years (Sequence change c.546delG (c.-44C>A, p. I183Ffs*95)), and Patient 3 at 13 years (Sequence change p.T155I (c.464C>T); c.806delCCCTG (p.A269Gfs*2)) and RPGRIP (Patient 4 at 11 years (Sequence change p.R890* (c.2668C>T); c.2532delC (p.Y846Tfs*12)) and Patient 5 at 18 years (Sequence change p.R814* (c.2440C>T) homozygous)). The RDH12 phenotype is associated with early funduscopic visible changes while the RPGRIP phenotype is not very revealing. (**b**) Corresponding fundus autofluorescence (FAF) images to (**a**). Patients 1–3 with sequence changes in *RDH12* develop an increase of parapapillary FAF. In line with the funduscopic appearance, FAF shows much more changes in *RDH12* compared to *RPGRIP*. (**c**) Corresponding SD-OCTs to (**a**) and (**b**) documenting the severe degeneration of the photoreceptor layers down to the RPE in advanced stages. Visual acuity (VA) is reported in logMAR

trate the early and severe retinal degeneration including the macula. Interestingly, the peripapillary retina appears relatively well preserved.

24.3.3.7 *RPGRIP* (Retinitis Pigmentosa GTPase Interacting Protein 1)

RPGRIP1 interacts with RPGR, the latter is encoded by the major X-linked RP (XLRP) gene, as it accounts for 70–80% of the XLRP patients and up to 13% of all RP patients. Both proteins co-localize to the photoreceptor connecting cilium and RPGRIP1 appears to be a structural component of the ciliary axoneme of the connecting cilium (which connects the inner to the outer segment of the photoreceptors) of both rods and cones and functions to anchor RPGR within the cilium [42–44]. Biallelic mutations have been shown to be associated with a severe rod and cone degeneration of the LCA type. Patients 4 and 5 in Fig. 24.10 illustrate the phenotype in the second decade of life. Different from *RDH12* sequence variations, the retinal structures particularly in the center are much better preserved but without the physiological foveal depression.

24.3.3.8 *RPE65* Phenotype (*RPE65* Mutation-Associated IRD)

Biallelic mutations in *RPE65* give rise to a spectrum of retinal diseases ranging from LCA to EOSRD, and to juvenile RP, now called *RPE65* mutation-associated IRD. *RPE65* codes for an isomerase in the RPE essential for retinol recycling [45, 46]. Some mutations have residual enzyme activity, the protein encoded by *RPE65,* which displays a much later phenotype, i.e., rod-cone-dystrophy (RCD) with juvenile onset [47]. In addition to severe or complete night blindness due to the enzymatic defect, lack of FAF in early years when the retina can look quite inconspicuous is a hallmark of the disease [48]. A recent multicenter cross-sectional natural history study describes phenotypic variability and clinical course in 70 patients [49]. Figure 24.11 shows a typical longitudinal course for patient 1 with a severe phenotype, and a milder phenotype for patient 2. Both patients experienced severe night blindness from infancy onward. FAF demonstrates the hallmark sign of lack of FAF. OCT shows some preservation of viable photoreceptor cells in patient 1, and very mild changes in patient 2. Knowledge of the natural history is of interest as the successful phase 3 study with the subretinal gene addition therapy [50] is now approved by the FDA, EMA, and other authorities, i.e., voretigene neparvovec-rzyl Luxturna®, is available in many countries (https://en.wikipedia.org/wiki/Voretigene_neparvovec; https://luxturna.com). The results are promising as the majority of patients experience a significant increase in vision at reduced light levels [50].

An even rarer entity is the autosomal dominant *RPE65*-associated disease due to monoallelic mutations. The age of onset is much later. The RPE atrophy is severe and may also involve the center or may resemble choroideremia with preserved central RPE islands [51, 52].

24.3.4 Childhood Onset Retinal Dystrophies

Mutations in genes discussed in the following chapter usually have a somewhat later onset than EOSRD.

24.3.4.1 *ABCA4* (ATP-Binding Cassette, Subfamily A, Member 4)

ABCA4 is a member of the superfamily of ATP-binding cassette (ABC) proteins that transports *N*-retinylidene-phosphatidylethanolamine (*N*-Ret-PE) across outer segment disc membranes thereby facilitating the removal of potentially toxic retinoid compounds from photoreceptor cells [53]. Biallelic mutations in *ABCA4* are associated with Stargardt disease, the most frequent juvenile macular dystrophy. The phenotypes range from early-onset STGD1, which clinically resembles severe cone-rod dystrophy, to intermediate STGD1 and late-onset STGD1. These different phenotypes can be correlated with different combinations of *ABCA4* variants that were classified according to their degree of functional loss as described in a recent review [54]. The authors also report that with expert clinical examination to distinguish STGD1 cases from other maculopathies, as well as in-depth genomics and transcriptomics data, it is now possible to identify both mutant *ABCA4* alleles in >95% of cases. Due to the high prevalence of *ABCA4* disease alleles in the population, different mutant alleles may be found in siblings and other relatives, possibly giving rise to intrafamilial phenotypic variability [55]. At a young age, patients may be misdiagnosed with amblyopia, myopia, optic disk pathology, mental health problems, tension headache, retrobulbar optic neuritis, and uveitis [56]. Figure 24.12 shows the spectrum of phenotypes in seven young patients including the natural course in siblings who were in the early disease course with variable disease severity. There were subtle abnormalities, such as lipofuscin accumulation seen in FAF, and that precede the ophthalmoscopic findings. On SD-OCT, a thickened external limiting membrane may indicate the beginning of the disease. To recognize such early signs becomes increasingly important in view of the development of gene-based therapeutic approaches as the therapeutic window is short with respect to the salvage of the macula, i.e., visual acuity. No gene replacement therapy is available to date due to the large size of *ABCA4*, which precludes the use of AAV vectors like in *RPE65*-associated IRDs. The specific challenges and problems are discussed in a published review [57]. Alternative approaches were also investigated [58]. Yet, no clinical treatment is available to date.

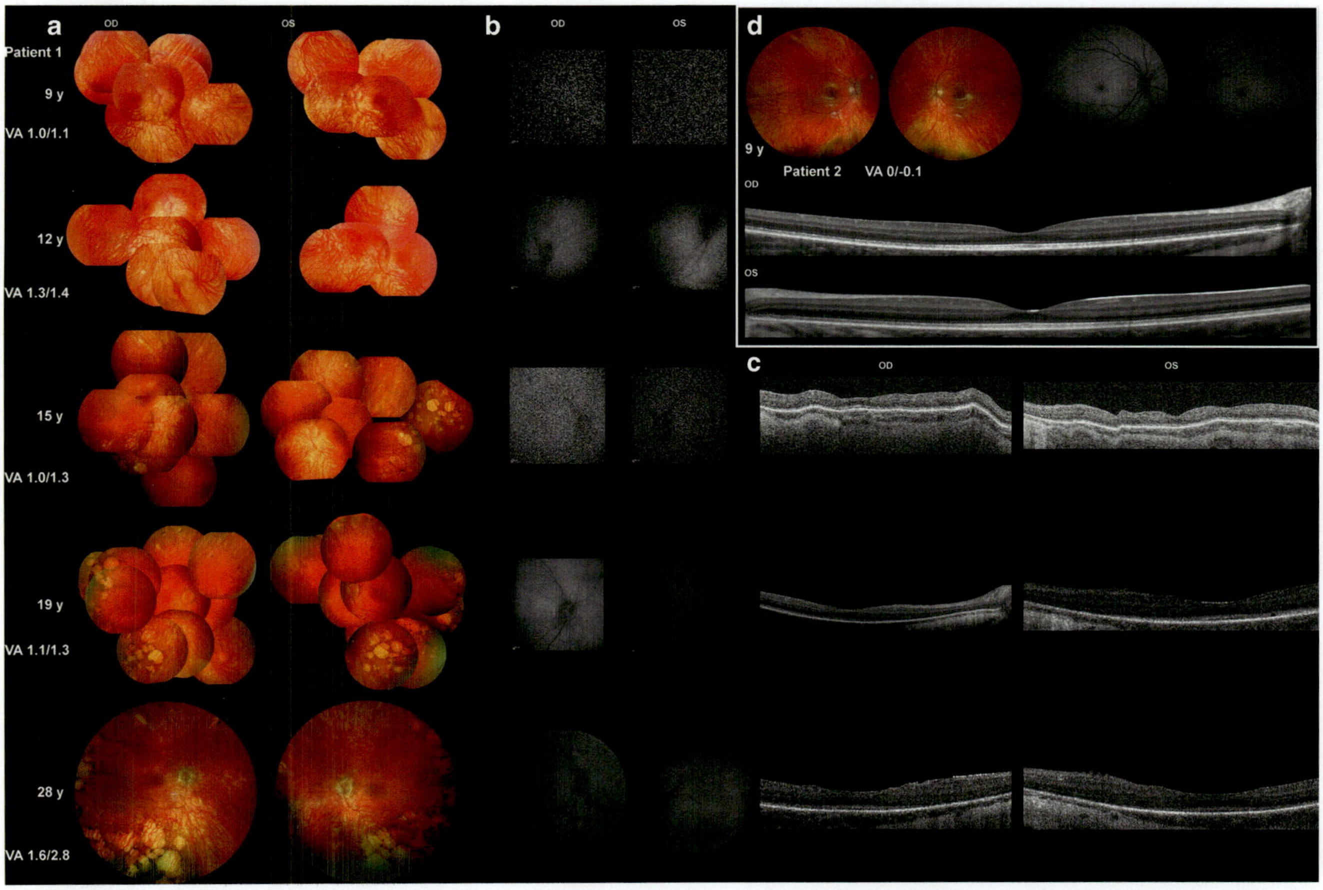

Fig. 24.11 *RPE65*. Natural course of Patient 1 with sequence changes in *RPE65* (c.11+5g>a; [p.T457N (c.1370C>A); c.1067delA (p. N356Mfs*17]). (**a**) Fundus photographs at 9 years, 12 years, 15 years, 19 years, and 28 years showing the progress of peripheral lesions toward the confluent chorioretinal degeneration. The macula is hypoplastic but the changes cannot be visualized throughout the observational period. (**b**) Corresponding fundus autofluorescence (FAF) images to (**a**). The strongly reduced FAF due to impaired supply of 11-cis retinol to the photoreceptors. (**c**) Optical Coherence Tomography (OCT) from the age of 16 years starting with time-domain (TD-OCT) followed by Spectral-domain (SD-OCT) recordings at 19 years and 28 years. The improvement of imaging techniques provided a major benefit for the documentation of the disease in these patients. The hypoplastic macula is obvious, as well as the clear reduction of the photoreceptor layer, and in particular the abnormal structure of the outer segments. The photoreceptor layers appear preserved in the fovea as an indicator of viability and hence treatable photoreceptor cells. (**d**) Age matched patient 2 at 9 years with two hypomorphic sequence changes (p.I115T (c.344T>C) and p.V443A (c.1328T>C)) in *RPE65* and almost unremarkable changes in fundus photograph, FAF and SD-OCT are presented in the white square to document the allelic heterogeneity of *RPE65* sequences changes causing a spectrum of expression. In this patient, outer and inner segment layers and photoreceptor layer appear relatively well preserved together with an identifiable RPE layer. The visual acuity in this patient is well preserved. Visual acuity (VA) is reported in logMAR

24.3.4.2 XLRP (RP3)-*RPGR* (Retinitis Pigmentosa GTPase Regulator)

The gene *RPGR* was cloned in 1996 [59]. Hemizygous mutations lead to a form of X-linked RP (RP3), with early central involvement and fast progression to legal blindness in the third to fourth decade. RPGR associated RP accounts for 10–20% of all RP cases. About 70% of mutations are located in ORF15 [60]. Most patients show a rod-cone degeneration, but cone-rod degeneration is also seen depending on mutation location. FAF shows a characteristic ring of increased fluorescence that can be quantified and used to document progression [61]. Carriers show fundus abnormalities in a high percentage of cases in addition to ERG changes. The radial pattern nicely seen on FAF is attributed to random X-inactivation [62]. Inactivation of the normal gene in the majority of photoreceptors in carriers can lead to functionally relevant retinal changes and mimic autosomal dominant RP [63]. However, clinical signs typically appear later in female carriers compared to male patients. A recent paper reviewed the present knowledge and described the actual gene therapeutic approach in a clinical trial through codon optimization [64]. Figure 24.13 shows the central involvement already in children best seen on FAF and OCT.

24.3.4.3 Choroideremia

Choroideremia is an X-linked chorioretinal degeneration caused by mutations in the *CHM* gene which encodes Rab escort protein 1 (REP1), a ubiquitously expressed protein

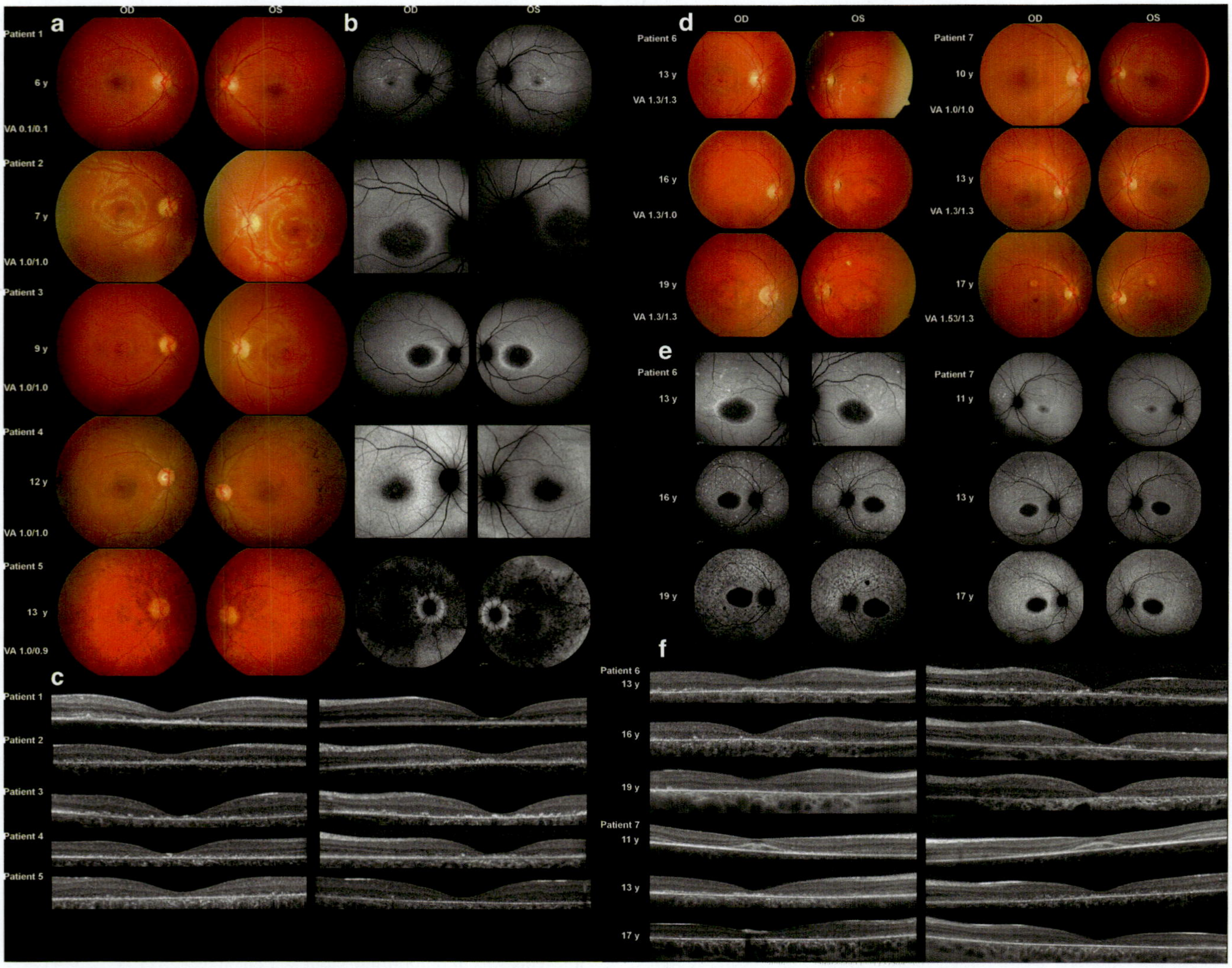

Fig. 24.12 *ABCA4*. (**a**) Fundus appearance of five age matched patients with different biallelic sequence variations in *ABCA4* presenting with the spectrum of phenotypes from fundus flavimaculatus (Patient 1, 6 years, sequence variations [p.L541P (c.1622T>C); p. A1038V (c.3113C>T)]; p.N1868I (c.5603A>T)) to typical juvenile macular Stargardt degeneration (Patient 2, 7 years, sequence variations c.768G>T; [p.L541P (c.1622T>C), p.A1038V (c.3113C>T)]; p. G1961E (c.5882G>A), c.5018+2T>A)) and wide-spread cone-rod degeneration (Patient 3, 9 years, changes Exon 1del, p.G65E (c.194G>A)). There was generalized cone-rod degeneration mimicking retinitis pigmentosa (although atypically with early loss of visual acuity) in a progressive fashion (Patient 4, 12 years, p.W41* (c.122G>A), [p.H1125L (c.3374A>T); p.Q1126L (c.3375AA>TT)] and Patient 5, 13 years, sequence variations p.F56V (c. 166T>G), [p.L541P (c.1622T>C), p.A1038V (c.3113C>T)]). (**b**) Corresponding fundus autofluorescence (FAF) images to (**a**). (**c**) Corresponding SD-OCT recordings to (**a**) presenting absence of outer segments in the macula and perimacular area even in early stages. Intrafamilial variability between siblings at matched ages. (**d**) Fundus appearance in Patient 6 vs. Patient 7 (sequence variations [p.L541P (c.1622T>C); p.A1038V (c.3113C>T)]; p.Q1412* (c.4234C>T)). (**e**) Increasing fluorescent spots in the retinal periphery in FAF (**d**). At more advanced stages, the phenotypes become almost similar. (**f**) Corresponding SD-OCTs illustrating macular photoreceptor degeneration. Visual acuity (VA) is reported in logMAR

involved in intracellular trafficking and prenylation activity [65]. In early stages, it may be confounded with X-linked RP. However, the chorioretinal atrophies differ from what is seen in RP. FAF shows a very characteristic pattern depending on progression [66]. Late in the disease, only a small island of central FAF from preserved RPE is present correlating with visual acuity and visual field as well as with OCT data. Several reviews have been published recently including detailed natural course studies [67–69] that are important in view of clinical trials with gene addition therapy, and reporting eventual beneficial effects such as preservation of visual acuity and slowing of visual field loss in a phase I/II study [70, 71]. Figure 24.14 shows a compilation of imaging data in young patients and in two older female carriers. Similar to RP3, *CHM* lyonization can also cause some pathologies in the fundus, and often asymptomatic. FAF differs from FAF in carriers for RPGR as it shows a stars-in-the-sky pattern, and not the radial pattern seen in carriers for RP3 (compare Fig. 24.13).

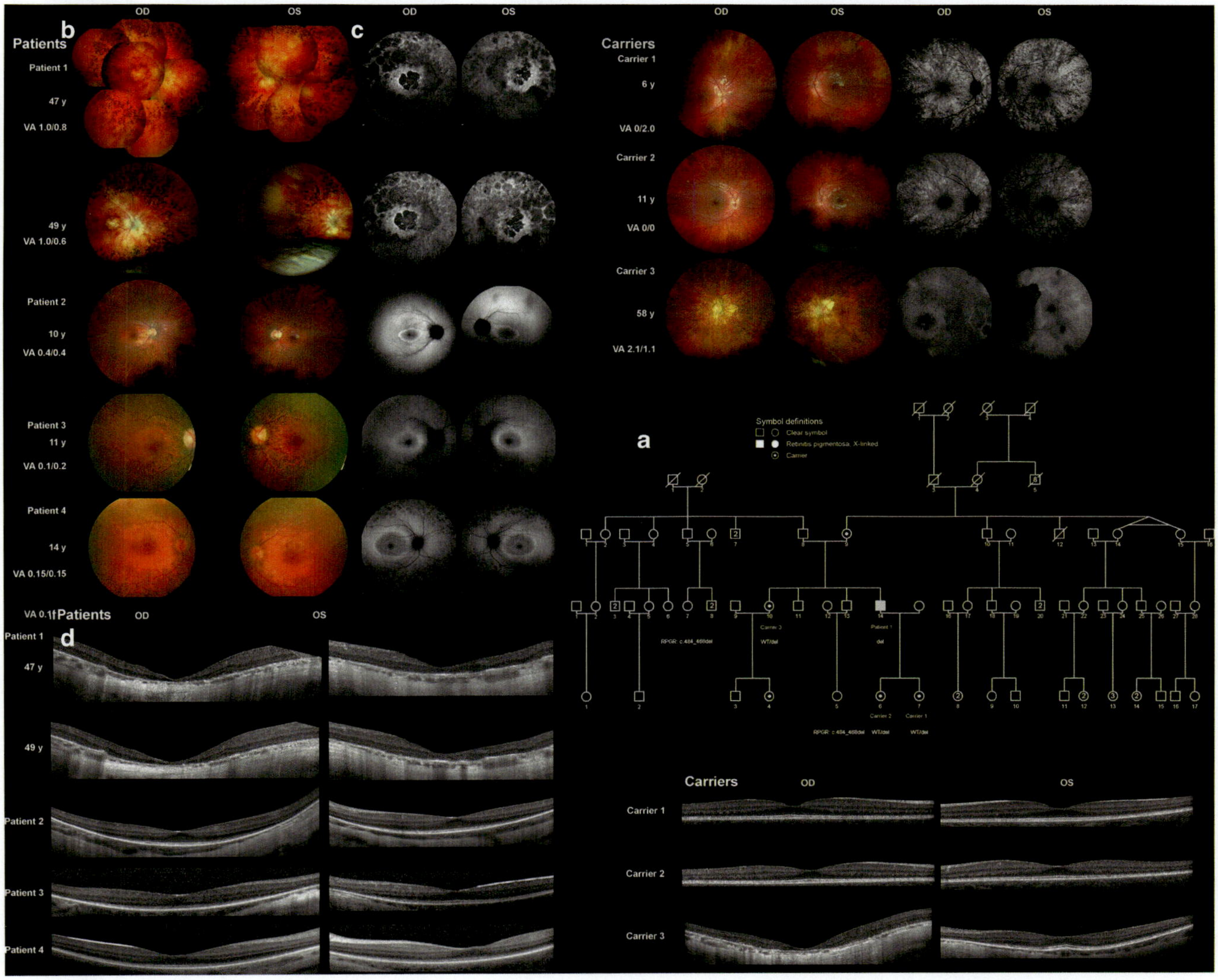

Fig. 24.13 X-linked Retinitis pigmentosa from *RPGR*. Characteristic phenotypes of mutant *RPGR*-gene in male patients and female carriers. (**a**) Pedigree of a family segregating sequence variant c.484_468delTTT (p.F162del) in *RPGR*. (**b**) Fundus photographs of Patient 1 at 47 years and 49 years, his daughter is carrier 1 at 6 years, and carrier 2 at 11 years, and his sister is carrier 3 at 58 years from pedigree in (**a**). Please note the bone spicules in the periphery and the progressed degeneration in the central retina of Patient 1 and severe changes in the macula which are common in X-linked RP. His sister presented as an affected carrier with advanced retinal degeneration. His daughters who are obligatory carriers, although still young already presented with subtle degenerative lesions in the retinal periphery. Three additional patients, independent from the family in (**a**) presented with common fundus appearance of male patients at childhood and adolescence. Patient 2 at 10 years (Sequence variant p.R449* (c.1345C>T)) was at the beginning of the disease. Patient 3 at 11 years (Sequence variant c.2363_2364delAG (p.E788Gfs*46)) was at a comparable stage. Both showed the beginning of degenerative changes in the periphery, but also already in the perimacular area. Patient 4 at 14 years (Sequence variant p.E778* (c.2332G>T)) was much more advanced in his disease. He already developed bone spicules in the retinal periphery and more advance degenerative changes in the macula. (**c**) FAF images corresponding to the fundus photographs in (**b**). The young Patients 2 and 3 presented with the characteristic circular increase of FAF surrounding the macula that is well known from rod-cone dystrophies. In Patient 4, in addition to the ring, the periphery showed already significantly reduced FAF indicating loss of RPE and the overlying photoreceptors. In the advanced state of patient 1, severely reduced FAF indicates large areas of RPE degeneration together with photoreceptor loss. These areas further enlarged within the 2 years of follow-up even though the disease was already in an advanced state. Already in young carriers (carriers 1 and 2), FAF may form a characteristic centrifugal pattern of increased and decreased FAF due to lyonization along the development lines of retinal cell division. In their aunt, the degeneration already led to areas of obvious RPE loss as a severe form of carrier phenotype in RP3. Of note, a normal fundus appearance including normal FAF does not exclude a carrier state. In this case, almost all chromosomes with the mutated gene have been inactivated. (**d**) Corresponding SD-OCT recordings to (**a**) and (**b**). Patient 1 and carrier 3 have clear loss of RPE and photoreceptor layers along with reduced FAF while the younger patients have photoreceptor layer loss only in the periphery, and only more subtle changes in the macula itself with structural changes mainly in the outer segments. The young carriers do no present with obvious changes in the retinal layers even though their FAF is highly indicative of degenerative effects throughout the retina. Visual acuity (VA) is reported in logMAR

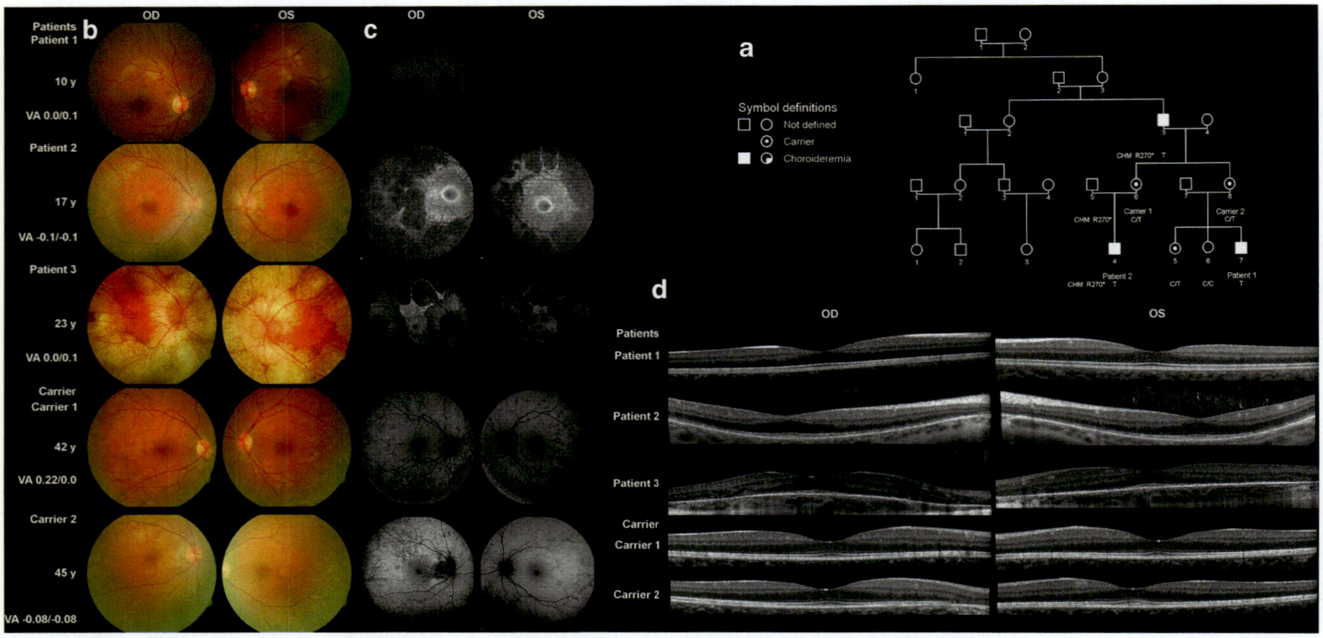

Fig. 24.14 *CHM*. Phenotypical spectrum of male patients and female carriers in choroideremia (CHM). (**a**) Pedigree of a family segregating the common sequence variation p.R270* (c.808C>T) in the Rab escort protein 1 gene (*CHM*) showing a typical X-linked inheritance pattern. (**b**) Fundus photographs of patient 1 at 10 years and Patient 2 (1984.03) at 17 years from pedigree in (**a**) and carrier 1 at 42 years and carrier 2 at 45 years. In addition, Patient 3 at 23 years (Sequence variation p.R267* (c.799C>T)) exemplifies a more advanced phenotype in early adulthood. Note the large areas of RPE destruction with choroid shining through the RPE in the males. The carriers present with small localized areas of RPE degeneration due to the lyonization mosaic in both photoreceptors and RPE. (**c**) The degeneration of the RPE is much more obvious in the males demonstrated by the absence of fundus autofluorescence (FAF) in the periphery and the remaining FAF in the area of residual function of the retina. Note the preserved and eventually increased FAF in the posterior pole in patient 2 associated with the highest density of rods peripheral to this area. The female carriers present with a spotty pattern of reduced FAF according to a mosaic of degenerated RPE cells from random inactivation of the unaffected copy of the *CHM*-gene. Comparing the carrier findings in the RPGR phenotype shown in Fig. 24.13 which is very different from the CHM carrier phenotype. Please note that also in CHM, a normal fundus appearance does not exclude the carrier state. (**d**) SD-OCT recordings corresponding to (**b**) and (**c**). Note the loss of photoreceptor and RPE layers which spares the fovea and covers the area of decreased FAF. In the very young patient aged 10 years, the OCT appears normal. Visual acuity (VA) is reported in logMAR

24.3.5 Bestrophinopathies

Mutations in bestrophin-1 (*BEST1* gene) cause autosomal dominant Best vitelliform macular dystrophy (VMD2, [72]), the second frequent macular dystrophy with childhood onset. Since then, other diseases have been associated with mutations in the same gene, now summarized as bestrophinopathies, i.e., autosomal dominant vitreoretinochoroidopathy ADVIRC, and autosomal recessive bestrophinopathy (for a review see [73]). Mutations in the gene affect anion transport through the plasma membrane of the RPE. Recently, Nachtigal et al. described mutation-dependent mechanisms that determine the phenotypes of bestrophinopathies [74]. The authors described five classes and proposed an explanation of why heterozygous mutation carriers in autosomal recessive bestrophinopathy (ARB) do not show any disease signs compared to heterozygous mutation carriers in autosomal dominant Best disease and in ADVIRC. These findings may allow the development of efficient therapies for the different forms of bestrophinopathies.

24.3.5.1 Vitelliform Macular Dystrophy (Best Disease, VMD2)

Autosomal dominant Best disease (VMD2) is characterized by highly variable expressivity and variable penetrance. Typically, the normal light rise is absent in the electrooculogram, and was the only way to identify mutation carriers before molecular testing of the gene became available. The disease typically progresses through five stages but not all patients show full progression. The vitelliform stage has been observed already in infancy. Visual acuity only declines when the vitelliform stage progresses to the pseudohypopyon and vitelliruptive stage. In the cicatricial stage, subretinal neovascularization may develop and require treatment. Figure 24.15 shows the five stages as seen by funduscopy, FAF, and OCT.

24.3.5.2 Autosomal Recessive Bestrophinopathy

Autosomal recessive bestrophinopathy has been described first in 2008 [75].

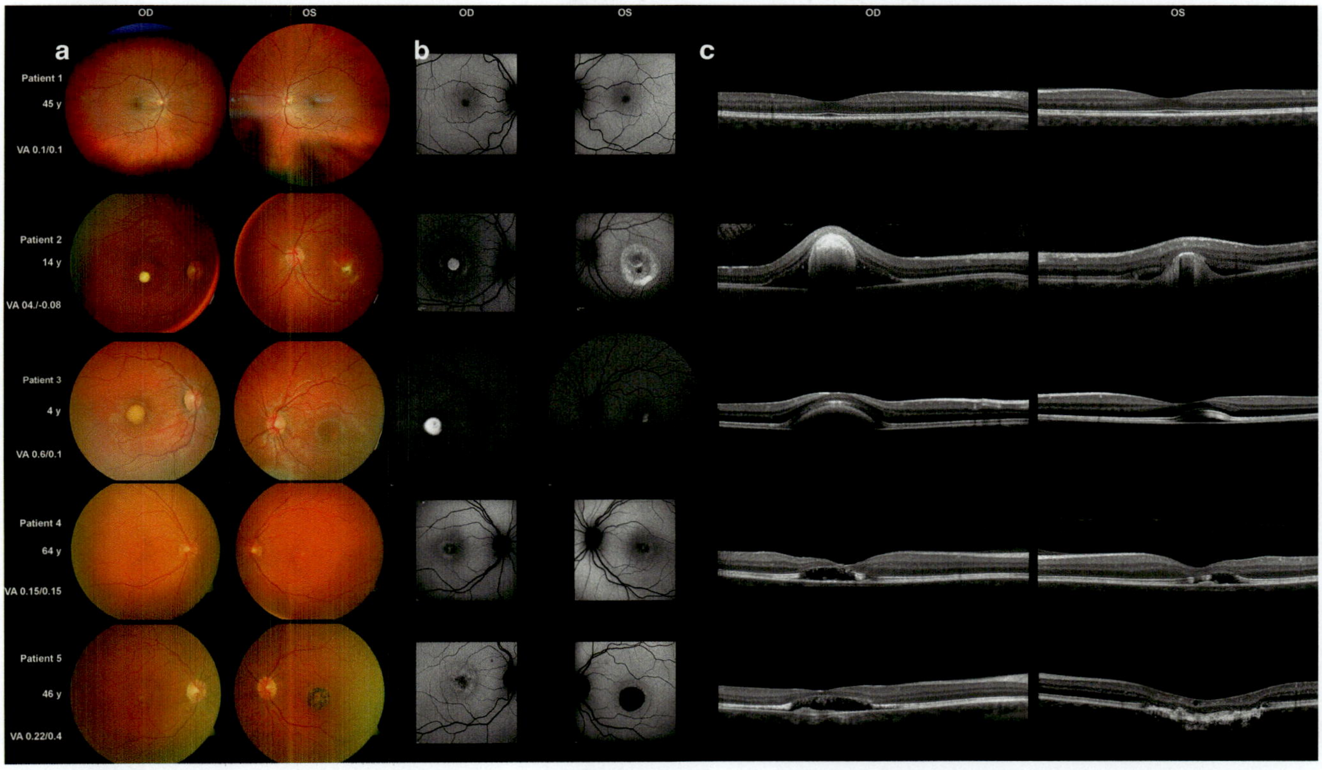

Fig. 24.15 Best disease. Comparison of phenotypes associated with sequence variations in the *BEST1*-gene (OMIM #607854). For all stages, the electrooculogram is pathognomonic with absent light rise of the signal. (**a**) Fundus photographs presenting the stages of autosomal dominant juvenile vitelliform macular dystrophy (VMD2, Best disease, OMIM #153700). Carriers of *BEST1* sequence variations may not develop morphological changes and remain in the pre-vitelliform state according to Gass et al. as Patient 1 at 45 years (sequence variation p. R25W (c.73C>T)). The pre-vitelliform stage is followed by the vitelliform stage as represented by the right eye of Patient 2 at 14 years (sequence variation p.Q96R (c.287A>G)) and Patient 3 at 4 years (sequence variation p.T2S (c.5C>G)). A prominent vitelliform lesion that expands to finally cover the macular area completely characterizes the vitelliform stage. The vitelliform stage usually persists for a long period of time before it starts progressing into the pseudohypopyon (left eye of Patient 2) and the vitelliruptive stage (left eye of Patient 3). Patients 2 and 3 present bilateral affection with independent progression in the contralateral eye as one frequent feature of VMD2. The disease finally develops from the vitelliruptive stage like in Patient 4 at 64 years (sequence variation [p.T536W (c.1696T>C); p.W24C (c.72G>C)] monoallelic) to the fibrotic stage in Patient 5 at 46 years (sequence variation p.W24C (c.72G>T)). (**b**) Corresponding fundus autofluorescent (FAF) images, (**a**). Note the characteristically increased macular FAF in the vitelliform stage in Patients 2 and 3 and how it progress into the vitelliruptive stage. (**c**) Corresponding SD-OCT recordings to (**a**) and (**b**). The vitelliform stage is characterized by a dome shape detachment of the neuroretina from the RPE corresponding to the area of increased FAF. In this stage, the photoreceptor layer is still present. With advanced loss of the RPE, the photoreceptor layers also degenerate and progress from the pseudohypopyon stage to the vitelliruptive stage and fibrotic stage. The latter is characterized by a fibrotic scar in the macular area at the level of the RPE and photoreceptor layers. Visual acuity (VA) is reported in logMAR

Biallelic mutations in *BEST1* are associated with a distinct retinopathy characterized by central visual loss, an absent EOG light-rise, and a reduced EOG. Yellowish blunt retinal deposits may be confused with an inflammatory uveitis-like condition, but FAF reveals them to be hyperfluorescent. An example is shown by patient 1 in Fig. 24.16.

24.3.5.3 VRCP (ADVIRC, Vitreoretinochoroidopathy, Autosomal Dominant)

In 2004, Yardley et al. reported [76] heterozygous mutations of *BEST1* splicing regulators causing nanophthalmos and autosomal dominant vitreoretinochoroidopathy (VRCP, ADVIRC). This was confirmed in 2008 by another group [75]. The consequences of this very special mutation type have been investigated and explained recently [74, 77]. Typical retinal findings over a follow-up of 3 years are shown in Fig. 24.16 and confirm progression described by others.

24.3.6 The Achromatopsias

Achromatopsias are autosomal recessive cone dysfunction disorders characterized by profound color vision deficiency and significant aversion to light. Visual acuity is usually reduced to logMAR 1, and cut-on filter glasses are usually very helpful.

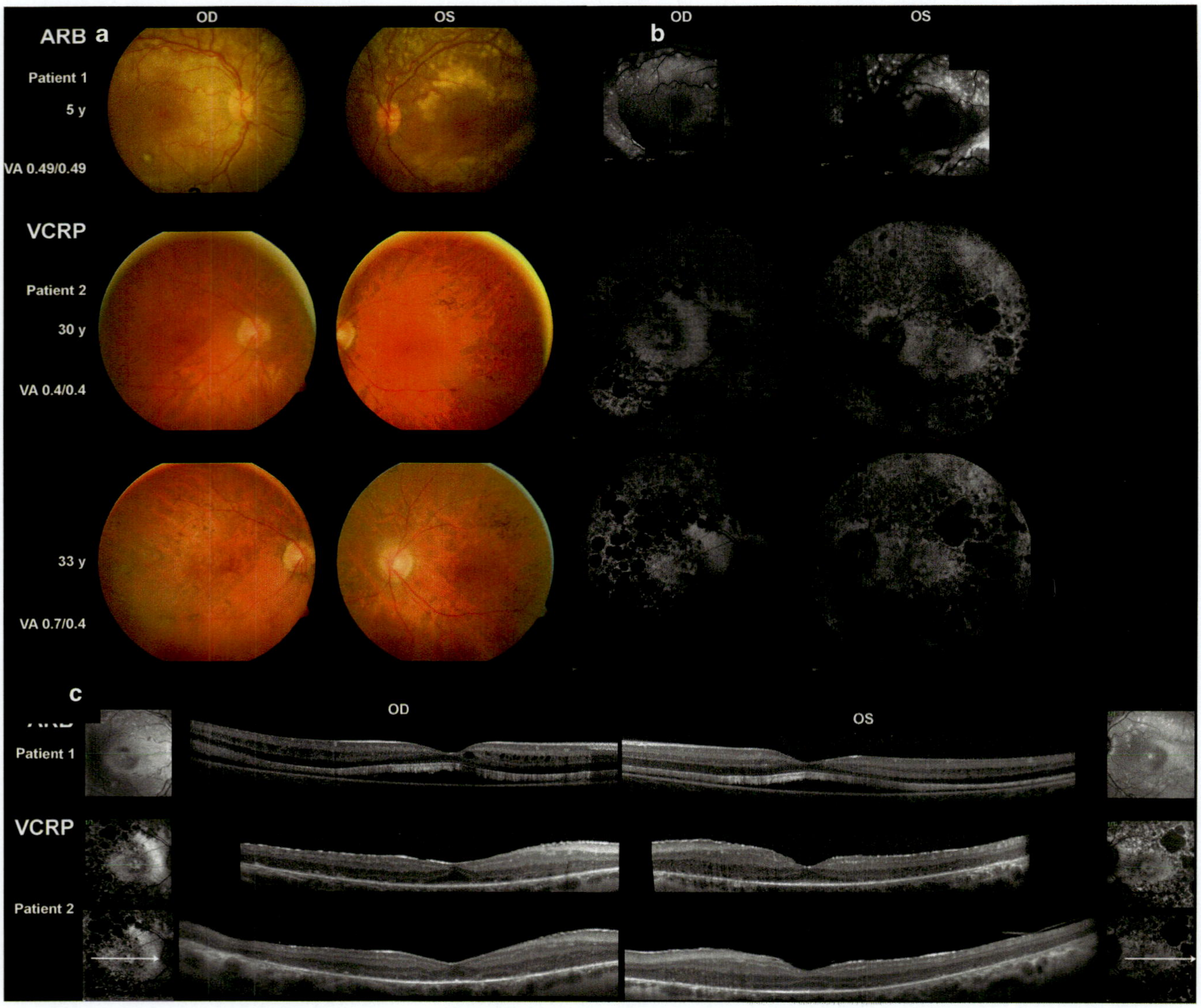

Fig. 24.16 Bestrophinopathies. Comparison of unusual phenotypes associated with sequence variations in the *BEST1*-gene (OMIM #607854). (**a**) Fundus photographs presenting autosomal recessive bestrophinopathy ARB as a pan-retinal degeneration. The characteristic distribution of ARB lesions throughout the retina is shown in patient 1 at 5 years (Sequence variation c.779delC (p.P260Qfs*29); p.L294F (c.880C>T)). Note the characteristic yellowish lesion outside the macula and in the periphery. A further phenotypic variation is autosomal dominant vitreochoroidal retinopathy VCRP (also called ADVIRC= autosomal dominant vitreoretinochoroidopathy ADVIRC). Patient 2 is shown at 30 years and 33 years (Sequence variation c.724+44c>t). Disease progression in the periphery can be seen on funduscopy (but best on FAF). (**b**) Corresponding FAF images to A are presented. The yellowish peripheral lesions in ARB seen on funduscopy present with increased FAF while VCRP is characterized by loss of FAF with progression. (**c**) Corresponding SD-OCT recordings to (**a**) and (**b**). Even though the macular lesion in ARB is not prominent in the fundus photographs and FAF images, SD-OCT reveals a corresponding detachment of the neuroretina in the macula accompanied by cystic spaces also in the inner nuclear layer. In VCRP, the RPE and the photoreceptor layer grossly degenerate in confluent spots in the periphery and toward the center. FAF is helpful in following this progression as shown in this figure. Visual acuity (VA) is reported in logMAR

24.3.6.1 Achromatopsia

To date, six genes have been associated with achromatopsia [78–82]. Although some progression has been reported, most patients with autosomal recessive achromatopsia have a relatively stable course. Nevertheless, achromatopsia is another disease where gene therapy has been started for two of the six genes identified so far. Recently, it was reported that an additional heterozygous mutation in *CNGA3* may alter the course of *CNGB3*-associated achromatopsia with biallelic mutations, giving rise to a more severe and more progressive phenotype [83]. Usually, OCT changes are mild and may show some minor defects of outer photoreceptor segments in the fovea. In the *ATF6* phenotype, the absence of OS is pathognomonic [82]. Semiquantitative FAF and Near-Infrared FAF may show typical patterns in some genes [84]. Figure 24.17 summarizes phenotypes for the more frequent genes *CNGA3*, *CNGB3*, *GNAT*, and *PED6C*. Gene augmentation therapy was successful in a naturally occurring sheep model with mutations

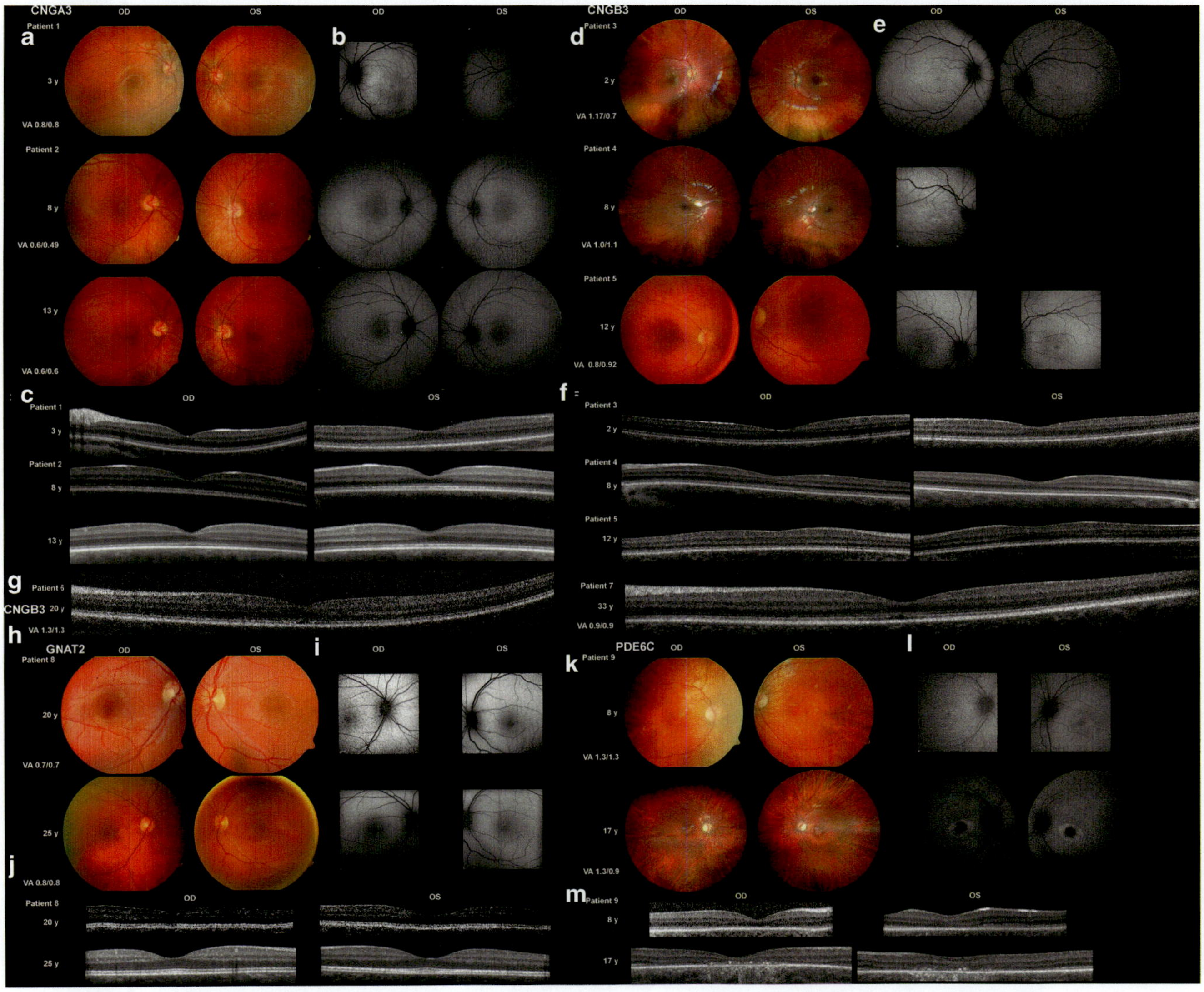

Fig. 24.17 ACHM: Phenotype of patients affected with achromatopsia (ACHM) caused by sequence variations in the four major ACHM genes. Fundus appearance in most cases is normal. FAF may show minor changes related to changes in outer segments. (**a**) Fundus photographs of two patients with sequence variations in *CNGA3* at 3 years (Patient 1, sequence variations p.R223Q (c.668G>A), p.R436W (c.1306C>T)), at 8 years, and 13 years (Patient 2 sequence variations p.F547L (c.1641C>A), p.T565M (c.1694C>T)). (**b**) Corresponding fundus autofluorescence (FAF) images to (**a**). (**c**) Corresponding SD-OCT recordings to (**a**). (**d**) Series of fundus photographs of patients carrying the homozygous *CNGB3* sequence variation c.1148delC (p.T383Ifs*13). The age of the patients is matched to (**a**) with Patient 3 at 2 years, Patient 4 at 8 years, and Patient 5 at 12 years. (**e**) Corresponding FAF images to (**d**). (**f**) Corresponding SD-OCT recordings to (**d**). (**g**) In addition Patient 6 at 20 years (Sequence change c.1148delC (p.T383Ifs*13), c.896_903+3delinsT) and Patient 7 at 33 years (Sequence change c.1148delC (p.T383Ifs*13) homozygous) presented with an advanced degeneration in the fovea that may occur in several patients contrary to the notion that ACHM from *CNGB3* sequence changes is stationary and not degenerative. (**h**) Fundus photographs, (**i**) corresponding FAF images, and (**j**) SD-OCT recordings in Patient 8 at 20 years and 25 years with sequence variations (p.R208T (c.623G>C); c.720+2t>c) in GNAT2. (**k**) Fundus photographs, (**l**) FAF images, and (**m**) TD-OCT (at 8 years) resp. SD-OCT (at 17 years) recordings in Patient 9 with a homozygous sequence change c.2449delG (p.R817Mfs*7) in PDE6C. Note the foveal degeneration is visible on fundus photograph, FAF, and SD-OCT in this patient. Visual acuity (VA) is reported in logMAR

in *CNGA3* [85]. The paper on the first gene augmentation trial for *CNGA3* conducted in Germany reported no major complications and some subjective improvement [86].

24.3.6.2 *KCNV2* (Potassium Channel, Voltage-Gated, Subfamily V, Member 2)

Early in childhood, the *KCNV2* phenotype maybe confounded with achromatopsia. Mutations in *KCNV2* cause a form of cone dystrophy with a very specific form of rod ERG, i.e., supernormal rod electroretinogram (CDSRR) [87]. The gene product is expressed in the outer retina as part of a tetrameric potassium channel controlling potassium flow in the photoreceptors [88]. The most obvious clinical feature in *KCNV2* mutations is the supranormal a-wave amplitude and increased latency of the scotopic ERG responses. Since cone responses are quick and depending on potassium clear-

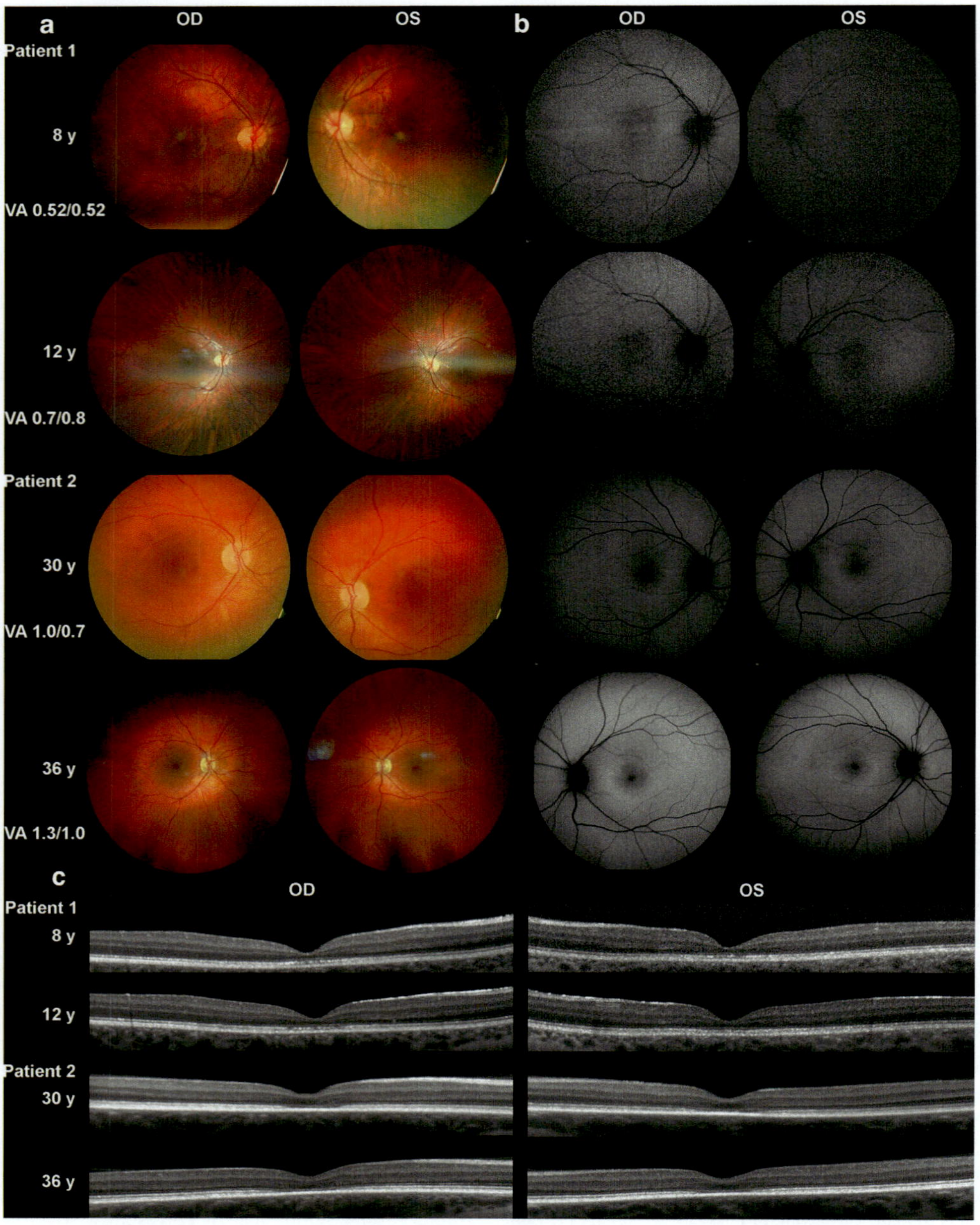

Fig. 24.18 *KCNV2*. Phenotype of patients affected with biallelic *KCNV2* mutations. Early on this phenotype may be confounded with achromatopsia. The characteristic test is the full-field ERG which shows typical changes in the b-wave (see [89]). (**a**) Fundus photographs of two patients with sequence variations in *KCNV2* at 8 years (Patient 1, sequence variations p.R223Q (c.668G>A), p.R436W (c.1306C>T)), and 12 years. Patient 2 (Sequence variations p.K260* (c.778A>T); c.1016_1024delACCTGGTGG (p.D339_V341del)) is shown at 30 years and 36 years. The fundus appearance is inconspicuous. (**b**) Corresponding fundus autofluorescence (FAF) images. Subtle changes in the center. (**c**) Corresponding SD-OCT recordings. The outer nuclear layer is thin, particularly in the center. In the younger patient, the ISE appears irregular; in the older patient, the ISE is missing in the center. Visual acuity (VA) is reported in logMAR

ing, the cone responses are severely reduced. Patients with *KCNV2* mutations present with a progressive cone degeneration in contrast to most achromatopsia patients as shown in Fig. 24.18.

24.3.7 X-Linked Retinoschisis

Juvenile X-linked retinoschisis is a juvenile progressive cone degeneration caused by mutations in *RS1* coding for the secreted protein retinoschisin in the synaptic space between photoreceptors and bipolar cells [90]. Retinoschisin connects photoreceptors and bipolar cells. Mutations in *RS1* lead to detachment of photoreceptors from bipolar cells thus leading to a schisis in the outer plexiform layer with large cavities in the inner nuclear layer (Fig. 24.19). The detachment blocks the transmission of the nerve impulse thus creating a characteristic electrophysiological response known as the "negative ERG" which exemplifies the inability of the bipolar cells to create the b-wave without excitation from the photoreceptors

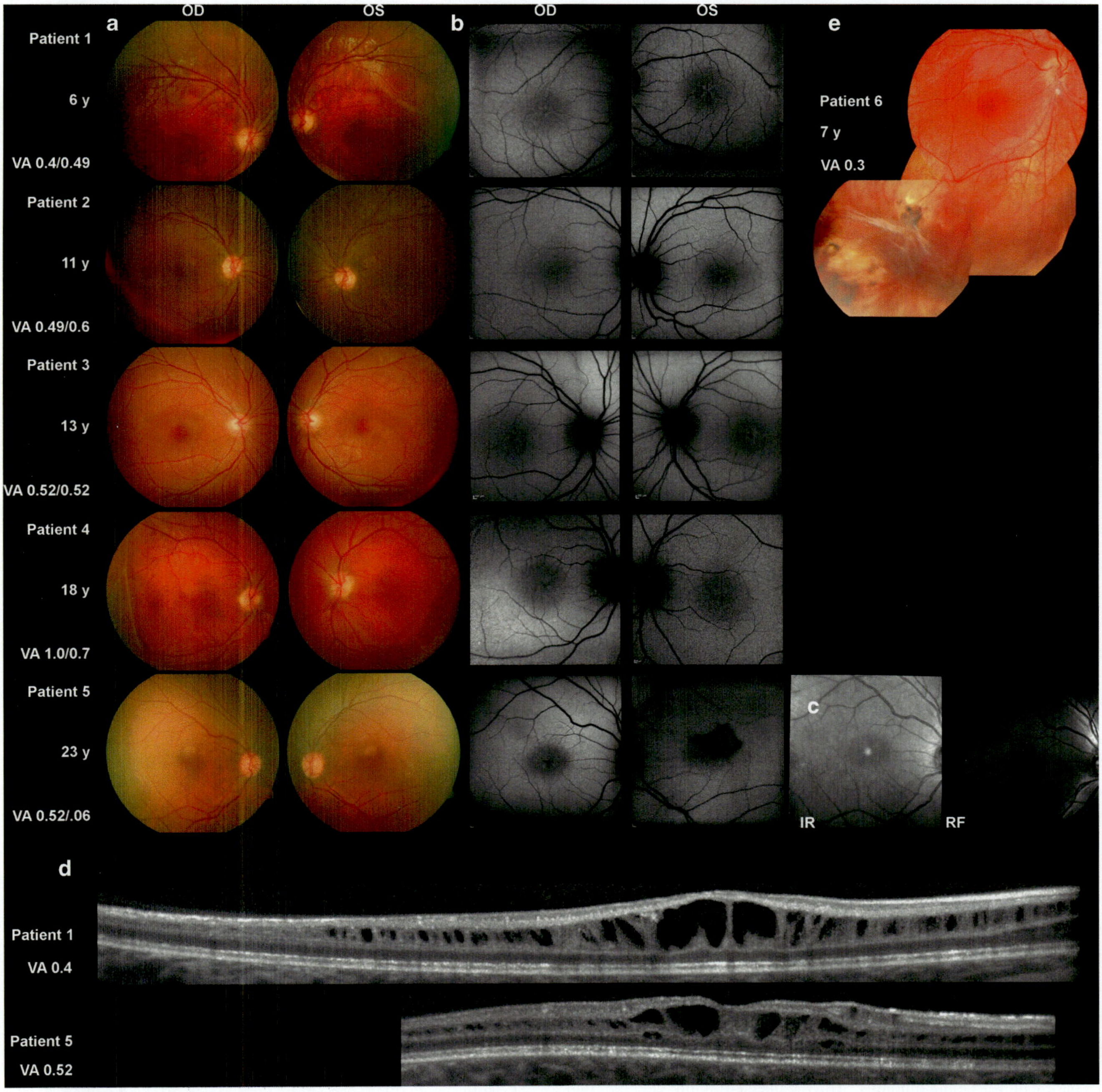

Fig. 24.19 *XLRS*. (**a**) and (**e**) Compilation of fundus photographs from patients with X-linked juvenile retinoschisis at various ages. Patient 1 (6 years, sequence variations p.R209H (c.626G>A)), Patient 2 (11 years, p.C142W (c.426T>G)), Patient 3 (13 years, p.R200C (c.598C>T)), Patient 4 (18 years, p.W163G (c.487T>G)), Patient 5 (23 years, p.R102W (c.304C>T)), Patient 4 shows peripheral retinoschisis. Patient 6 shows peripheral schisis with additional retinal detachment post-surgery at age 7 years (mutation p.P193L (c.578C>T)). The fellow eye had a complete retinal detachment. For an overview of the clinical spectrum, see Pimenides et al. [91], and Bowles et al. [92]. (**b**) Compilation of corresponding fundus autofluorescence images (FAF) from patients in (**a**). In some patients, the spoke-like appearance of the macula is evident just like on funduscopy. Patients with XLRS are usually extremely photophobic during fundus examination, which in the past led to undiagnosed patients by ophthalmoscopy. Nowadays OCT is an easy and very revealing test. As it uses infrared light, patient compliance is much better than with funduscopy. (**c**) Corresponding infrared (IR) image and red-free (RF) image of Patient 5, right eye from (**a**) and (**b**). (**d**) Corresponding SD-OCT recordings from the right eye of Patient 1 and Patient 5. Note the characteristic schisis in the INL and the beginning schisis in the ONL in Patient 5. At later ages, the schisis may disappear and the disease confounded with age-related macular degeneration. Visual acuity (VA) is reported in logMAR

[93]. The phenotype can be very variable with some genotype–phenotype correlation [91, 92, 94]. Infantile presentation may be severe [95, 96].

Different from other X-linked degenerations, female carriers do not show any symptoms or signs.

A recent phase I/II AAV-mediated intravitreal gene therapy approach [97] led to short time closure of the schisis but had no long-term effect either on morphology or on function. The same group reported interocular symmetry and stability over time of visual acuity and ERG which would allow to use the fellow eye as a control in gene therapy studies [98]. The attempt to control the schisis with carbonic anhydrase inhibitors is successful at short application and therefore an option to prepare the patient for gene therapy [99]. Unfortunately, the effect is lost on long-term application preventing carbonic anhydrase inhibitors from being a suitable drug-based treatment option [100].

24.3.8 Summary

Genetic ophthalmology and particularly retinal pediatric ophthalmogenetics are constantly evolving. New methods such as NGS (new generation sequencing) have revolutionized molecular genetic research and diagnostics. Tests have become much more affordable and give a higher yield of genetically solved cases (e.g., [101]). An excellent overview by Drack et al. summarizes currently available tests, the role of the pediatric ophthalmologist and the retinal specialist in identifying patients amenable to testing, the importance of genetic testing for counseling families and patients, recruiting patients suitable for clinical trials, detecting patients for whom treatment is already available, and actual limitations of genetic testing [102]. Widely available databases allow the clinician to stay updated and to check the most recent advancements when a new patient presents.

Acknowledgments The images presented in this chapter were recorded with informed consent taken from the patients or legal custodian at the Department of Ophthalmology, Universitaetsklinikum Giessen und Marburg GmbH, Justus-Liebig University Giessen (Head: Prof. Birgit Lorenz from 2007 till 2019) and the Department of Pediatric Ophthalmology, Strabismology and Ophthalmogenetics, University of Regensburg (Head Prof. Birgit Lorenz from 1996 till 2007) and with approval from the ethical review boards at both institutions (Approval 00/106 and 149/07).

All cases were genetically genotyped in the Laboratory of Molecular Ophthalmology at both institutions and in collaboration with Prof. Hanno Bolz at Bioscientia GmbH Ingelheim, Germany and Senckenberg Centre for Human Genetics, Frankfurt, Germany, Prof. Bernd Wissinger and Dr. Susanne Kohl at the Institute for Ophthalmic Research Centre for Ophthalmology, University of Tuebingen, Germany.

The authors thank the German Research Foundation (DFG) for financial support (DFG Lo457-3, Lo457-5), and the patients and their families for taking part in extensive phenotyping.

References

1. Sergouniotis PI, Maxime E, Leroux D, et al. An ontological foundation for ocular phenotypes and rare eye diseases [published correction appears in Orphanet J Rare Dis. 2019 Aug 15;14(1):200]. Orphanet J Rare Dis. 2019;14(1):8. https://doi.org/10.1186/s13023-018-0980-6.
2. Bertsch M, Floyd M, Kehoe T, Pfeifer W, Drack AV. The clinical evaluation of infantile nystagmus: what to do first and why. Ophthalmic Genet. 2017;38(1):22–33. https://doi.org/10.1080/13816810.2016.1266667.
3. Lorenz B, Gampe E. Analyse von 180 Patienten mit sensorischem Defektnystagmus (SDN) und kongenitalem idiopathischen Nystagmus (CIN) [Analysis of 180 patients with sensory defect nystagmus (SDN) and congenital idiopathic nystagmus (CIN)] [published correction appears in Klin Monatsbl Augenheilkd 2001 Apr;218(4):208]. Klin Monbl Augenheilkd. 2001;218(1):3–12. https://doi.org/10.1055/s-2001-11254.
4. Tavares J, Lorenz B, van den Born I, Marques JP, Lacey S, Scholl H, EVICR.net. Current management of Inherited Retinal Degenerations (IRD) subjects in Europe. Results of an international survey by the EVICR.net. IOVS Abstracts. 2020.
5. Holder GE, Robson AG. Paediatric electrophysiology: a practical approach. In: Lorenz B, Moore AT, editors. Pediatric ophthalmology, neuro-ophthalmology, genetics. Essentials in ophthalmology. Berlin: Springer; 2006.
6. Preising MN, Görg B, Friedburg C, et al. Biallelic mutation of human *SLC6A6* encoding the taurine transporter TAUT is linked to early retinal degeneration. FASEB J. 2019;33(10):11507–27. https://doi.org/10.1096/fj.201900914RR.
7. Traboulsi EI, editor. Genetic diseases of the eye. 2nd ed. New York: Oxford University Press; 2012. 994 pages
8. Preising MN, Stieger K, Lorenz B. Genetik ophthalmologischer Erkrankungen. Teil 1: Genetische Grundlagen und Phänotypen [Inherited ophthalmological disorders. Part 1: Genetic fundamentals and phenotypes]. Klin Monbl Augenheilkd. 2014;231(2):177–91. https://doi.org/10.1055/s-0033-1346933.
9. Preising MN, Stieger K, Lorenz B. Genetik ophthalmologischer Erkrankungen. Teil 2: Diagnostik und Therapiekonzepte [Inherited ophthalmological disorders. Part 2: Diagnostics and therapeutic concepts]. Klin Monbl Augenheilkd. 2014;231(2):e1–e17. https://doi.org/10.1055/s-0033-1346935.
10. Preising MN, Forster H, Gonser M, Lorenz B. Screening of TYR, OCA2, GPR143, and MC1R in patients with congenital nystagmus, macular hypoplasia, and fundus hypopigmentation indicating albinism. Mol Vis. 2011;17:939–48. Published 2011 Apr 15.
11. Grønskov K, Brøndum-Nielsen K, Lorenz B, Preising MN. Clinical utility gene card for: oculocutaneous albinism. Eur J Hum Genet. 2014;22(8) https://doi.org/10.1038/ejhg.2013.307.
12. Lima Cunha D, Arno G, Corton M, Moosajee M. The spectrum of *PAX6* mutations and genotype-phenotype correlations in the eye. Genes (Basel). 2019;10(12):1050. https://doi.org/10.3390/genes10121050.
13. Wang X, Gregory-Evans K, Wasan KM, Sivak O, Shan X, Gregory-Evans CY. Efficacy of postnatal in vivo nonsense suppression therapy in a Pax6 mouse model of aniridia. Mol Ther Nucleic Acids. 2017;7:417–28. https://doi.org/10.1016/j.omtn.2017.05.002.
14. Meindl A, Berger W, Meitinger T, et al. Norrie disease is caused by mutations in an extracellular protein resembling C-terminal globular domain of mucins. Nat Genet. 1992;2(2):139–43. https://doi.org/10.1038/ng1092-139.
15. Meindl A, Lorenz B, Achatz H, Hellebrand H, Schmitz-Valckenberg P, Meitinger T. Missense mutations in the NDP gene

in patients with a less severe course of Norrie disease. Hum Mol Genet. 1995;4(3):489–90. https://doi.org/10.1093/hmg/4.3.489.

16. Wang Z, Liu CH, Huang S, Chen J. Wnt Signaling in vascular eye diseases. Prog Retin Eye Res. 2019;70:110–33. https://doi.org/10.1016/j.preteyeres.2018.11.008.
17. Walsh MK, Drenser KA, Capone A Jr, Trese MT. Early vitrectomy effective for Norrie disease. Arch Ophthalmol. 2010;128(4):456–60. https://doi.org/10.1001/archophthalmol.2009.403.
18. Preising MN, Abura M, Jäger M, Wassill KH, Lorenz B. Ocular morphology and function in juvenile neuronal ceroid lipofuscinosis (CLN3) in the first decade of life. Ophthalmic Genet. 2017;38(3):252–9. https://doi.org/10.1080/13816810.2016.1210651.
19. Reiter JF, Leroux MR. Genes and molecular pathways underpinning ciliopathies. Nat Rev Mol Cell Biol. 2017;18(9):533–47. https://doi.org/10.1038/nrm.2017.60.
20. Cideciyan AV, Jacobson SG, Drack AV, et al. Effect of an intravitreal antisense oligonucleotide on vision in Leber congenital amaurosis due to a photoreceptor cilium defect. Nat Med. 2019;25(2):225–8. https://doi.org/10.1038/s41591-018-0295-0.
21. Valkenburg D, van Cauwenbergh C, Lorenz B, et al. Clinical characterization of 66 patients with congenital retinal disease due to the deep-intronic c.2991+1655A>G mutation in CEP290. Invest Ophthalmol Vis Sci. 2018;59(11):4384–91. https://doi.org/10.1167/iovs.18-24817.
22. Preising MN, Schneider U, Friedburg C, Gruber H, Lindner S, Lorenz B. Das phänotypische Spektrum der Augenveränderungen bei CEP290-Sequenzvariationen [The Phenotypic Spectrum of Ophthalmic Changes in CEP290 Mutations]. Klin Monbl Augenheilkd. 2019;236(3):244–52. https://doi.org/10.1055/a-0842-3250.
23. Rohrschneider K, Bolz HJ. Bardet-Biedl-Syndrome – Diagnose und klinischer Verlauf [The Bardet-Biedl Syndrome - Diagnosis and Follow-up]. Klin Monbl Augenheilkd. 2020;237(3):239–47. https://doi.org/10.1055/a-1118-3748.
24. Weihbrecht K, Goar WA, Pak T, et al. Keeping an eye on Bardet-Biedl syndrome: a comprehensive review of the role of Bardet-Biedl syndrome genes in the eye. Med Res Arch. 2017;5:9. https://doi.org/10.18103/mra.v5i9.1526.
25. Henderson R, Lorenz B, Moore AT. Clinical and molecular genetic aspects of Leber's congenital amaurosis. In: Lorenz B, Moore AT, editors. Pediatric ophthalmology, neuro-ophthalmology, genetics. Essentials in ophthalmology. Berlin: Springer; 2006.
26. Sharon D, Wimberg H, Kinarty Y, Koch KW. Genotype-functional-phenotype correlations in photoreceptor guanylate cyclase (GC-E) encoded by GUCY2D. Prog Retin Eye Res. 2018;63:69–91. https://doi.org/10.1016/j.preteyeres.2017.10.003.
27. Aguirre GK, Butt OH, Datta R, et al. Postretinal structure and function in severe congenital photoreceptor blindness caused by mutations in the GUCY2D gene. Invest Ophthalmol Vis Sci. 2017;58(2):959–73. https://doi.org/10.1167/iovs.16-20413.
28. Bouzia Z, Georgiou M, Hull S, et al. GUCY2D-associated Leber congenital amaurosis: a retrospective natural history study in preparation for trials of novel therapies. Am J Ophthalmol. 2020;210:59–70. https://doi.org/10.1016/j.ajo.2019.10.019.
29. Perdigao PRL, van der Spuy J. Gene and cell therapy for AIPL1-associated Leber congenital amaurosis: challenges and prospects. Adv Exp Med Biol. 2019;1185:97–101. https://doi.org/10.1007/978-3-030-27378-1_16.
30. Garafalo AV, Cideciyan AV, Héon E, et al. Progress in treating inherited retinal diseases: early subretinal gene therapy clinical trials and candidates for future initiatives [published online ahead of print, 2019 Dec 30]. Prog Retin Eye Res. 2019:100827. https://doi.org/10.1016/j.preteyeres.2019.100827.
31. den Hollander AI, Roepman R, Koenekoop RK, Cremers FP. Leber congenital amaurosis: genes, proteins and disease mechanisms. Prog Retin Eye Res. 2008;27(4):391–419. https://doi.org/10.1016/j.preteyeres.2008.05.003.
32. Gu S, Lennon A, Li Y, Lorenz B, Fossarello M, North M, Gal A, Wright A. Tubby-like protein-1 mutations in autosomal recessive retinitis pigmentosa. Lancet. 1998;351(9109):1103–4. https://doi.org/10.1016/S0140-6736(05)79384-3.
33. Ikeda A, Nishina PM, Naggert JK. The tubby-like proteins, a family with roles in neuronal development and function. J Cell Sci. 2002;115(Pt 1):9–14.
34. Bujakowska K, Audo I, Mohand-Saïd S, et al. CRB1 mutations in inherited retinal dystrophies. Hum Mutat. 2012;33(2):306–15. https://doi.org/10.1002/humu.21653.
35. Papadopoulou Laiou C, Preising MN, Bolz HJ, Lorenz B. Genotyp-Phänotyp-Korrelation bei Patienten mit CRB1-Mutationen [Genotype-Phenotype Correlations in Patients with CRB1 Mutations]. Klin Monbl Augenheilkd. 2017;234(3):289–302. https://doi.org/10.1055/s-0043-103961.
36. Talib M, van Schooneveld MJ, van Genderen MM, et al. Genotypic and phenotypic characteristics of CRB1-associated retinal dystrophies: a long-term follow-up study. Ophthalmology. 2017;124(6):884–95. https://doi.org/10.1016/j.ophtha.2017.01.047.
37. Mackay DS, Henderson RH, Sergouniotis PI, et al. Novel mutations in MERTK associated with childhood onset rod-cone dystrophy. Mol Vis. 2010;16:369–77. Published 2010 Mar 9.
38. Audo I, Mohand-Said S, Boulanger-Scemama E, et al. MERTK mutation update in inherited retinal diseases. Hum Mutat. 2018;39(7):887–913. https://doi.org/10.1002/humu.23431.
39. Ramsden CM, Nommiste B, R Lane A, et al. Rescue of the MERTK phagocytic defect in a human iPSC disease model using translational read-through inducing drugs. Sci Rep. 2017;7(1):51. https://doi.org/10.1038/s41598-017-00142-7.
40. Sarkar H, Moosajee M. Retinol dehydrogenase 12 (RDH12): role in vision, retinal disease and future perspectives. Exp Eye Res. 2019;188:107793. https://doi.org/10.1016/j.exer.2019.107793.
41. Fahim AT, Thompson DA. Natural history and genotype-phenotype correlations in RDH12-associated retinal degeneration. Adv Exp Med Biol. 2019;1185:209–13. https://doi.org/10.1007/978-3-030-27378-1_34.
42. Gerber S, Perrault I, Hanein S, et al. Complete exon-intron structure of the RPGR-interacting protein (RPGRIP1) gene allows the identification of mutations underlying Leber congenital amaurosis. Eur J Hum Genet. 2001;9(8):561–71. https://doi.org/10.1038/sj.ejhg.5200689.
43. Dryja TP, Adams SM, Grimsby JL, et al. Null RPGRIP1 alleles in patients with Leber congenital amaurosis. Am J Hum Genet. 2001;68(5):1295–8. https://doi.org/10.1086/320113.
44. Koenekoop RK. RPGRIP1 is mutated in Leber congenital amaurosis: a mini-review. Ophthalmic Genet. 2005;26(4):175–9. https://doi.org/10.1080/13816810500374441.
45. Gu SM, Thompson DA, Srikumari CR, Lorenz B, Finckh U, Nicoletti A, Murthy KR, Rathmann M, Kumaramanickavel G, Denton MJ, Gal A. Mutations in RPE65 cause autosomal recessive childhood-onset severe retinal dystrophy. Nat Genet. 1997 Oct;17(2):194–7.
46. Lorenz B, Gyürüs P, Preising M, Bremser D, Gu S, Andrassi M, Gerth C, Gal A. Early-onset severe rod-cone dystrophy in young children with RPE65 mutations. Invest Ophthalmol Vis Sci. 2000 Aug;41(9):2735–42.
47. Lorenz B, Poliakov E, Schambeck M, Friedburg C, Preising MN, Redmond TM. A comprehensive clinical and biochemical functional study of a novel RPE65 hypomorphic mutation. Invest Ophthalmol Vis Sci. 2008;49(12):5235–42. https://doi.org/10.1167/iovs.07-1671.
48. Lorenz B, Wabbels B, Wegscheider E, Hamel CP, Drexler W, Preising MN. Lack of fundus autofluorescence to 488

nanometers from childhood on in patients with early-onset severe retinal dystrophy associated with mutations in RPE65. Ophthalmology. 2004;111(8):1585–94. https://doi.org/10.1016/j.ophtha.2004.01.033.
49. Chung DC, Bertelsen M, Lorenz B, et al. The natural history of inherited retinal dystrophy due to biallelic mutations in the RPE65 gene. Am J Ophthalmol. 2019;199:58–70. https://doi.org/10.1016/j.ajo.2018.09.024.
50. Russell S, Bennett J, Wellman JA, et al. Efficacy and safety of voretigene neparvovec (AAV2-hRPE65v2) in patients with RPE65-mediated inherited retinal dystrophy: a randomised, controlled, open-label, phase 3 trial [published correction appears in Lancet. 2017 Aug 26;390(10097):848]. Lancet. 2017;390(10097):849–60. https://doi.org/10.1016/S0140-6736(17)31868-8.
51. Hull S, Mukherjee R, Holder GE, Moore AT, Webster AR. The clinical features of retinal disease due to a dominant mutation in RPE65. Mol Vis. 2016;22:626–35. Published 2016 Jun 10.
52. Jauregui R, Cho A, Oh JK, Tanaka AJ, Sparrow JR, Tsang SH. Phenotypic expansion of autosomal dominant retinitis pigmentosa associated with the D477G mutation in RPE65. Cold Spring Harb Mol Case Stud. 2020;6(1):a004952. . Published 2020 Feb 3. https://doi.org/10.1101/mcs.a004952.
53. Molday LL, Wahl D, Sarunic MV, Molday RS. Localization and functional characterization of the p.Asn965Ser (N965S) ABCA4 variant in mice reveal pathogenic mechanisms underlying Stargardt macular degeneration. Hum Mol Genet. 2018;27(2):295–306. https://doi.org/10.1093/hmg/ddx400.
54. Khan M, Cremers FPM. ABCA4-associated Stargardt disease. ABCA4-assoziierter Morbus Stargardt. Klin Monbl Augenheilkd. 2020;237(3):267–74. https://doi.org/10.1055/a-1057-9939.
55. Michaelides M, Chen LL, Brantley MA Jr, et al. ABCA4 mutations and discordant ABCA4 alleles in patients and siblings with bull's-eye maculopathy. Br J Ophthalmol. 2007;91(12):1650–5. https://doi.org/10.1136/bjo.2007.118356.
56. Bax NM, Lambertus S, Cremers FPM, Klevering BJ, Hoyng CB. The absence of fundus abnormalities in Stargardt disease. Graefes Arch Clin Exp Ophthalmol. 2019;257(6):1147–57. https://doi.org/10.1007/s00417-019-04280-8.
57. Auricchio A, Trapani I, Allikmets R. Gene therapy of ABCA4-associated diseases. Cold Spring Harb Perspect Med. 2015;5(5):a017301. Published 2015 Jan 8. https://doi.org/10.1101/cshperspect.a017301.
58. Sabirzhanova I, Lopes Pacheco M, Rapino D, et al. Rescuing trafficking mutants of the ATP-binding cassette protein, ABCA4, with small molecule correctors as a treatment for Stargardt eye disease. J Biol Chem. 2015;290(32):19743–55. https://doi.org/10.1074/jbc.M115.647685.
59. Meindl A, Dry K, Herrmann K, et al. A gene (RPGR) with homology to the RCC1 guanine nucleotide exchange factor is mutated in X-linked retinitis pigmentosa (RP3). Nat Genet. 1996;13(1):35–42. https://doi.org/10.1038/ng0596-35.
60. Bader I, Brandau O, Achatz H, et al. X-linked retinitis pigmentosa: RPGR mutations in most families with definite X linkage and clustering of mutations in a short sequence stretch of exon ORF15. Invest Ophthalmol Vis Sci. 2003;44(4):1458–63. https://doi.org/10.1167/iovs.02-0605.
61. Tee JJL, Kalitzeos A, Webster AR, Peto T, Michaelides M. Quantitative analysis of hyperautofluorescent rings to characterize the natural history and progression in RPGR-associated retinopathy. Retina. 2018;38(12):2401–14.
62. Wegscheider E, Preising MN, Lorenz B. Fundus autofluorescence in carriers of X-linked recessive retinitis pigmentosa associated with mutations in RPGR, and correlation with electrophysiological and psychophysical data. Graefes Arch Clin Exp Ophthalmol. 2004;242(6):501–11.
63. Churchill JD, Bowne SJ, Sullivan LS, et al. Mutations in the X-linked retinitis pigmentosa genes RPGR and RP2 found in 8.5% of families with a provisional diagnosis of autosomal dominant retinitis pigmentosa. Invest Ophthalmol Vis Sci. 2013;54(2):1411–6. . Published 2013 Feb 19. https://doi.org/10.1167/iovs.12-11541.
64. Cehajic Kapetanovic J, McClements ME, Martinez-Fernandez de la Camara C, MacLaren RE. Molecular Strategies for RPGR Gene Therapy. Genes (Basel). 2019;10(9):674. Published 2019 Sep 4. https://doi.org/10.3390/genes10090674.
65. Cremers FP, van de Pol DJ, van Kerkhoff LP, Wieringa B, Ropers HH. Cloning of a gene that is rearranged in patients with choroideraemia. Nature. 1990;347(6294):674–7. https://doi.org/10.1038/347674a0.
66. Preising MN, Wegscheider E, Friedburg C, Poloschek CM, Wabbels BK, Lorenz B. Fundus autofluorescence in carriers of choroideremia and correlation with electrophysiologic and psychophysical data. Ophthalmology. 2009;116(6):1201–9.e92. https://doi.org/10.1016/j.ophtha.2009.01.016.
67. Dimopoulos IS, Radziwon A, St Laurent CD, MacDonald IM. Choroideremia. Curr Opin Ophthalmol. 2017;28(5):410–5. https://doi.org/10.1097/ICU.0000000000000392.
68. Aleman TS, Han G, Serrano LW, et al. Natural history of the central structural abnormalities in choroideremia: a prospective cross-sectional study. Ophthalmology. 2017;124(3):359–73. https://doi.org/10.1016/j.ophtha.2016.10.022.
69. Mitsios A, Dubis AM, Moosajee M. Choroideremia: from genetic and clinical phenotyping to gene therapy and future treatments. Ther Adv Ophthalmol. 2018;10:2515841418817490. . Published 2018 Dec 27. https://doi.org/10.1177/2515841418817490.
70. Xue K, Jolly JK, Barnard AR, et al. Beneficial effects on vision in patients undergoing retinal gene therapy for choroideremia. Nat Med. 2018;24(10):1507–12. https://doi.org/10.1038/s41591-018-0185-5.
71. Cehajic Kapetanovic J, Barnard AR, MacLaren RE. Molecular therapies for choroideremia. Genes (Basel). 2019;10(10):738. . Published 2019 Sep 23. https://doi.org/10.3390/genes10100738.
72. Marquardt A, Stohr H, Passmore LA, Kramer F, Rivera A, Weber BH. Mutations in a novel gene,VMD2, encoding a protein of unknown properties cause juvenile-onset vitelliform macular dystrophy (Best's disease). Hum. Mol. Genet. 1998;7:1517–25.
73. Pasquay C, Wang LF, Lorenz B, Preising MN. Bestrophin 1–phenotypes and functional aspects in bestrophinopathies. Ophthalmic Genet. 2015;36(3):193–212. https://doi.org/10.3109/13816810.2013.863945.
74. Nachtigal AL, Milenkovic A, Brandl C, et al. Mutation-dependent pathomechanisms determine the phenotype in the bestrophinopathies. Int J Mol Sci. 2020;21(5):1597. . Published 2020 Feb 26. https://doi.org/10.3390/ijms21051597.
75. Burgess R, Millar ID, Leroy BP, et al. Biallelic mutation of BEST1 causes a distinct retinopathy in humans. Am J Hum Genet. 2008;82(1):19–31. https://doi.org/10.1016/j.ajhg.2007.08.004.
76. Yardley J, Leroy BP, Hart-Holden N, et al. Mutations of VMD2 splicing regulators cause nanophthalmos and autosomal dominant vitreoretinochoroidopathy (ADVIRC). Invest Ophthalmol Vis Sci. 2004;45(10):3683–9. https://doi.org/10.1167/iovs.04-0550.
77. Burgess R, MacLaren RE, Davidson AE, et al. ADVIRC is caused by distinct mutations in BEST1 that alter pre-mRNA splicing. J Med Genet. 2009;46(9):620–5. https://doi.org/10.1136/jmg.2008.059881.
78. Wissinger B, Gamer D, Jägle H, et al. CNGA3 mutations in hereditary cone photoreceptor disorders. Am J Hum Genet. 2001;69(4):722–37. https://doi.org/10.1086/323613.
79. Kohl S, Varsanyi B, Antunes GA, et al. CNGB3 mutations account for 50% of all cases with autosomal recessive achromatopsia. Eur J Hum Genet. 2005;13(3):302–8. https://doi.org/10.1038/sj.ejhg.5201269.

80. Felden J, Baumann B, Ali M, et al. Mutation spectrum and clinical investigation of achromatopsia patients with mutations in the GNAT2 gene. Hum Mutat. 2019;40(8):1145–55. https://doi.org/10.1002/humu.23768.
81. Weisschuh N, Stingl K, Audo I, et al. Mutations in the gene PDE6C encoding the catalytic subunit of the cone photoreceptor phosphodiesterase in patients with achromatopsia. Hum Mutat. 2018;39(10):1366–71. https://doi.org/10.1002/humu.23606.
82. Mastey RR, Georgiou M, Langlo CS, et al. Characterization of retinal structure in ATF6-associated achromatopsia. Invest Ophthalmol Vis Sci. 2019;60(7):2631–40. https://doi.org/10.1167/iovs.19-27047.
83. Burkard M, Kohl S, Krätzig T, et al. Accessory heterozygous mutations in cone photoreceptor CNGA3 exacerbate CNG channel-associated retinopathy. J Clin Invest. 2018;128(12):5663–75. https://doi.org/10.1172/JCI96098.
84. Matet A, Kohl S, Baumann B, et al. Multimodal imaging including semiquantitative short-wavelength and near-infrared autofluorescence in achromatopsia. Sci Rep. 2018;8(1):5665. . Published 2018 Apr 4. https://doi.org/10.1038/s41598-018-23919-w.
85. Ofri R, Averbukh E, Ezra-Elia R, et al. Six years and counting: restoration of photopic retinal function and visual behavior following gene augmentation therapy in a sheep model of CNGA3 achromatopsia. Hum Gene Ther. 2018;29(12):1376–86. https://doi.org/10.1089/hum.2018.076.
86. Kahle NA, Peters T, Zobor D, et al. Development of methodology and study protocol: safety and efficacy of a single subretinal injection of rAAV.hCNGA3 in patients with CNGA3-linked achromatopsia investigated in an exploratory dose-escalation trial. Hum Gene Ther Clin Dev. 2018;29(3):121–31. https://doi.org/10.1089/humc.2018.088.
87. Wissinger B, Dangel S, Jägle H, et al. Cone dystrophy with supernormal rod response is strictly associated with mutations in KCNV2. Invest Ophthalmol Vis Sci. 2008;49(2):751–7. https://doi.org/10.1167/iovs.07-0471.
88. Wu H, Cowing JA, Michaelides M, et al. Mutations in the gene KCNV2 encoding a voltage-gated potassium channel subunit cause "cone dystrophy with supernormal rod electroretinogram" in humans. Am J Hum Genet. 2006;79(3):574–79. PMID:16909397.
89. Friedburg C, Wissinger B, Schambeck M, Bonin M, Kohl S, Lorenz B. Long-term follow-up of the human phenotype in three siblings with cone dystrophy associated with a homozygous p.G461R mutation of KCNV2. Invest Ophthalmol Vis Sci. 2011;52(12):8621–9. . Published 2011 Nov 7. https://doi.org/10.1167/iovs.11-8187.
90. Sauer CG, Gehrig A, Warneke-Wittstock R, Marquardt A, Ewing CC, Gibson A, Lorenz B, Jurklies B, Weber BH. Positional cloning of the gene associated with X-linked juvenile retinoschisis. Nat Genet. 1997;17(2):164–70. https://doi.org/10.1038/ng1097-164.
91. Pimenides D, George ND, Yates JR, et al. X-linked retinoschisis: clinical phenotype and RS1 genotype in 86 UK patients. J Med Genet. 2005;42(6):e35. https://doi.org/10.1136/jmg.2004.029769.
92. Bowles K, Cukras C, Turriff A, et al. X-linked retinoschisis: RS1 mutation severity and age affect the ERG phenotype in a cohort of 68 affected male subjects. Invest Ophthalmol Vis Sci. 2011;52(12):9250–6. . Published 2011 Nov 29. https://doi.org/10.1167/iovs.11-8115.
93. Bradshaw K, George N, Moore A, Trump D. Mutations of the XLRS1 gene cause abnormalities of photoreceptor as well as inner retinal responses of the ERG. Doc Ophthalmol. 1999;98(2):153–73. https://doi.org/10.1023/a:1002432919073.
94. Vincent A, Robson AG, Neveu MM, et al. A phenotype-genotype correlation study of X-linked retinoschisis. Ophthalmology. 2013;120(7):1454–64. https://doi.org/10.1016/j.ophtha.2012.12.008.
95. George ND, Yates JR, Bradshaw K, Moore AT. Infantile presentation of X linked retinoschisis. Br J Ophthalmol. 1995;79(7):653–7. https://doi.org/10.1136/bjo.79.7.653.
96. Lee JJ, Kim JH, Kim SY, Park SS, Yu YS. Infantile vitreous hemorrhage as the initial presentation of X-linked juvenile retinoschisis. Korean J Ophthalmol. 2009;23(2):118–20. https://doi.org/10.3341/kjo.2009.23.2.118.
97. Cukras C, Wiley HE, Jeffrey BG, et al. Retinal AAV8-RS1 gene therapy for X-linked retinoschisis: initial findings from a phase I/IIa trial by intravitreal delivery. Mol Ther. 2018;26(9):2282–94. https://doi.org/10.1016/j.ymthe.2018.05.025.
98. Cukras CA, Huryn LA, Jeffrey BG, Turriff A, Sieving PA. Analysis of anatomic and functional measures in X-linked retinoschisis [published correction appears in Invest Ophthalmol Vis Sci. 2018 Aug 1;59(10):3868]. Invest Ophthalmol Vis Sci. 2018;59(7):2841–7. https://doi.org/10.1167/iovs.17-23297.
99. Testa F, Di IV, Gallo B, Marchese M, Nesti A, De RG, Melillo P, Simonelli F. Carbonic anhydrase inhibitors in patients with X-linked retinoschisis: effects on macular morphology and function. Ophthalmic Genet. 2019;40(3):207–12.
100. Galantuomo MS, Fossarello M, Cuccu A, Farci R, Preising MN, Lorenz B, Napoli PE. Rebound macular edema following oral acetazolamide therapy for juvenile X-linked retinoschisis in an Italian family. Clin. Ophthalmol. 2016;10:2377–82.
101. Eisenberger T, Neuhaus C, Khan AO, et al. Increasing the yield in targeted next-generation sequencing by implicating CNV analysis, non-coding exons and the overall variant load: the example of retinal dystrophies [published correction appears in PLoS One. 2014;9(11):e108840]. PLoS One. 2013;8(11):e78496. Published 2013 Nov 12. https://doi.org/10.1371/journal.pone.0078496.
102. Drack AV, Lambert SR, Stone EM. From the laboratory to the clinic: molecular genetic testing in pediatric ophthalmology. Am J Ophthalmol. 2010;149(1):10–7. https://doi.org/10.1016/j.ajo.2009.08.038.

Familial Exudative Vitreoretinopathy

25

Boontip Tipsuriyaporn, Harald Gjerde,
and Yoshihiro Yonekawa

Abstract

Familial exudative vitreoretinopathy (FEVR) is a hereditary retinal vascular anomaly characterized by incomplete peripheral retinal vascularization during development. The vascular abnormalities exhibit varying degrees of severity: from minor changes in peripheral retinal vessels to severe retinal detachments leading to blindness. FEVR has been shown to have autosomal dominant, autosomal recessive, and X-linked recessive inheritance patterns, with numerous genes implicated in the condition. Wide-field fluorescein angiography is essential for early detection, diagnosis, and management. Laser photocoagulation is used to treat sequelae from the avascular retina, and retinal detachments are managed with vitreoretinal surgery. Visual prognosis depends on the severity of the disease, and lifelong follow-up is recommended.

Keywords

Angiogenesis · Familial exudative vitreoretinopathy
Inherited retinal diseases · Pediatric retina · Retina
Vitrectomy

B. Tipsuriyaporn
Retina Service, Massachusetts Eye and Ear, Harvard Medical School, Boston, MA, USA

Pediatric Retina Service, Boston Children's Hospital, Harvard Medical School, Boston, MA, USA

Department of Ophthalmology, Faculty of Medicine, Ramathibodi Hospital, Mahidol University, Bangkok, Thailand

H. Gjerde
Department of Ophthalmology and Visual Sciences, Dalhousie University, Halifax, NS, Canada

Y. Yonekawa (✉)
Retina Service, Massachusetts Eye and Ear, Harvard Medical School, Boston, MA, USA

Pediatric Retina Service, Boston Children's Hospital, Harvard Medical School, Boston, MA, USA

25.1 Introduction and Epidemiology

Familial exudative vitreoretinopathy (FEVR) was first described by Criswick and Schepens in 1969 as an inherited condition that appeared similar to retinopathy of prematurity (ROP), but occurring in patients without prematurity or oxygen supplementation, and the disease continued to progress several years after birth. Clinical features included vitreous membranes, retinal traction, temporal dragging of the macula, subretinal and intraretinal exudates in the periphery, and peripheral neovascularization [1].

The phenotype in FEVR tends to be asymmetric between eyes, and variable penetrance and expressivity is seen within the same family. Vascular abnormalities vary in severity: from asymptomatic peripheral vascular changes to poor vision from severe retinal detachments [2]. FEVR is associated with significant visual impairment [3]. The prevalence of FEVR is unknown due to its rarity, but studies have shown that between 58 and 90% of individuals with FEVR may be asymptomatic [4, 5], so it is likely an under-diagnosed condition.

FEVR can be differentiated from other pediatric retinal vascular diseases, such as ROP and persistent fetal vasculature (PFV), by performing a complete ophthalmic examination together with wide-field fluorescein angiography. The retinal abnormalities of FEVR can progress over time without treatment, resulting in diagnostic and treatment challenges. Identification of asymptomatic family members can aid in diagnosis as well as genetic counseling. Continued follow-up and examinations with retina specialists are essential for patients, since FEVR is a lifelong condition that can reactivate at any age (although young children are usually burdened with the most progressive disease).

25.2 Pathophysiology

FEVR is an inherited disorder characterized by abnormal peripheral avascular retina due to dysfunction in retinal angiogenesis. The incomplete development of retinal vascu-

W.-C. Wu, W.-C. Lam (eds.), *A Quick Guide to Pediatric Retina*, https://doi.org/10.1007/978-981-15-6552-6_25

lature causes retinal ischemia that induces neovascularization and other sight-threatening complications, such as vitreoretinal traction, retinal falciform folds, macular traction, retinal exudates, and retinal detachments. Studies have suggested that abnormal membranes originating from abnormal vitreous are formed, causing traction in the form of hyaloidal contraction [6].

FEVR is most commonly inherited in an autosomal dominant (AD) pattern, but can also be autosomal recessive (AR) or X-linked recessive. FEVR genes show 100% penetrance but variable in expressivity, even between eyes in the same person or within the same family [7].

The normal vascular development of the eye is regulated by the Wnt signaling pathway.

There are two types of Wnt signaling pathways: the canonical Wnt/β-catenin pathway, which uses β-catenin as a transcriptional co-factor that enables cell proliferation and differentiation; and the non-canonical Wnt pathway that mediates cell migration and cytoskeletal organization [8]. The vascular angiogenic abnormalities associated with FEVR occur when the Wnt signaling pathway becomes dysfunctional.

Many genes that have been implicated in FEVR and FEVR-like phenotypes: Frizzled-4 (*FZD4*: 11q14.2; AD), norrin (*NDP*: Xp11.3; X-linked recessive), exudative vitreoretinopathy 3 (*EVR3:* 11p13-p12; AD), low density lipoprotein receptor-related protein 5 (*LRP5*: 11q13.2; AD or AR), tetraspanin (*TSPAN12*: 7q31.31; AD), zinc finger protein (*ZNF408*: 11p11.2; AD), β-catenin 1 (*CTNNB1*: 3p22.1; AD), and kinesin family member 11 (*KIF11* 10q23.33; AD).

FZD4, *NDP*, *LRP5*, and *TSPAN12* are the classic FEVR genes, and they are linked to the canonical Wnt/β-catenin pathway. At the cell surface of vascular endothelium, Wnt ligands and Norrin proteins bind to the FZD4 and LRP5 receptors on the plasma membrane to form the receptor complex. This results in the release of β-catenin into the cytoplasm. In addition, to amplify the Wnt signal, Norrin/FZD4 signaling requires the membrane protein TSPAN12 to increase FZD4 multimerization. Cytoplasmic β-catenin then translocates into the nucleus, leading to transcription of Wnt target genes. An abnormality of one of these genes will affect the normal angiogenesis of the eyes [9]. ZNF408 is thought to be a transcription factor in ocular vascular development. Defects in *ZNF408* genes have been reported to be associated with autosomal recessive retinitis pigmentosa. Collin et al. [10] identified a mutation in the *ZNF408* genes in a large Dutch pedigree with exudative vitreoretinopathy.

KIF11 is in the kinesin family, of which the relation to the Wnt/β-catenin signaling pathway is still unknown. Mutations in *KIF11* exhibit an autosomal dominant inheritance pattern that have been associated with microcephaly with or without intellectual disability, lymphedema, and chorioretinopathy [11]. Robitaille et al. [12] identified *KIF11* mutations in patients with FEVR-like phenotypes; and Hu et al. [13] reported that 8.3% of FEVR patients had *KIF11* mutations, with these patients showing ocular signs of FEVR with or without the systemic associations of KIF11.

25.3 Histopathology

Pathological results of two enucleated eyes from two patients with angle-closure glaucoma secondary to FEVR showed retinal detachment, abnormal peripheral retinal vascular proliferation, intraocular hemorrhage, fibrovascular formation, and intraretinal infiltration of inflammatory cells [14]. In 1995, Benson [15] reported histopathological results from intraocular fluid and fibrous tissue samples that were collected during vitrectomies from three patients with FEVR. The specimens showed the infiltration of lymphocytes, plasma cells, and macrophages. The retinal tissue segments showed retinal degeneration, vessel wall thickening, and areas of avascular retina. All findings were not specific for the diagnosis of FEVR, however.

25.4 Clinical Presentation

FEVR is a rare, hereditary, congenital vitreoretinal disorder, which can cause significant visual impairment, but many patients are also asymptomatic. Most patients present younger than 7–10 years of age [16–19], without a history of preterm birth or supplemental oxygen, and with normal birth weight—the typical considerations for ROP, which is at the top of the differential diagnosis. A positive family history of FEVR can be found in 10–50% [1, 16, 19, 20]. FEVR typically progresses during childhood, especially before age 3. Progression of the disease is rare after age 20 [16] but does occur.

FEVR is a bilateral condition, but the severity can be very asymmetric between eyes in the same patients [15]. There is a wide range of clinical presentations, such as being asymptomatic, refractive errors, nystagmus, strabismus, microphthalmia, and phthisis bulbi. Mild forms of the disease show peripheral avascular retina with a line of vascular buds at the vascular and avascular junction, venous-venous anastomoses, and extensive vascular branching. In more severe cases, neovascularization, dragged disc and macula, radial falciform retinal folds, tractional retinal detachments (alone or combined with rhegmatogenous retinal detachments), vitreous hemorrhage, and secondary glaucoma can occur [1, 2, 16]. Exudation can occur concurrently with any stage of FEVR, manifesting as intraretinal or subretinal lipid exudates on fundus examination, or leakage on fluorescein angiography [17].

In 1998, Pendergast and Trese [21] proposed a five-stage FEVR classification that was subsequently modified in 2011 [16] and 2014 [17] (Table 25.1). The modified classifications were based on long-term observations of large case series using wide-field angiography, which improved disease recognition, clinical staging consensus, and management of patients and affected family members. Table 25.1 describes the details of the most recent 2014 classification system by Kashani and Trese [17]: Stage 1—peripheral avascular retina or anomalous intraretinal vascularization without (1A) or with (1B) exudates on fundus examination or angiographic leakage (Fig. 25.1); Stage 2—avascular peripheral retina with extraretinal neovascularization, without (2A) or with (2B) exudates or leakage (Fig. 25.2); Stage 3—extramacular retinal detachment; Stage 4—macula-involving retinal detachment (Fig. 25.3); Stage 5—total retinal detachment (Fig. 25.4).

Table 25.1 Staging system for familial exudative vitreoretinopathy

Stage	Clinical features	A	B
1	Avascular periphery or anomalous intraretinal vascularization	Without exudate or leakage	With exudate or leakage
2	Avascular retinal periphery with extraretinal vascularization	Without exudate or leakage	With exudate or leakage
3	Extramacular retinal detachment	Without exudate or leakage	With exudate or leakage
4	Macula-involving retinal detachment	Without exudate or leakage	With exudate or leakage
5	Total retinal detachment	Open funnel	Closed funnel

25.5 Multimodal Imaging

25.5.1 Fluorescein Angiography

Fluorescein angiography (FA) is the most important imaging modality for diagnosis of FEVR, and it can also be used to reveal abnormalities in asymptomatic patients and family members. FA in FEVR was first used by Canny and Oliver in 1976 [22], and they showed telangiectatic vessels at the border of vascularized and avascular retina, retinal capillary buds at that junction, and retinal feeder vessels to the temporal fibrovascular mass associated with fluorescein leakage. Ober et al. [19] reported the FA findings in 12 patients, showing increased number and caliber of retinal vessels, straightening of the vessels, arteriovenous anastomoses, temporal retinal vascular nonperfusion with scalloped borders, and leakage of vessels, optic disc, and macula.

FA demonstrates an avascular zone classically described as a V-shaped pattern in the temporal periphery, but this can extend 360 degrees [15]. Kashani et al. [17] describes a variety of retinal vascular anomalies in FEVR by using wide-field angiography (Fig. 25.5c, d), including telangiectasias in the macula or periphery, optic disc head leakage, arterial tortuosity, capillary agenesis, anomalous vascularization, aberrant circumferential vessels, delayed arteriovenous transit time, delayed or absent choroidal perfusion, venous-venous shunting, and central macular edema. They found that more than 50% of asymptomatic family members also showed peripheral vascular nonperfusion and vascular abnormalities indicative of a FEVR phenotype. The angiographic findings help with the management of these patients, as laser ablation of the retinal avascular areas to prevent complications can be considered.

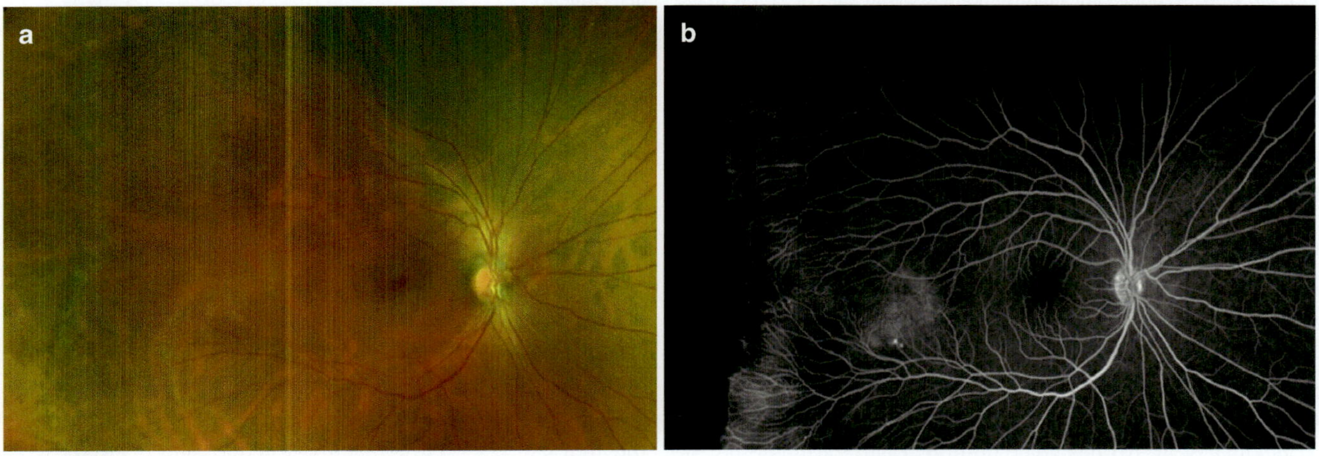

Fig. 25.1 Wide-field color fundus image and fluorescein angiography (FA) of a patient with stage 1A FEVR. (**a**) Color fundus imaging showing peripheral avascular retina with a line of vascular buds at the vascular and avascular junction and extensive vascular branching. (**b**) Midphase FA reveals a V-shaped avascular zone in the temporal periphery, increased number of retinal vessels (called "supernumerary vessels")

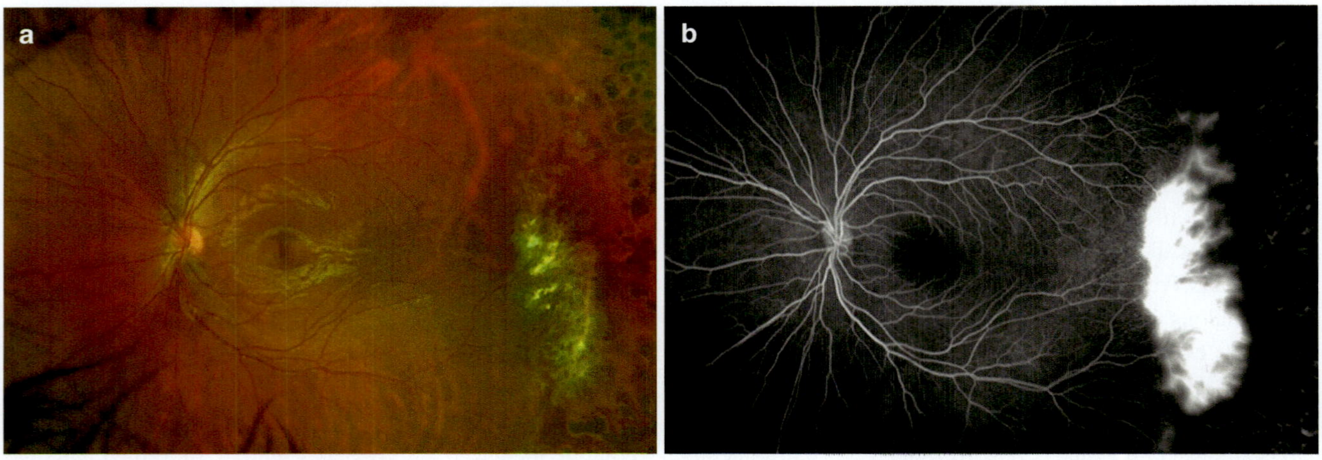

Fig. 25.2 Wide-field color fundus image and fluorescein angiography (FA) of a patient with stage 2B FEVR. (**a**) Color fundus imaging shows temporal extraretinal fibrovascular proliferation and laser scars from previous treatment. (**b**) FA shows extensive leakage from the fibrovascular proliferation, temporal peripheral nonperfusion, and staining of the laser-treated areas

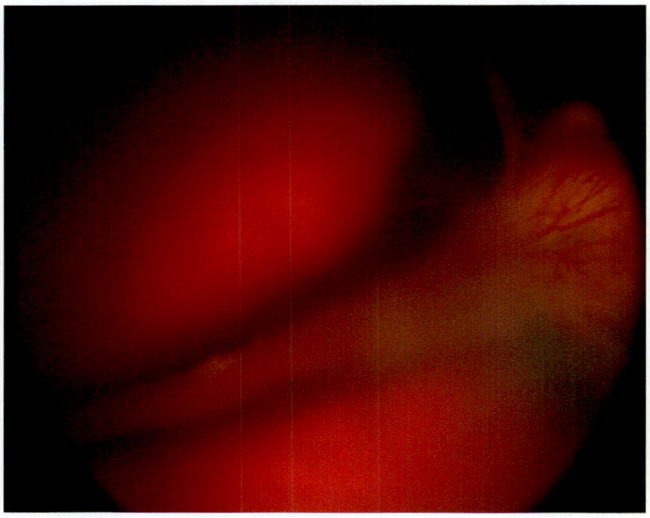

Fig. 25.3 Wide-field color fundus photography of stage 4 FEVR in the left eye showing a temporal falciform retinal fold with macula-involving retinal detachment, and overlying hyaloidal organization

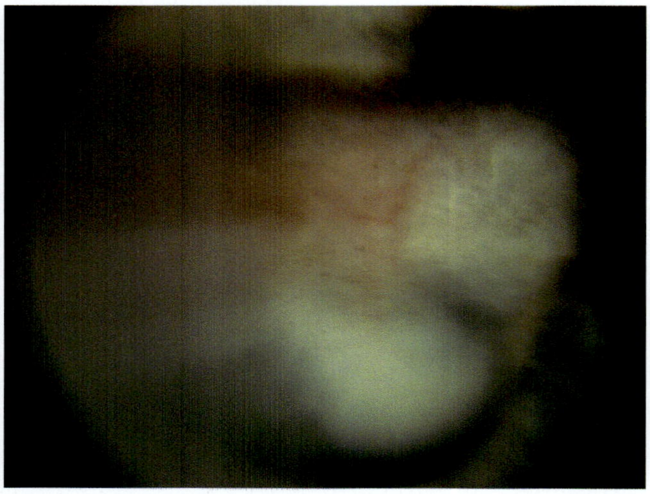

Fig. 25.4 Stage 5 FEVR is characterized by complete retinal detachment

25.5.2 Optical Coherence Tomography

Optical coherence tomography (OCT) is a non-invasive test that provides cross-sectional images of retinal microstructure. Shimouchi et al. [23] reported two cases of early-stage FEVR, with vitreoretinal interface abnormalities showing perifoveal posterior vitreous detachment (PVD) and epiretinal hyperreflective material deposited at the parafoveal area. Yonekawa et al. [6] has since demonstrated various types of vitreomacular interface abnormalities including posterior hyaloid organization, abnormal vitreous traction at the macula and optic disc (Fig. 25.5a, b), and vitreoadhesion at old peripheral retinal scars. Microstructural changes of the retina, such as loss of normal foveal contour, persistence of inner retinal layers, cystoid macular edema, intraretinal and subretinal lipid exudation, and disruption of the ellipsoid zone were also reported. Poor visual function was associated with disruption of ellipsoid zone, cystoid macular edema, macular exudates, vitreomacular traction, and posterior hyaloidal organization.

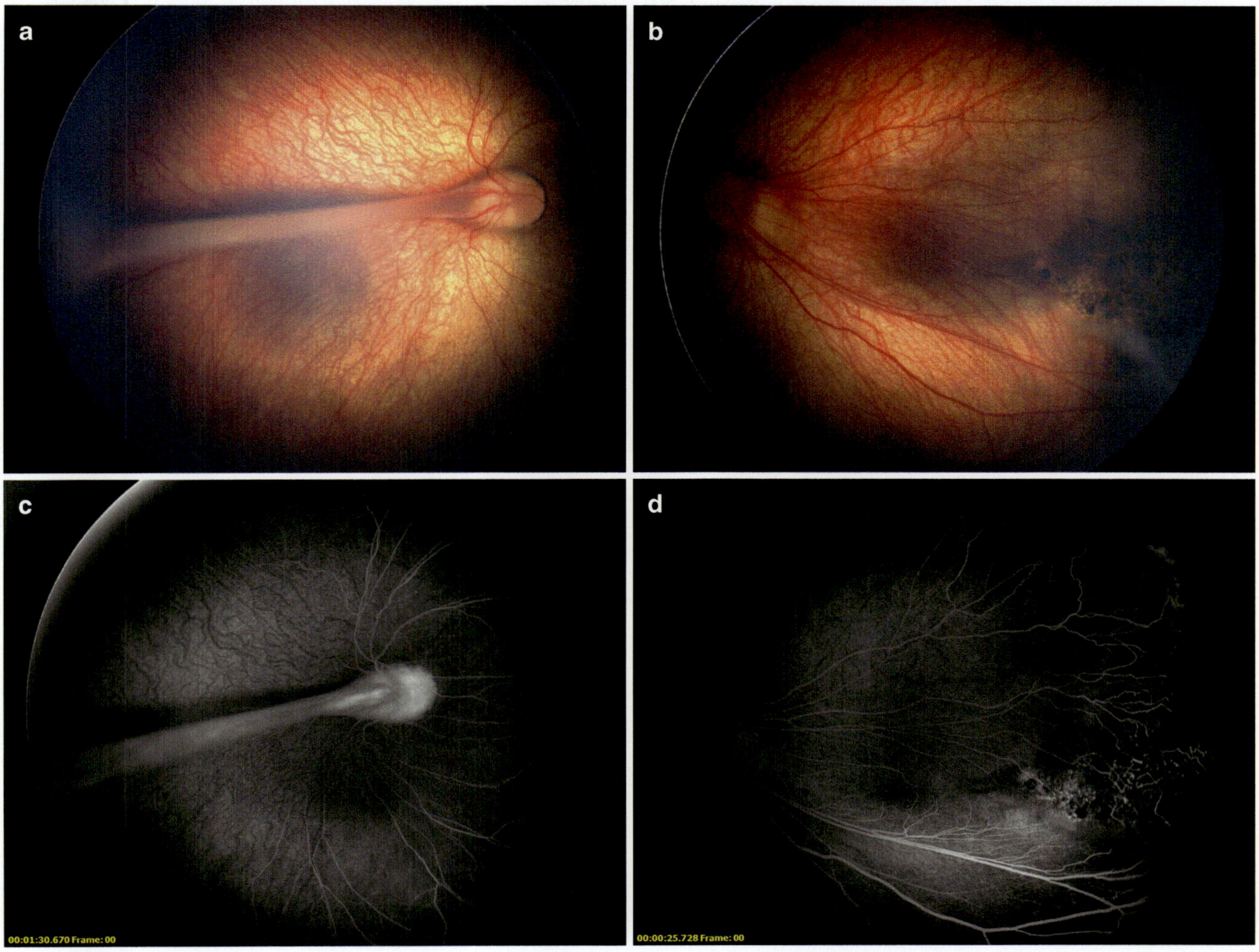

Fig. 25.5 FEVR is a bilateral condition but can be very asymmetric in presentation. (**a**, **b**) This patient has a tight radial retinal fold in the right eye, while the retinal traction is milder in the left eye. (**c**, **d**) Fluorescein angiography shows that the right eye's vasculature is relatively quiet, but the left eye has more leakage. The angiogram highlights the nonperfusion and anomalous vasculature ends

25.5.3 Optical Coherence Tomography Angiography (OCTA)

Chen et al. [24] reported the microstructural changes of the fovea in 41 FEVR patients compared to normal controls using optical coherence tomography angiography (OCTA): one-third of patients had small foveal avascular zones, and almost 50% of patients showed abnormal persistence of fetal foveal structures and decreased density of vascularization in parafoveal areas.

25.6 Differential Diagnosis

The clinical findings of FEVR can mimic other vitreoretinal disorders, such as ROP, Norrie's disease, Coats' disease, incontinentia pigmenti, toxocara infection, and PFV.

Unlike ROP, patients with FEVR are born full-term, with normal birth weights, and without having received significant oxygen supplement therapy. History of retinal diseases in family members might help in diagnosis, but because many affected are asymptomatic, FEVR should be considered on the differential of childhood vitreoretinopathy. Careful and complete ophthalmic examination of family members is important and helpful in terms of diagnosis, treatment, and counseling, especially when access to genetic testing is difficult. Both ROP and FEVR are bilateral diseases, but asymmetrical involvement between the eyes are frequently found in FEVR patients. Active ROP cases rarely develop exudates and tend to have circumferential, elevated fibrovascular ridges at the vascular–avascular junction, which then regress over time, especially after treatment [15]. On the other hand, FEVR usually does not develop circumferential elevated ridges, and the condition can progress despite treatment.

FEVR can be associated with both intraretinal and subretinal exudation, which mimics Coats' disease. However, FEVR frequently develops fibrous membranes and retinal traction, and commonly affects both eyes. Coats' disease is an idiopathic retinal telangiectatic condition. There is unilateral involvement in 95% of cases, and patients may present with exudative retinal detachments from actively leaking abnormal vessels. Unlike FEVR, neovascularization and tractional membranes are not usually seen in Coats' disease [25, 26].

Norrie disease and incontinentia pigmenti (IP) are X-linked conditions that can exhibit ocular findings that resemble FEVR, but they both tend to have systemic involvement. Many patients with Norrie disease are associated with developmental delay, and one-third develop progressive sensorineural hearing loss in the second decade of life [9, 27]. Note though that Norrie disease is caused by severe mutations in *NDP* and can be thought of as an extreme phenotype of FEVR. Indeed, children with Norrie disease often present with severe traction retinal detachment in both eyes. IP, or Bloch–Sulzberger syndrome, is an X-linked dominant neurocutaneous disorder and is usually lethal in males. Female infants can be born with characteristic skin lesions, along with developmental delay and seizures, and peripheral retinal avascularity and neovascular complications [28–30].

Toxocariasis is a rare infection caused by roundworms, *Toxocara canis* and *Toxocara cati*. As in FEVR, temporal dragging of the optic disc and macula can occur, though 90% of cases are unilateral and most patients present with posterior uveitis and vitritis.

Persistent fetal vasculature (PFV) is an idiopathic congenital ocular abnormality resulting from a failure of regression of fetal vasculature. PFV is most frequently unilateral, occurring in full-term infants. Ocular findings vary from mild persistent pupillary membranes to severe tractional retinal detachments which can mimic FEVR. Infants with PFV usually have anterior segment abnormalities, such as microcornea, ciliary body elongation, cataracts, or colobomas—all uncommonly found in FEVR [31, 32].

25.7 Treatment

Treatment of FEVR depends on the clinical stage of the disease. Earlier stages may be managed with careful observation or laser photocoagulation. More advanced disease usually requires complex surgical intervention. Early and appropriate interventions often lead to better outcomes and can be vision preserving.

25.7.1 Long-Term Ocular Examinations and Screening

FEVR is a progressive disease that requires lifelong management. Regular fundus examinations with fluorescein angiography are advised, especially in very young patients who can have rapid progression to advanced stages, causing severe loss of vision. Family members should be screened with full eye examinations, and genetic testing should be offered if possible to identify the genomic abnormalities, aiding in genetic counseling and family planning.

25.7.2 Non-surgical Treatment

For Stage 1 disease, patients can be observed carefully, as they have a lower likelihood of progressing to advanced stages. Treatment of avascular zones with laser photocoagulation can be considered though, in patients with moderate or severe avascularity. In patients with Stage 2 disease, laser photocoagulation is recommended to help regress neovascularization. Anti-VEGF therapy can help reduce neovascular regression but may aggravate fibrovascular contraction, causing severe traction to the retina. Further studies for the use of anti-VEGF treatment in FEVR are required, but at the moment, its role is limited.

25.7.3 Surgical Treatment

Vitreous traction from hyaloidal organization is the cause of tractional retinal detachments in FEVR. Areas of peripheral avascular retina are atrophic, which predisposes the eyes to retinal breaks and rhegmatogenous retinal detachments also [33]. The surgical options for retinal detachments in FEVR include scleral buckling, vitrectomy with or without lens removal, and combined procedures [20, 21, 34, 35]. The results of the surgery vary depending on patient age, the severity of detachments, macular involvement, and type of surgery.

Scleral buckling can be considered in patients who have peripheral traction anterior to the equator, as patients with Stage 3 disease or partial exudative retinal detachments can have favorable outcomes with scleral buckling alone [21]. Vitrectomy with hyaloidal resection is essential for severely active fibrovascular proliferation, and lensectomy may be done in cases that have membranes attached anteriorly to the lens. Recurrences of membranous proliferation and retinal detachments can occur, necessitating the need for subsequent procedures. Complications, such as secondary cataract formation, glaucoma, vitreous hemorrhage, and iatrogenic retinal breaks have been reported and should be avoided. Visual rehabilitation after treatment is crucial, especially in younger patients to prevent amblyopia.

25.8 Prognosis

FEVR tends to be a slow, progressive disease [36], yet rapid progression can occur, especially in children. Patients may not progress through the stages in a stepwise manner [18]. Progression mostly happens during the first decade of life. In patients who have useful visual function after age 20, the visual acuity usually remains stable throughout life [2, 18, 19]. Some causes of late-onset visual loss include progressive retina traction involving the macula, large exudates, retinal detachment, cataract, vitreous hemorrhage, and secondary glaucoma [34]. Further studies that look at long-term outcomes of FEVR patients are needed.

25.9 Conclusion

FEVR is a rare, yet likely very under-diagnosed, genetic disorder that affects retinal angiogenesis during eye development resulting in avascular peripheral retina. The phenotype is asymmetric between eyes, variable penetrance and expressivity is seen within the same family, and vascular abnormalities vary in severity. Numerous genes have been implicated in the condition. Careful and complete ocular examination with wide-field fluorescein angiography is essential for early detection, diagnosis, and management. Early treatment with laser photocoagulation may help prevent disease progression, and carefully planned surgical intervention is used to manage retinal detachments. Visual prognosis depends on the severity of the disease, and lifelong follow-up is important to reduce morbidity.

Disclosures Consultant for Alcon, Alimera, Allergan, Regeneron (YY)

References

1. Criswick VG, Schepens CL. Familial exudative vitreoretinopathy. Am J Ophthalmol. 1969;68(4):578–94.
2. Gow J, Oliver GL. Familial exudative vitreoretinopathy. An expanded view. Arch Ophthalmol. 1971;86(2):150–5.
3. Robitaille JM, Zheng B, Wallace K, Beis MJ, Tatlidil C, Yang J, Sheidow TG, Siebert L, Levin AV, Lam WC, Arthur BW, Lyons CJ, Jaakkola E, Tsilou E, Williams CA, Weaver RG Jr, Shields CL, Guernsey DL. The role of Frizzled-4 mutations in familial exudative vitreoretinopathy and Coats disease. Br J Ophthalmol. 2011;95(4):574–9. https://doi.org/10.1136/bjo.2010.190116.
4. Toomes C, Downey L. Familial exudative vitreoretinopathy, autosomal dominant. GeneReviews® [Internet]. Seattle, WA: University of Washington; 2005. Seattle; 1993–2019.
5. Kashani AH, Learned D, Nudleman E, Drenser KA, Capone A, Trese MT. High prevalence of peripheral retinal vascular anomalies in family members of patients with familial exudative vitreoretinopathy. Ophthalmology. 2014;121(1):262–8. https://doi.org/10.1016/j.ophtha.2013.08.010.
6. Yonekawa Y, Thomas BJ, Drenser KA, Trese MT, Capone A Jr. Familial exudative vitreoretinopathy: spectral-domain optical coherence tomography of the vitreoretinal interface, retina, and choroid. Ophthalmology. 2015;122(11):2270–7. https://doi.org/10.1016/j.ophtha.2015.07.024.
7. van Nouhuys CE. Signs, complications, and platelet aggregation in familial exudative vitreoretinopathy. Am J Ophthalmol. 1991;111(1):34–41.
8. Tauqeer Z, Yonekawa Y. Familial exudative vitreoretinopathy: pathophysiology, diagnosis, and management. Asia Pac J Ophthalmol (Phila). 2018;7(3):176–82. https://doi.org/10.22608/APO.201855.
9. Wang Z, Liu CH, Huang S, Chen J. Wnt Signaling in vascular eye diseases. Prog Retin Eye Res. 2018; https://doi.org/10.1016/j.preteyeres.2018.11.008.
10. Collin RW, Nikopoulos K, Dona M, Gilissen C, Hoischen A, Boonstra FN, Poulter JA, Kondo H, Berger W, Toomes C, Tahira T, Mohn LR, Blokland EA, Hetterschijt L, Ali M, Groothuismink JM, Duijkers L, Inglehearn CF, Sollfrank L, Strom TM, Uchio E, van Nouhuys CE, Kremer H, Veltman JA, van Wijk E, Cremers FP. ZNF408 is mutated in familial exudative vitreoretinopathy and is crucial for the development of zebrafish retinal vasculature. Proc Natl Acad Sci U S A. 2013;110(24):9856–61. https://doi.org/10.1073/pnas.1220864110.
11. Jones GE, Ostergaard P, Moore AT, Connell FC, Williams D, Quarrell O, Brady AF, Spier I, Hazan F, Moldovan O, Wieczorek D, Mikat B, Petit F, Coubes C, Saul RA, Brice G, Gordon K, Jeffery S, Mortimer PS, Vasudevan PC, Mansour S. Microcephaly with or without chorioretinopathy, lymphoedema, or mental retardation (MCLMR): review of phenotype associated with KIF11 mutations. Eur J Hum Genet. 2014;22(7):881–7. https://doi.org/10.1038/ejhg.2013.263.
12. Robitaille JM, Gillett RM, LeBlanc MA, Gaston D, Nightingale M, Mackley MP, Parkash S, Hathaway J, Thomas A, Ells A, Traboulsi EI, Heon E, Roy M, Shalev S, Fernandez CV, MacGillivray C, Wallace K, Fahiminiya S, Majewski J, McMaster CR, Bedard K. Phenotypic overlap between familial exudative vitreoretinopathy and microcephaly, lymphedema, and chorioretinal dysplasia caused by KIF11 mutations. JAMA Ophthalmol. 2014;132(12):1393–9. https://doi.org/10.1001/jamaophthalmol.2014.2814.
13. Hu H, Xiao X, Li S, Jia X, Guo X, Zhang Q. KIF11 mutations are a common cause of autosomal dominant familial exudative vitreoretinopathy. Br J Ophthalmol. 2016;100(2):278–83. https://doi.org/10.1136/bjophthalmol-2015-306878.
14. Boldrey EE, Egbert P, Gass JD, Friberg T. The histopathology of familial exudative vitreoretinopathy. A report of two cases. Arch Ophthalmol. 1985;103(2):238–41.
15. Benson WE. Familial exudative vitreoretinopathy. Trans Am Ophthalmol Soc. 1995;93:473–521.
16. Ranchod TM, Ho LY, Drenser KA, Capone A Jr, Trese MT. Clinical presentation of familial exudative vitreoretinopathy. Ophthalmology. 2011;118(10):2070–5. https://doi.org/10.1016/j.ophtha.2011.06.020.
17. Kashani AH, Brown KT, Chang E, Drenser KA, Capone A, Trese MT. Diversity of retinal vascular anomalies in patients with familial

exudative vitreoretinopathy. Ophthalmology. 2014;121(11):2220–7. https://doi.org/10.1016/j.ophtha.2014.05.029.
18. Tasman W, Augsburger JJ, Shields JA, Caputo A, Annesley WH Jr. Familial exudative vitreoretinopathy. Trans Am Ophthalmol Soc. 1981;79:211–26.
19. Ober RR, Bird AC, Hamilton AM, Sehmi K. Autosomal dominant exudative vitreoretinopathy. Br J Ophthalmol. 1980;64(2):112–20.
20. Shukla D, Singh J, Sudheer G, Soman M, John RK, Ramasamy K, Perumalsamy N. Familial exudative vitreoretinopathy (FEVR). Clinical profile and management. Indian J Ophthalmol. 2003;51(4):323–8.
21. Pendergast SD, Trese MT. Familial exudative vitreoretinopathy. Results of surgical management. Ophthalmology. 1998;105(6):1015–23. https://doi.org/10.1016/S0161-6420(98)96002-X.
22. Canny CL, Oliver GL. Fluorescein angiographic findings in familial exudative vitreoretinopathy. Arch Ophthalmol. 1976;94(7):1114–20.
23. Shimouchi A, Takahashi A, Nagaoka T, Ishibazawa A, Yoshida A. Vitreomacular interface in patients with familial exudative vitreoretinopathy. Int Ophthalmol. 2013;33(6):711–5. https://doi.org/10.1007/s10792-012-9707-1.
24. Chen C, Liu C, Wang Z, Sun L, Zhao X, Li S, Luo X, Zhang A, Chong V, Lu L, Ding X. Optical coherence tomography angiography in familial exudative vitreoretinopathy: clinical features and phenotype-genotype correlation. Invest Ophthalmol Vis Sci. 2018;59(15):5726–34. https://doi.org/10.1167/iovs.18-25377.
25. Shields JA, Shields CL, Honavar SG, Demirci H, Cater J. Classification and management of Coats disease: the 2000 Proctor Lecture. Am J Ophthalmol. 2001;131(5):572–83.
26. Shields JA, Shields CL, Honavar SG, Demirci H. Clinical variations and complications of Coats disease in 150 cases: the 2000 Sanford Gifford Memorial Lecture. Am J Ophthalmol. 2001;131(5):561–71.
27. Andersen SR, Warburg M. Norrie's disease: congenital bilateral pseudotumor of the retina with recessive X-chromosomal inheritance; preliminary report. Arch Ophthalmol. 1961;66:614–8.
28. Gilmour DF. Familial exudative vitreoretinopathy and related retinopathies. Eye (Lond). 2015;29(1):1–14. https://doi.org/10.1038/eye.2014.70.
29. Narayanan MJ, Rangasamy S, Narayanan V. Incontinentia pigmenti (Bloch-Sulzberger syndrome). Handb Clin Neurol. 2015;132:271–80. https://doi.org/10.1016/B978-0-444-62702-5.00020-2.
30. Greene-Roethke C. Incontinentia pigmenti: a summary review of this rare ectodermal dysplasia with neurologic manifestations, including treatment protocols. J Pediatr Health Care. 2017;31(6):e45–52. https://doi.org/10.1016/j.pedhc.2017.07.003.
31. Goldberg MF. Persistent fetal vasculature (PFV): an integrated interpretation of signs and symptoms associated with persistent hyperplastic primary vitreous (PHPV). LIV Edward Jackson Memorial Lecture. Am J Ophthalmol. 1997;124(5):587–626.
32. Chen C, Xiao H, Ding X. Persistent fetal vasculature. Asia Pac J Ophthalmol (Phila). 2018; https://doi.org/10.22608/APO.201854.
33. van Nouhuys CE. Juvenile retinal detachment as a complication of familial exudative vitreoretinopathy. Fortschr Ophthalmol. 1989;86(3):221–3.
34. Ikeda T, Fujikado T, Tano Y, Tsujikawa K, Koizumi K, Sawa H, Yasuhara T, Maeda K, Kinoshita S. Vitrectomy for rhegmatogenous or tractional retinal detachment with familial exudative vitreoretinopathy. Ophthalmology. 1999;106(6):1081–5. https://doi.org/10.1016/S0161-6420(99)90268-3.
35. Yamane T, Yokoi T, Nakayama Y, Nishina S, Azuma N. Surgical outcomes of progressive tractional retinal detachment associated with familial exudative vitreoretinopathy. Am J Ophthalmol. 2014;158(5):1049–55. https://doi.org/10.1016/j.ajo.2014.08.009.
36. Slusher MM, Hutton WE. Familial exudative vitreoretinopathy. Am J Ophthalmol. 1979;87(2):152–6.

Persistent Fetal Vasculature

26

Limei Sun, Chonglin Chen, and Xiaoyan Ding

Abstract

Persistent fetal vasculature (PFV), previously called as persistent hyperplastic vitreous (PHPV), is a congenital ocular anomaly in which the fetal hyaloid vasculature network fails to regress partially or completely. Ninety-five percent of PFV cases are unilateral. The clinical manifestations of PFV are highly diverse, including glaucoma, cataract, falciform retinal folds, funnel or stalk-shaped retinal detachment, spontaneous fundus hemorrhage, and a congenitally small eye. In this chapter, we describe the diversity of various clinical manifestations.

Keywords

Persistent fetal vasculature · Glaucoma · Cataract
Falciform retinal folds · Stalk-shaped retinal detachment

Intraocular fetal vascular system is critical for the development of the eye. During early embryogenesis, the intraocular fetal vascular system arises from the optic nerve head, extends through the central vitreous, surrounds the developing crystalline lens, reaches and finally, nourishes the anterior segment of the eye. Timely regression of the fetal vascular system before birth is critical for the development of a clear optical pathway. Only an acellular hyaloid canal, which is called as the Cloquet's canal, in the center of the vitreous cavity from the optic disc to the posterior capsule of the lens, could be left [1].

Persistent fetal vasculature (PFV), previously called as persistent hyperplastic vitreous (PHPV), is a congenital ocular anomaly in which the fetal hyaloid vasculature network fails to regress partially or completely [1, 2]. This disease was first reported by Cloquet in 1818 [3] and since then it has been called by various names, including persistent posterior fetal fibrovascular sheath of the lens, persistent tunica vasculosalentis, congenital retinal septum, and ablation falciform [1, 4]. It was divided into three categories based on the location of the vascular abnormalities—anterior, posterior, and combined PHPV. In 1997, Goldberg proposed to place all the anterior, posterior, and combined manifestations into the same category with a general name—Persistent fetal vasculature (PFV) [4]. This novel term has gradually replaced the older PHPV in recent years, since it reflects a more accurate description of anatomic and pathologic features of this disease.

26.1 Classification of PFV

26.1.1 Laterality of PFV

PFV accounts for about 5% of blindness in childhood in the United States [5]. Notably, 95% of PFV cases are affected unilaterally. Although rare, bilateral cases have been noted in some cases (Figs. 26.1 and 26.2). This unilateral onset is an important clue in distinguishing it from other bilateral diseases, such as retinopathy of prematurity (ROP) or familial exudative vitreoretinopathy (FEVR).

26.1.2 Anterior, Posterior, and Combined PFV

PFV could be divided into three categories based on the location of the vascular abnormalities. Anterior PFV is relatively common, accounting for approximately 25% of cases, and is characterized by a shallow anterior chamber, elongation of ciliary processes, cataracts, and retrolental opacity (Figs. 26.3 and 26.4). Posterior PFV mainly involves the vitreous and the retina and accounts for 12% of PFV patients. It may manifest as a stalk from the optic nerve, retinal proliferative membrane, retinal fold, retinal detachment, or optic nerve

L. Sun · C. Chen · X. Ding (✉)
State Key Laboratory of Ophthalmology, Zhongshan Ophthalmic Center, SunYat-Sen University, Guangzhou, China
e-mail: dingxiaoyan@gzzoc.com

W.-C. Wu, W.-C. Lam (eds.), *A Quick Guide to Pediatric Retina*, https://doi.org/10.1007/978-981-15-6552-6_26

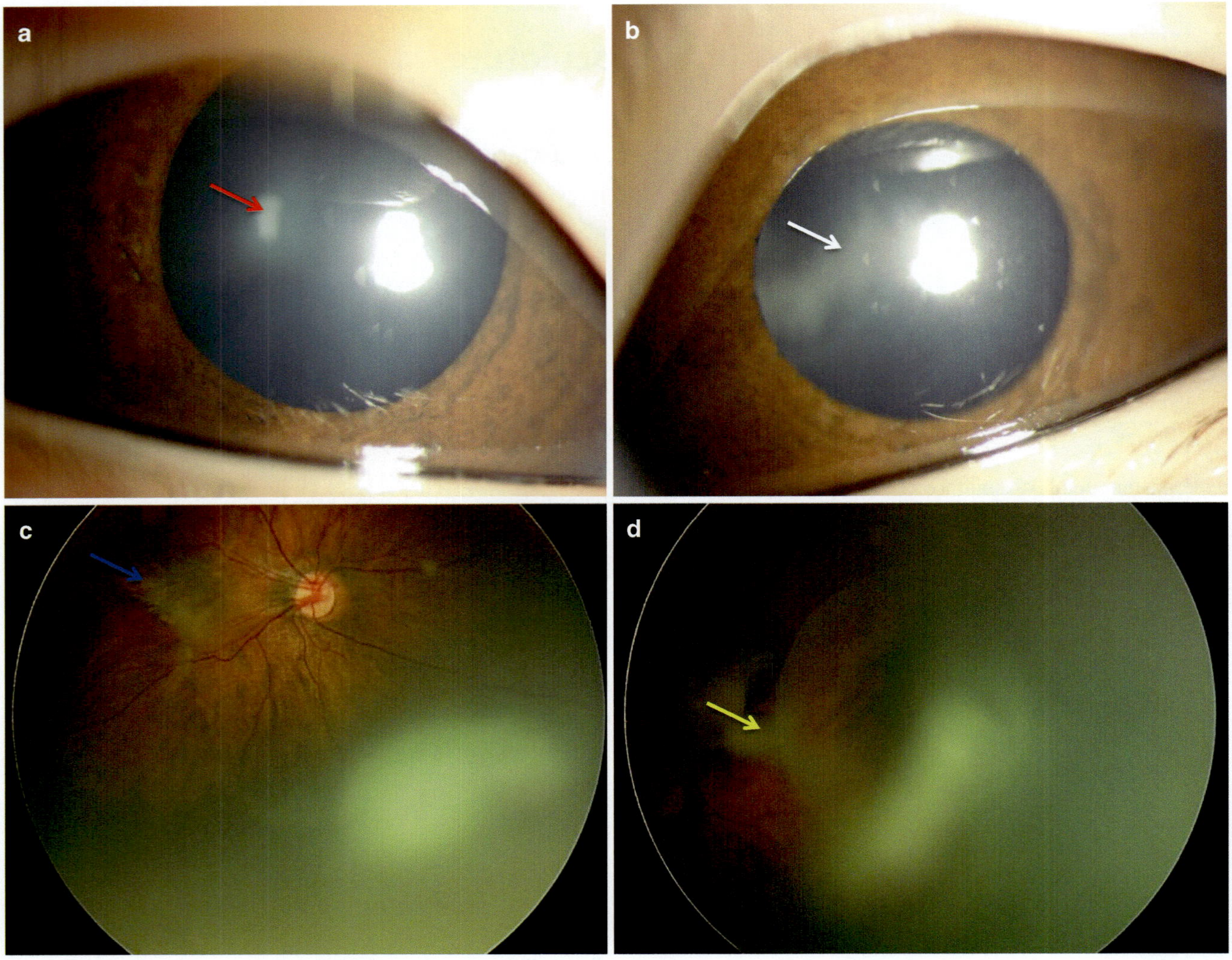

Fig. 26.1 Bilateral PFV. A 4-month-old boy with bilateral PFV. No other systemic syndromes were found. The genetic screening failed to identify any known genetic mutation. Focal (**a**, red arrow) and diffuse (**b**, white arrow) opacity on the posterior capsule of lens could be noted in his right (**a**) and left (**b**) eyes, respectively. A wide (**d**, yellow arrow) stalk from the optic disc to the posterior capsule of lens is remarkable. Note that in his right eye, a thick preretinal membrane is present in the macular area (**c**, blue arrow)

hypoplasia. Combined PFV, which is the most common type involving both the anterior and posterior segments, accounts for about 60% of all cases.

26.2 Clinical Manifestations of PFV

The clinical manifestations of PFV are highly diverse. Each of the anatomic abnormalities is associated with partial or complete persistence of the fetal vasculature and thus can be considered a limited expression of the complete PFV syndrome [4–7]. The defects include glaucoma, cataract, falciform retinal folds, funnel or stalk-shaped retinal detachment, spontaneous fundus hemorrhage, a congenitally small eye.

26.2.1 Anterior PFV

1. *Persistent pupillary membranes*

Remnants of the capillaries may persist as small strands attached to the iris, or the membrane-like lesion located in the pupillary area (Fig. 26.3). These loops, strands, or membranes are remnants of the anterior tunica vasculosalentis, which is the blood supply during lens development of the fetus. Visual acuity is compromised only when the membrane becomes thick or intact (Fig. 26.4), which causes deprivational amblyopia. It should be noted that in some cases, the lens behind the membrane might be totally transparent, presenting without any opacity of the lens itself. Lens should be gently protected when removing the pupillary

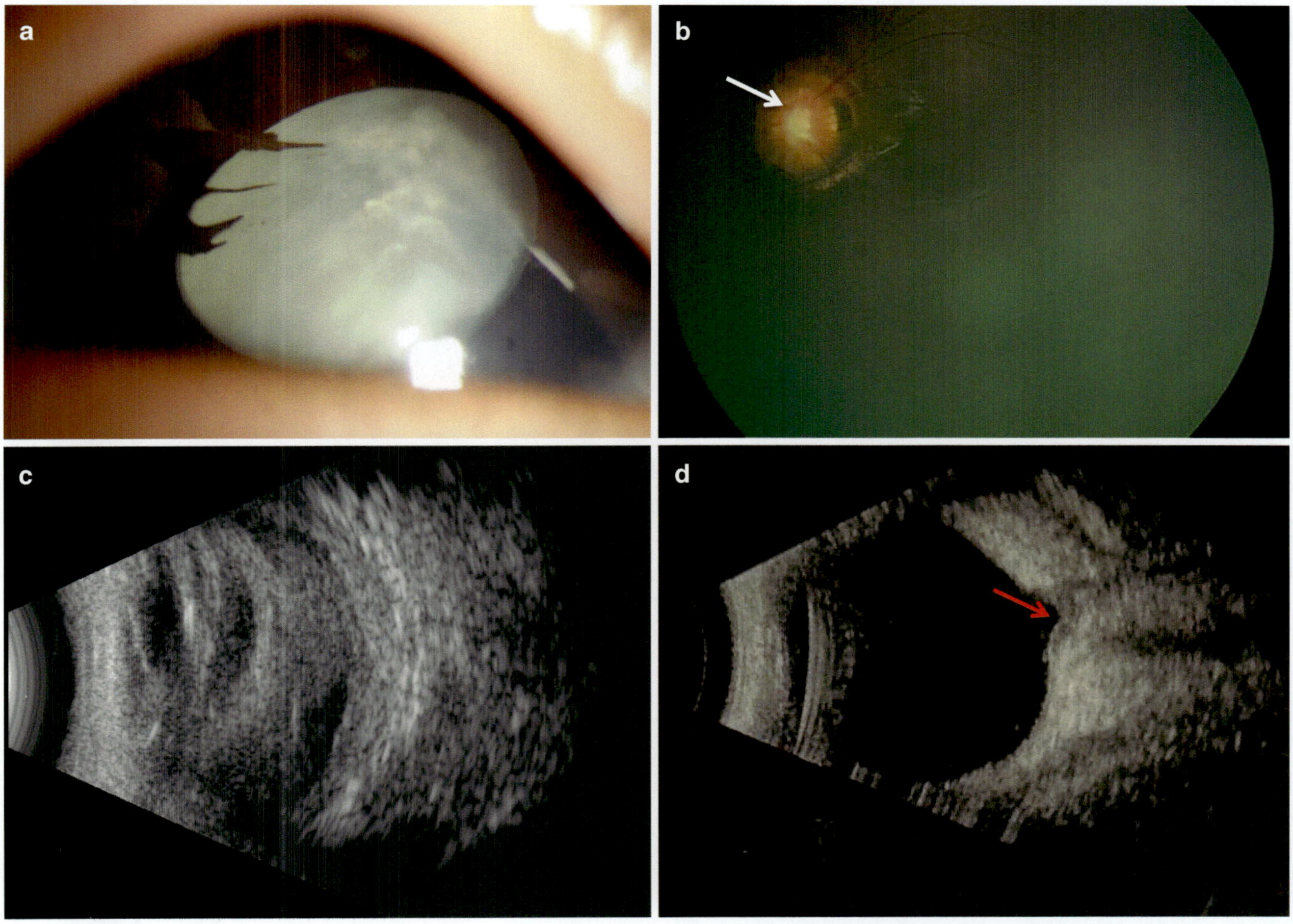

Fig. 26.2 Bilateral PFV manifested with cataract and morning glory syndrome. A 7-month-old girl presented with posterior fetal fibrovascular membrane posterior to the lens (**a**) and retrolental fibrovascular stalk (**c**) in her right eye. The optic nerve appears large and funneled and straight retinal vessels arise from the disc margin in the left eye (**b**, white arrow). Ultrasonography shows a conical excavation of the dysplastic optic disc (**d**, red arrow)

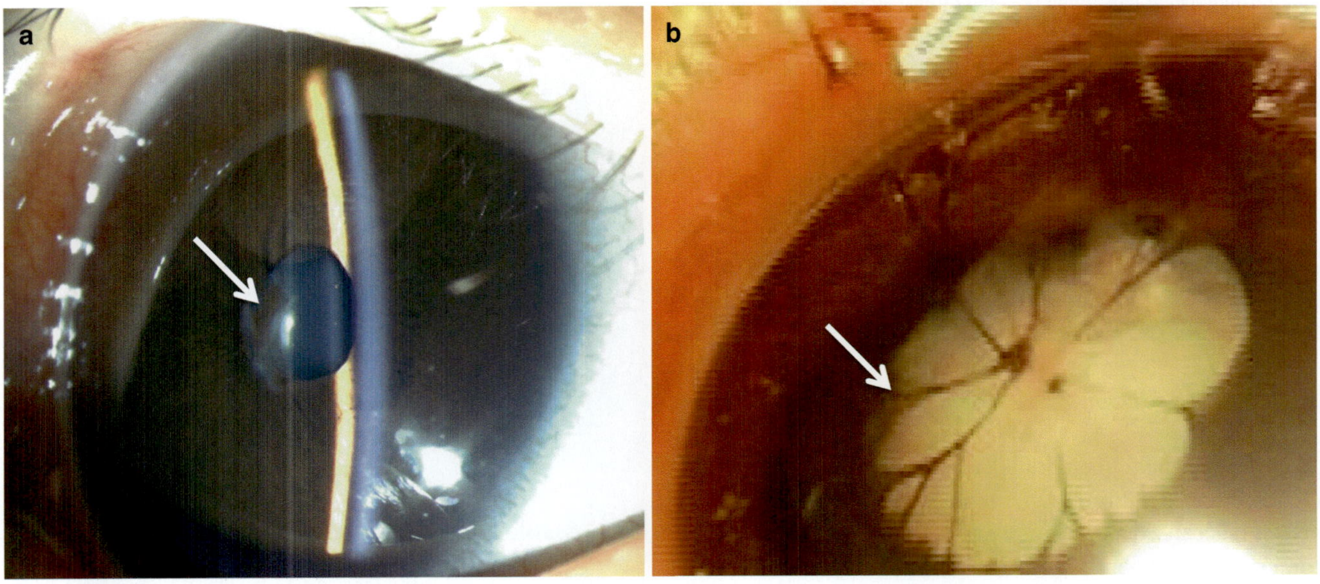

Fig. 26.3 Partial persistent pupillary membranes in two PFV patients. A 5-month-old boy presented with a visible papillary membrane at the nasal side of his left eye (**a**, white arrow). A 2-year-old boy presented with a visible papillary membrane, iris dysplasia, and cataract in his left eye (**b**, white arrow)

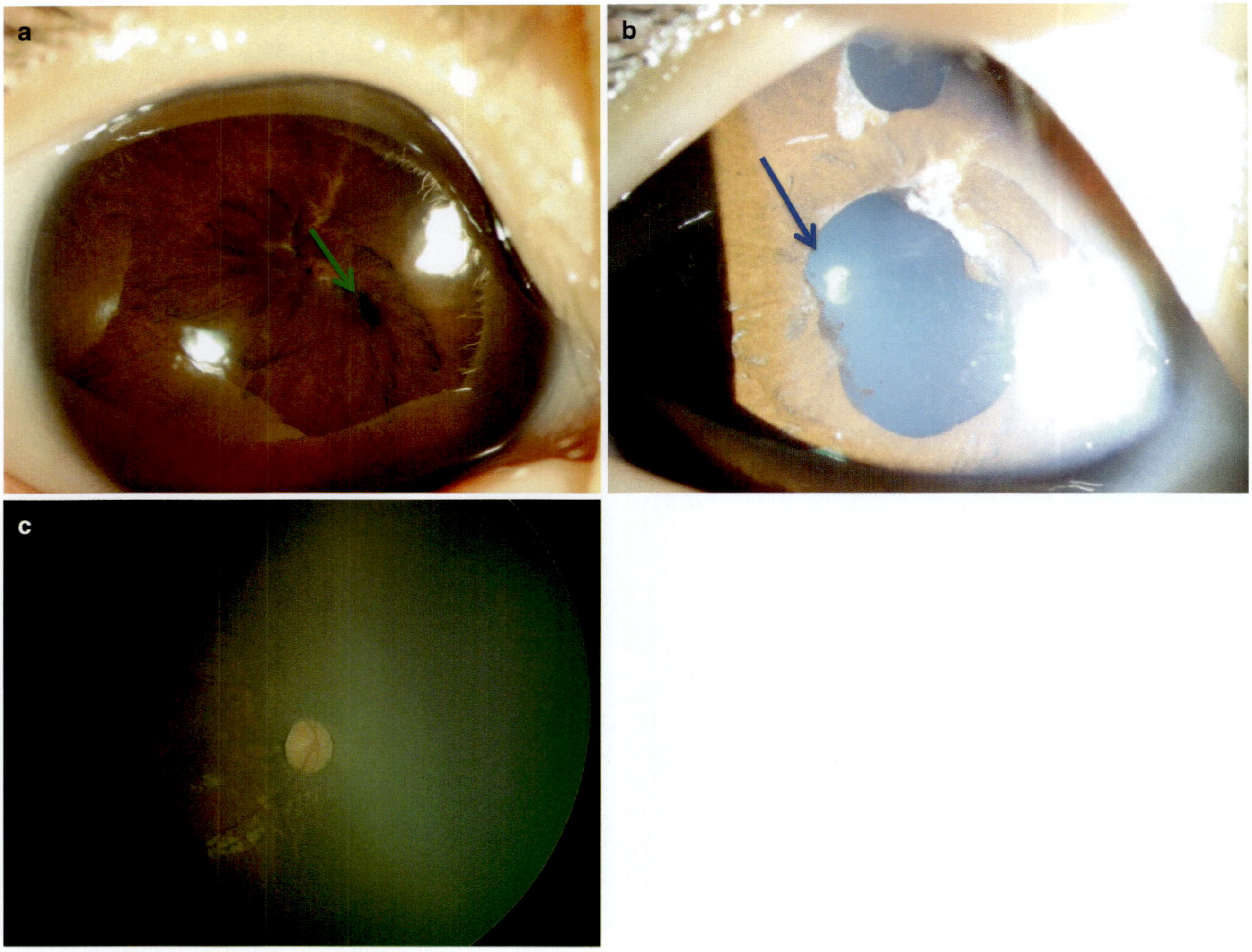

Fig. 26.4 Persistent pupillary membranes. A 6-month-old girl with a papillary membrane covered the pupil area in her right eye (green arrow, **a**). The pupil is as small as a pinhole, and ectopic. It is notable that the underneath lens might be totally transparent. Gently manipulations are highly recommended during the surgery. Figure (**b**) showed the enlarged pupil (blue arrow) 1 month after the surgery. Wide-field funduscopy showed that the fundus is unremarkable (**c**)

membrane during the surgery. In some cases, congenital cataract or retrolental fibrous tissue could be seen.

2. *Mittendorf dot*

The Mitterndorf dot is a local white dot located on the posterior lens capsule, usually about 0.5 mm nasal to the posterior pole. It is caused by the remnants of the regression hyaloid artery.

3. *Retrolental Membrane*

The retrolental membrane, classically called PHPV, is characterized by fibrous membranes located in retrolental space. It is caused by the failure of regression of the posterior tunica vasculosa lentis (Fig. 26.5). Typically, the retrolental membrane is a white membrane with vessels. Elongated ciliary processes can be found, which is due to the proliferation

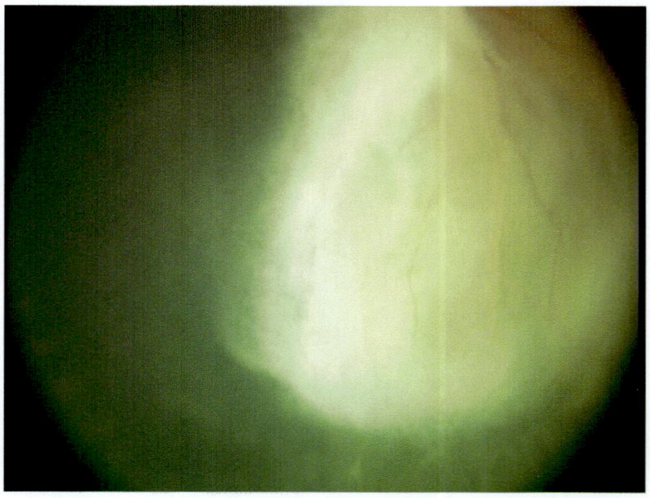

Fig. 26.5 Retrolental membrane. An 11-month-old boy with a white fibrous membrane covering the entire posterior surface of the lens in his left eye. There are vessels on the membrane. The fundus is invisible

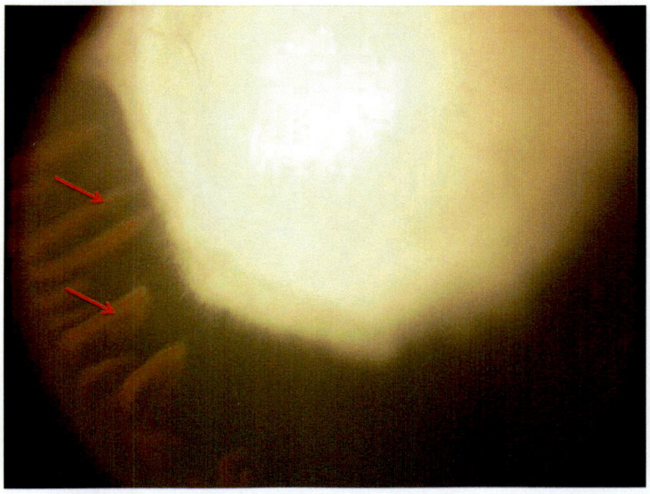

Fig. 26.6 Retrolental membrane with elongated ciliary processes. A 1.5-year-old girl presented with a yellowish-white retrolenticular fibrovascular membrane in her right eye, and the ciliary processes are centrally dragged and elongated (red arrows) shown by Retcam wide-field funduscopy

and concentric traction of the remnant posterior tunica vasculosa lentis (Fig. 26.6).

4. *Leukocoria*

Leukocoria is one of the most commonly reported symptoms by the parents of children with PFV. The white pupil is due to cataract (minority of patients, Fig. 26.7) or the retrolental membrane (majority of the patients). In most cases, the proliferating fibrous membrane is attached to the posterior lens capsule, leading to the appearance of cataract (Fig. 26.8).

5. *Spontaneous intralenticular bleeding*

Spontaneous intralenticular bleeding is reported as a rare manifestation of anterior PFV. The underlying mechanism is not clear. In some patients, the hallmark stalk could be identified; however, in other cases, no intraocular stalks or tractions are found (Fig. 26.9).

26.2.2 Posterior PFV

6. *Bergmeister papilla*

A Bergmeister papilla manifests as a membranous or short band-like lesion attached to the optic disc, which is the incomplete regression of the posterior part of the hyaloid artery [5]. The Bergmeister papilla itself will not affect visual function, if the remnant causes no macula traction.

26.2.3 Combined PFV

7. *Congenital hyaloid stalk*

The primary vitreous, containing the hyaloid artery, locates between the optic disc and lens posterior capsule (Figs. 26.10 and 26.11).

8. *Tent-shaped retinal detachment*

The remnant hyaloid artery and the vicinity proliferates and adheres to the retina, causing partial retinal traction and thus leading to tent-shaped retinal detachment (Fig. 26.12). Macular abnormalities are secondary to tent-shaped or other tractional retinal detachments.

9. *Morning Glory syndrome*

Optic nerve abnormalities were also found in children with combined PFV. In about 25% of children who were diagnosed with Morning Glory syndrome, the remnants of persistent fetal vasculature could be identified (Figs. 26.13 and 26.14). However, the falciform retinal detachment in retinopathy of prematurity or familial exudative vitreoretinopathy should be distinguished from the tent-shaped retinal detachment more typical of PFV.

10. *Microophthalmia/phthisis bulbi and buphthalmia*

End stage of PFV is usually accompanied by the arrested development of the eyeball. Microphthalmia and *buphthalmia* are severe complications of combined PFV.

Without treatment, the majority of the combined PFV is stable with a lack of visual function (Fig. 26.15). However, in some cases, PFV can lead to corneal opacification, shallowing of the anterior chamber, spontaneous intraocular bleeding, and secondary glaucoma. These complications usually occur suddenly within the first 3 years of life. In the progressive cases, the prognosis is quite poor (Fig. 26.16). Sometimes, enucleation of the eyeball is required due to either painful, uncontrolled intraocular pressure or phthisis bulbi.

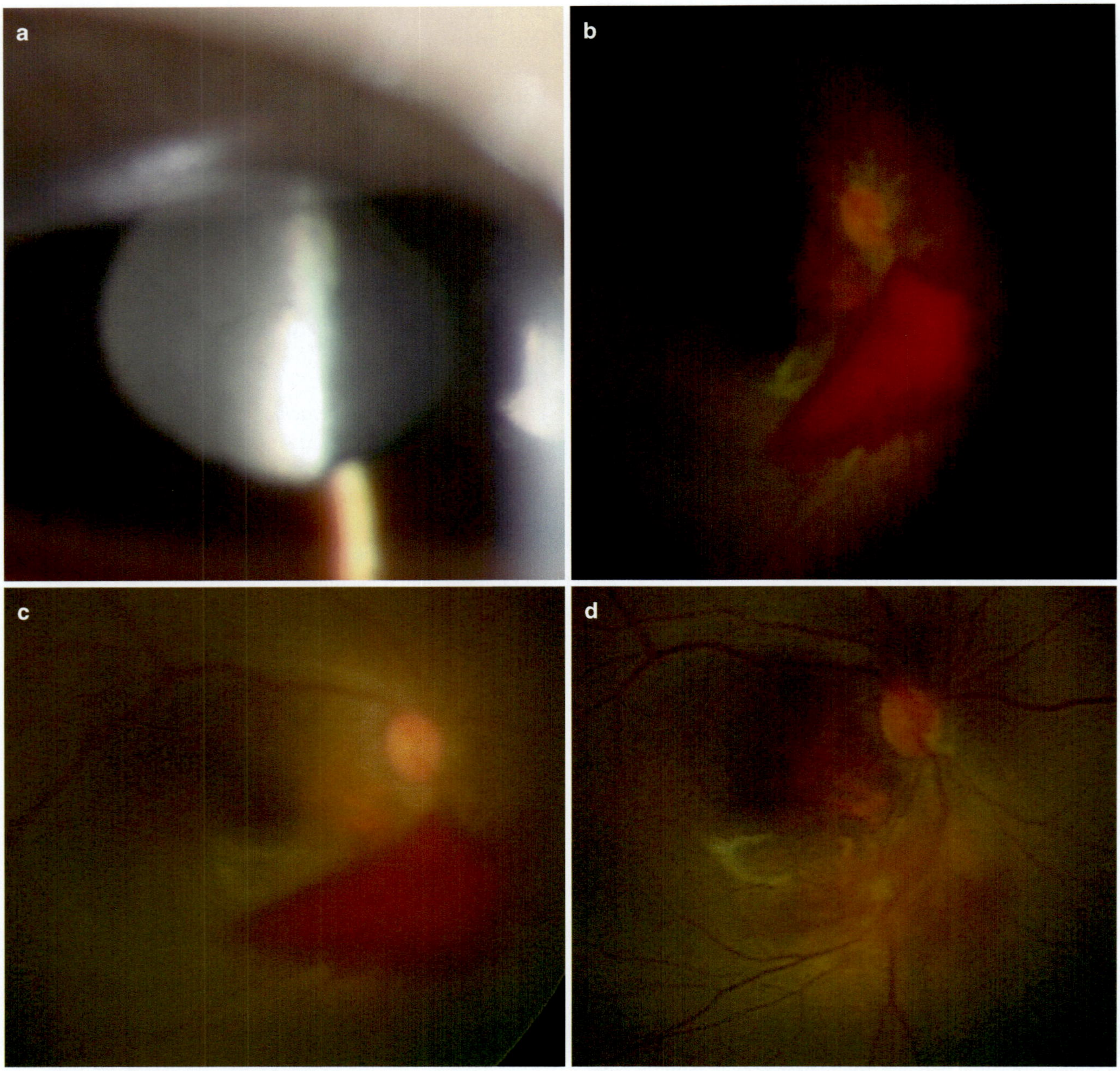

Fig. 26.7 Vitreous hemorrhage after the cataract removal in PFV. A 4-month-old girl presented with unilateral cataract associated with PFV in her right eye (**a**). The axial length is 16 mm, which is shorter than that of her left eye (18 mm). The depth of right anterior chamber is 0.9 mm, but 1.3 mm in her left eye. However, the lens was thicker (3.9 mm) in her right eye when compared to that of her left eye (3.6 mm). After removing the cataract, mild hemorrhage from the regressed stalk was observed during the surgery. The hemorrhage was well-demarcated on the 1st day postoperatively (**b**). However, the bleeding was gradually resolved after 2 weeks (**c**) and completely disappeared after 3 months (**d**)

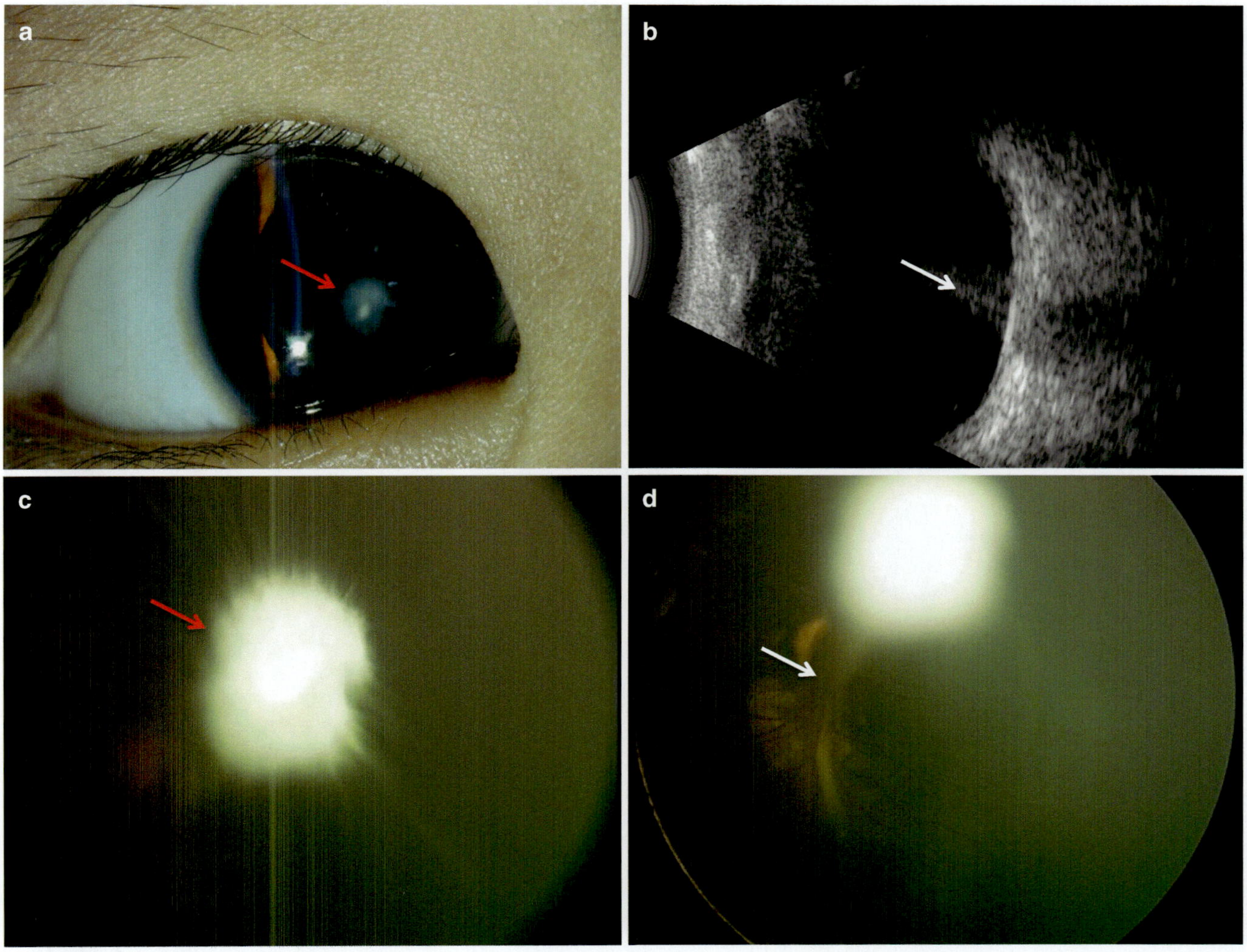

Fig. 26.8 Retrolental membrane and vitreous stalk in PFV. A 3-year-old girl presented with unilateral PFV in her right eye. The hyaloid artery and proliferative tissues were seen between the posterior lens capsule and the optic papilla. Notably, the lens itself is transparent (**a**). The stalk reached the posterior lens capsule (**c**, red arrow); The posterior pole retina is tractionally detached (**d**, white arrow); a tent-shaped lesion was located inferior to the optic disc (**b**, **d**, white arrow)

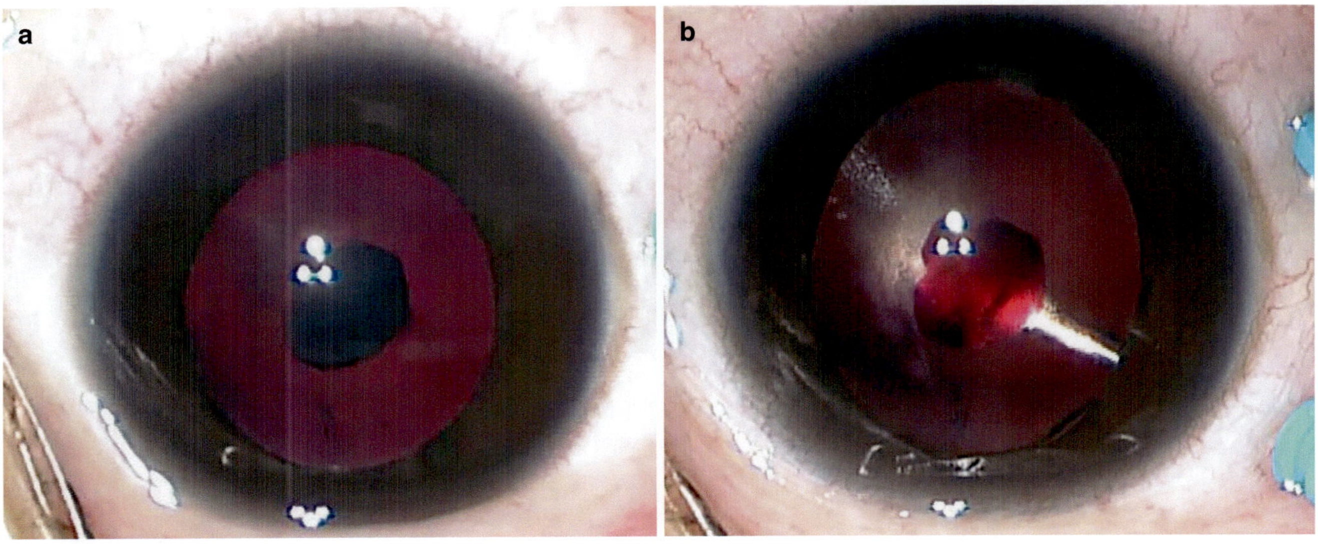

Fig. 26.9 Spontaneous intralenticular hemorrhage. A 3-year-old boy presented with visual decrease in his left eye for 1 month. The intralenticular central bleeding was noted (**a**). The bleeding is located between the posterior capsule and the lens cortex (**b**). These pictures are snapshots from surgery video

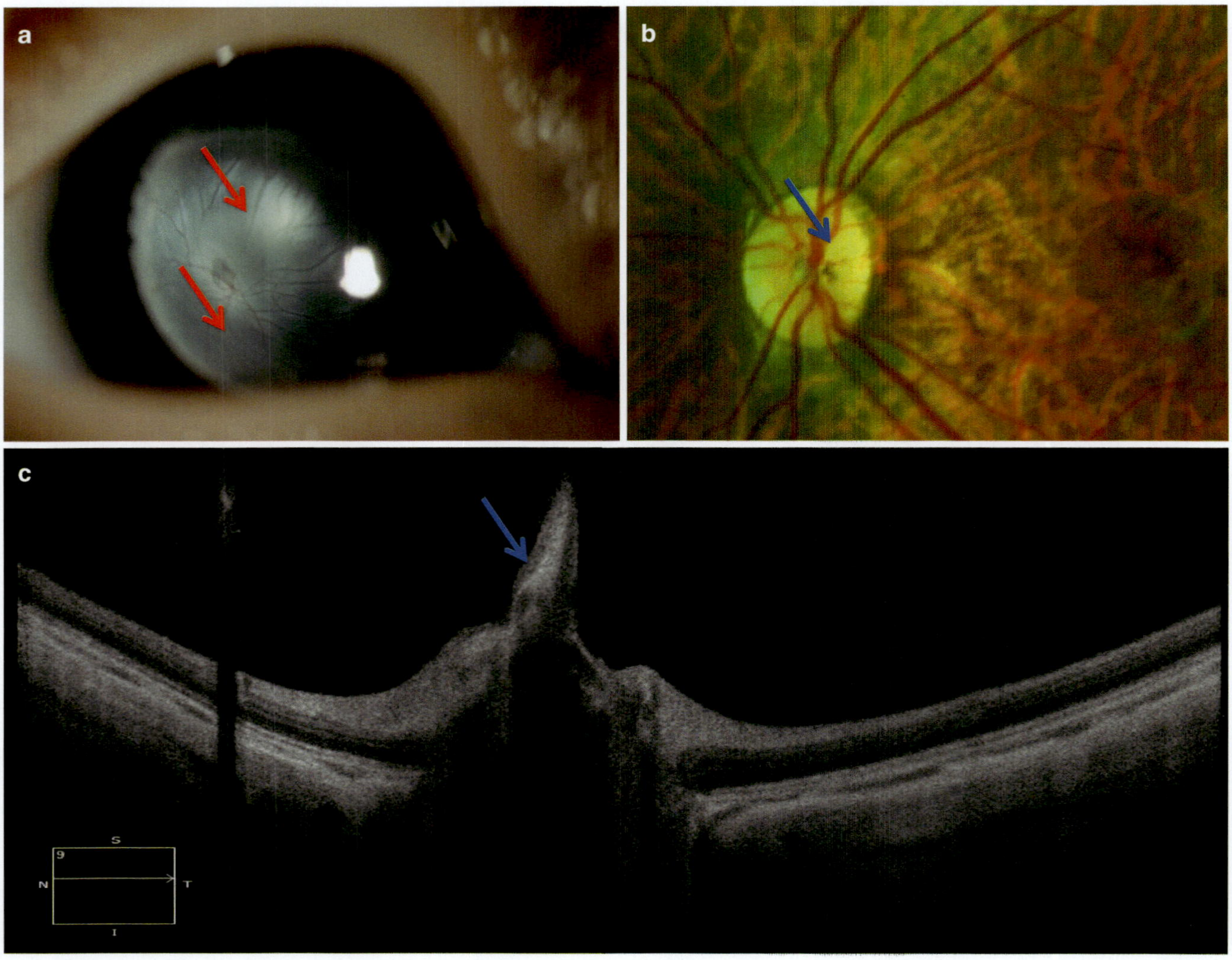

Fig. 26.10 Remnant of hyaloid artery arising from the optic nerve. A 1-year-old girl with unilateral retrolenticular vascular fibrotic membrane in her left eye (red arrows, **a**) After cataract removal, a remnant from the optic nerve (blue arrow) could be found (**b**) and could be detected with OCT (**c**). This patient was diagnosed as combined PFV

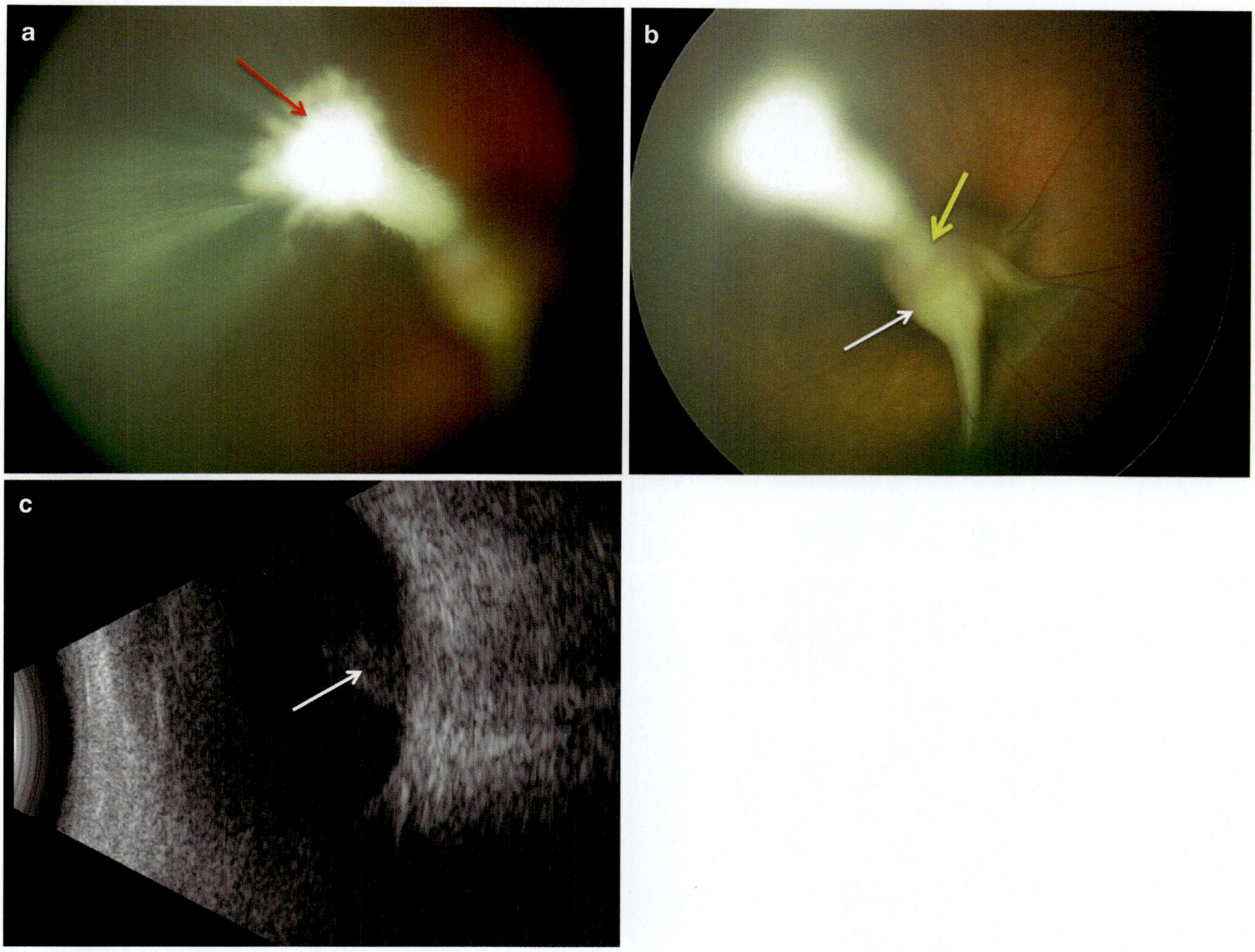

Fig. 26.11 Combined PFV with a vitreous stalk and tractional detached retina. A 6-month-old boy presented with the primary vitreous which contained the hyaloid artery and was located between lens posterior capsule (**a**, red arrow) the optic disc. Retinal traction leads to tent-shaped retinal detachment (**b**, **c**, white arrows). The yellow arrow indicated the junction of the remnant vessels and the detached retina

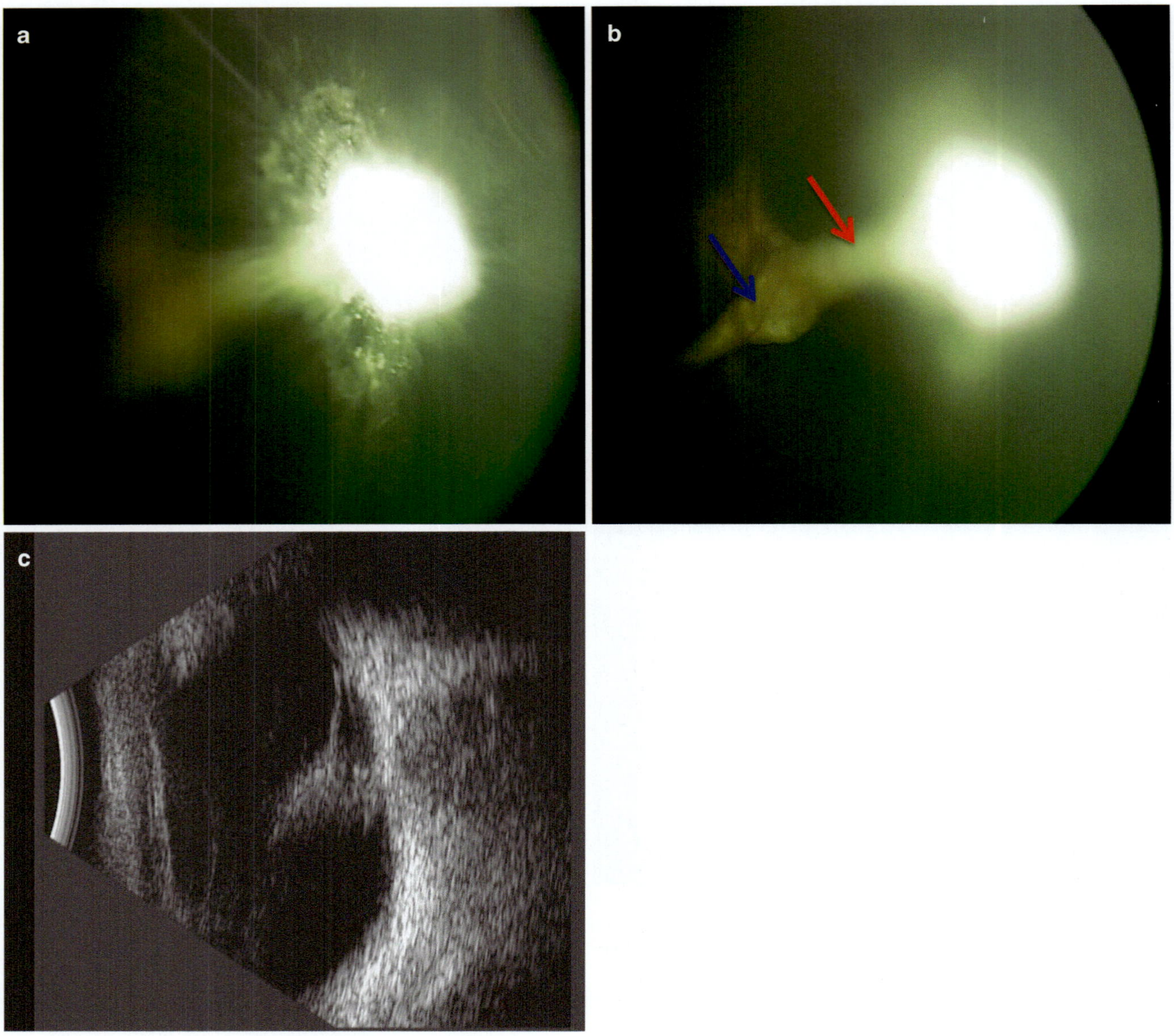

Fig. 26.12 Combined PFV with phthisis bulbi. A 1-year-old boy presented with partial retrolenticular opacity. Radial traction of the anterior vitreous cortex was noted (**a**). A stalk was noted between the optic nerve and the lens (**c**). There are two components in the stalk: the remnant hyaloid vessels with proliferative tissues (red arrow) and the tent-shaped detached retina (**b**, blue arrow). The macula was also tractional detached, indicating poor visual function. The axial length was very short shown on B-scan

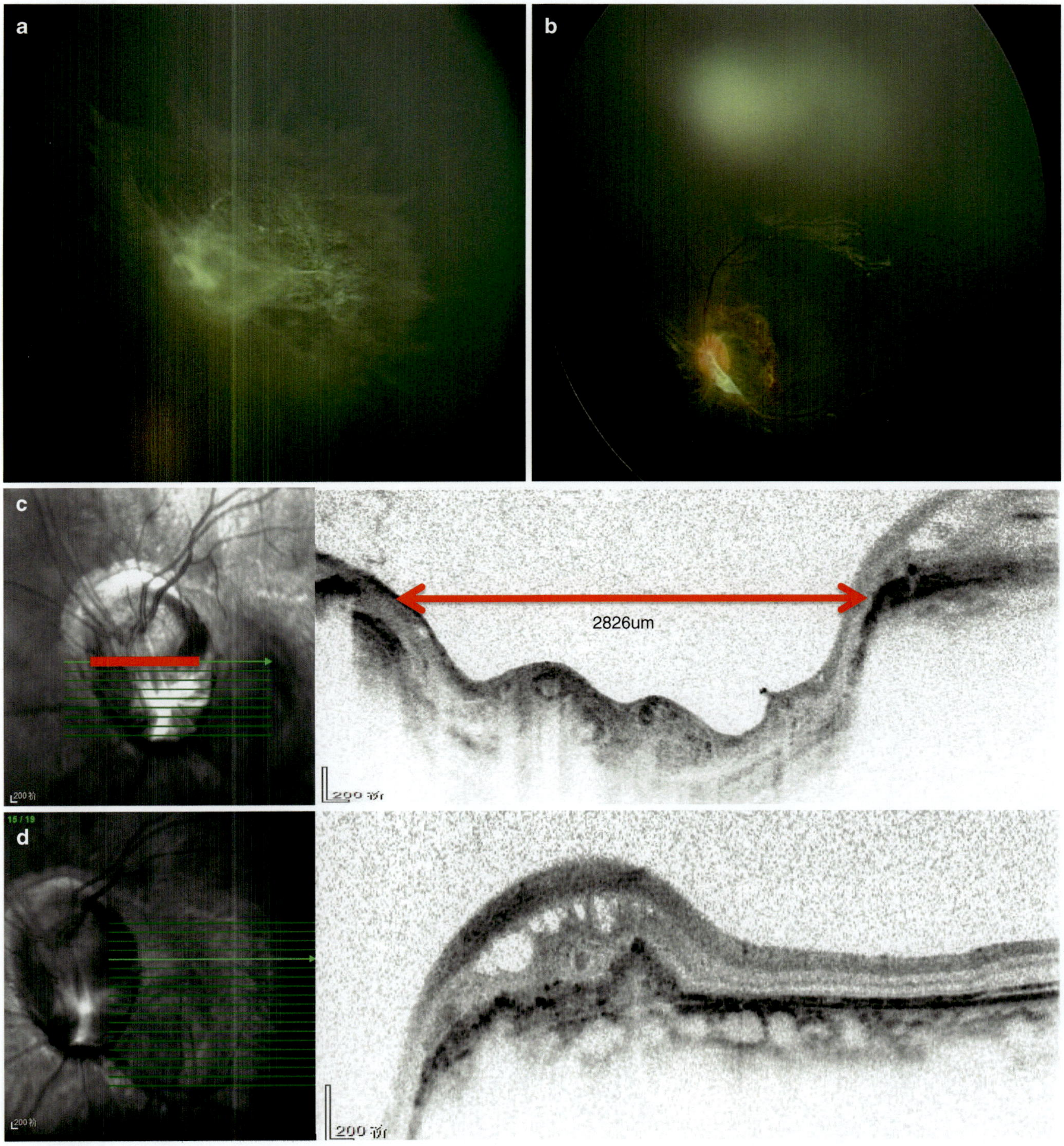

Fig. 26.13 Combined PFV with morning glory syndrome (MGS). Figure (**a**) is focusing the posterior lenticular membrane, which is thin, gray, and irregular. Figure (**b**) is focusing on the optic disc, which is abnormally enlarged. (**c**) The optic disc is dented and enlarged, which with a horizontal diameter of 2800 μm. (**d**) There was some intraretinal fluid (space) in the inner layers of the retina. The mechanisms and the clinical significance of this intraretinal fluid are still not elucidated

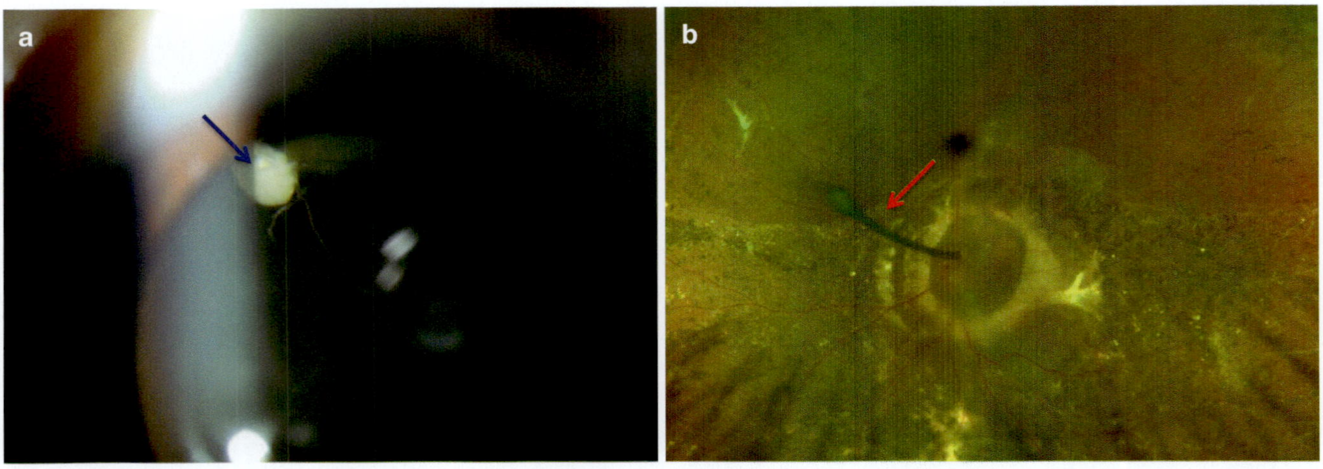

Fig. 26.14 Combined PFV with morning glory syndrome (MGS). The left eye of a 26-year-old male presented with a stalk adherent between the posterior capsule of lens (**a**, blue arrow) and the optic disc where his disc is enlarged and excavated like a morning glory (**b**, red arrow)

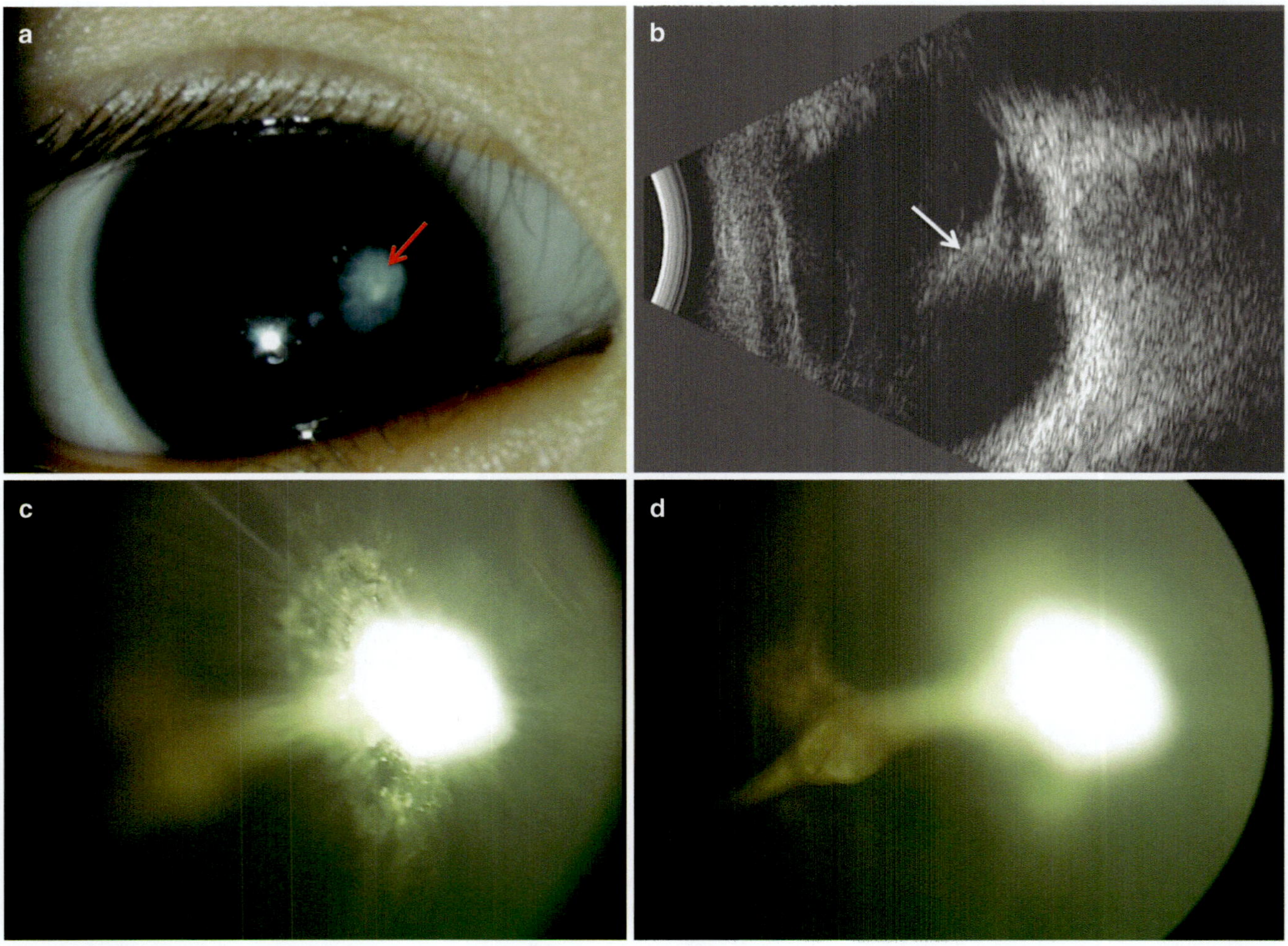

Fig. 26.15 Stable PFV. An 11-month-old boy with the primary vitreous located between the posterior lens capsule (**a**, red arrow) and the optic papilla (**b**, white arrow) in his left eye. Figure (**c**) focuses on the posterior capsule cataract and figure and Figure (**d**) focuses on the tent-like retinal detachment, in which the macula is involved. With the wide-field photography, shadow retinal detachment with profound sub-retinal fibrosis is noted (**e**). The lesion is stable, nonprogressive during the follow-up of 3 years

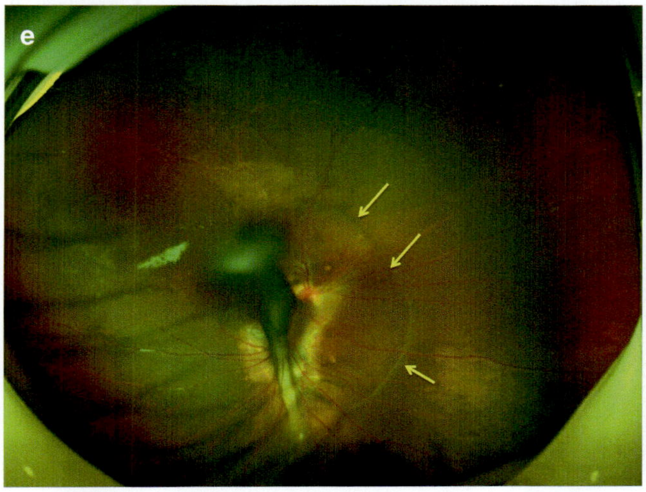

Fig. 26.15 (continued)

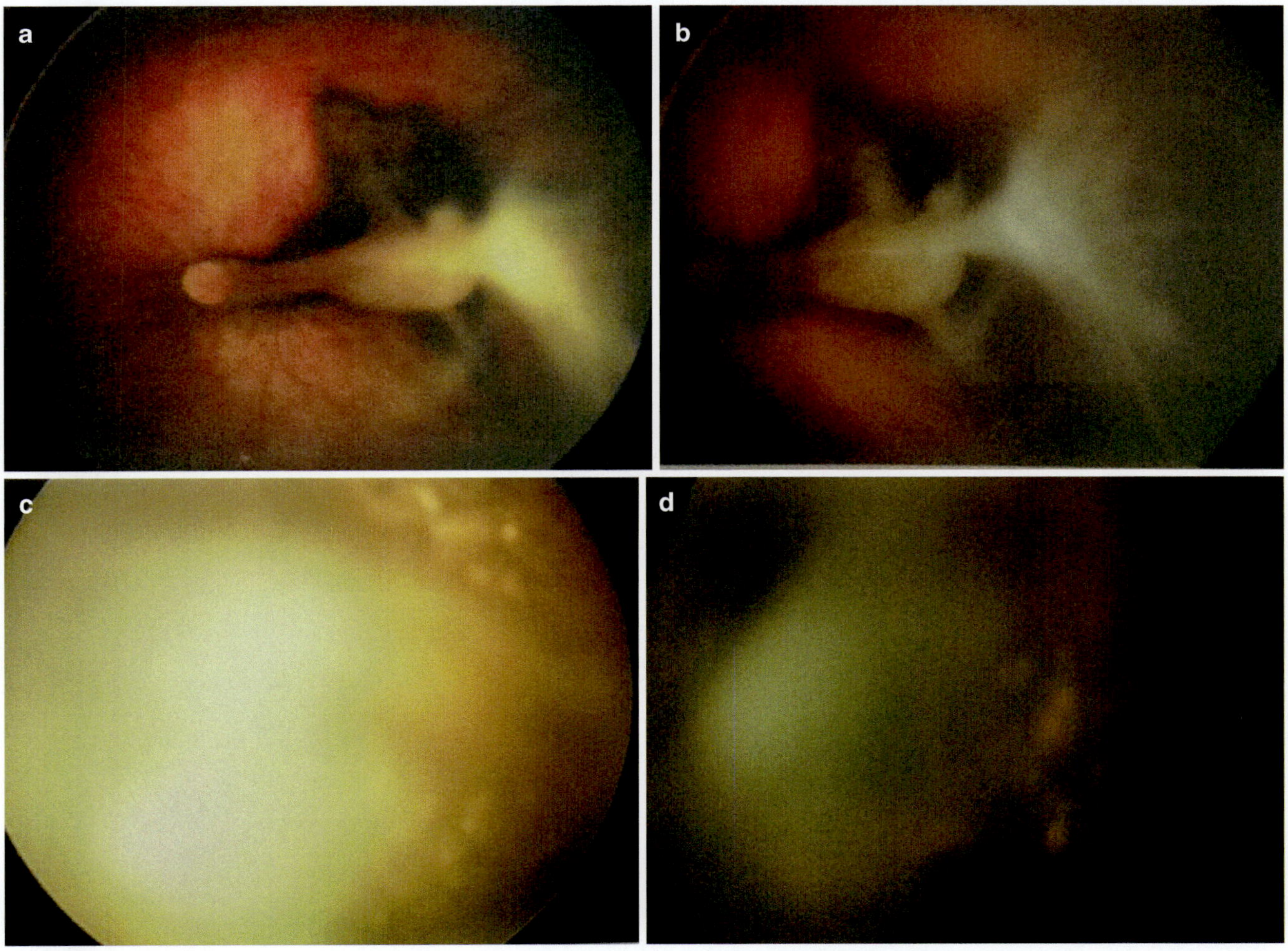

Fig. 26.16 Progressive PFV. A 10-month-old girl with combined PFV from the optic disc to the posterior capsule of lens in her right eye (**a**, **b**). This girl suffered eye pain after 18 months. End-stage lesions including disappearance of the anterior chamber, vitreous hemorrhage, and total retinal detachment was noted (**c**, **d**)

References

1. Reese AB. Persistent hyperplastic primary vitreous. Trans Am Acad Ophthalmol Otolaryngol. 1955;59(3):271–95.
2. Sanghvi DA, Sanghvi CA, Purandare NC. Bilateral persistent hyperplastic primary vitreous. Australas Radiol. 2005;49(1):72–4.
3. Gulati N, Eagle RC Jr, Tasman W. Unoperated eyes with persistent fetal vasculature. Trans Am Ophthalmol Soc. 2003;101:59–64; discussion 5.
4. Goldberg MF. Persistent fetal vasculature (PFV): an integrated interpretation of signs and symptoms associated with persistent hyperplastic primary vitreous (PHPV). LIV Edward Jackson Memorial Lecture. Am J Ophthalmol. 1997;124(5):587–626.
5. Santos-Bueso E, Asorey-Garcia A, Vinuesa-Silva JM, Garcia-Sanchez J. Bergmeister's papilla. Arch Soc Esp Oftalmol. 2015;90(8):395–6.
6. Manschot WA. Persistent hyperplastic primary vitreous; special reference to preretinal glial tissue as a pathological characteristic and to the development of the primary vitreous. AMA Arch Ophthalmol. 1958;59(2):188–203.
7. Anteby I, Cohen E, Karshai I, BenEzra D. Unilateral persistent hyperplastic primary vitreous: course and outcome. J AAPOS. 2002;6(2):92–9.

Pediatric Uveitis

27

Koh-Hei Sonoda

Abstract

Pediatric uveitis differs from adult-onset uveitis and needs special attention to its diagnosis and therapies. Children with uveitis are often asymptomatic and the uveitis is often chronic and persistent.

Keywords

Juvenile idiopathic arthritis · Tubulointerstitial nephritis and uveitis syndrome · Brau syndrome · Ocular toxoplasmosis · Cat-scratch disease

27.1 Juvenile Idiopathic Arthritis

Juvenile idiopathic arthritis (JIA) is the common rheumatic disease in children and there are several subtypes (such as oligoarticular, polyarticular, and systemic) that are classified based on the clinical presentation and laboratory markers. Chronic uveitis is a common manifestation and is potentially sight-threatening and thus carries a considerable risk of reduction in quality of life. "Oligoarticular JIA" is a major form of JIA, which occurs typically in pre-school girls with single knee or ankle involvement. Although blood tests including rheumatoid factor and radiographs are often normal, this is a high-risk group of "uveitis."

JIA-associated uveitis is non-granulomatous inflammation which is sometimes asymptomatic in the initial stage. The ocular inflammation is initially limited in the anterior part in most of the case (Fig. 27.1), but eventually expands to the posterior part, and sometimes cause significant damage (Fig. 27.2). Complications may include band keratopathy in the visual axis (Fig. 27.1c, d), posterior synechiae (Fig. 27.1a, b), cataract (Fig. 27.1a–d), hypotony, secondary glaucoma, epiretinal membrane, cystoid macular edema, and optic nerve edema (Fig. 27.2).

The cooperation of ophthalmologists with rheumatologists will help perform accurate diagnosis and define the best treatment plan. Methotrexate is recommended in patients with severe uveitis [1]. The ophthalmic therapeutic regimen includes mydriatic and topical corticosteroid, while systemic corticosteroid and biological drugs are introduced in severe cases. Surgical treatment for ocular complications such as cataract and epiretinal membrane is sometimes needed. Systemic glucocorticoid is used for severe complications such as severe refractory uveitis and macrophage activation syndrome as bridging therapy while waiting for the full effect of disease-modifying anti-rheumatic drugs (DMARDs).

The tumor necrosis factor-α inhibitors are the most commonly employed biological drugs for JIA-associated uveitis. Adalimumab has been proven very successful in aiding corticosteroid therapy in different non-infectious uveitis. A recently published randomized controlled trial provides convincing evidence for the use of Adalimumab in patients who fail to respond to methotrexate [2]. Other biological agents that have been investigated to treat the disease include drugs that target lymphocyte co-stimulation and signals cytokine receptors. Tocilizumab and abatacept are considered to alternatives in children inadequately treated with TNFα inhibitors [3].

27.2 Tubulointerstitial Nephritis and Uveitis Syndrome

Tubulointerstitial nephritis and uveitis (TINU) syndrome is an important cause of uveitis in children. Dobrin et al. initially reported it as an inflammatory granulomatous syndrome [4]. Classically, patients present renal impairment due to acute interstitial nephritis, combined with bone marrow granuloma, bilateral anterior uveitis, and an increased erythrocyte sedimentation rate. A hypersensitivity reaction

K.-H. Sonoda (✉)
Department of Ophthalmology, Graduate School of Medical Sciences, Kyushu University, Fukuoka, Japan
e-mail: sonodak@med.kyushu-u.ac.jp

W.-C. Wu, W.-C. Lam (eds.), *A Quick Guide to Pediatric Retina*, https://doi.org/10.1007/978-981-15-6552-6_27

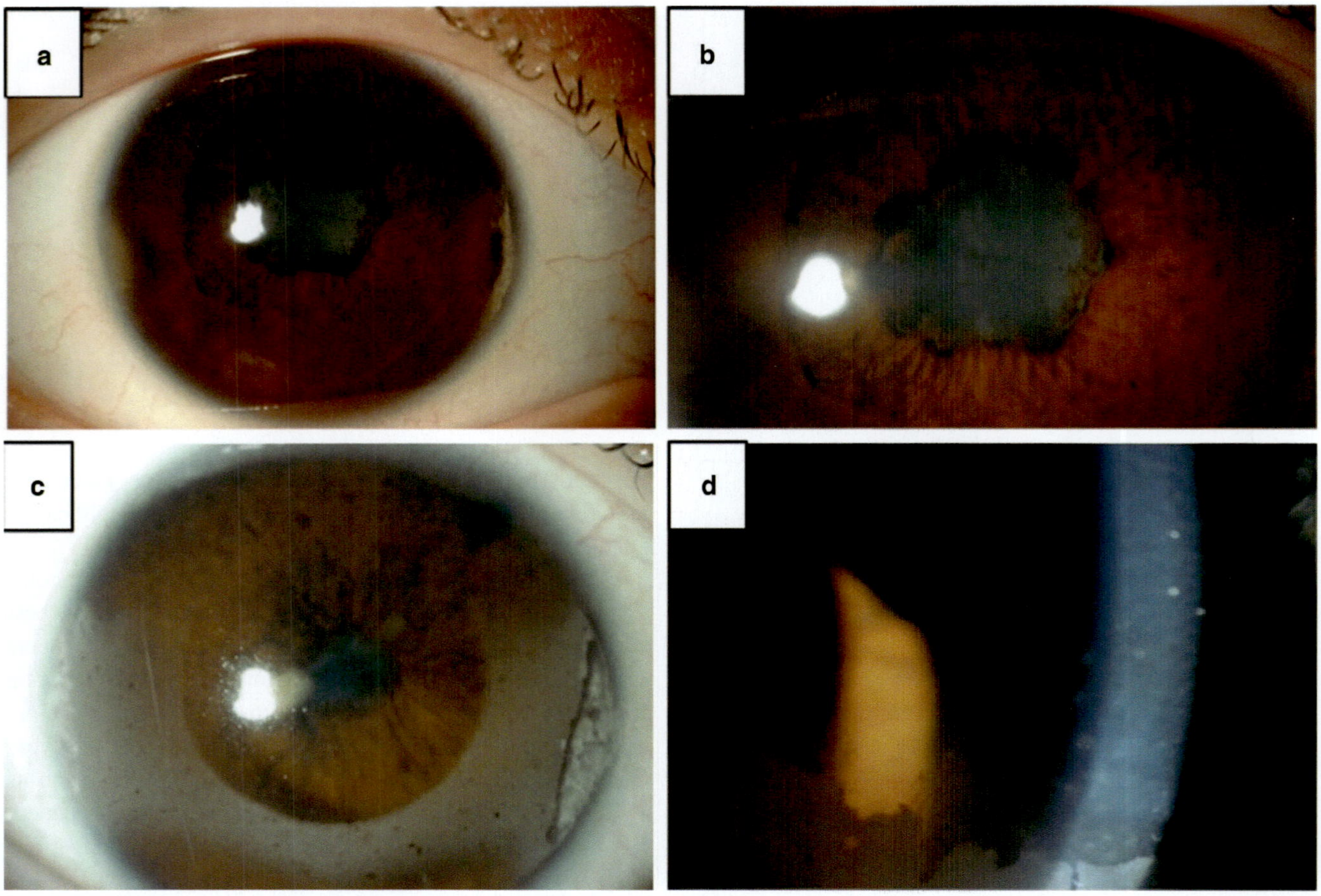

Fig. 27.1 Juvenile idiopathic arthritis (JIA), anterior uveitis. (**a**) Relatively early stage of JIA. Eight years old girl diagnosed as JIA. She had been suffering from bilateral uveitis for 4 years. Despite anterior uveitis was controlled, band keratopathy, anterior synechia, and cataract have developed. (**b**) Higher magnification of (**a**). (**c**) Advanced stage of JIA. Twelve-year-old girl diagnosed as JIA. She had been suffering from bilateral uveitis for 5 years. She had ongoing fibrinoid inflammation. Her band keratopathy was treated by excimer laser but had severe anterior synechia, cataract, and secondary glaucoma. (**d**) She had mutton-fat keratic precipitates and showed active anterior inflammation

is suspected, especially when a medication reaction or an infection can initiate such an event.

Patients with this syndrome frequently experienced bilateral anterior uveitis of sudden onset. Fortunately, the prognosis for vision is generally good. Patients are usually treated with systemic corticosteroids and with some immunosuppressive drugs. Systemic steroid therapy results in prompt renal recovery and may provide the benefit of reduced uveitis recurrence in most cases. There are some reports resulted in poor visual prognosis, if the patients combined with macular edema (Fig. 27.3) and choroidal neovascularization. In those cases, uveitis became relapsing and chronic.

TINU syndrome is rare and still unfamiliar to most ophthalmologists. Diagnostic criteria for TINU syndrome were published [5], and it provided levels of certainty ranging from "definite," "probable," and "possible." While renal biopsy is considered the gold standard for diagnosis, "definite" TINU can be diagnosed without biopsy as long as other major clinical findings are present.

Matsumoto et al. summarized the findings from 102 Japanese patients with TINU syndrome [6] and demonstrated that TINU showed a female predominance and was more likely to develop in younger patients.

TINU patients show elevated serum creatinine, low-grade proteinuria, and microscopic hematuria by urinalysis. Elevated urinary beta-2-microglobulin (β $2m$) has emerged as a sensitive test useful in the diagnosis of TINU syndrome [7] and the levels can correlate to histologic grade of interstitial nephritis. β2M is a small protein excreted by glomeruli and resorbed by healthy tubular epithelium. However, its resorption is reduced in tubulointerstitial nephritis, leading to elevated levels in the urine. Further workup of an elevated urinary β2M includes refer-

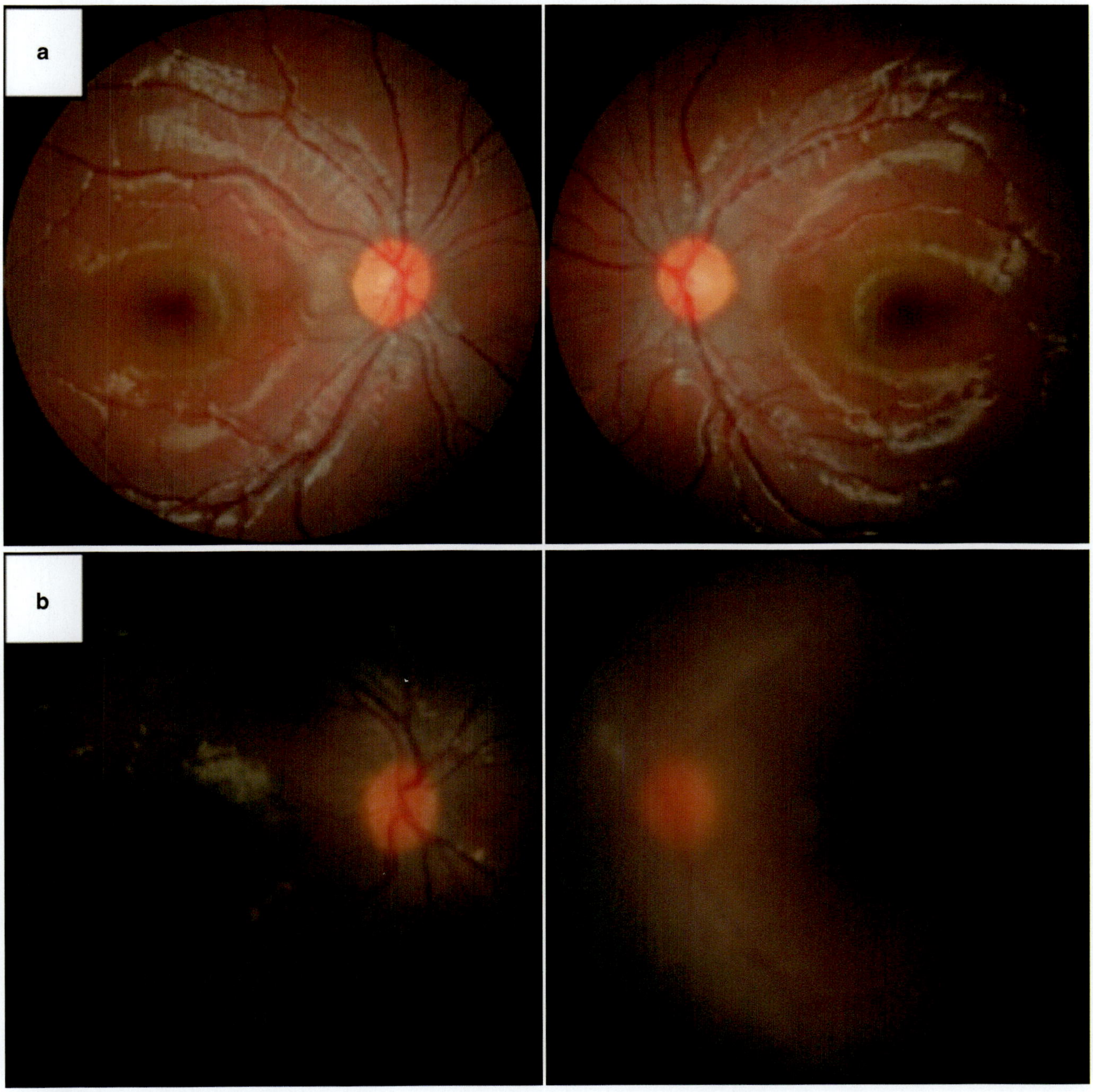

Fig. 27.2 Juvenile idiopathic arthritis (JIA), posterior uveitis. (**a**) Early stage of JIA. Four-year-old girl was diagnosed as JIA, with positive antinuclear antibodies. She has bilateral mild anterior inflammation and optic disc swelling. She was treated with methotrexate. (**b**) Advanced stage of JIA. Eight-year-old girl was diagnosed as JIA, with positive antinuclear antibodies. She had been treated for 4 years with methotrexate and topical corticosteroid. She had swollen optic disc and vitreous opacity

ral to a nephrologist for consideration of renal biopsy and to determine renal indication for systemic treatment. Additionally, N-acetyl-beta-glucosaminidase (NAG) urine activity is another screening marker for detecting renal dysfunction in TINU syndrome [8].

27.3 Brau Syndrome

Blau syndrome (BS) is a rare autosomal dominant, autoinflammatory disease characterized by the clinical triad of dermatitis, granulomatous uveitis, and symmetric arthritis.

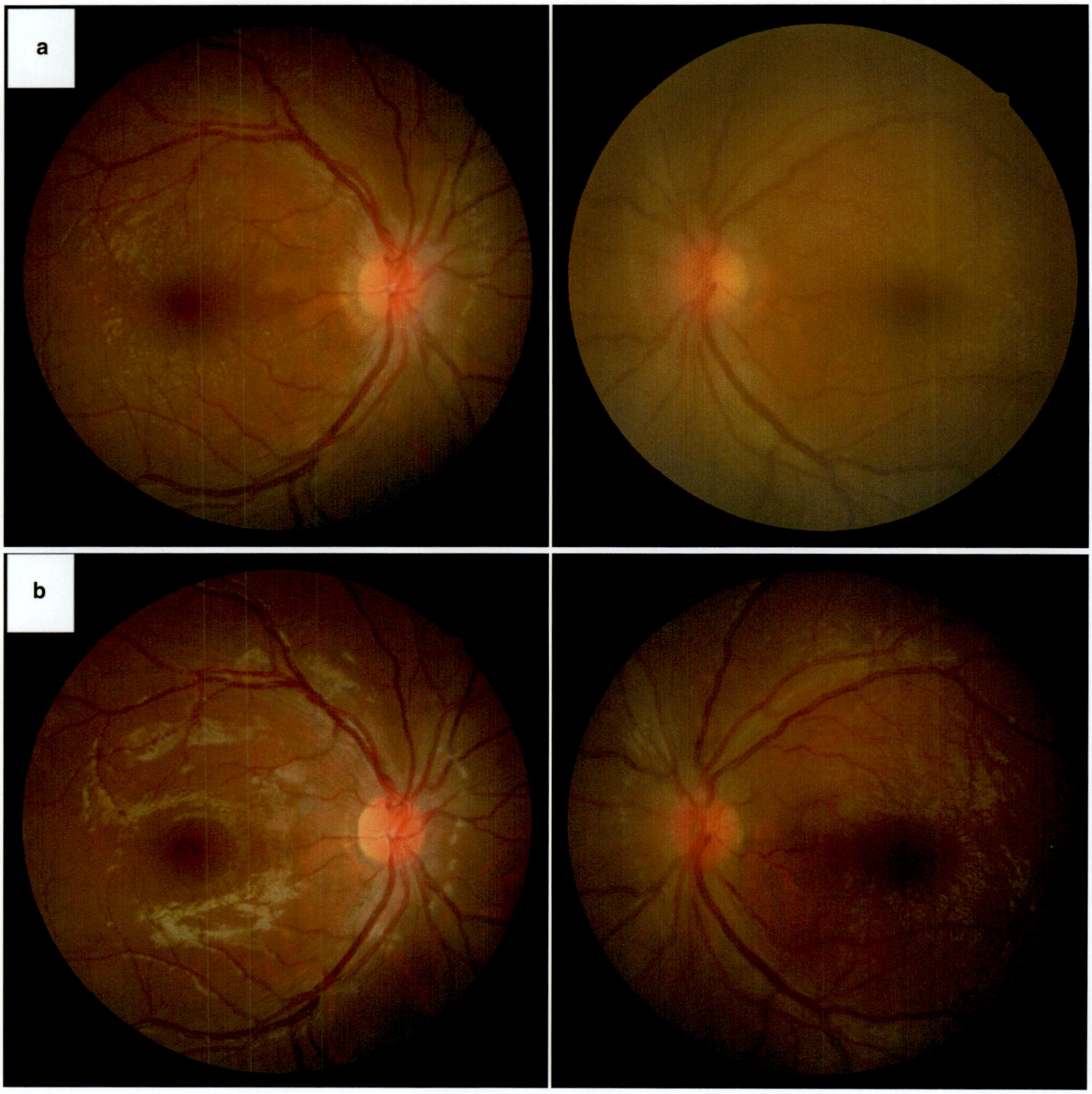

Fig. 27.3 Tubulointerstitial nephritis and uveitis (TINU) syndrome. (**a**) 13-year-old girl diagnosed with TINU syndrome. Her urinary β2M and N-acetyl-beta-glucosaminidase (NAG) were positive. She had been treated with systemic and topical corticosteroid for 3 years. She showed bilateral optic disc swelling and vitreous haze on the left eye. (**b**) 15 years old girl diagnosed as TINU syndrome. Her urinary β2M was positive and she had biopsy-proven tubulointerstitial nephritis. She had been treated by topical + systemic corticosteroid for 8 years, but still has bilateral optic swelling and macular edema in her left eye

The gene responsible for this syndrome has been identified in the caspase recruitment domain gene CARD15/NOD2. In many cases, the disease is characterized by early onset, usually before 4 years of age. Since that time, the phenotype has been expanded to include fever, granulomas of the liver and kidney, cardiovascular abnormalities, and cranial neuropathies. The ocular inflammation often occurs later in the disease course but carries the greatest morbidity in BS.

Monogenic "auto-inflammatory syndromes" are a new group of distinct hereditable disorders characterized by unprovoked inflammation in the absence of a high titer of auto-antibodies or auto-reactive T cells, and a congenital

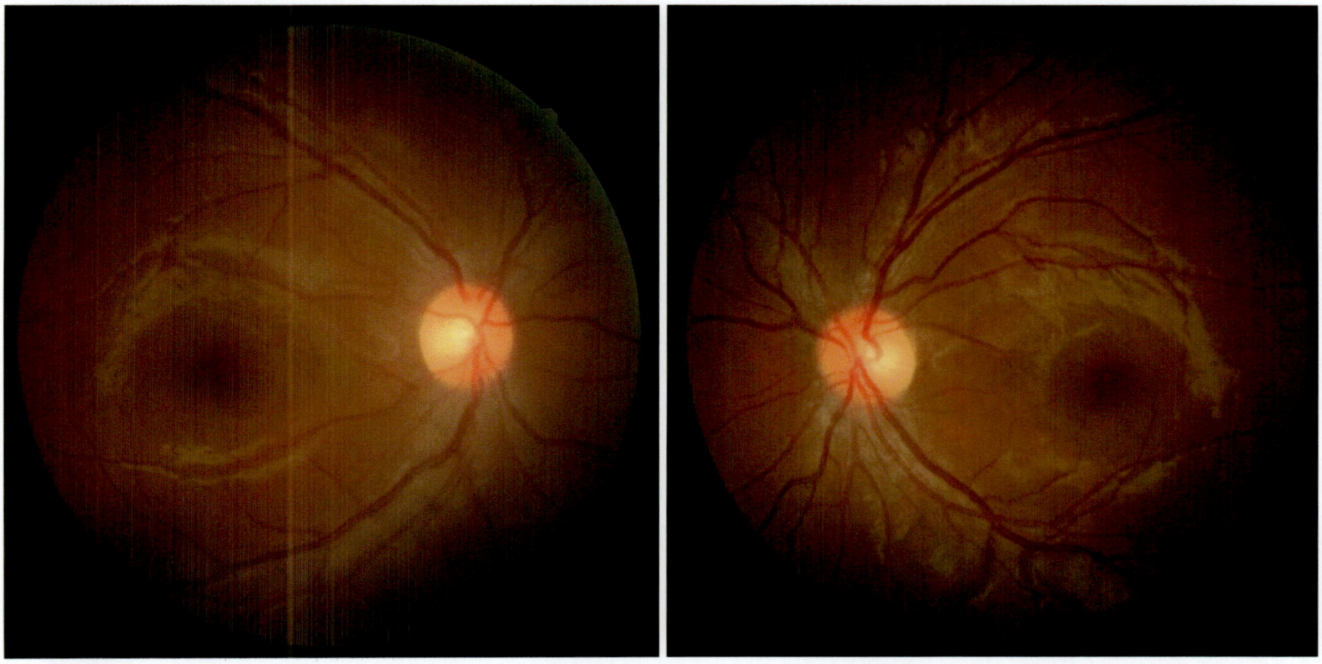

Fig. 27.4 Early stage of Brau syndrome. Ten-year-old girl diagnosed with Brau syndrome. Mutation of NOD2 gene was detected. She had photophobia and bilateral anterior uveitis. Her optic disc was swollen. Vitreous haze was observed in the right eye

error of innate immunity. The main monogenic autoinflammatory syndromes are Blau syndrome, mevalonate kinase deficiency (MKD), TNF receptor-associated periodic syndrome (TRAPS), familial Mediterranean fever (FMF), cryopyrin-associated periodic syndrome (CAPS), and pyogenic arthritis with pyoderma gangrenosum and acne (PAPA) [9]. These disorders are mediated by excessive IL-1 secretion activated by monocytes and macrophages.

The cytosolic pattern recognition receptor NOD2 is activated by the peptidoglycan fragment to contribute host defense against invaded microorganisms. Downstream effects include the secretion of proinflammatory cytokines such as IL-8, the upregulation of pro-IL-1β, the production of antimicrobial peptides and defensin, and the induction of autophagy.

Uveitis in BS is originally characterized by progressive panuveitis with multifocal choroiditis. Kurokawa T et al. summarized the ocular manifestation in BS, which are anterior and posterior synechiae, corneal opacities, iris bombe, secondary glaucoma, cataract, disc swelling (Fig. 27.4), cystoid macular edema, anterior ischemic optic neuropathy, and multifocal choroiditis (Fig. 27.5) [10].

There is no established therapy for BS in general, and the main aim in ophthalmic care is to manage ocular inflammations to prevent blindness. On-demand nonsteroidal anti-inflammatory drugs can be effective for pain control, but they have limited efficacy in the prevention of disease progression. Steroid sparing immunosuppressants, such as azathioprine or methotrexate, may be helpful. Low-dose glucocorticoids can maintain the quiescent stage, but high-dose corticosteroids are necessary in acute flare up. When patients are unresponsive to the combination of immunosuppressant agents and corticosteroid, the tumor necrosis factor-α inhibitor infliximab should be considered. Data on anti-IL-1 inhibition with anakinra and canakinumab are still limited and further investigation is required [11].

27.4 Ocular Toxoplasmosis

Ocular toxoplasmosis is the common cause of posterior uveitis in children. Toxoplasma gondii is an obligate intracellular parasite that is known to infect one-third of the world population chronically though it is asymptomatic in immunocompetent patients. Geography, ethnicity, and socioeconomic factors are influencing the prevalence of ocular toxoplasmosis in specific areas and countries.

The parasite may cross the placenta of an infected mother and then infect the fetus. Congenital toxoplasmosis may result in non-specific consequences like abortion, jaundice, hepatosplenomegaly, intrauterine growth retardation, or even intrauterine death. It may also result in ocular manifestations like retinochoroiditis.

The most common ocular finding of toxoplasmosis is an acute focal-necrotizing retinochoroiditis adjacent to an old chorioretinal scar (Fig. 27.6). Some of the children affected with congenital toxoplasmosis present with a healed punched out scar in the macula. Although the inner retina is the pri-

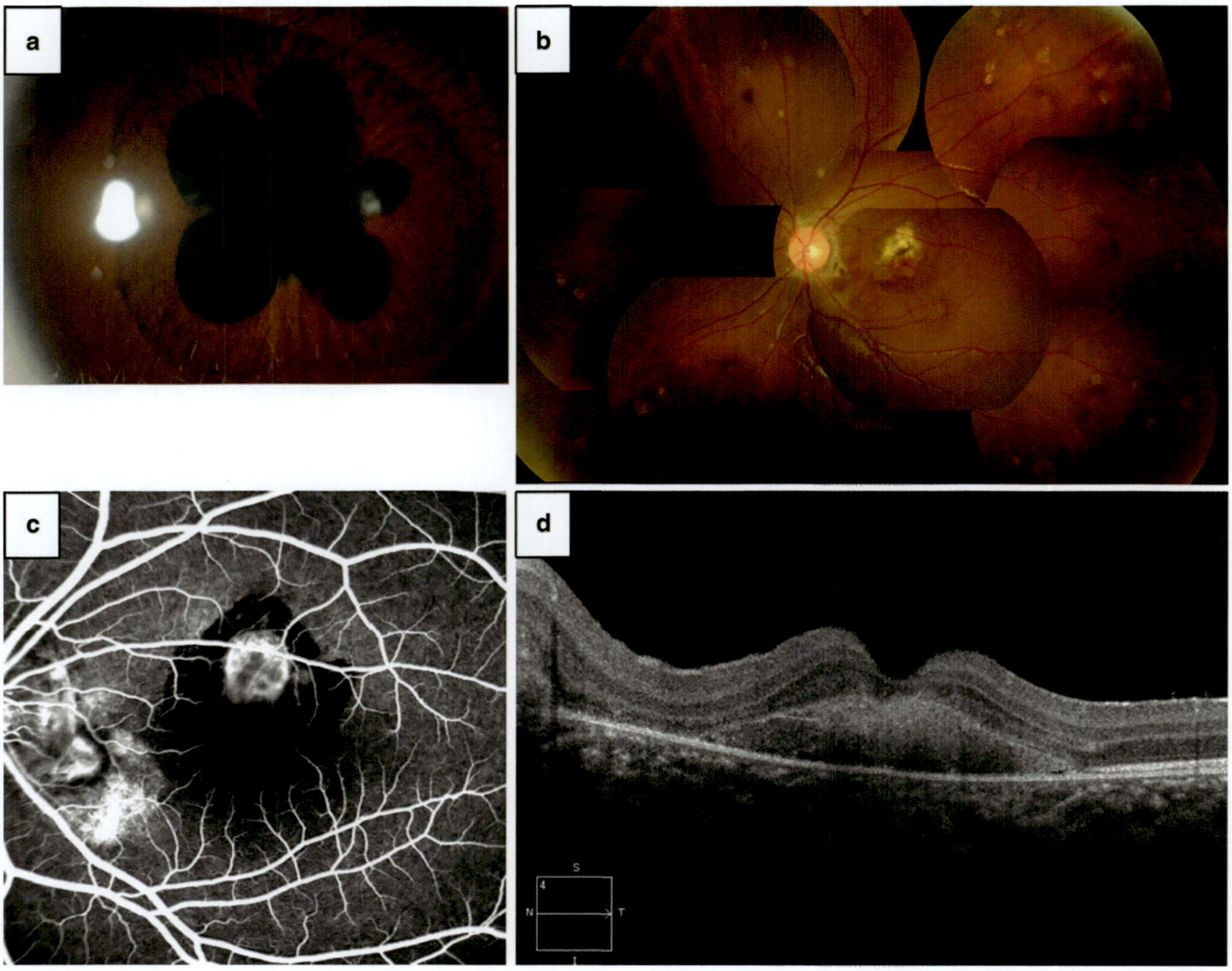

Fig. 27.5 Advanced stage of Brau syndrome. Nine-year-old girl diagnosed with Brau syndrome. Mutation of NOD2 gene was detected, while her parents were not. She had blurred vision and red eye for 5 years, had been treated with topical steroid. (**a**) Anterior segment of the patient. She presented bilateral anterior inflammation, with posterior synechia. (**b**) Progressive panuveitis with multifocal choroiditis. Macula area was severely damaged. (**c**) Choroidal neovascular membranes (juxtapapillary and extrafoveal) were observed in the fluorescein angiography. (**d**) Subretinal scar and hemorrhage were observed beneath the fovea

mary site of infection, vitreous, choroid, and sometimes sclera are secondarily affected. Foci of inflammation within or directly adjacent to the optic disc can result in papillitis and neuroretinitis. Rare presentations include granulomatous anterior uveitis, retinal vasculitis (Fig. 27.7), branch retinal vascular obstruction, and intermediate uveitis. It is important that ocular toxoplasmosis is commonly diagnosed during the inactive stage in children. The major symptoms were strabismus and reduced visual acuity with an inactive chorioretinal scar [12].

The diagnosis may be based on the titer of anti-toxoplasma antibodies (IgM and IgG). Accurate diagnosis depends on the characteristic clinical features of this disease, but atypical presentations, especially in immunocompromised patients, may sometimes lead to misdiagnosis and inappropriate treatment. Molecular biology techniques to diagnose ocular toxoplasmosis have been available are now accessible in many countries. Aqueous humor or vitreous fluid evaluation to detect parasite DNA by polymerase chain reaction is useful for rapid diagnosis [12, 13].

Oral pyrimethamine and sulfadiazine plus systemic corticosteroids are an effective therapy for ocular toxoplasmosis. Recent data supports the use of other treatment approaches, including intravitreal clindamycin. For other treatment regimens, spiramycin is used to prevent congenital transmission from an infected mother, while pyrimethamine, sulfadoxine, and folinic acid are used to treat the infected fetus.

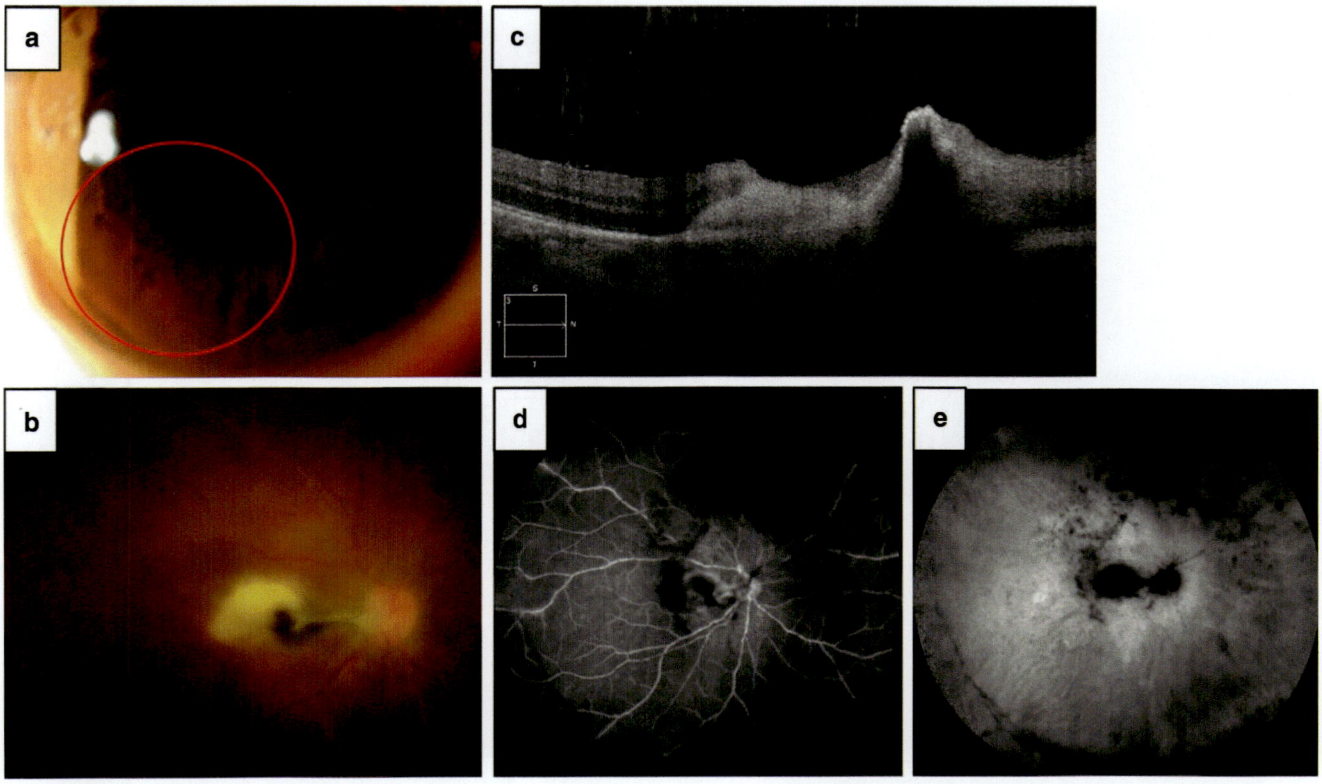

Fig. 27.6 Ocular toxoplasmosis showing focal-necrotizing retinochoroiditis. Nine-year-old boy suffered from sudden visual loss in the right eye. The patient was found to have significantly elevated serum titers of anti-Toxoplasma gondii IgG, followed by an appearance of a focal retinal lesion typical of ocular toxoplasmosis. (**a**) Anterior segment of the patient. Presence of mutton-fat keratic precipitates and active inflammation. (**b**) Exudative retinochoroiditis at macular area adjacent to an old chorioretinal scar. (**c**) The structure of fovea was severely damaged, suggesting necrotizing inflammation. (**d**) Fluorescein angiography revealed active inflammation at fovea, optic disc, and peripheral retinal artery. (**e**) Indocyanine green angiography revealed choroidal structure was also damaged in this patient

27.5 Ocular Cat-Scratch Disease

Bartonella henselae are facultative intracellular Gram-negative rods, and its infection has local or systemic features and related to cat-scratch disease [14]. The diagnosis is based on laboratory tests and clinical findings.

Bartonella infections sometimes cause uveitis with ophthalmic manifestations ranging from neuroretinits, vascular occlusion, to choroidal granulomas [15]. Cat-scratch disease causes a febrile illness with subacute regional lymphadenopathy. In many cases, there is a spontaneous resolution within 4 weeks. However, severe and disseminated disease can occur in both immunocompetent and immunocompromised hosts. Prominent optic disc swelling (neuroretinitis) and vascular leakage have been reported as common manifestations of ocular bartonellosis (Fig. 27.8). The use of several antigens for serodiagnosis and real-time PCR assays for molecular diagnosis have been described. Despite the lack of a standard treatment, good visual outcomes were generally reported.

Parainfectious disorders of the nervous system include conditions that are temporally associated with antigenic stimuli or toxin exposure in the absence of direct invasion

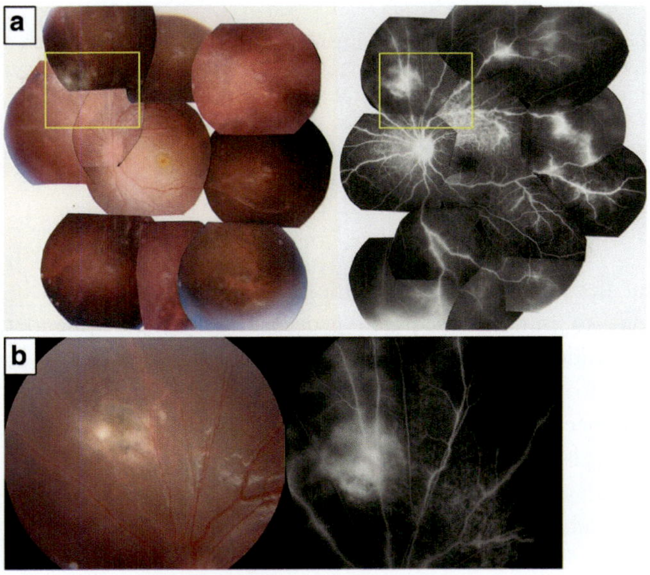

Fig. 27.7 Ocular toxoplasmosis mainly showing retinal vasculitis (by courtesy of Dr. Yoh-Ichi Kawano). Ten-year-old boy suffered from foggy vision in the left eye. The right eye was normal showing no sign of inflammation. The anterior chamber of his left eye presented slight cell infiltration. (**a**) The panorama fundus photo and fluorescein angiography showed marked and multiple retinal vasculitis on the left eye. (**b**) He had an old scar lesion in the upper nasal retina (yellow rectangle), and inflammation expanding from there

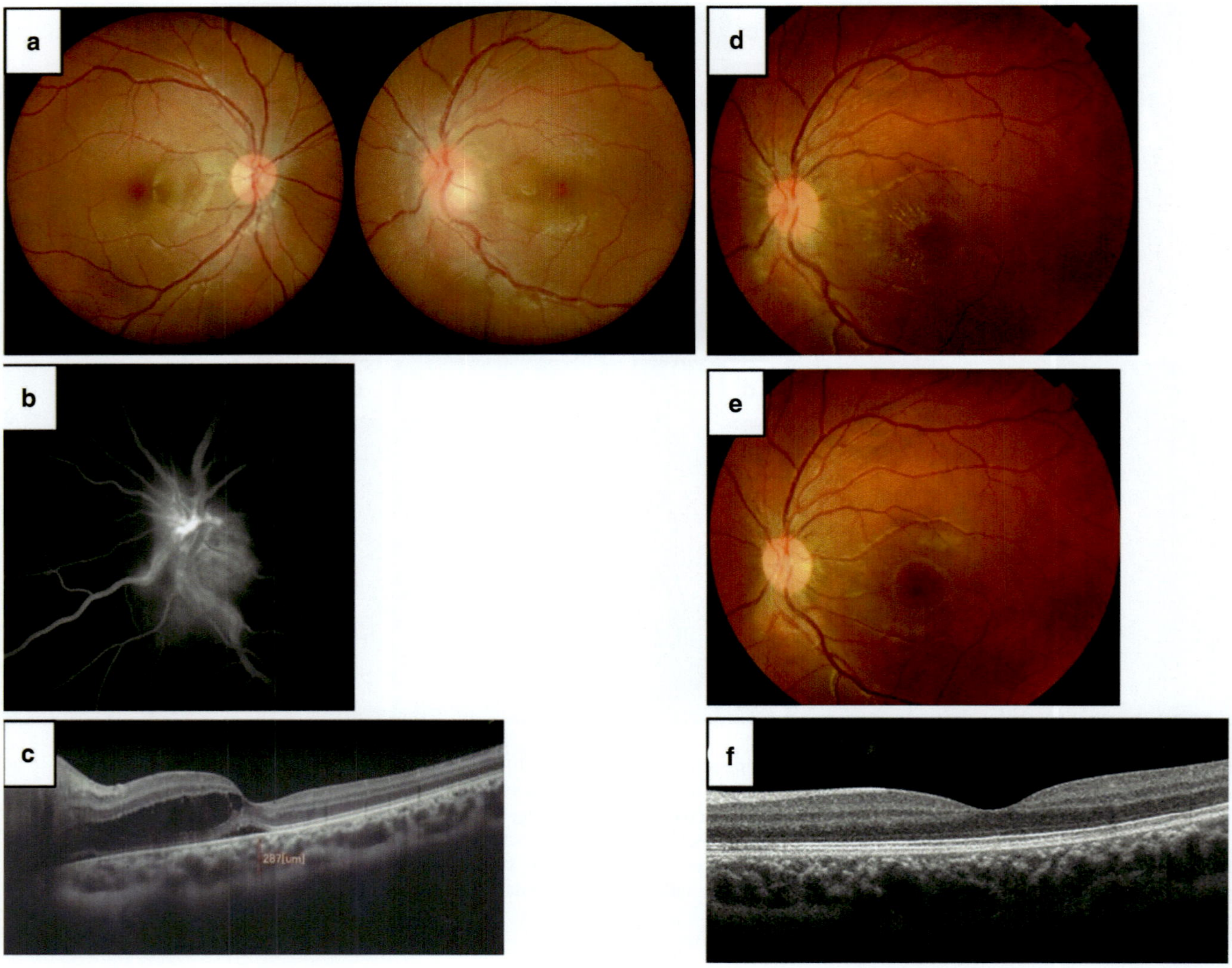

Fig. 27.8 Ocular cat-scratch disease. Fourteen-year-old girl suffered from sudden visual loss in the left eye. She had long-lasting fatigue and fever for a month. She had a cat for 5 years. She showed positive anti-*B. henselae* IgM and IgG antibodies detected by enzyme immunoassay and diagnosed as cat-scratch disease. She thus was treated with minocycline hydrochloride. (**a**)–(**c**) Fundus photo, Fluorescein angiography, and OCT at initial visit. Prominent optic disc swelling (neuroretinitis), vascular leakage, and retinal detachment/retinoschisis. (**d**) Fundus photo, a month later. Showing partial macular star. (**e, f**) Fundus photo, 3 months later. Showing normal optic disc and macula structure

of the nervous system. Pathogenetic mechanisms can be due to immune-mediated processes (such as bystander activation, molecular mimicry) or the inciting insult can be due to toxic factors. A myriad of clinical manifestations can occur including seizures, headaches, and mental status changes.

Diagnosis is based not only on the history, examination, and laboratory but also on epidemiological factors. Other parainfectious disorders such as legionellosis, Lyme borreliosis, botulism, brucellosis, pertussis, and mycoplasma, each is associated with a distinct organism, has both systemic and neurological manifestations, and has a different epidemiological profile.

The indication of antibiotic therapy depends on the severity of manifestation and the host immune status. Immunocompetent patients sometimes do well for ocular complications without antimicrobial therapy. Immunocompromised patients usually show a dramatic response to treatment with either erythromycin or doxycycline.

References

1. Papadopoulou C, Kostik M, Böhm M, Nieto-Gonzalez JC, Gonzalez-Fernandez MI, Pistorio A, et al. Methotrexate therapy may prevent the onset of uveitis in juvenile idiopathic arthritis. J Pediatr. 2013;163:879–84.

2. Ramanan AV, Dick AD, Jones AP, McKay A, Williamson PR, Compeyrot-Lacassagne S, et al. Adalimumab plus methotrexate for uveitis in juvenile idiopathic arthritis. N Eng J Med. 2017;376:1637–46.
3. Tappeiner C, Mesquida M, Adán A, Anton J, Ramanan AV, Carreno E, et al. Evidence for tocilizumab as a treatment option in refractory uveitis associated with juvenile idiopathic arthritis. J Rheumatol. 2016;43:2183–8.
4. Dobrin RS, Vernier RL, Fish AL. Acute eosinophilic interstitial nephritis and renal failure with bone marrow-lymph node granulomas and anterior uveitis. A new syndrome. Am J Med. 1975;59:325–33.
5. Mandeville JT, Levinson RD, Holland GN. The tubulointerstitial nephritis and uveitis syndrome. Surv Ophthalmol. 2001;46:195–208.
6. Matsumoto K, Fukunari K, Ikeda Y, Miyazono M, Kishi T, Matsumoto R, et al. A report of an adult case of tubulointerstitial nephritis and uveitis syndrome, with a review of 102 Japanese cases. Am J Case Rep. 2015;16:119–23.
7. Hettinga YM, Scheerlinck LM, Lilien MR, Rothova A, de Boear JH. The value of measuring urinary b2-microglobulin and serum creatinine for detecting tubulointerstitial nephritis and uveitis syndrome in young patients with uveitis. JAMA Ophthalmol. 2015;133:140–5.
8. Kwiatkowska E, Domanski L, Bober J, Kłoda K, Safranow K, Szymanska-Pasternak J, et al. N-acetyl-beta-glucosaminidase urine activity as a marker of early proximal tubule damage and a predictor of the long-term function of the transplanted kidneys. Acta Biochem Pol. 2014;61:275–80.
9. Vitale A, Rigante D, Lucherini OM, Caso F, Muscari I, Magnotti F, et al. Biological treatments: new weapons in the management of monogenic autoinflammatory disorders. Mediators Inflamm. 2013;2013:93984. https://doi.org/10.1155/2013/939847.
10. Kurokawa T, Kikuchi T, Ohta K, Imai H, Yoshimura N. Ocular manifestations in Blau syndrome associated with a CARD15/Nod2 mutation. Ophthalmology. 2003;110:2040–4.
11. Simonini G, Xu Z, Caputo R, De Libero C, Pagnini I, Pascual V, et al. Clinical and transcriptional response to the long-acting interleukin-1 blocker canakinumab in Blau syndrome-related uveitis. Arthritis Rheum. 2013;65:513–8.
12. Padhi TR, Das S, Sharma S, Rath S, Rath S, Tripathy D, et al. Ocular parasitoses: a comprehensive review. Surv Ophthalmol. 2017;62:161–89.
13. Nakano S, Sugita S, Tomaru Y, Hono A, Nakamuro T, Kubota T, et al. Establishment of multiplex solid-phase strip PCR test for detection of 24 ocular infectious disease pathogens. Invest Ophthalmol Vis Sci. 2017;58:1553–9.
14. Biancardi AL, Curi AL. Cat-scratch disease. Ocul Immunol Inflamm. 2014;22:148–54.
15. Mabra D, Yeh S, Shantha JG. Ocular manifestations of bartonellosis. Curr Opin Ophthalmol. 2018;29:582–7.

Coats' Disease

28

Michael J. Wan, Jingyi Ma, Hannah H. Chiu, and Wai-Ching Lam

Abstract

Coats' disease is an idiopathic condition characterized by peripheral retinal telangiectasia with intraretinal and subretinal exudation. Isolated Coats' disease is non-hereditary and the majority of cases are unilateral and affect young males, although bilateral and adult-onset cases do occur. Young children tend to present with leukocoria or strabismus, while older children and adults usually present with subjective vision loss or as an incidental finding. The clinical severity at presentation can range widely from retinal telangiectasia only to total retinal detachment with secondary ocular complications. Treatment is indicated in most cases and is effective at achieving good structural outcomes. However, the long-term visual prognosis remains poor, especially in advanced cases.

Keywords

Coats disease · Retinal detachment · Telangiectasia Retinoblastoma · Leukocoria · Enucleation

M. J. Wan
Department of Ophthalmology and Vision Sciences, University of Toronto, Toronto, ON, Canada

Department of Ophthalmology and Vision Sciences, The Hospital for Sick Children, Toronto, ON, Canada

J. Ma
Department of Ophthalmology and Vision Sciences, The Hospital for Sick Children, Toronto, ON, Canada

Faculty of Medicine and Dentistry, University of Alberta, Edmonton, AB, Canada

H. H. Chiu
Department of Ophthalmology and Vision Sciences, University of Toronto, Toronto, ON, Canada

W.-C. Lam (✉)
Department of Ophthalmology and Vision Sciences, University of Toronto, Toronto, ON, Canada

Department of Ophthalmology and Vision Sciences, The Hospital for Sick Children, Toronto, ON, Canada

Department of Ophthalmology, The University of Hong Kong, Hong Kong, Hong Kong

28.1 Introduction

Coats' disease is an idiopathic condition characterized by abnormal development of the retinal vasculature. The retinal findings are characteristic, ranging in severity from peripheral retinal telangiectasia to massive subretinal exudation with retinal detachment [1]. It is important to accurately diagnose Coats' disease as the clinical findings can overlap with other serious, potentially life-threatening conditions such as retinoblastoma. There are also effective therapies available for the abnormal retinal blood vessels in Coats' disease which can improve clinical outcomes. As such, it is imperative to recognize the clinical manifestations of Coats' disease in order to make a prompt diagnosis and optimize management.

28.2 Pathogenesis

Coats' disease was first described in 1908 by Scottish ophthalmologist George Coats [2], who recognized the massive yellowish intraretinal and subretinal exudation, which is characteristic of the condition. Coats proposed that retinal hemorrhages were the primary lesion of the disease. Subsequent histopathological studies of Coats' disease have revealed that the actual cause of the disease is likely congenital retinal telangiectasia (i.e., abnormal retinal vasculature) [3]. Leakage of serum, plasma, and blood cells from the abnormal retinal vasculature leads to the degeneration of retinal cells and the accumulation of lipid deposits and exudation [4]. The disease is progressive, and subretinal exudates can progress to retinal detachment, eventually leading to severe complications such as neovascular glaucoma and pthisis bulbi. Despite significant advancements in the understanding of Coats' disease, it remains an idiopathic condition and an underlying etiology for the development of the congenital retinal telangiectasia has yet to be identified.

W.-C. Wu, W.-C. Lam (eds.), *A Quick Guide to Pediatric Retina*, https://doi.org/10.1007/978-981-15-6552-6_28

28.3 Epidemiology

Coats' disease is uncommon, with an estimated incidence of approximately 1 in 100,000 [5]. The vast majority of cases are unilateral, although rare bilateral cases have been reported [6, 7]. Approximately 80–90% of affected patients are male [5, 8]. The mean age of presentation is around 12 years old, but this is biased by a small number of cases presenting late in life. In general, most cases present in the first 15 years of life (with a peak between the ages 5 and 10), with a much smaller number of cases presenting well into adulthood [9]. Isolated Coats' disease is not an inherited condition and there are no known risk factors. In rare cases, Coats' disease can be associated with other abnormalities of the brain, bones, and gastrointestinal system (i.e., Coats' plus syndrome), which is caused by mutations in the *STN1* gene and inherited in an autosomal recessive manner [10].

28.4 Presentation

The presentation of Coats' disease depends on the age of the affected individual and severity of the disease. Young children with advanced disease typically present with leukocoria (Fig. 28.1) or strabismus [5]. In less severe cases, Coats' disease may be detected incidentally through school vision screening programs or during routine dilated eye examinations. Older children and adults with Coats' disease most commonly present with subjective changes in their visual acuity or visual field [5, 11].

28.5 Clinical Findings at Presentation

Coats' disease can have a myriad of different clinical manifestations at presentation, relating to the severity of disease and the presence of ocular complications. A classification for disease severity at presentation has been described by Shields et al. based on a large case series of over 150 patients (Table 28.1) [1]. This widely used classification system can be readily applied based on clinical examination findings and has been shown to have important prognostic value in several studies [8, 12]. In the classification system, all stages of Coats' disease involve retinal telangiectasia. Stage 1 is the least severe with retinal telangiectasia only. In stage 2, there are retinal telangiectasia with exudation, either extrafoveal exudation (2A—Fig. 28.2) or foveal exudation (2B—Fig. 28.3). In stage 3, there is associated retinal detachment, either subtotal (3A—Fig. 28.4) or total (3B—Fig. 28.5). Stage 4 involves total retinal detachment with secondary glaucoma (Fig. 28.6) and stage 5 is advanced end-stage disease with no chance for visual recovery (e.g., phthisis—Fig. 28.7). While Coats' disease can present with any stage of severity, the majority of newly diagnosed cases fall into either stage 2 or stage 3 [5].

Table 28.1 Classification system for severity of Coats' disease at presentation [1]

Stage	Definition
1	Retinal telangiectasia only
2	Retinal telangiectasia and exudation A. Extrafoveal exudation B. Foveal exudation
3	Exudative retinal detachment A. Subtotal retinal detachment B. Total retinal detachment
4	Total retinal detachment and secondary glaucoma
5	Advanced end-stage disease (blind eyes with retinal telangiectasia, exudation, total retinal detachment, and anterior chamber involvement or phthisis)

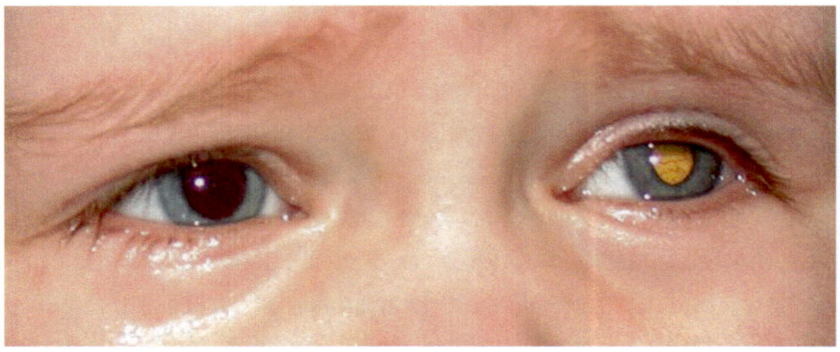

Fig. 28.1 Anterior photo showing advanced Coats' disease, with leukocoria of the left eye and a total retinal detachment visible just posterior to the crystalline lens

Although the stage of disease can usually be identified on clinical examination, fluorescein angiography is often very useful in assessing the full extent of vascular changes and identifying areas of capillary non-perfusion, which are important factors in directing treatment (see Figs. 28.2–28.4). In young children, fluorescein angiography generally necessitates general anesthesia. In order to minimize the duration of anesthesia and the time from diagnosis to treatment, a fluorescein angiogram should be performed in the operating room and then immediately followed by treatment if possible.

28.6 Differentiation from Retinoblastoma

The most important condition to differentiate from Coats' disease in infants and young children is retinoblastoma. This is a common diagnostic dilemma as both conditions often present with the same chief complaint (i.e., leukocoria and/or strabismus) and the clinical appearance and neuro-imaging findings can overlap [13–16]. It is imperative to try to avoid misdiagnosing retinoblastoma as Coats' disease as this can directly lead to the death of a young child [17].

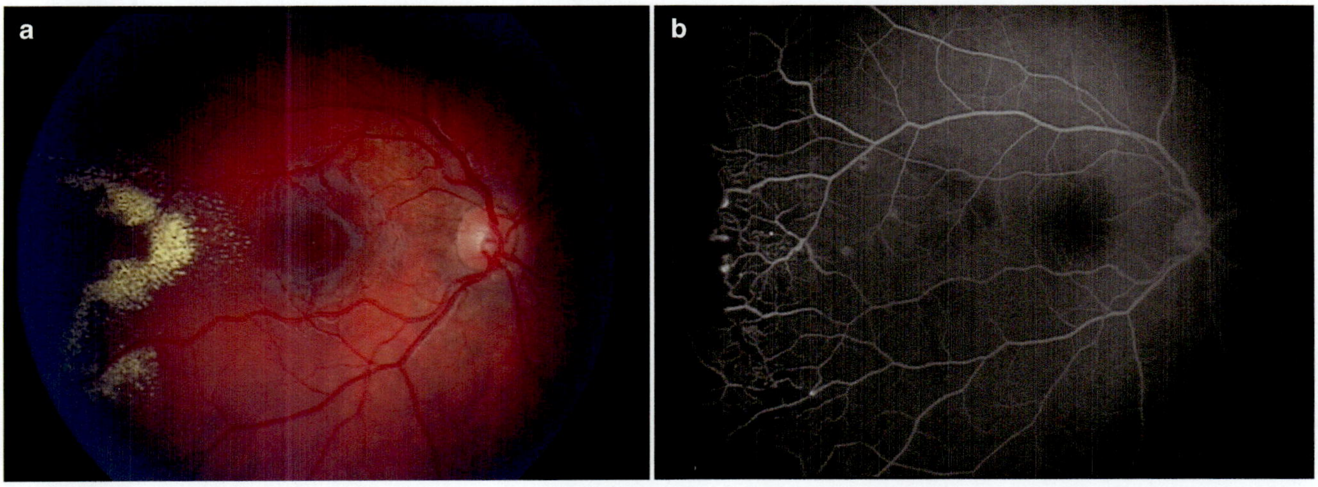

Fig. 28.2 Fundus photo (**a**) and fluorescein angiography (**b**) showing peripheral telangiectasia with extrafoveal exudation (Stage 2A)

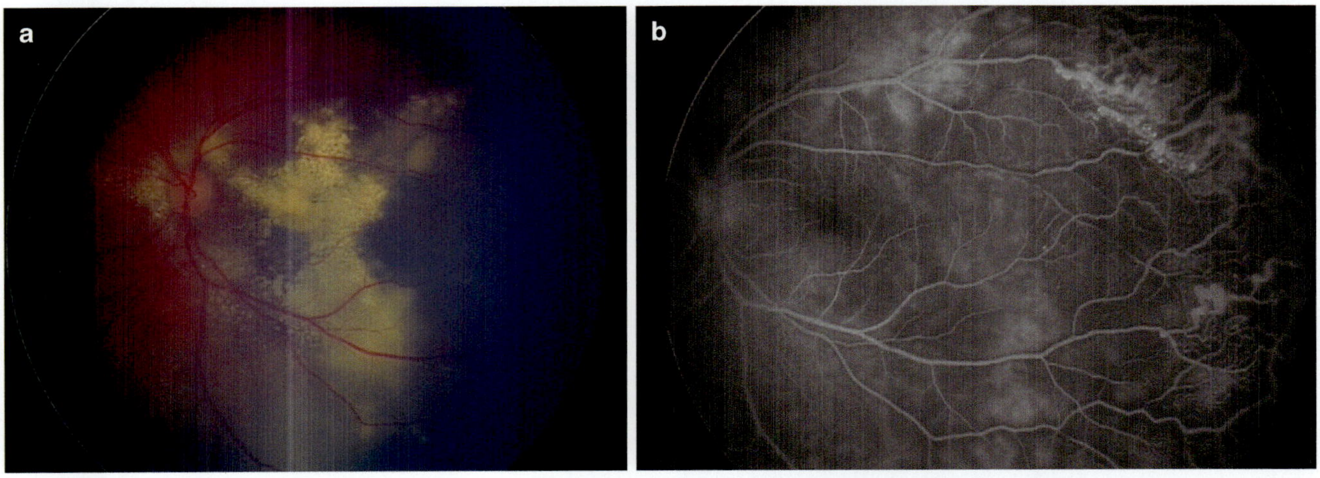

Fig. 28.3 Fundus photo (**a**) and fluorescein angiography (**b**) showing extensive, leaking peripheral telangiectasia with foveal exudation (Stage 2B)

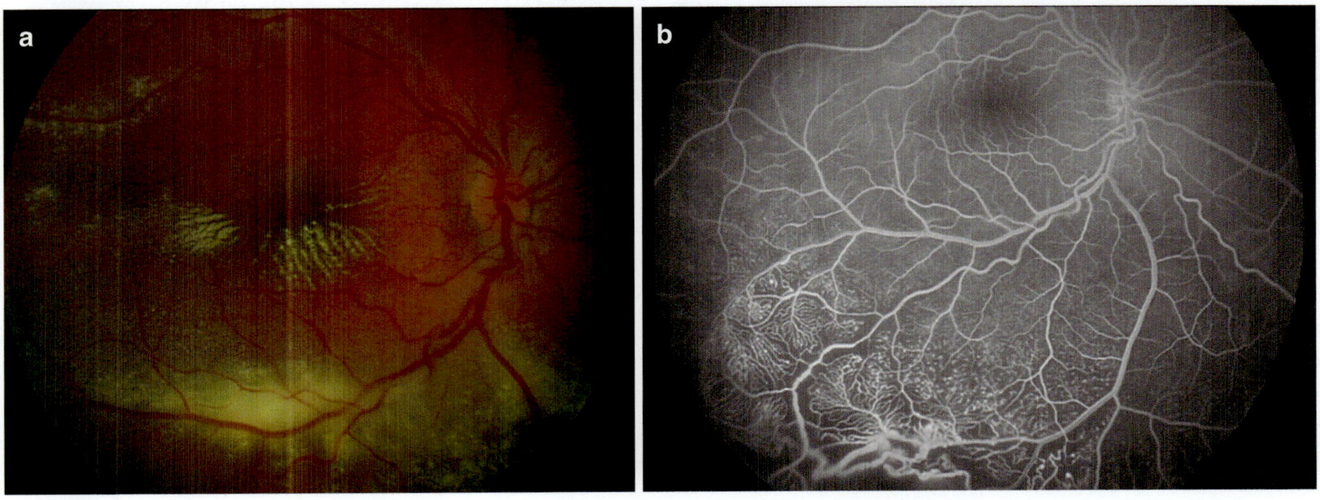

Fig. 28.4 Fundus photo (**a**) and fluorescein angiography (**b**) showing an inferior exudative retinal detachment with inferior retinal telangiectasia and both foveal and extrafoveal exudation (Stage 3A)

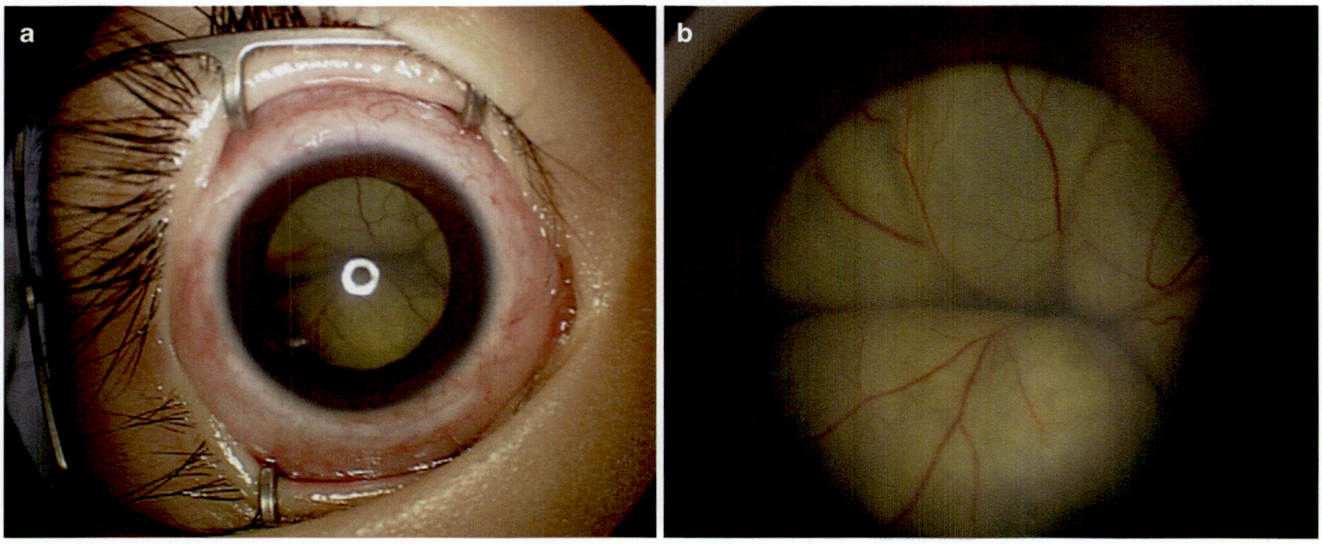

Fig. 28.5 External (**a**) and anterior segment (**b**) photos showing a total funnel retinal detachment with massive subretinal exudate (Stage 3B)

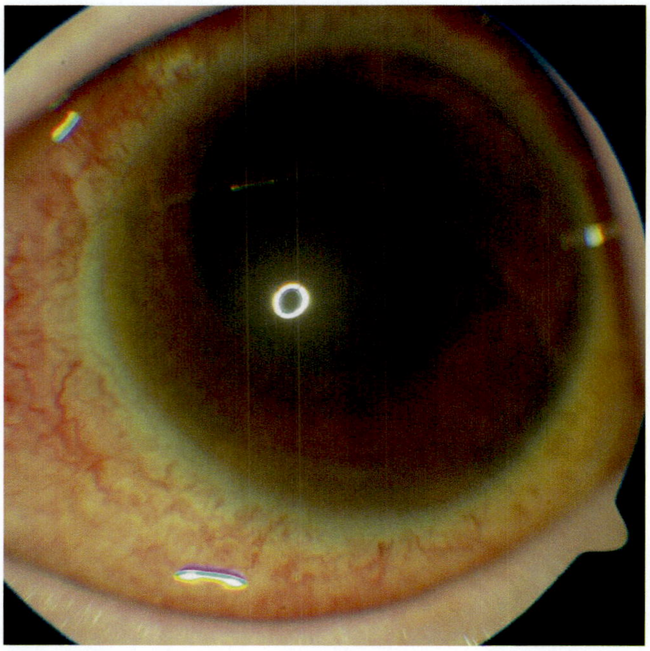

Fig. 28.6 Anterior segment photo showing neovascularization of the iris and mild corneal edema in a child with neovascular glaucoma due to advanced Coats' disease with a chronic total retinal detachment (Stage 4)

In differentiating Coats' disease from retinoblastoma, careful clinical examination is crucial. Both conditions can cause retinal detachment, dilated vasculature, and subretinal exudates/masses. In Coats' disease, the subretinal exudates are typically more yellow compared to a white mass in retinoblastoma. The presence of anterior segment cells is suggestive of advanced retinoblastoma, as is the presence of vitreous seeds (Fig. 28.8). Calcification is more typical of retinoblastoma, although there are reports of calcification in advanced Coats' disease [18]. Retinal telangiectasia is more classic for Coats' disease, but can also be present in both conditions. Neuroimaging with MRI and an examination under anesthesia with fluorescein angiography is often helpful in clarifying the diagnosis (Fig. 28.9). However, if the diagnosis remains uncertain, primary enucleation must be considered [19]. Although enucleation is certainly not the preferred primary treatment for Coats' disease, the prognosis for useful vision in advanced cases of Coats' disease is very poor. Therefore, if advanced retinoblastoma cannot be excluded, primary enucleation is the safest treatment

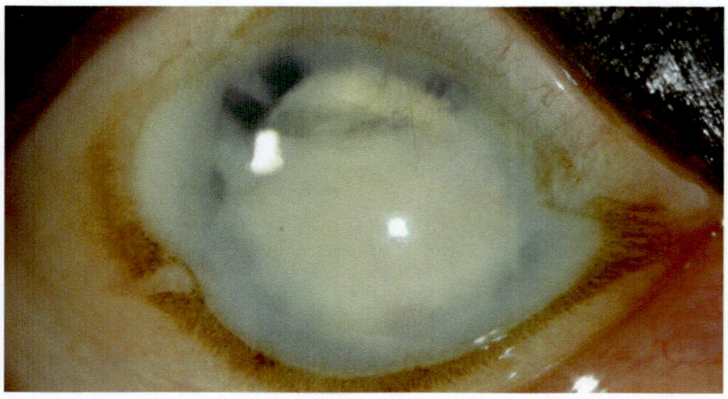

Fig. 28.7 External photo showing end-stage advanced Coats' disease (i.e., phthisis bulbi) with a dense cataract and corneal neovascularization and opacification (Stage 5)

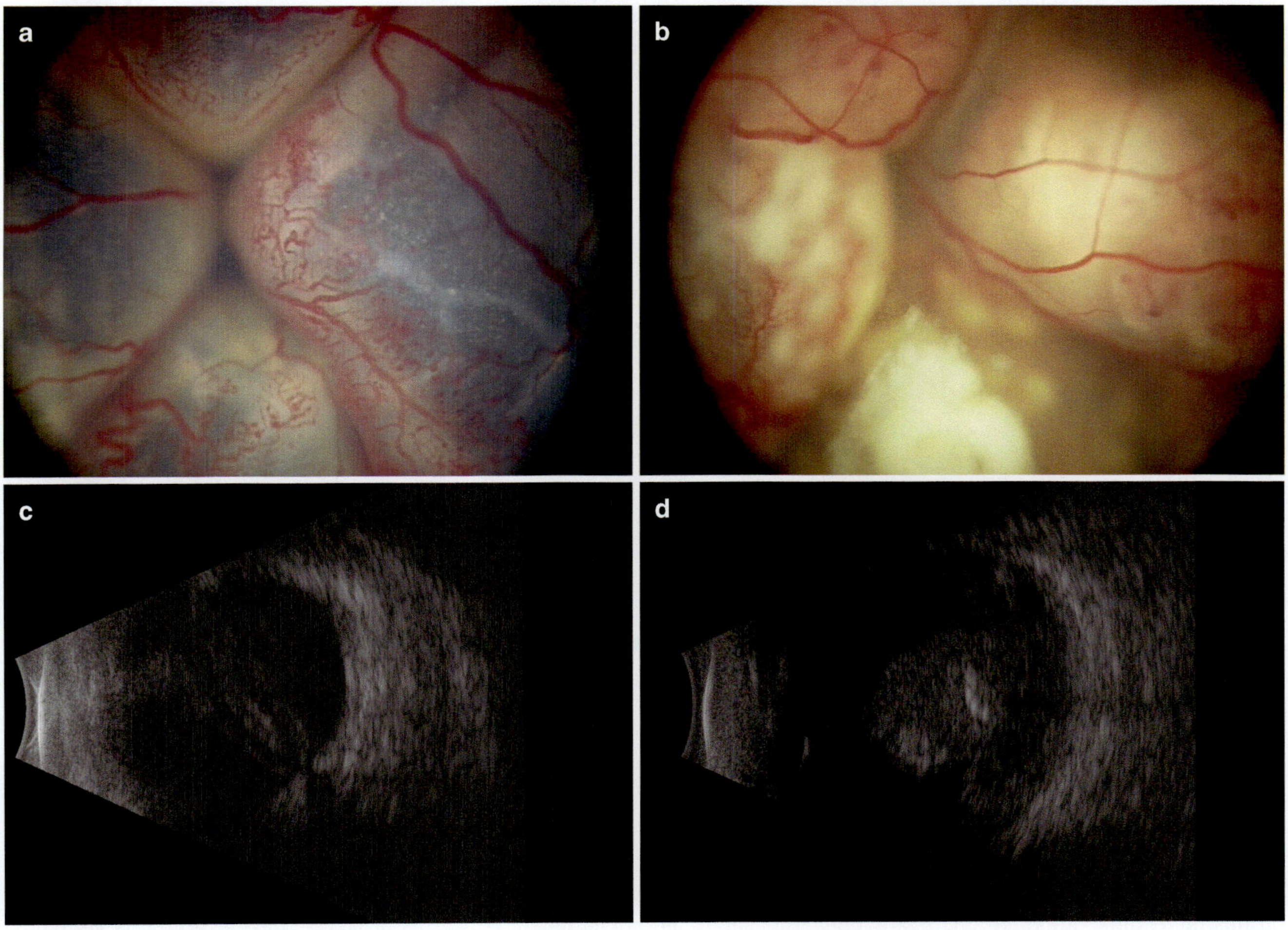

Fig. 28.8 Comparison of Coats' disease and retinoblastoma with fundus photos and B Scan ultrasounds. Fundus photo of advanced Coats' disease (**a**) shows many telangiectatic vessels with a funnel retinal detachment. Fundus photo of advanced retinoblastoma (**b**) showing fewer retinal telangiectasia, a white subretinal mass and inferior vitreous seeds. B Scan ultrasound shows a funnel retinal detachment in Coats' disease (**c**) compared to a solid mass with calcifications in retinoblastoma (**d**)

option in order to minimize risk to the child's life, while sacrificing an eye that was very unlikely to ever have meaningful vision.

28.7 Treatment

The majority of cases of Coats' disease can benefit from treatment. In very mild cases (stage 1), treatment may be unnecessary, and in very advanced cases (stage 5), treatment is likely futile. However, for a large majority of Coats' disease cases, the severity is in stages 2–4 at diagnosis, so treatment is indicated. Given the poor prognosis for vision with or without treatment, the main benefit of therapy is to treat leaking retinal telangiectatic vessels and resolve exudate and retinal detachment in order to minimize the risk of long-term complications such as neovascular glaucoma, rubeosis iridis, cataract, and phthisis bulbi [8].

Primary treatment is usually with either cryotherapy or laser photocoagulation, both of which can be effective at treating leaking telangiectatic vessels and resolving exudates. At most centers, the preferred current treatment modality is laser photocoagulation (Fig. 28.10). However, peripheral retinal telangiectasia in the setting of total retinal detachment may preclude effective laser photocoagulation, so cryotherapy may still be useful in this setting [20]. In advanced cases of Coats' disease with a total exudative retinal detachment, posterior sclerotomy or pars plana vitrectomy may be needed to try to achieve an acceptable structural result (Fig. 28.11) [21, 22]. Following primary treatment, patients need to be monitored long term as recurrent disease is common and repeat treatment is often necessary [23].

A recent trend in treatment is the use of intravitreal anti-VEGF (vascular endothelial growth factor) agents as an adjunct to primary treatment. The underlying concept is that anti-VEGF agents can decrease the vascular permeability of

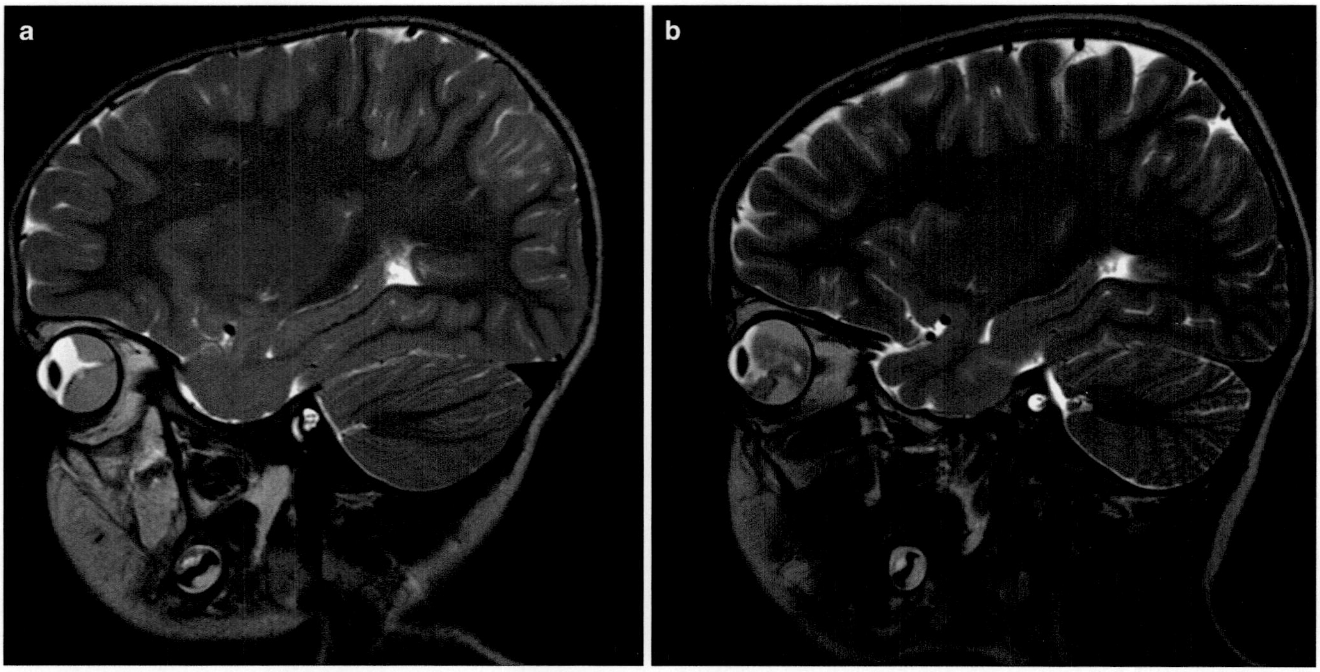

Fig. 28.9 MRI (Sagittal, T2-weighted) comparison of Coats' disease to retinoblastoma. MRI of Coats' disease (**a**) showing a funnel-shaped retinal detachment, a cystic and slightly thickened appearance of the detached retina, and no discernable mass. MRI of retinoblastoma (**b**) showing a funnel-shaped retinal detachment, significant retinal thickening, and a solid mass originating from the inferior/anterior aspect of the retina

capillary endothelial cells, thereby improving the effectiveness of laser ablation [24]. Several case series have reported promising results, although there are concerns about an increased risk of vitreous fibrosis and tractional retinal detachment [24–27].

28.8 Prognosis

The visual prognosis of Coats' disease has been historically quite poor [1, 28]. However, with more aggressive use of laser ablative therapy, surgical intervention for retinal detachment, and the recent introduction of intravitreal anti-VEGF agents, there has been a gradual trend of improving outcomes [29]. Structural outcomes in particular have improved with aggressive treatment. Even in cases with total retinal detachment, treatment can usually achieve anatomic success, which decreases the risk of phthisis bulbi and enucleation [21, 30–32].

Unfortunately, functional outcomes remain poor, especially in advanced disease [1]. The disease severity at presentation is the most important prognostic factor in the final visual outcome [33]. Eyes that present with a total retinal detachment (stage 3B or worse) have essentially no chance of achieving useful vision and most end up with no light perception vision despite aggressive treatment [28]. Eyes with extensive foveal exudation at diagnosis (stage 2B) also have a high rate of subfoveal fibrosis and a very poor prognosis for visual acuity. Young age at diagnosis has been associated with a worse visual outcome, although this may be due to the fact that young children usually present with leukocoria or strabismus, which only occurs once the disease is advanced and vision is poor [5]. If Coats' disease is detected at an early stage, good long-term visual outcomes are possible. Approximately 50% of stage 2 eyes ultimately achieve a visual acuity of better than 20/200 and a smaller proportion have normal visual acuity, generally if the telangiectatic vessels can be treated prior to foveal involvement [1]. Ultimately, improving the long-term visual outcomes of Coats' disease will likely require advancements in treatment as well as methods of consistently detecting the condition at an early stage.

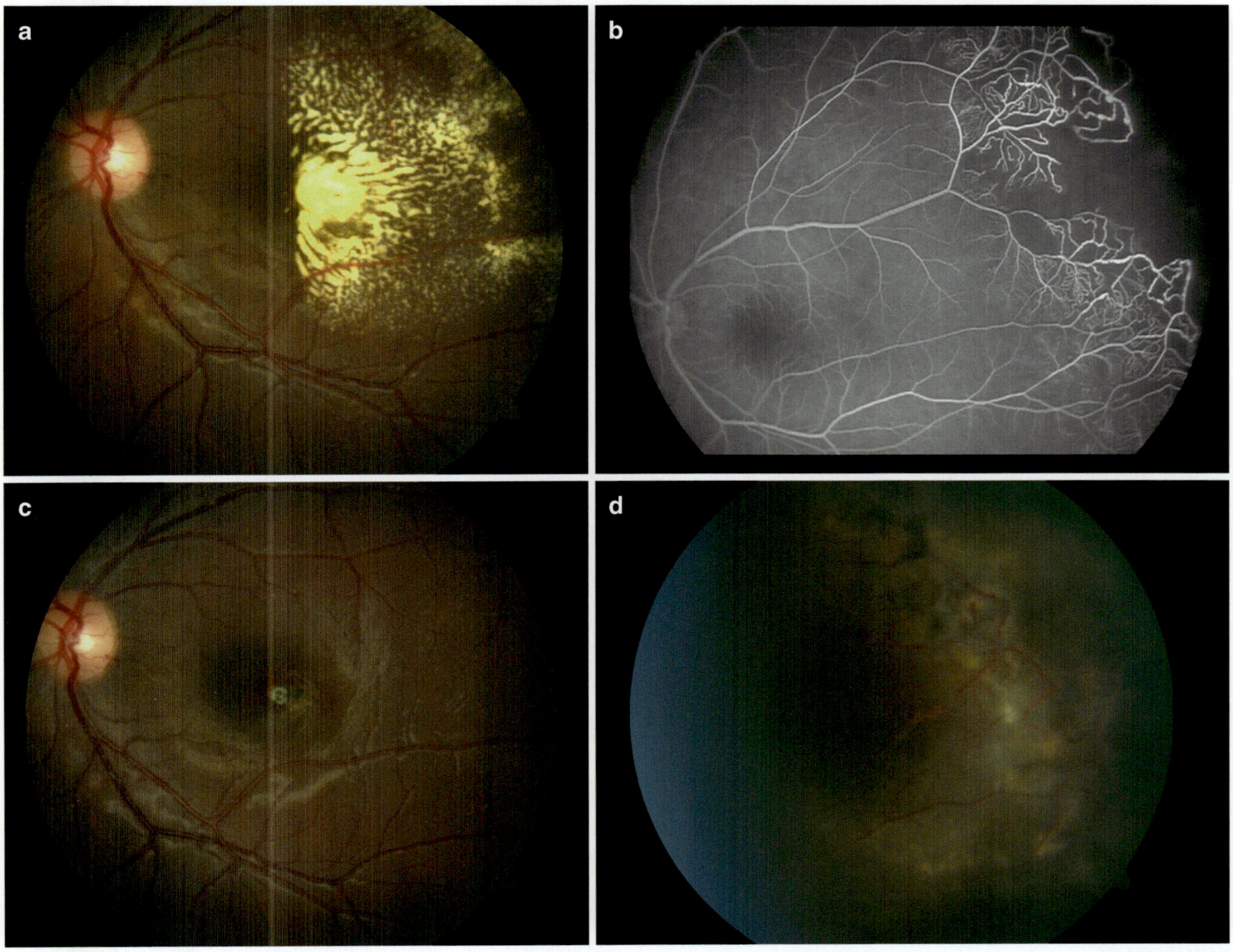

Fig. 28.10 Laser photocoagulation treatment of Coats' disease. A fundus photo of the left eye (**a**) shows foveal exudation and a fluorescein angiogram (**b**) shows peripheral telangiectasia with capillary non-perfusion. A single session of laser photocoagulation to the peripheral telangiectatic vessels and areas of non-perfusion was performed. Following treatment, the foveal exudates gradually resolved with a small area of subfoveal fibrosis (**c**). Peripheral fundus photo (**d**) several months after treatment shows scarring of the abnormal peripheral retinal vessels

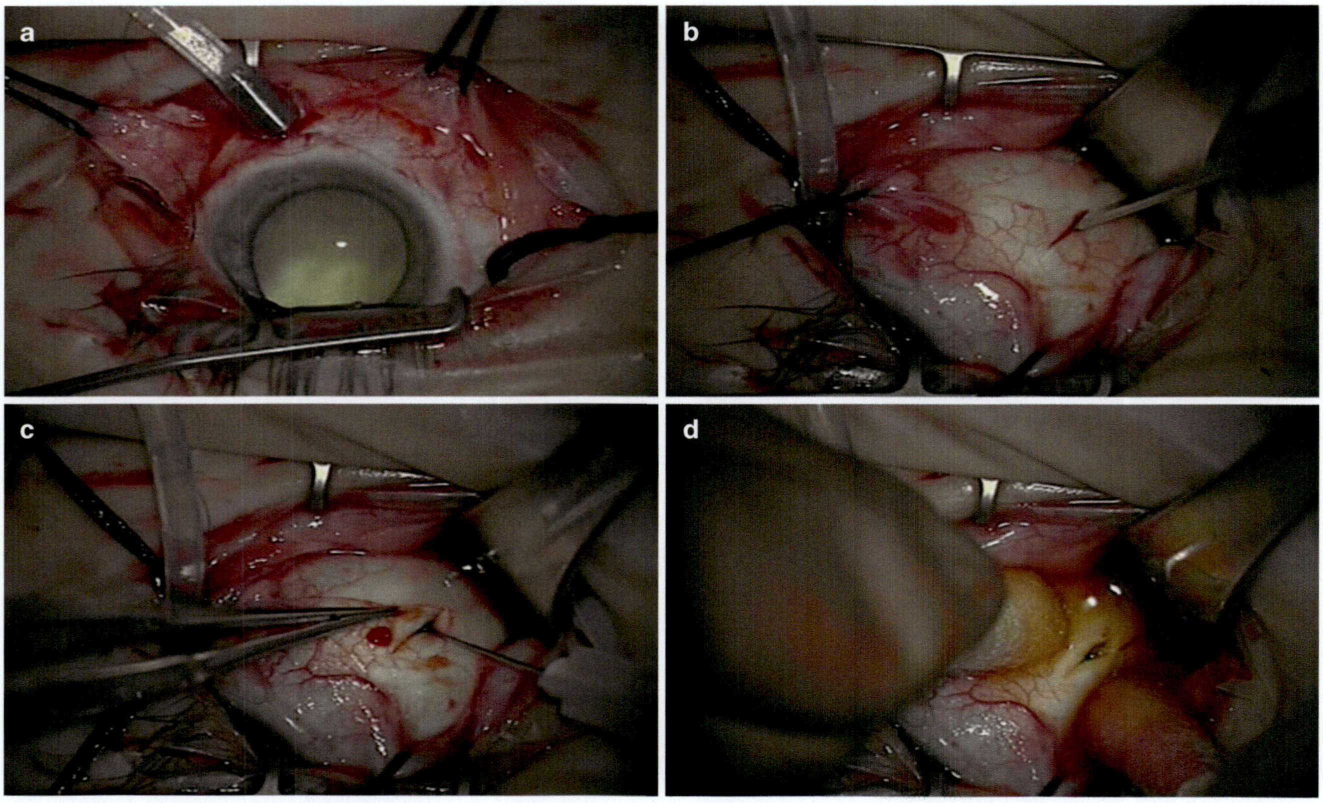

Fig. 28.11 Treatment of an exudative retinal detachment with posterior sclerotomy and drainage of subretinal fluid. (**a**) A 180-degree conjunctival peritomy is made and the rectus muscles are bridled with silk sutures. (**b**) A sclerotomy is made near the equator with a Beaver blade until the uvea is exposed. (**c**) The subretinal space is entered with a 30-gauge needle until subretinal fluid is expressed. (**d**) Cotton-tip applicators are used to gap the sclerotomy opening to facilitate drainage of the straw-colored subretinal fluid

References

1. Shields JA, Shields CL, Honavar SG, Demirci H, Cater J. Classification and management of Coats disease: the 2000 Proctor Lecture. Am J Ophthalmol. 2001;131(5):572–83.
2. Coats G. Forms of retinal disease with massive exudation. Roy Lond Ophth Hosp Rep. 1908;17:440–525.
3. Manschot WA, de Bruijn WC. Coats's disease: definition and pathogenesis. Br J Ophthalmol. 1967;51(3):145–57.
4. Duke JR. The role of cholesterol in the pathogenesis of Coats' disease. Trans Am Ophthalmol Soc. 1963;61:492–544.
5. Morris B, Foot B, Mulvihill A. A population-based study of Coats disease in the United Kingdom I: epidemiology and clinical features at diagnosis. Eye. 2010;24(12):1797–801.
6. Alexandridou A, Stavrou P. Bilateral Coats' disease: long-term follow up. Acta Ophthalmol Scand. 2002;80(1):98–100.
7. De Blauwe A, Van Ginderdeuren R, Casteels I. Bilateral Coats' disease with unusual presentation–a case report. Bulletin de la Societe belge d'ophtalmologie. 2005(295):35–9.
8. Rishi P, Rishi E, Uparkar M, et al. Coats' disease: an Indian perspective. Indian J Ophthalmol. 2010;58(2):119–24.
9. Smithen LM, Brown GC, Brucker AJ, Yannuzzi LA, Klais CM, Spaide RF. Coats' disease diagnosed in adulthood. Ophthalmology. 2005;112(6):1072–8.
10. Simon AJ, Lev A, Zhang Y, et al. Mutations in STN1 cause Coats plus syndrome and are associated with genomic and telomere defects. J Exp Med. 2016;213(8):1429–40.
11. Otani T, Yasuda K, Aizawa N, Sakai F, Nakazawa T, Shimura M. Over 10 years follow-up of Coats' disease in adulthood. Clin Ophthalmol. 2011;5:1729–32.
12. Al-Qahtani AA, Almasaud JM, Ghazi NG. Clinical characteristics and treatment outcomes of coats disease in a Saudi Arabian population. Retina. 2015;35(10):2091–9.
13. Grabowska A, Calvo JP, Fernandez-Zubillaga A, Rios JC, Gomez JA. A magnetic resonance imaging diagnostic dilemma: diffuse infiltrating retinoblastoma versus Coats' disease. J Pediatr Ophthalmol Strabismus. 2010; 47 Online:e1-3.
14. Shields JA, Shields CL. Differentiation of coats' disease and retinoblastoma. J Pediatr Ophthalmol Strabismus. 2001;38(5):262–6; quiz 302-263.
15. Shields CL, Uysal Y, Benevides R, Eagle RC Jr, Malloy B, Shields JA. Retinoblastoma in an eye with features of Coats' disease. J Pediatr Ophthalmol Strabismus. 2006;43(5):313–5.
16. Lam HD, Samuel MA, Rao NA, Murphree AL. Retinoblastoma presenting as Coats' disease. Eye. 2008;22(9):1196–7.
17. Shen T, Liu R, Lin J, Huang H, Li X, Yan J. Pars plana vitrectomy and evisceration resulting in death due to misdiagnosis of retinoblastoma in children: a review of 3 cases. Medicine. 2015;94(32):e1338.
18. Haik BG. Advanced Coats' disease. Trans Am Ophthalmol Soc. 1991;89:371–476.
19. Soliman SE, Wan MJ, Heon E, Hazrati LN, Gallie B. Retinoblastoma versus advanced Coats' disease: is enucleation the answer? Ophthalmic Genet. 2016;1–3.

20. Sigler EJ, Randolph JC, Calzada JI, Wilson MW, Haik BG. Current management of Coats disease. Surv Ophthalmol. 2014;59(1):30–46.
21. Muftuoglu G, Gulkilik G. Pars plana vitrectomy in advanced Coats' disease. Case Rep Ophthalmol. 2011;2(1):15–22.
22. Adam RS, Kertes PJ, Lam WC. Observations on the management of Coats' disease: less is more. Br J Ophthalmol. 2007;91(3):303–6.
23. Schefler AC, Berrocal AM, Murray TG. Advanced Coats' disease. Management with repetitive aggressive laser ablation therapy. Retina. 2008;28(3 Suppl):S38–41.
24. Giannakopoulos M, Drimtzias E, Panteli V, Vasilakis P, Gartaganis SP. Intravitreal ranibizumab as an adjunctive treatment for Coats disease (6-year follow-up). Retinal Cases Brief Rep. 2016.
25. Villegas VM, Gold AS, Berrocal AM, Murray TG. Advanced Coats' disease treated with intravitreal bevacizumab combined with laser vascular ablation. Clin Ophthalmol. 2014;8:973–6.
26. Gaillard MC, Mataftsi A, Balmer A, Houghton S, Munier FL. Ranibizumab in the management of advanced Coats disease Stages 3B and 4: long-term outcomes. Retina. 2014;34(11):2275–81.
27. Ramasubramanian A, Shields CL. Bevacizumab for Coats' disease with exudative retinal detachment and risk of vitreoretinal traction. Br J Ophthalmol. 2012;96(3):356–9.
28. Budning AS, Heon E, Gallie BL. Visual prognosis of Coats' disease. J AAPOS. 1998;2(6):356–9.
29. Ong SS, Buckley EG, McCuen BW II, et al. Comparison of visual outcomes in Coats' disease: a 20-year experience. Ophthalmology. 2017;124(9):1368–76.
30. Mrejen S, Metge F, Denion E, Dureau P, Edelson C, Caputo G. Management of retinal detachment in Coats disease. Study of 15 cases. Retina. 2008;28(3 Suppl):S26–32.
31. Kiratli H, Eldem B. Management of moderate to advanced Coats' disease. Ophthalmologica Journal international d'ophtalmologie/Int J Ophthalmol Zeitschrift fur Augenheilkunde. 1998;212(1):19–22.
32. Silodor SW, Augsburger JJ, Shields JA, Tasman W. Natural history and management of advanced Coats' disease. Ophthalmic Surg. 1988;19(2):89–93.
33. Chiu HH, Wan MJ, Kertes PJ, Muni RH, and Lam WC. Visual outcomes after treatment in pediatric patients with Coats' disease. Can J Ophthalmol. 2019;54(6):647–652.

Stickler Syndrome and Associated Collagenopathies

29

Michael J. Shapiro, Michael P. Blair, Sidney A. Schechet, Boleslav Kotlyar, Lisa L. Leishman, Mark A. Solinski, and David L. Zhang

Abstract

Stickler Syndrome (SS) is a hereditary disease of the vitreous collagen matrix that is composed of collagen Types II, XI/V, and IX. SS is a major contributor to nontraumatic rhegmatogenous retinal detachment (RD) in children. 50–70% of SS patients develop RD. The authors describe both the ocular and the non-ocular expressions of the SS collagen mutations. They focus on the diagnosis and management of SS, including phenotypic features and variations. Special attention is given to identification of Type I (membranous) vitreous anomaly because it is the gateway to expert management of ocular complications of SS. Other key topics include recommendations for Stickler suspects as well as the efficient diagnosis for genetic and retina consultants, proper patient surveillance, the role of prophylaxis, and advanced surgical techniques for repair of retinal detachment associated with giant retinal tear.

Keywords

Vitreous anomaly · Giant retina tear · Pediatric retinal detachment · Prophylaxis · Collagen mutation

M. J. Shapiro (✉)
Retina Consultants, Ltd., Des Plaines, IL, USA

Department of Ophthalmology and Visual Science, University of Illinois at Chicago, Chicago, IL, USA

M. P. Blair
Retina Consultants, Ltd., Des Plaines, IL, USA

Department of Ophthalmology and Visual Science, University of Chicago, Chicago, IL, USA

S. A. Schechet
Department of Ophthalmology and Visual Science, University of Chicago, Chicago, IL, USA

B. Kotlyar · L. L. Leishman · M. A. Solinski · D. L. Zhang
Retina Consultants, Ltd., Des Plaines, IL, USA

29.1 History

In June of 1965 Gunnar Stickler et al. reported on a family pedigree of 6 generations and 64 members [1]. In affected family members, they found myopia ranging from 8 to 18 diopters with a large proportion showing retinal detachment (RD) and blindness. They found that all affected members showed joint abnormalities. The long bones findings included hypermobility, stiffness, abnormal articular surfaces, and degeneration. The pedigree suggested an autosomal dominant pattern. The condition was termed hereditary progressive arthro-ophthalmopathy. The joint findings suggested defective cartilage. Finally, three members of the pedigree were also noted to have cleft palate.

After this initial report further features were identified: midfacial hypoplasia, low nasal bridge, low bulbous nasal tip, cleft palate [2] (full or partial), bifid uvula, Pierre Robin sequence (PRS) [2, 3], disorder of teeth, including crowding, hearing disorder (conductive and sensorineural), mild spondyloepiphyseal dysplasia, vitreous anomaly, early cortical cataract, RD, giant retinal tear (GRT), retina breaks, lattice and perivascular lattice and perivascular pigment [2, 4–10].

The constellation of findings pointed toward connective tissue disorder involving the cartilage and vitreous. As the molecular biology of collagen advanced, the importance of type II collagen in both vitreous and cartilage was clarified, and it became a very strong candidate for this disorder. In 1987, Francamono et al. [11] found a linkage between the affected patients and their COL2A locus. In 1991 Ahmad [12] identified a linked polymorphism in COL2A with a single base mutation causing a stop codon and a truncated type 2 procollagen protein. This abnormal protein leads to disruption in the assembly of the vitreous fibrllar structure (Fig. 29.1).

W.-C. Wu, W.-C. Lam (eds.), *A Quick Guide to Pediatric Retina*, https://doi.org/10.1007/978-981-15-6552-6_29

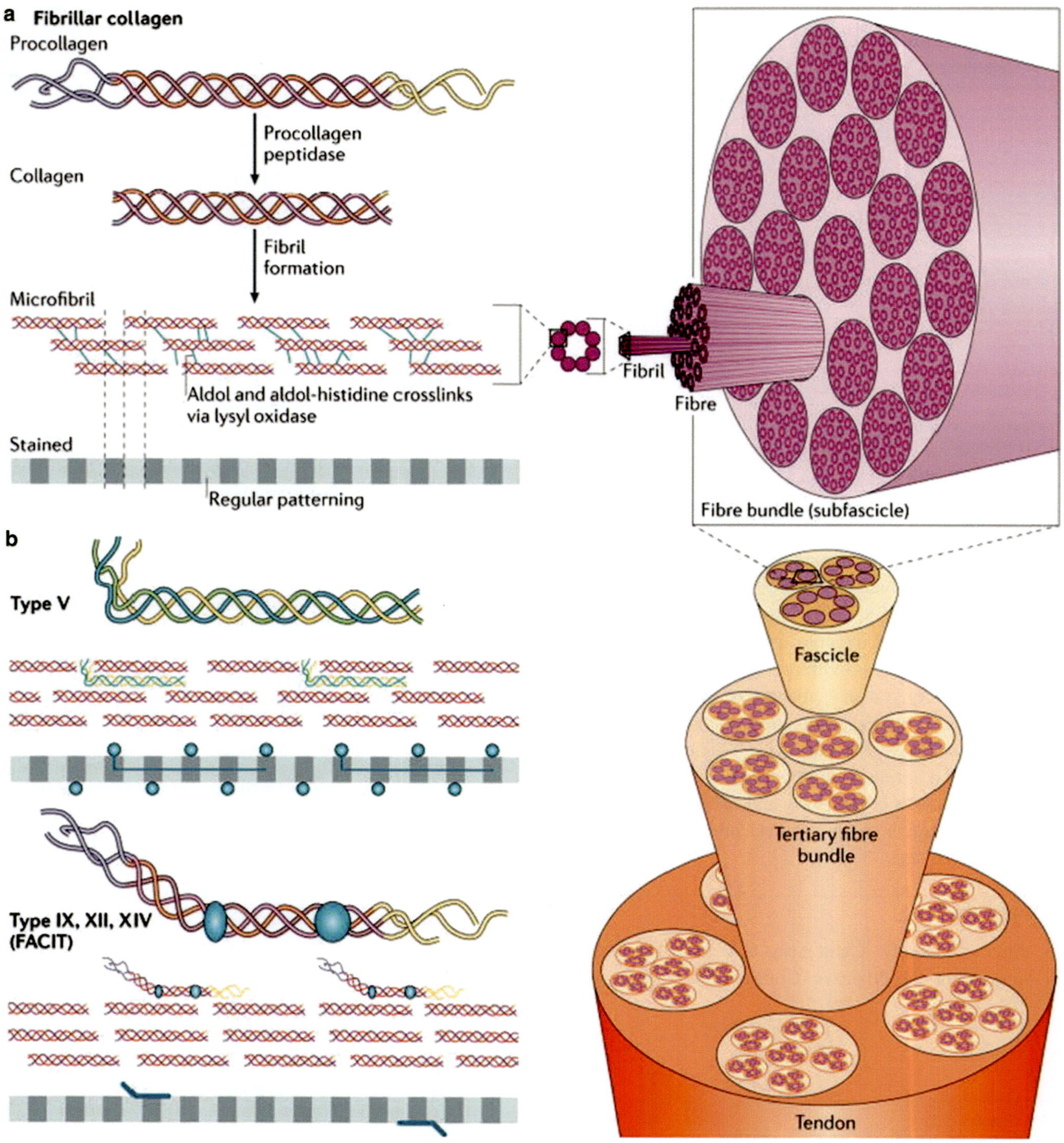

Fig. 29.1 Process of Collagen Fiber assembly. (**a**) Depicts fibrillar collagen assembly in the vitreous for type II and type XI. (**b**) Depicts insertion of type V and type IX collagen within the fibril structure of the vitreous. Vitreous collagen constituents include type II, a hybrid of type V and type XI, and type IX (Reproduced with permission from Mouw JK, Ou G, Weaver VM. Extracellular matrix assembly: a multiscale deconstruction. Nature Reviews Molecular Cell Biology. 2014;15(12):771-785. PubMed PMID: 25370693)

29.2 Genetics and Clinical Categories

Currently, Online Mendelian Inheritance in Man (OMIM) identifies four forms of Stickler Syndrome (SS). Stickler Syndrome type I (STL1) is caused by heterozygous mutation in the COL2A1 gene (OMIM 120140) on chromosome 12q13. Stickler Syndrome type II (STL2) is caused by heterozygous mutation in the COL11A1 gene (OMIM 120280) on chromosome 1p21. Stickler Syndrome type IV (STL4) is caused by a homozygous mutation in the COL9A1 gene OMIM 120210) on chromosome 6q13. Stickler Syndrome type V (STL5) is caused by a homozygous mutation in the COL9A2 gene (OMIM 120260) on chromosome 1p34.

This numbering of the types of SS reflects that formerly, there were five forms of SS. This included "non-ocular stickler disease" as Stickler syndrome type III. It was renamed autosomal dominant otospondylomegaepiphyseal dysplasia (OSMEDA), also known as Weissenbacher–Zweymuller syndrome (WZS). It is caused by heterozygous mutation in the COL11A2 gene (OMIM 120290) on chromosome 6p21. The vitreous is not affected in OSMEDA because collagen type V from the COL5A2 gene replaces collagen type XI from the COL11A2 gene in the vitreous [13].

Currently, the type I SS has two phenotypes; the predominantly ocular stickler (non-syndromic) and the syndromic subgroup with both eye and non-ocular features. This occurs either from mutations causing alternate splicing abnormalities related to exon 2 mutations [14] or "mild" mutations that lead proteins with reduced biophysical impact on the resulting collagen function [15].

Aside from SS, there are quite a large number of COL2A1 syndromes, each of which has a particular phenotypic description (Table 29.1) (OMIM 120140). Since they affect the same type 2 procollagen product that is shared by cartilage and vitreous there is significant overlap. Spondyloepiphysial Dysplasia Congenita and Kniest Dysplasia are relatively large groups. These more common syndromes have established RD risk [16, 17], and patients with these phenotypes should be treated similar to SS. Although in some rare phenotypes, RD has not been described, we consider it biologically likely that a set of COL2A1 mutations with significant cartilage abnormality result in abnormal vitreous fibrillar structures and, therefore, a increased risk of RD. As a result we treat all these key collagen gene syndromes similair to SS. We recommend this biology based approach as a practical solution for uncertainty regarding the rare COL2A1 and COL11A1 syndromes until we have relevant patient experience, and directly observe the presence or absence of vitreous anomaly and retinal disease. We also look forward to communication with other specialists on this topic in order to test our biologically based practice.

29.3 Diagnosis: Patient Presentation Categories, and Key Clinical Features

We see four categories of patients among new patient referrals. The examinations of these patients are both diagnostic and therapeutic. In the office, our exam emphasizes SS (Tables 29.3 and 29.4) features and the associated family history of RD. The first group, and least surprising, are patients sent because of newly diagnosed SS by a geneticist usually because of a defined family history or a genetics work up of PRS or cleft palate. In these patients, the central question is the presence of RD or RD risk. The most troubling subset within this group of patients are those with developmental

Table 29.1 COL2A1 phenotypes (OMIM 120140)

Location	Phenotype	Phenotype MIM number	Inheritance	Phenotype mapping key
12q13.11	Achondrogenesis, type II or hypochondrogenesis	200610	AD	3
	Avascular necrosis of the femoral head	608805	AD	3
	Czech dysplasia	609162	AD	3
	Epiphyseal dysplasia, multiple, with myopia and deafness	132450	AD	3
	Kniest dysplasia	156550	AD	3
	Legg–Calve–Perthes disease	150600	AD	3
	Osteoarthritis with mild chondrodysplasia	604864	AD	3
	Platyspondylic skeletal dysplasia, Torrance type	151210	AD	3
	SED congenita	183900	AD	3
	SMED Strudwick type	184250	AD	3
	Spondyloepiphyseal dysplasia, Stanescu type	616583	AD	3
	Spondyloperipheral dysplasia	271700	AD	3
	Stickler syndrome, type I, nonsyndromic ocular	609508	AD	3
	Stickler syndrome, type I	108300	AD	3
	Vitreoretinopathy with phalangeal epiphyseal dysplasia			3

delay and self-injurious behavior, many of whom may have tracheostomies. This behavior simultaneously induces RD and obscures its discovery.

The second group of new referrals are patients (children and adults) with *Rhegmatogenous* RD (RRD). Clearly, the primary response is surgical repair. However, we also emphasize a careful SS-oriented family history (Table 29.2) and trauma history.

Then, we study both eyes looking for the special SS findings (Table 29.3); cortical cataract (Figs. 29.2a, b and 29.3a, b) vitreous anomaly (Figs. 29.4a–c, 29.5, 29.6, 29.7, 29.8), GRT (Figs. 29.9, 29.10, 29.11, 29.12a–d) and perivascular lattice (Fig. 29.13) are most specific. While taking the history of trauma it is important to consider its role in the RD: was trauma the sole cause, a contributor in the context of underlying genetic risk, or an occasion to discover a preexisting RD. We observe that in a healthy pediatric eye with well-formed vitreous (Figs. 29.14 and 29.15) there is often a slow, insidious course with a long delay from traumatic event to clinical detection of RD. Therefore, the state of the anterior vitreous will again help in assessing the contribution of the trauma described. Finally, we will also observe and examine for some non-ocular signs of SS (Table 29.4). Taken together, this careful evaluation will help determine whether the second eye has high risk or normal risk of RD. After the repair, we examine as many family members as possible and begin surveillance of the members with probable clinical SS (Table 29.5). We attempt to clarify the diagnosis and offer prophylaxis to patients with significant risk. This will include all eyes contralateral to GRT as well as clinical SS. If they have any of the SS molecular pathologic mutations we will recommend prophylaxis. Our prophylaxis targets the retina in the region of the vitreous base and just posterior to it, it will be described below. We will also limit contact sports and very high impact activities. The surveillance of children who are preverbal and/or unaware is especially important.

Table 29.2 Questions for children with retinal detachment

Family history of SS
Family history early-onset myopia
Family history of RD or blindness
Family history of early or childhood cataract
Family history of cleft palate
Family history of congenital airway problems
Family history of early-onset hearing impairment
Family history of joint pain join replacement or early arthritis

Key: *SS* Stickler syndrome, *RD* retinal detachments S1

Table 29.3 Eye examination for ocular findings of Stickler Syndrome

Myopia
Vitreous anomaly: anterior slit lamp membranous (type 1), beaded (type 2), empty (atypical)
OPTOS vitreous opacity in sheets
OCT dense cortical vitreous
Cataracts (especially cortical and wedge-shaped)
Perivascular lattice or pigment disruption
Typical lattice
Posterior staphyloma
RD (especially GRT)

Key: OPTOS = Ultra-wide field retinal imaging (Optos P200Tx, Optos, Scotland, UK)
OCT optical coherence tomography, *RD* retinal detachment, *GRT* giant retinal tear

Table 29.4 Characteristic non-ocular findings for diagnosis of Stickler Syndrome

Midfacial hypoplasia ranges of malar hypoplasia, broad or flat nasal bridge, indistinct nasal structure.
Incomplete palate: ranges from open cleft, submucous cleft, to bifid uvula.
Mandibular hypoplasia: micrognathia, PRS.
Auditory: high-frequency sensorineural hearing loss.
Skeletal: mild spondyloepiphesia dysplasia, Slipped epiphysis, scoliosis, spondylolisthesis, or Scheuermann-like kyphotic deformity, osteoarthritis before age 40. Hyperextensibility.

Key: *PRS* Pierre Robin sequence

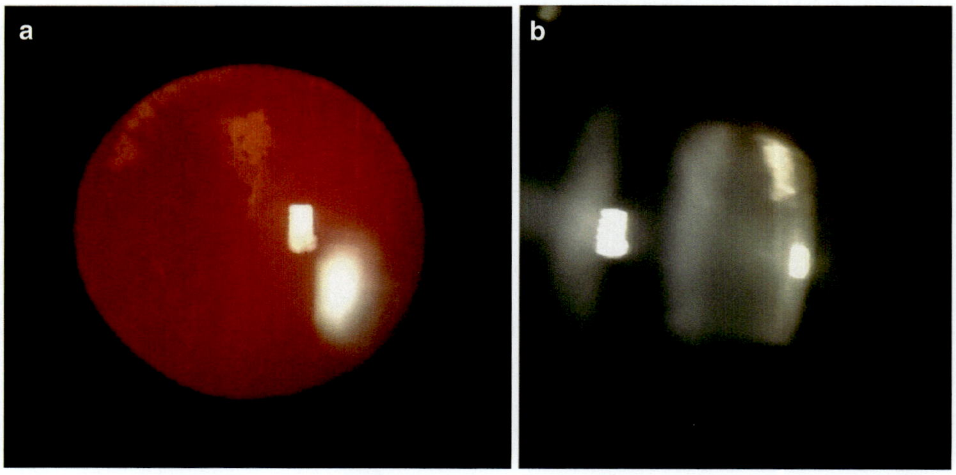

Fig. 29.2 (**a**, **b**) Figure shows a small off-axis posterior cataract. The exam also found anomalous vitreous, cataract and EOHM. This is a SS suspect because the findings are very suggestive and referral to genetics and surveillance are recommended. An additional criterion would be needed before recommending prophylaxis, see text

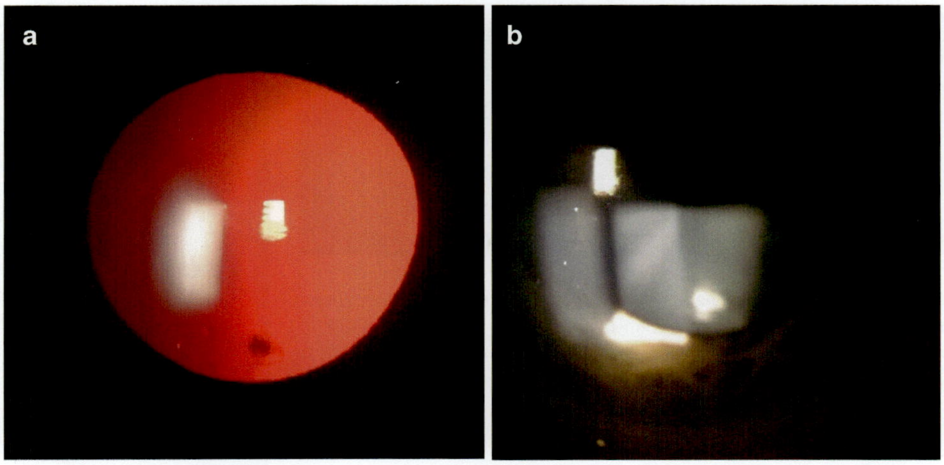

Fig. 29.3 (**a**, **b**) Figure shows a small teardrop-shaped off-axis cataract in and otherwise clear lens

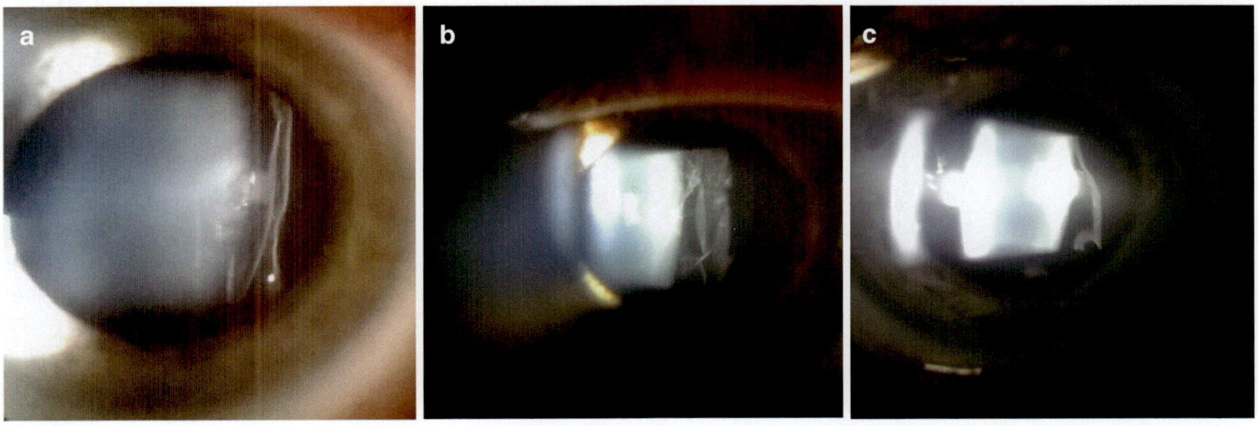

Fig. 29.4 (**a**–**c**) These are Type 1 vitreous anomaly from three different families. The patients were young with clear lenses. They show membranous interface reflections with folding and scant vitreous. Absence of or minimal fibrillar structure. In children this is a strong finding for SS and makes the patient a SS suspect and referral to genetics, surveillance, and eye protection would be started. See text for a detailed discussion of our practice pattern

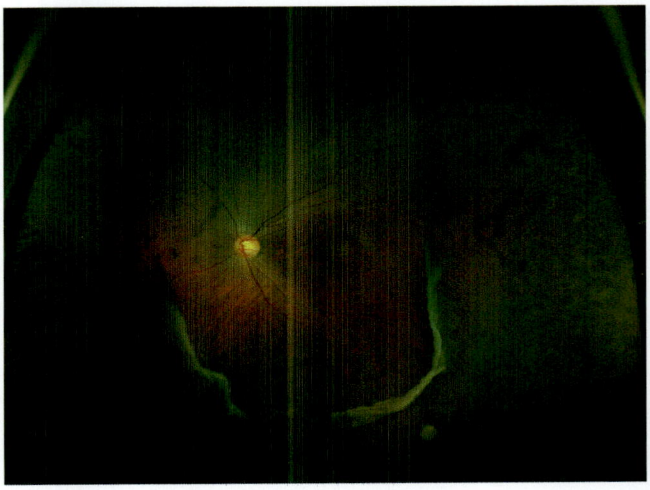

Fig. 29.5 Wide-field fundus image (OPTOS) shows an anomalous vitreous that we have not seen in non-SS cases even among adults

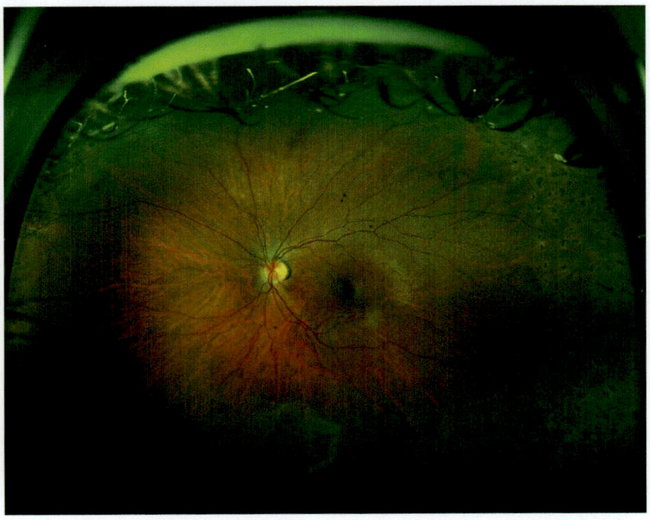

Fig. 29.6 Wide-field fundus image (OPTOS) shows an anomalous vitreous with sheets of folded vitreous

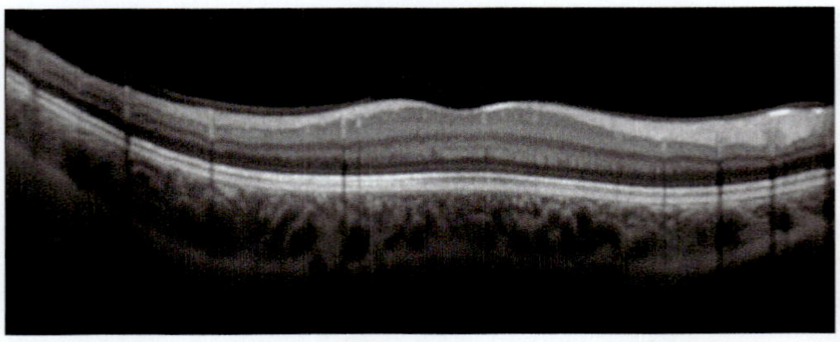

Fig. 29.7 OCT shows a band of cortical attached to retina. Our experience indicates that this is common in SS but not in normal eyes or in myopic children and warrants a particularly careful slit-lamp exam. It can be seen in myopic adults, therefore, this is more suggestive than definitive

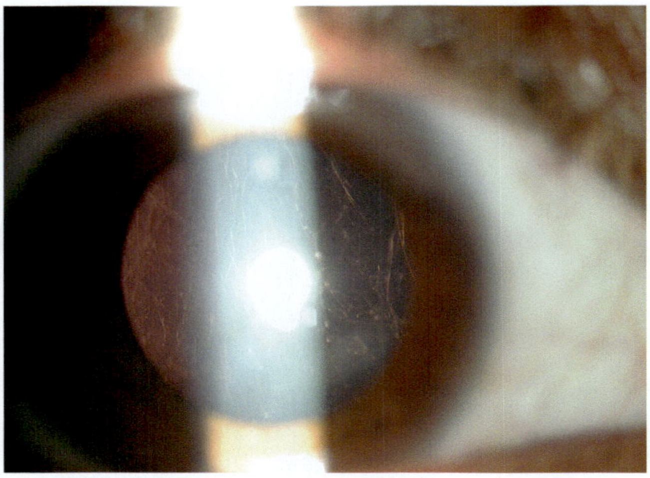

Fig. 29.8 Retroillluminated view of a beaded vitreous anomaly. This anomaly is more often seen with COL11A2 mutations or Type 2 Vitreous Anomaly

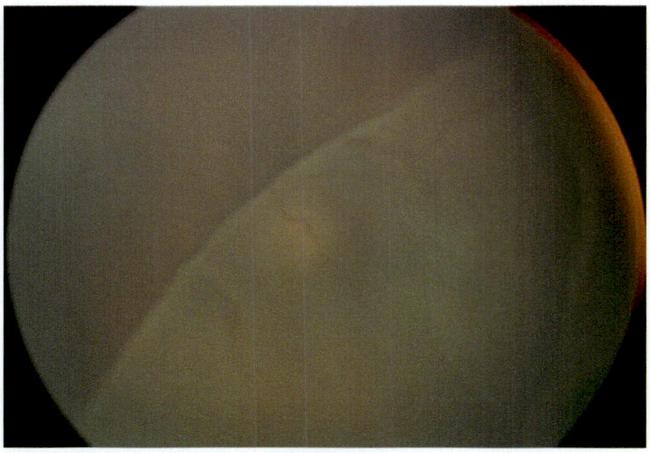

Fig. 29.9 Figure shows a fresh GRT without PVR. The disc can be seen through a partially transparent folded flap of retina

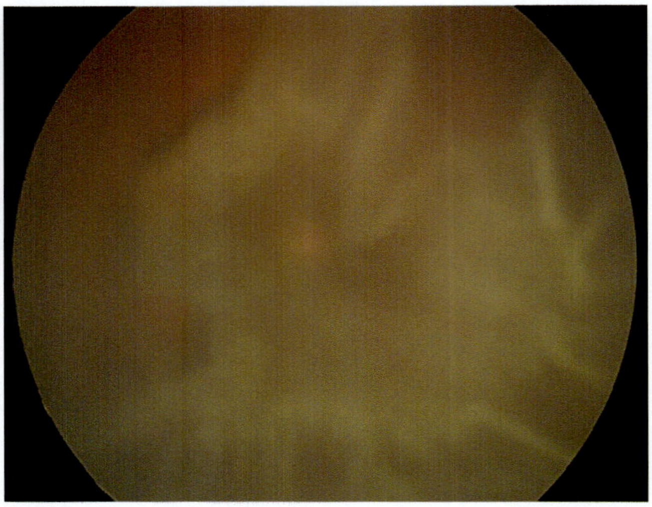

Fig. 29.10 Figure shows a moderate funnel and GRT. The funnel shows moderated fixed folds and the superior nasal GRT flap edge is scrolled. Because of PVR and GRT, there is poor countertraction. The scrolling has a membrane on the inner retina surface and requires patient work. The posterior PFCL and anterior bimanual surgery may open and mobilized the edge with careful effort. Often there is pigment that marks the membranes

Table 29.5 Surveillance: A program of examinations for children with Stickler Syndrome to detect retinal detachments before severe proliferative vitreoretinopathy occurs

Examinations begin at 6 months.
Follow-up examinations at 3–4-month intervals until reaching developmental states that allow clear and reliable communication.
Between examinations, the parents are instructed to perform home examinations to detect change in *uni*lateral vision (cover each eye and test for age-appropriate responses to visual stimuli).
Ultrasound may help augment incomplete examinations and probably detect posterior RD in 85–90% of cases.
Perform EUA at risk estimate 15%: indicated to follow-up on suspicion and when no examination beyond ultrasound is possible.
Special examinations after eye trauma events.

Key: *RD* retinal detachments, *EUA* examination under anesthesia

The third group of new referrals are patients with early-onset high myopia (EOHM). We have been passively accepting these referrals without a specific indication. Zhou et al. proved the value of a criterion for EOHM of −6 diopters at 7 years for molecular study and discovery of SS [18]. EOHM does not require specialized retina equipment and is a sensitive and easy feature to trigger investigation for SS. In that sense, it has potential as a useful indication for SS screening. However, since it is seen in many other circumstances and is not present in all SS with molecular proven mutations, it is

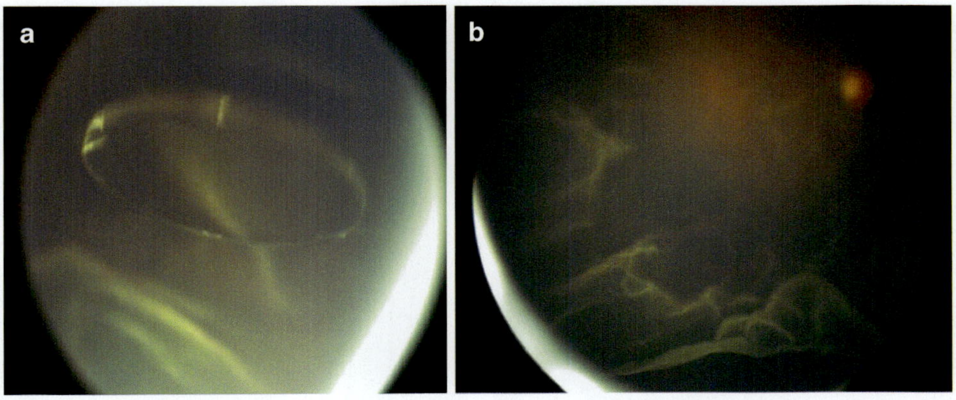

Fig. 29.11 (**a**, **b**) Top shows a dislocated PCIOL with RD. Right shows inferior GRT with very mild edge rolling. This child had a tracheostomy, developmental delay, and was non-verbal. She banged her head against surfaces when frustrated or upset. This activity was evident in the office during the exam. The PVR was mild. The mildness of the PVR allowed surgery without the use of bimanual active instruments. However, the inferior GRT required a face-down position. The IOL was removed. Postoperative she was admitted to the ICU for sedated, face down-position

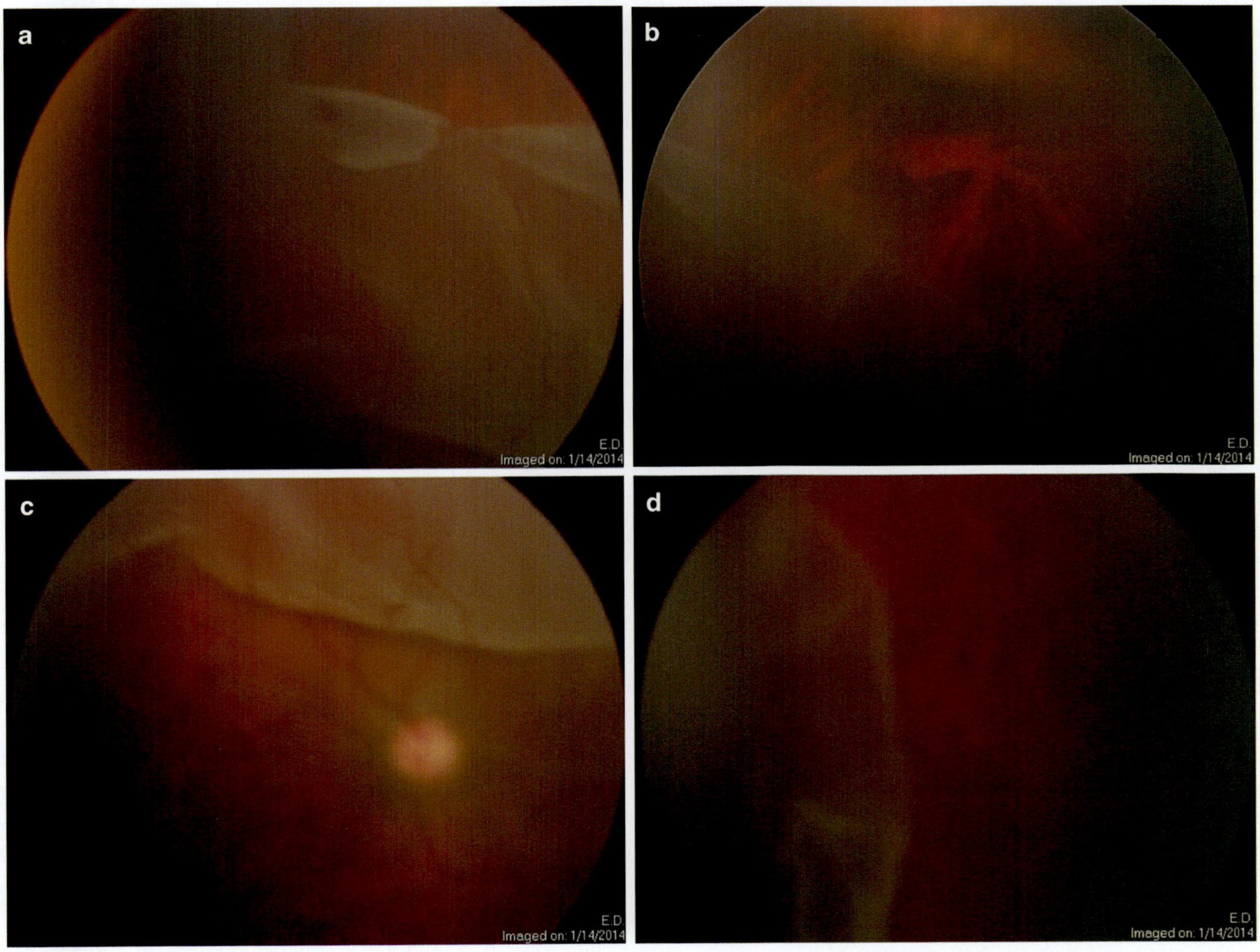

Fig. 29.12 (**a–d**) This is a GRT after ineffective Scleral Buckle prophylaxis. We found no areas of chorioretinal adhesion. This treatment had no effect on the prognosis and shows the importance of treating the vitreous base to induce chorioretinal adhesion. The secondary goal of prophylaxis is to reduce the failure rate by changing the RD from configuration from GRT to RD with single or multiple small breaks. These latter detachments have lower PVR rates

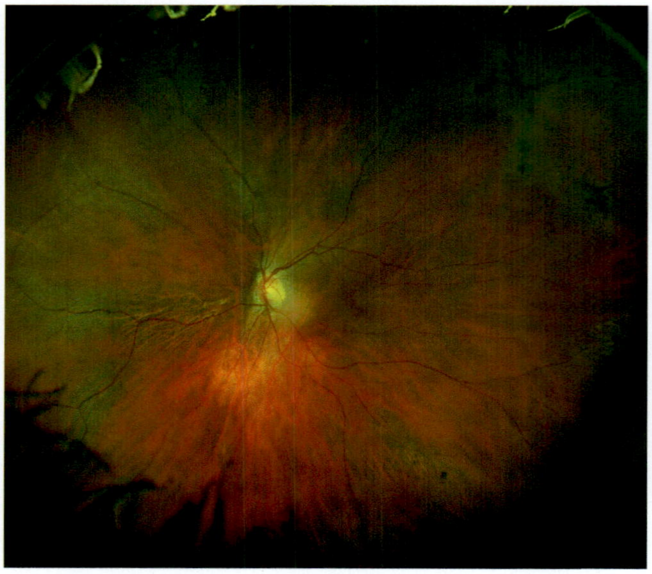

Fig. 29.13 Figure shows perivascular lattice with pigmentation. This is a highly specific finding for SS. When added to vitreous anomaly we will consider this combination adequate for the clinical diagnosis of SS. We prefer more clinical criteria, family history, or molecular confirmation and will refer this patient to genetics. However, this combination of vitreous anomaly and perivascular lattice is the minimum criteria for an informed discussion and recommendation of prophylaxis laser. We speculate that there may be rare masquerades without SS but have not yet encountered that case. This possibility might be part if of the informed discussion

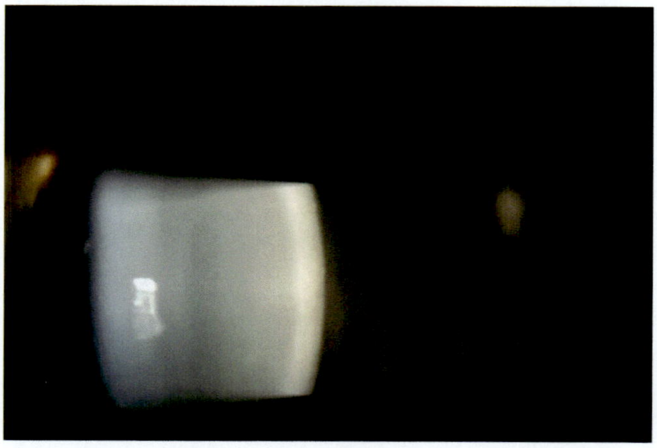

Fig. 29.14 This is an example of an early-onset high myopia (EOHM) referral who displayed a well-formed anterior vitreous with continuous fibrils and no bright interfaces. We have never seen a well-formed vitreous in our cohort of stickler patients. Therefore, we consider this finding an exclusion criterion for SS

not specific enough to function as a strong inclusion or exclusion diagnostic criterion. Seven years old is quite a late moment for diagnosis, since a significant percentage will have already suffered a retinal detachment at that point. Therefore, −3 diopters under the age of 5 years seems a more useful screening threshold.

Finally, a fourth group of patients are referred because of a family history of RRD. This history is a clinical indication

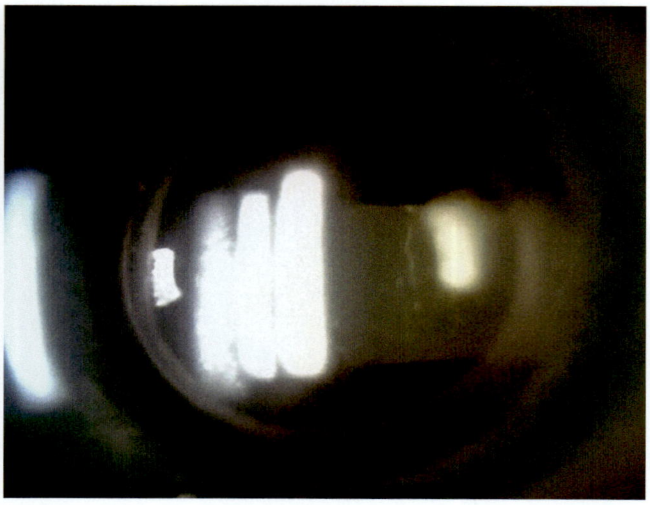

Fig. 29.15 This figure shows a well-formed vitreous in a myopic woman in her 50s with PCIOLG. The PCIOL allows an enhanced view of the anterior vitreous. Syneresis is common in this age group without Stickler and there are indeterminate exams. However, a normal well-formed vitreous has not been seen or reported in ocular or combined ocular and systemic stickler syndrome

for continued observation of patients with or without EOHM. In order to provide evidence for an inherited risk, a family history of RD requires a minimum is two family members. Of course, in case of a suspected inherited risk of RD, for example, a sibling or parent with RRD, they should also be examined for vitreous anomaly and other SS findings, and the pedigree should be invited for retina care. Indeed, all these children with non-specific features such as EOHM or RRD pedigree are examined for ocular (Table 29.3) and non-ocular signs (Table 29.4) of SS.

29.4 Diagnostic Criteria for SS and Clinical Practice Pattern

There is a proposed formal diagnostic schema geared to pediatric geneticists and pediatricians that emphasizes the non-ocular findings [19] (Table 29.6).

Although some criteria are based on direct observations, others are based on testing performed by radiology and audiology. Although published in 2005, the ease of molecular testing has probably supplanted the diagnostic motivation for radiology. Nonetheless, they remain important tests for therapeutic evaluation of patients with SS. Moreover, this diagnostic schema may not detect the ocular predominant form of STL1 who will be found especially among our patients. Therefore, it would be counterproductive to require five points if there is a strong ocular phenotype.

The pediatric retina specialist's tools to directly examine the vitreous structure provide wonderful opportunities for both clinical and experimental study of type II collagen. It takes a short time to learn to differentiate normal well-formed vitreous from abnormal vitreous. A more sustained effort is

Table 29.6 Diagnostic criteria for Type 1 Stickler Syndrome (Reproduced with permission from Rose PS, Levy HP, Liberfarb RM, Davis J, Szymko-Bennett Y, et al. Stickler syndrome: clinical characteristics and diagnostic criteria. Am J Med Genet A. 2005 Oct 15;138A(3):199-207. PubMed PMID: 16152640)

Orofacial abnormalities (2 points maximum)	
2 points	Cleft palate (open cleft, submucous cleft, or bifid uvula) (major)
1 point	Characteristic face (malar hypoplasia, broad or flat nasal bridge, and micro/retrognathia)
Ocular abnormalities (2 points maximum)	
2 points	Characteristic vitreous changes or retinal abnormalities (lattice degeneration, retinal hole, retinal detachment or retinal tear) (major)
Auditory abnormalities (2 points maximum)	
2 points	High frequency sensorineural hearing loss (major)
	Age < 20: threshold ≥20 dB at 4–8 kHz
	Age 20–40: threshold ≥30 dB at 4–8 kHz
	Age >40: threshold ≥40 dB at 4–8 kHz
1 point	Hypermobile tympanic membranes
Skeletal abnormalities (2 points maximum)	
1 point	Femoral head failure (slipped epiphysis or Legg–Perthes-like disease)
1 point	Radiographically demonstrated osteoarthritis before age 40
1 point	Scoliosis, spondylolisthesis, or Scheuermann-like kyphotic deformity
Family history/molecular data	
1 point	Independently affected first degree relative in a pattern consistent with autosomal dominant inheritance or presence of *COL2A1*. *COL11A1*, or *COL11A2* mutation associated with Stickler syndrome
Diagnosis requires	
	5 or more points
	At least one major 2-point manifestation
	Absence of features suggestive of a more severe skeletal dysplasia or other syndrome (e.g., stature <5th percentile)

needed to identify vitreous anomaly as a subtype of abnormal vitreous. The tools we use clinically include slit-lamp biomicroscopy, optical coherence tomography (OCT), ultrasound, and wide-field laser fundus photography. We included multiple examples to help model a range of vitreous phenotypes (Figs. 29.4–29.7, 29.14, 29.15). The vitreous is the best in-vivo subject for the detection of the collagen abnormality of SS [20].

The diagnostic criteria used by Snead and Yeats for research purposes are: (1) congenital vitreous anomaly and, any three of the following: (2) myopia with onset before 6 years of age, usually stable, (3) RRD or para-vascular pigmented lattice degeneration, (4) joint hypermobility with abnormal Beighton score, with or without radiological evidence of joint degeneration, (5) audiometric confirmation of sensorineural hearing defect, and (6) midline clefting [21]. They also suggest a vitreous-based algorithm for efficient molecular testing (Fig. 29.16).

In our clinical practice, the diagnostic criteria for SS evolved organically since our first identified case in 1994 and was influenced by Snead and Yeats [21] as well as Rose et.al. [19]. Our clinical criteria are: (A) congenital vitreous anomaly (typical) and two (B) items: (1) Family history of RD, (2) perivascular lattice, (3) GRT, (4) systemic findings in the patient or in the pedigree, (5) oro-facial hypoplasia (nasal hypoplasia, cleft, mandibular (PRS) hearing impairment, or (6) joint findings of dysplasia. The basic oro-facial exam is within our experience. We accept the presence of a hearing aid in a child as a sign of impairment. The single most helpful eye finding is a normally formed vitreous (Figs. 29.14 and 29.15). Since we have never seen a normal patient among our SS pedigrees, we consider a normal vitreous structure the most definitive exclusion criterion for clinical SS.

Discovering any one of the specific eye findings would lead us to consider the patient a SS suspect, and we would refer to genetics expecting a more complete systemic evaluation as well as molecular confirmation. Discovery of three criteria (vitreous anomaly plus two items from the B list) will lead to clinical SS diagnosis that includes high-grade surveillance, recommendation of prophylaxis, and activity precautions. GRT alone without any other findings will lead to contralateral eye prophylaxis because of the influence of H. Mackenzie Freeman [22]. Otherwise, in suspect-only cases we do high-grade surveillance and study the pedigree; we will discuss prophylaxis, but not recommend it pending further evidence.

Finally, we also discuss the importance of the SS for pregnant mothers and children and recommend notification of the primary care physician and obstetrician. Timely prenatal referral and diagnosis is very important because it allows preparation for airway difficulties and can avoid cerebral anoxia with potential neurologic implications [23].

29.5 Management

29.5.1 Surveillance

Once a patient is diagnosed with SS, we recommend a program of monitoring in order to detect a new RD within 3 months (Table 29.5). This is likely to allow an efficient repair of GRT detachments before the development of severe proliferative vitreoretinopathy (PVR). PVR reduces the structural and visual outcomes of GRT repairs [24, 25].

We consider this guideline a work in progress that will change as more data is collected. Since we have repaired a SS patient at 8 months with a GRT (Fig. 29.21), we suggest a first exam at 6 months. After the initial exam, we recommend follow-up examinations every 3–4 months. Under the age of 1 year, the exam would be with a papoose constraint and using indirect ophthalmoscopy (IO) with scleral depressor and speculum. At ages 1–3, the child sits on the parent's lap without constraint, and IO set at the lowest light intensity. Additionally, we supplement the IO exam with a B-scan ultrasound study. We recommend EUA annually until the

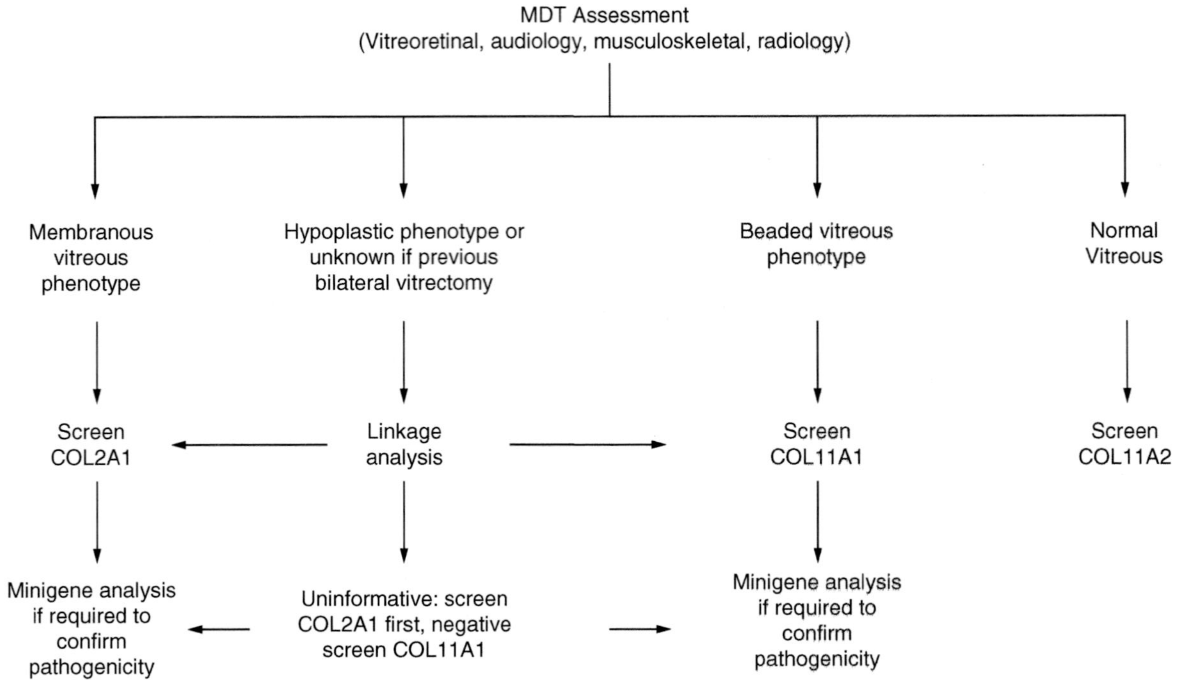

Fig. 29.16 Algorithm for gene selection and mutation analysis in Stickler Syndrome based on vitreous phenotype (Reproduced with permission from Snead MP, Mcninch AM, Poulson AV, et al. Stickler syndrome, ocular-only variants and a key diagnostic role for the ophthalmologist. Eye. 2011;25(11):1389–1400. PubMed PMID: 21921955)

child allows an exam of the posterior and anterior retina, or, in cases where prophylaxis has been performed, until the zone of chorioretinal atrophy can be seen. Wide-field office imaging (e.g., Optos) can also be quite useful in viewing the peripheral retina in young and partially cooperative children since the imaging laser has a rapid capture with low-intensity and is less bothersome. EUA is recommended for suspicion of break or RD or in event of significant trauma. At 3 years or when the child is able to communicate and follow instructions, we attempt to train the child with frequent friendly exams that are rewarded. The office exams and annual EUAs continue until around 7 years old or when the child can fully cooperate with the parents and demonstrate clear communication skills. As young as possible, we ask the parents to test each eye for "normal" vision on a monthly basis. We instruct them to cover each eye separately and elicit a verbal or behavioral response to age-appropriate visual stimuli.

29.5.2 Prophylaxis and Degrees of Uncertainty

The controversy about prophylaxis is not about whether it is better to prevent an RD or treat it after it occurs, but rather what is an effective and safe preventative treatment. The discussion of prophylaxis has a few sources of complexity. First, there is a definitional variability of retina prophylaxis. For example, the prophylaxis for RD as described by the American Academy of Ophthalmology (AAO) surrounds the retina break and areas of lattice of fellow eyes with three rows of laser [26], while the Cambridge stickler prophylaxis data shows a single row of cryotherapy spots around the retina just behind the ora serrata [27, 28]. Our general sense is that prophylaxis is learned during training and therefore the procedure is highly influenced by each surgeon's particular educational lineage. For example, MJS was a fellow under Dr. Charles Schepens and H. Mackenzie Freeman. Both were masters of the peripheral retina and treated the retina contralateral to GRT with 360-degree anterior extensive cryotherapy or scleral buckle with diathermy (Fig. 29.17). Thus, the term "retina prophylaxis" refers to very different treatments both in modality of adhesion and target of adhesion.

Second, even with a similar intention of treatment, there is a difference in implementation from physician to physician and case to case; clearly, the effect of pupil size and lens opacity will influence the visualization of the target tissue, consequently changing the settings for treatment and the visual feedback. Third, there may be a difference in response among the different phenotypes and subtypes. This complexity may be a source of variability in outcomes which leads to different practice patterns. While we have seen a very low rate of failure after GRT prophylaxis with our protocol. We have occasional cases that present after other treatments (Figs. 29.12a–d and 29.18). We are not in a position to know the ratio of success to failure for other practices. However, practitioners that have seen poor outcomes after prophylaxis ought not to adopt it as a standard treatment [29, 30].

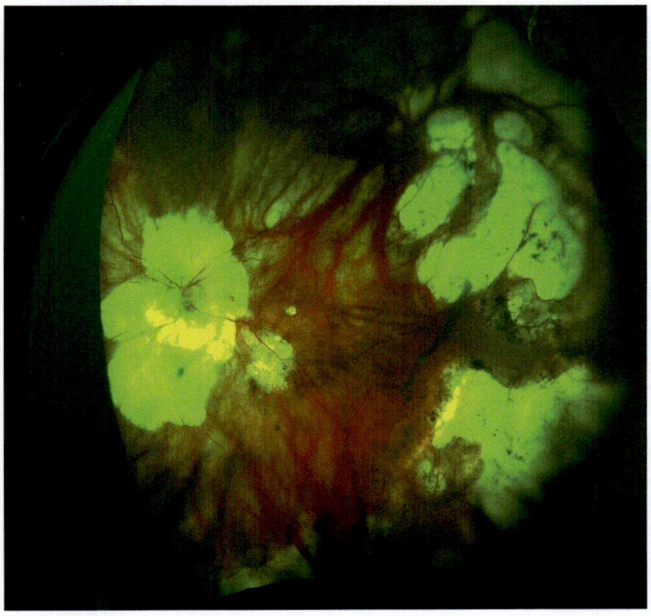

Fig. 29.17 Wide-angle photo of eye of monocularly functional SS syndrome patient treatment by Schepens. The cryotherapy extended 360 degrees from ora to equator without reference to lattice degeneration. The daughter's retina detachment was treated by T. Hirose and diagnosed clinical SS

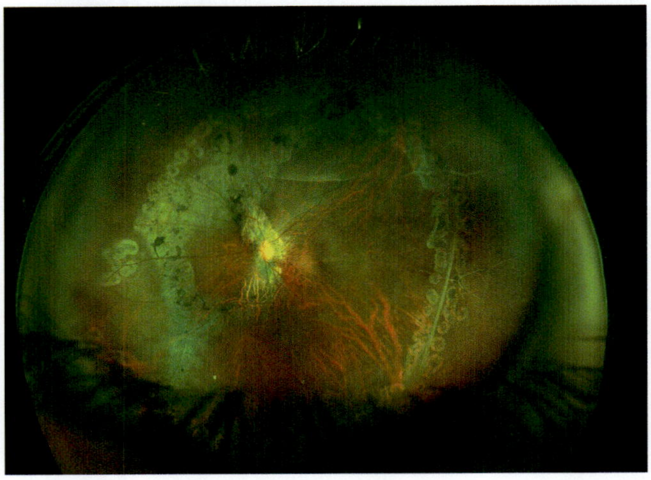

Fig. 29.18 This is a case of (spondyloepipesia dysplasia congenita) the right eye was phthisical and in the left widefield photography showed a lattice centered prophylaxis and no treatment targeted to area of GRT formation. We completed the treatment to the ora serratta before cataract surgery in the left eye. The figure also shows perivascular pigment atrophy and mild vitreous sheets superior to macula

The Cambridge group has taken an effort to standardize and describe their treatment and have presented data that supports its use [27, 28]. Although there is no identifiable bias, some bias may exist in the absence of a randomized controlled trial (RCT), and an RCT is not possible without a very large multi-center study. At this time, it remains the best evidence on which to base treatment. A review of other series reporting no benefit after prophylaxis seems significantly less persuasive because of ill-defined selection criteria and treatment patterns [29, 30].

We recommend the reader study the video in the supplementary material section of the Cambridge paper as a guide for surgeons interested in performing prophylaxis [28]. The targeting of the area of the GRT has a biologic basis. The collagen fibrillar orientation (Fig. 29.19) and vitreoretinal interface are different at the vitreous base when compared to the equatorial retina. Chorioretinal adhesion in the area that is vulnerable to GRT tears is more likely to prevent GRT than treatments that induce adhesions in other parts of the retina [27]. The preference of cryotherapy over other forms of chorioretinal adhesion (i.e., diathermy or laser) might be an important difference [29, 30]. However, it does not have an obvious compelling historical or biophysical basis [22, 31, 32].

Our only concern about the Cambridge protocol is that the skill needed for using cryotherapy may not be easy to transfer, confirm, or document. The precise application of contiguous cryotherapy applications, as seen in the supplemental video of the Cambridge Protocol report [28], requires strong cryotherapy experience and skill that was more common in previous generations. Generally, laser treatment is an easier skill because it provides better defined and more immediate visual feedback to the surgeon. Laser is the most common and effective method of inducing chorioretinal adhesion throughout vitreoretinal surgery, including the surgical repair of GRTs. Based on evidence for the equivalence of laser and cryotherapy [31, 32], in our center, we target the area of GRT extending from the ora posterior to the anterior part of the equator. Applying about 10 rows of laser, more or less to the equator. We use Laser Indirect Ophthalmoscope (LIO). The well-defined photocoagulation spot guides the treatment and helps the surgeon determine the adequacy of the treatment. Figure 29.20 shows our pattern of treatment.

While SS prophylaxis is targeted to the GRT, typical circumferential lattice may also be present and its treatment may be helpful. The treatment of circumferential lattice is standard for our practice; however, *perivascular* lattice is an uncertain target. Since it often extends to the posterior retina, we choose to treat it only anterior to the equator, within or near the usual target area for GRT prophylaxis. The most posterior areas are observed for development of breaks.

We feel that a large percentage of failures (n = 4) in our group were associated with developmental delay and tracheostomy scars. Most of the patients are clearly observed as self-injurious patients. We speculate that the late development of verbal communication or brain injury contributes to this behavior. This behavior remains an important area to investigate in order to prevent blindness. Avoidance of brain hypoxia at birth through prenatal diagnosis of cleft palate, PRS, and SS may also have an impact on this behavior.

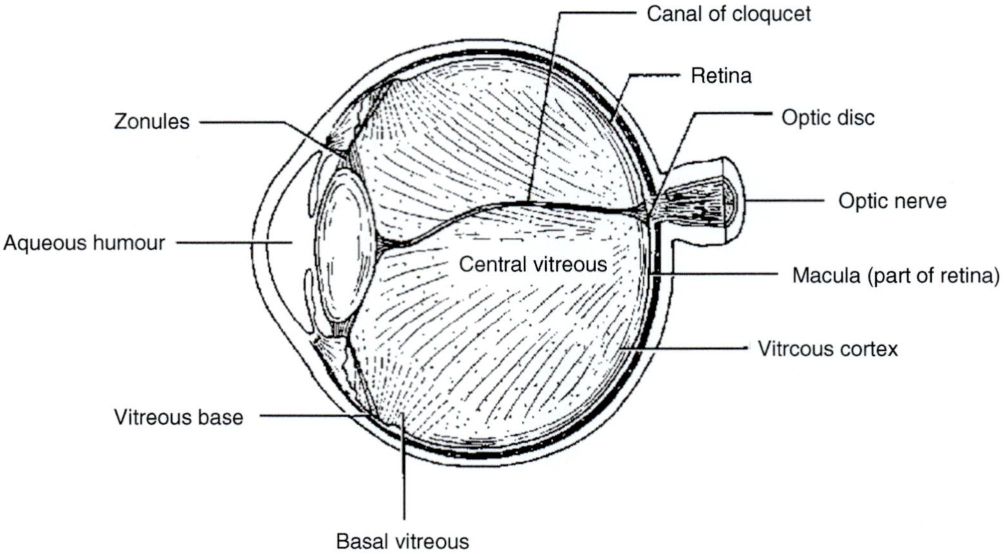

Fig. 29.19 Schematic of normal vitreous shows the importance of the vitreous base (Reproduced with permission from Bishop PN. Structural macromolecules and supramolecular organization of the vitreous gel. Progress in Retinal and Eye Research. 2000;19(3):323-344. PubMed PMID: 10749380)

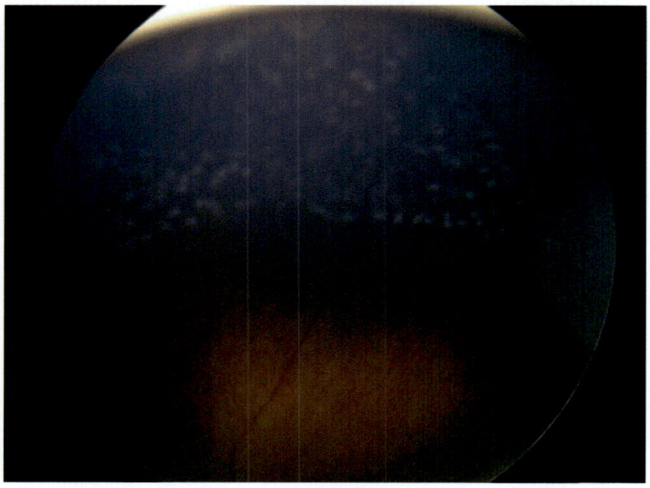

Fig. 29.20 Figure shows laser prophylaxis that targets the zone of the GRT from the ora serrata to the equatorial zone. Using the Retcam with scleral depression intraoperatively provided a confirmation of the treatment. The ora teeth and bays can be seen at the 12 o'clock position

29.5.3 Limiting High-Risk Behaviors

The data for limiting sport and other physical activity is absent, and we therefore depend on our experience and understanding of the biology of the disease. It seems to make sense to limit activities that could result in a direct and indirect impact on the eye or vigorous vitreous traction through repetitive jerky motion. These may include ball sports, contact sports, trampoline, martial arts, and roller-coaster. At the same time, other physical activities should be encouraged so as not to induce a sedentary lifestyle and associated morbidities.

29.5.4 Surgical Planning

In adults, the technique for repair of GRT is well established [33], and since the approval of perfluorocarbon liquid (PFCL), good results are the rule even with mild PVR [33–36]. However, the outcomes in children are significantly worse [24]. The increased failures revolve around the later diagnosis (with worse PVR) and the normal exploring and adaptive behaviors of children.

In vitreoretinal surgery cooperation between surgeon and patient is key to successful outcome. Needless to say, patients without cognitive ability or emotional endurance are at increased risk for failure. Children require extra effort, and it is very helpful when parents have an enthusiastic engagement in the process. In order to recruit the parents' effort, they must first understand the importance of postoperative patient cooperation. We routinely explain the key postoperative goal using an analogy. First we give a surgical overview: during surgery we attach the retina to the eye wall and apply laser which is the glue that is needed to keep the retina attached. However, the adhesion does not occur immediately but rather develops in the post-operative period. Therefore, during this period, the retina must stay in contact with the eye wall in order for the glue to work, and in order to stick the retina down permanently. It is like gluing 2 pieces of paper if you spread glue on two sheets of paper but does not keep them together in direct contact, the glue will work. Similarly, in the post-operative period we need to keep the retina in contact with the eye wall, or it will not stay glued. We do this by positioning the gas bubble or oil globule in the eye. The gas bubble floats above the fluid, and it moves with the head position. Therefore parents must give attention to keeping the correct head and eye position during the post-operative 2 weeks. We further set expectations for the the parents, and tell them they often need to stay awake every night depending on the position of the break, and actively promote the cooperation of the child. This post-operative-component is often unexpected and difficult. Therefore, it must be part of the preoperative part of the plan for surgery. Some family situations are chaotic, underresourced, or unsupervised, and this is also a high risk for failure and blindness. There is reduced value to surgery with poor postoperative cooperation.

In the infant and very young child, face-down positioning is reasonably achievable. The parents can hold the child on the lap, the chest or organize a bed position (Fig. 29.21). However, as the child becomes larger from 18 months to 4 years old, face-down positioning can be quite difficult. Beyond age 3, some parents seem capable of achieving face-down while others are not. One strategy is to use a computer tablet or smartphone for entertainment while in the face-down position. This can be done if the child holds it in the lap against the abdomen. Alternatively, playing with toys that are on the floor while the child is sitting will encourage at least partial face-down behavior (e.g., pushing toy cars). These adjustments can have a major effect on outcomes with inferior breaks.

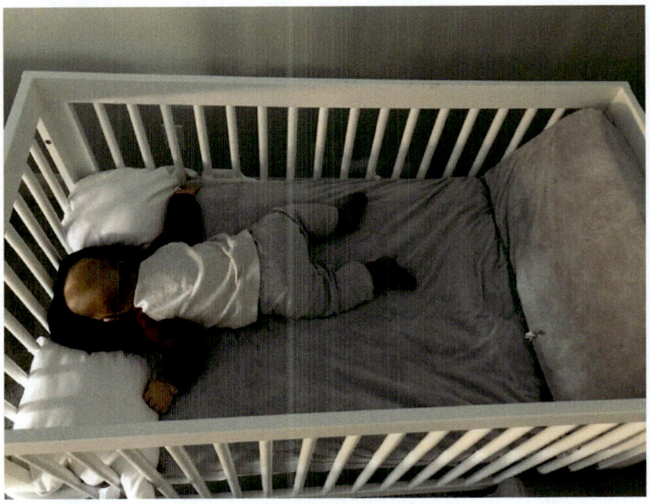

Fig. 29.21 This was an 8-month-old male with COL2A1 mutation (c. 1299_1302delCCCT) who presented with strabismus and was found to have a giant retina tear. The family was able to maintain his face-down position asleep in this created apparatus. The mattress was folded and moved toward the foot and a travel neck pillow held the face. The child was monitored from below. The repair was successful

Because the examination is often very brief in toddlers and young children, there is a balance between the number of EUAs and the tolerance of uncertainty about the retinal status. Also, the option to inject or remove gas in the office to adjust the gas fill is unrealistic; therefore, silicone oil is a frequent choice for children. Silicone oil allows an optically clear postoperative view of the retina and a reliable and persistent tamponade fill of the vitreous cavity. The reliable fill is especially reassuring when day 1 post operative exam is limited to the anterior segment. Another very helpful advantage of silicone oil over gas tamponade for children with complex RD is the delay of hypotony, ocular collapse, and phthisis in the case of RD recurrence. This feature allows multiple interventions. Both gas and silicone oil have an increased risk of failure from an incorrect eye position. However, the complication of elevated pressure from face-up position is generally less severe with gas than with silicone oil. Both situations can result in closure of the angle and cause pain and loss of vision. The elevated pressure with gas can be quite high, but with silicone oil, extremely high pressure can occur from a malignant glaucoma configuration with aqueous accumulated into a space posterior the silicone oil. Strict face-down position should resolve the pressure elevation with gas tamponade and help in eyes with silicone oil unless the oil has migrated into the anterior chamber around an IOL or crystalline lens [37]. When silicone oil migrates across the zonule into the anterior chamber (AC), an urgent reoperation for elevated IOP may be required to remove the oil completely and then replace it with either gas or new oil. The lens may need to be removed and an inferior peripheral iridectomy created in cases of zonular compromise. Although in most cases surgery to remove all the oil advised, it is possible to remove the AC oil selectively at the slit lamp. This requires two ports because the AC infusion is needed in order to maintain the AC pressure above the vitreous chamber throughout the removal. One port enters horizontally near the base and a second allows egress of the oil at the anti-dependent position. This procedure requires an exceptional patient. Selective removal of AC silicone oil is essentially impossible in a supine position because the BSS used to maintain the AC pressure is heavier than oil and therefore, will migrate posteriorly into the vitreous cavity when gravity is greater than surface tension and raise the vitreous cavity pressure. In the end, the oil removed from the AC is invariably replace with oil from the vitreous cavity. Complete removal and replacement of the silicone oil is more effective.

Despite possible complications, we consider silicone to be an effective tool for tamponade in children and monitor it closely. We plan its removal in 3–6 months in most situations. However, we may leave it in situ long term or indefinitely in two situations: the self-injurious patient, and the patient with persistent hypotony. In the self-injurious patient, long-term oil can protect against future breaks and detachments from trauma through tamponade. It seems to reduce the extent of ocular deformation that results from traumatic compressive force. Removing oil in an already hypotonous eye can accelerate phthisis. In eyes where the pressure is elevated but not immediately threatening, we will monitor and, if reasonably safe, try to keep it for 4–6 weeks.

In the past, we had two cases of patients with RD in the only seeing eye, for whom positioning was critical because of inferior breaks, but impossible (both were self-injurious, developmentally delayed patients), we took unusual measures to achieve retina attachment. We admitted them to the intensive care unit in order to allow 5 days of sedated face-down positioning. Both eyes had successful attachment; however, the second patient developed bacterial sepsis that required a week of intravenous antibiotics. Since then we have used an expansile gas in order to overfill the vitreous cavity, followed by anti-glaucoma drops, pressure monitoring, and EUA for gas fill adjustment during the first week and replacement with silicone oil after 2 weeks. This has also worked. Other options are heavy PFCL for a week of postoperative tamponade. This can lead to a significant inflammatory reaction, so the family needs to be aware that the PFCL needs to be removed within 1 week. Heavy silicone oil may also have a role for postoperative inferior retinal tamponade. We have no recent experience with heavy oils.

29.5.5 Giant Retinal Tear Surgery

The repair of GRT with*out* PVR is mildly technical, but it is more challenging if more severe PVR is present. First, we will describe our technique for the *basic* GRT repair. In children and phakic adults, we use an adjuvant scleral buckle for GRT. Cerclage can also be considered in pseudophakic patients. It can reduce the slippage of retina and reduce the effect of contractile elements that may develop in the residual vitreous base, since this can be impossible to completely remove in Stickler anomaly. We place a 240-band at the equator approximately 12 mm from the limbus 360 degrees and form an encirclement with a 4-0 nylon suture clove-hitch tightened and secured with a square knot. The buckle is secured to the sclera in each quadrant with a 4-0 nylon anchoring, circumferential mattress suture. Then three pars plana vitrectomy ports are placed normal to the sclera rather than beveled, in a manner to allow direct access to the vitreous cavity. The vitreous is removed and the retina mobilized. Because of the large break, the retina is more mobile and countertraction is reduced. In many cases, the retina may become dangerously hypermobile and PFCL may be injected posterior to the vitreous in order to weigh down the retina and help separate the vitreous from the retinal surface. This provides increased retinal stability and "counter traction" facilitating removal of the vitreous and membranes. The use of PFCL is monitored in order to avoid its migration into the subretinal space over an elevated edge or through a posterior break. The anterior flap and vitreous should be cleaned thoroughly to improve retinal mobility and remove vitreous that has prolapsed into the subretinal space that may prevent the retina from reattaching to the RPE. Special attention is given to the posterior retinal edge since this tends to roll. PFCL helps unroll this edge and helps to limit slippage during fluid–air exchange which may frequently occur due to lack of anterior tethering in the area of GRT.

In cases of GRT with PVR, a bimanual approach will likely be needed to remove the membranes. We use a chandelier in a fourth port. A lighted pick and/or forceps may also be used in conjunction with the chandelier to better illuminate areas requiring fine dissection. Occasionally, it may be necessary for an assistant to direct the chandelier for optimal illuminating conditions in the area of interest. The strategies for PVR mainly require experience, careful observation, and patient peeling to reach retina mobilization. Although published before the use of PFCL, Zivoijnovic's monogram *Silicone Oil in Vitreoretinal Surgery* (available as ebook) provides the best description of PVR surgery [38]. Any pigment on the surface represents a PVR membrane, and the membranes on inspection are often shiny and transparent and often are difficult to visualize. Their effects are often appreciated by the irregular response to smooth manipulations using a Tano diamond-dusted brush or flex-loop with micro-serrations, and the immobility during fluid drainage from the subretinal space is also a sign. Peeling off the disc and maintaining large sheets of membranes leads to more effective work. Elevating membranes with a forceps and undermining adhesion with a second instrument, such as a pick, "light-pipe" or scissors, works well. Frequently, gently sliding the second instrument (back and forth) against the junction of the retina and PVR membrane allows them to separate. In GRT, the subretinal space can also be inspected and treated as needed. Caution must be taken when addressing subretinal PVR, as bands and sheets may insert at distant locations. Lysing and dissecting subretinal PVR, rather than attempting complete removal by pulling on exposed ends, may avoid distant retinal breaks or choroidal bleeding. In reoperations, the fibrous membranes are more likely to arise from the choroid and need to be cut rather than removed with traction. In cases of choroidal hemorrhage, hemostasis is obtained without touching the tissue using a laser set at low energy and long duration. Using a bipolar cautery may cause the treated choroid to adhere to the probe leading to re-bleeding with movement of the probe. Subretinal PVR may also be left in-situ if it does not elevate the breaks. Often, the pump action of retinal pigment epithelium (RPE) may flatten the PVR or retina around the PVR in the postoperative period, assuming adequate tamponade. Posterior radial buckle elements may also be placed to counter subretinal PVR traction if complete removal of subretinal PVR is judged to be risky. Avoidance of posterior breaks makes the PFCL injection safer and avoids ablating posterior retina while creating laser-induced adhesion around these breaks.

If the media are compromised and the membranes are not well seen, we will remove the opacities, whether capsule, lens, intraocular lens (IOL), or band keratopathy. If the view is suboptimal because of corneal edema, we will use 50% glucose as an osmotic agent. In some cases, we may be forced to return for more complete repair as part of a staged second sitting because of media and time constraints. Retinectomy should be absolutely minimal or preferably avoided. We will prefer to abort a case, hoping for some reattachment and countertraction that may aid in subsequent surgeries, rather than to reduce the retina to a "postage stamp," except as a last resort in the only eye. Our experience with the large retinectomy is that it results in hypotony, induces PVR admixed with a fibrinous response, requires reoperation to avoid contraction and detachment, and does not add visual function if the fellow eye has more than count fingers vision. Therefore, we reserve this as a last resort for monocular patients for whom the low vision may add function and quality of living. In other cases, the radical retinotomy that reduced the retina to a posterior "postage stamp," allows the surgeon to report successful retinal attachment, but the middle and long-term prognosis is grave. Moreover, retinal removal is not reversible and may preclude visual rehabilitation in the event that new technologies are developed.

The subretinal fluid removal and exchange to PFCL is performed when the membrane peeling, release of pleats and folds, and subsequent retina mobilization is adequate. This mobility can be tested by subretinal drainage in the fluid-infused eye. The eye is filled with PFCL while the eye rotated away from the GRT, toward a zone of intact peripheral retina. In this rotated position, the vitreous cavity is filled to a few millimeters below the GRT edge. The eye is rotated smoothly toward the GRT in a manner that rolls the PFCL posterior and across the GRT gap, displacing the subretinal fluid and closing the posterior edge of the GRT without subretinal migration. Then the laser is performed with minimal movement for eight rows. The most common error in GRT surgery is in the fluid-to-air exchange. This is done very differently than in the usual RRD repair. The intraocular fluids, both residual BSS and PFCL, are removed anterior to posterior. One uses an extrusion (or backflush cannula) removing fluid as it is "walked" down along the eye wall from behind the lens anterior-to-posterior to the GRT edge. This requires the break to be high, rather than dependent. The most critical moments are at the level of the break edge and just anterior. No fluid should be allowed under the GRT edge. The edge is dried completely against the choroid before continuing posteriorly. This maneuver requires meticulous attention. In case of an irregular GRT, the extrusion must dry all the fluid under the GRT starting along the anterior-most edge of the posterior flap of the GRT and continue to the posterior edge of the posterior flap in order to lock it in place and avoid slippage.

At this point, PFCL–air exchange can be continued posteriorly. After the fluid is removed to a couple of millimeters below the posterior GRT edge, it is no longer critical to use this "walking along the eye wall" technique, and the residual PFCL can be removed from the vitreous cavity over the disc. Prior to the air–fluid exchange the vitreous fluid and PFCL hold up the subretinal pocket of BSS. During the air–fluid exchange, that mass is replaced with air of much lower mass and the pocket falls posterior in the subretinal space causing the GRT to slip down the eye wall. Slippage occurs when BSS fluid migrates under the retina and forms a subretinal fluid pocket that is rolled forward with the air–fluid exchange resulting in a fold. A small fold from minor slippage away from the macula may be tolerated. However, once the GRT dries it is very difficult to open a dry fold. After the PFCL-to-air exchange, tamponade choice is usually silicone oil, but gas may be considered in selected cases.

One of us (MPB) prefers bimanual, direct PFCL–oil exchange as it seems to avoid further slippage that can occasionally occur as fluid from the AC or dehydrating vitreous base region run posterior. In this technique, PFCL is brought above the GRT. Then oil is infused above the PFCL while removing air. Once most of the air is removed, then bimanual, direct PFCL–oil exchange is performed under visualization using a chandelier for illumination, with oil injection cannula in one port and extrusion or back flush in the other. The extrusion tip is placed just beneath the oil to remove the thin layer of fluid (water and salts) that is between the PFCL and the oil. Once the two hydrophobic substances touch, the water layer is excluded from the interface and from the break as long as the eye pressure is low (i.e., low or now air infusion and extruding PFO faster than injecting oil). Bimanual PFCL–oil exchange is continued, walking the extrusion tip down the eyewall until the oil is below the posterior aspect of the break at which point extrusion can be performed above the nerve, keeping the intraocular pressure low and monitoring the perfusion of the retinal vessels and nerve.

We prefer high viscosity (5000cs) silicone oil since it reduces the emulsification complications. It is frequent for children to have extensive emulsification which can lead to pressure elevation. Oil can be removed between 3 and 6 months unless there are pressure issues that require earlier removal. Leaving oil for too long may predispose to more extensive peri-silicone proliferation and potential subsequent issues such as epiretinal membrane formation over the macula with peripheral traction, particularly in these eyes that likely have some vitreous remnant (given anomalous adhesions in SS) and large areas of exposed RPE. However, oil may need to be left in-situ long-term in hypotonous eyes and in children that have self-injurious behavior.

In conclusion, Stickler Syndrome is a key disease for pediatric retina specialists. The patients present in a variety of ways, and the pediatric retina specialist must expand the standard diagnostic role with a thorough family history, nonocular findings, and a more sophisticated vitreous and retina examination in order to identify patients at high risk. Pediatric retina specialists have a critical role in continued surveillance of SS patients, and they need to know the evidence and techniques of the potentially important role of prophylaxis as mentioned earlier. Finally, the techniques of GRT repair may pose a challenge that requires some mastery, but ultimately are very satisfying. In our practice, the behavioral modification of the developmentally delayed, self-injurious patients in order to stop self-hitting and head-banging is unresolved, and we would appreciate input from colleagues that read this chapter.

References

1. Stickler GB, Belau PG, Farrell FJ, Jones JD, Pugh DG, et al. Hereditary progressive arthro-ophthalmopathy. Mayo Clin Proc. 1965 Jun;40:433–55.
2. Hall JG, Herrod H. The Stickler syndrome presenting as a dominantly inherited cleft palate and blindness. J Med Genet. 1975 Dec;12(4):397–400.
3. Izumi K, Konczal LL, Mitchell AL, Jones MC. Underlying genetic diagnosis of Pierre Robin sequence: retrospective chart review at two children's hospitals and a systematic literature review. J Pediatr. 2012 Apr;160(4):645–650.e2.
4. Donoso LA, Edwards AO, Frost AT, Ritter R 3rd, Ahmad N, et al. Clinical variability of Stickler syndrome: role of exon 2 of the collagen COL2A1 gene. Surv Ophthalmol. 2003;48(2):191–203.
5. Opitz JM, France T, Herrmann J, Spranger JW. The Stickler syndrome. N Engl J Med. 1972 Mar 9;286(10):546–7.
6. Hall J. Stickler syndrome presenting as a syndrome of cleft palate, myopia and blindness inherited as a dominant trait. Birth Defects Orig Artic Ser. 1974;10(8):157–71.
7. Herrmann J, France TD, Spranger JW, Opitz JM, Wiffler C. The Stickler syndrome (hereditary arthroophthalmopathy). Birth Defects Orig Artic Ser. 1975;11(2):76–103.
8. Herrmann J, France TD, Opitz JM. The Stickler syndrome. Birth Defects Orig Artic Ser. 1975;11(6):203–4.
9. Beals RK. Hereditary arthro-ophthalmopathy (the Stickler syndrome) Report of a kindred with protrusio acetabuli. Clin Orthop Relat Res. 1977 Jun;125:32–5.
10. Blair NP, Albert DM, Liberfarb RM, Hirose T. Hereditary progressive arthro-ophthalmopathy of Stickler. Am J Ophthalmol. 1979 Nov;88(5):876–88.
11. Francomano CA, Liberfarb RM, Hirose T, Maumenee IH, Streeten EA, et al. The Stickler syndrome: evidence for close linkage to the structural gene for type II collagen. Genomics. 1987 Dec;1(4):293–6.
12. Ahmad NN, Ala-Kokko L, Knowlton RG, Jimenez SA, Weaver EJ, et al. Stop codon in the procollagen II gene (COL2A1) in a family with the Stickler syndrome (arthro-ophthalmopathy). Proc Natl Acad Sci U S A. 1991 Aug 1;88(15):6624–7.
13. Mayne R, Brewton RG, Mayne PM, Baker JR. Isolation and characterization of the chains of type V/type XI collagen present in bovine vitreous. J Biol Chem. 1993 May 5;268(13):9381–6.
14. Richards AJ, Laidlaw M, Whittaker J, Treacy B, Rai H, et al. High efficiency of mutation detection in type 1 stickler syndrome using a two-stage approach: vitreoretinal assessment coupled with exon sequencing for screening COL2A1. Hum Mutat. 2006;27(7):696–704.
15. Richards AJ, Meredith S, Poulson A, Bearcroft P, Crossland G, et al. A novel mutation of COL2A1 resulting in dominantly inherited rhegmatogenous retinal detachment. Invest Ophthalmol Vis Sci. 2005 Feb;46(2):663–8.
16. Sergouniotis PI, Fincham GS, McNinch AM, Spickett C, Poulson AV, et al. Ophthalmic and molecular genetic findings in Kniest dysplasia. Eye (Lond). 2015 Apr;29(4):475–482. PubMed PMID: 25592122.
17. Terhal PA, Nievelstein RJ, Verver EJ, Topsakal V, van Dommelen P, et al. A study of the clinical and radiological features in a cohort of 93 patients with a COL2A1 mutation causing spondyloepiphyseal dysplasia congenita or a related phenotype. Am J Med Genet A. 2015 Mar;167A(3):461–75.
18. Zhou L, Xiao X, Li S, Jia X, Zhang Q. Frequent mutations of RetNet genes in eoHM: further confirmation in 325 probands and comparison with late-onset high myopia based on exome sequencing. Exp Eye Res. 2018 Jun;171:76–91.
19. Rose PS, Levy HP, Liberfarb RM, Davis J, Szymko-Bennett Y, et al. Stickler syndrome: clinical characteristics and diagnostic criteria. Am J Med Genet A. 2005 Oct 15;138A(3):199–207.
20. Snead MP, McNinch AM, Poulson AV, Bearcroft P, Silverman B, et al. Stickler syndrome, ocular-only variants and a key diagnostic role for the ophthalmologist. Eye (Lond). 2011 Nov;25(11):1389–400.
21. Snead MP, Yates JR. Clinical and molecular genetics of Stickler syndrome. J Med Genet. 1999 May;36(5):353–9.
22. Freeman HM. Fellow eyes of giant retinal breaks. Trans Am Ophthalmol Soc. 1978;76:343–82.
23. Shapiro MJ, Blair MP, Solinski MA, Zhang DL, Jabbehdari S. The importance of early diagnosis of Stickler syndrome: finding opportunities for preventing blindness. Taiwan J Ophthalmol. 2018 Oct-Dec;8(4):189–95.
24. Scott IU, Flynn HW Jr, Azen SP, Lai MY, Schwartz S, et al. Silicone oil in the repair of pediatric complex retinal detachments: a prospective, observational, multicenter study. Ophthalmology. 1999;106(7):1399–407; discussion 1407-8.
25. Reddy DN, Yonekawa Y, Thomas BJ, Nudleman ED, Williams GA. Long-term surgical outcomes of retinal detachment in patients with Stickler syndrome. Clin Ophthalmol. 2016;10:1531–4.
26. Silva RA, Blumenkranz MS. Prophylaxis for retina detachment; AAO Clinical Education. https://www.aao.org/munnerlyn-laser-surgery-center/prophylaxis-retinal-detachments. Accessed 23 Oct 2018.
27. Ang A, Poulson AV, Goodburn SF, Richards AJ, Scott JD, et al. Retinal detachment and prophylaxis in type 1 Stickler syndrome. Ophthalmology. 2008 Jan;115(1):164–8.
28. Fincham GS, Pasea L, Carroll C, McNinch AM, Poulson AV, et al. Prevention of retinal detachment in Stickler syndrome: the Cambridge prophylactic cryotherapy protocol. Ophthalmology. 2014 Aug;121(8):1588–97.
29. Alshahrani ST, Ghazi NG, Al-Rashaed S. Rhegmatogenous retinal detachments associated to Stickler syndrome in a tertiary eye care center in Saudi Arabia. Clin Ophthalmol. 2016;10:1–6.
30. Monin C, Van Effenterre G, Andre-Sereys P, Haut J. Prevention of retinal detachment in Wagner-Stickler disease comparative study of different methods Apropos of 22 cases. J Fr Ophtalmol. 1994;17(3):167–74.
31. Zauberman H. Tensile strength of chorioretinal lesions produced by photocoagulation, diathermy, and cryopexy. Br J Ophthalmol. 1969 Nov;53(11):749–52.

32. Kita M, Negi A, Kawano S, Honda Y, Maegawa S. Measurement of retinal adhesive force in the in vivo rabbit eye. Invest Ophthalmol Vis Sci. 1990 Apr;31(4):624–8.
33. Berrocal MH, Chenworth ML, Acaba LA. Management of giant retinal tear detachments. J Ophthalmic Vis Res. 2017 Jan-Mar;12(1):93–7.
34. Chang S, Lincoff H, Zimmerman NJ, Fuchs W. Giant retinal tears Surgical techniques and results using perfluorocarbon liquids. Arch Ophthalmol. 1989 May;107(5):761–6.
35. Scott IU, Murray TG, Flynn HW Jr, Feuer WJ, Schiffman JC. Outcomes and complications associated with giant retinal tear management using perfluoro-n-octane. Ophthalmology. 2002 Oct;109(10):1828–33.
36. Kertes PJ, Wafapoor H, Peyman GA, Calixto N Jr, Thompson H. The management of giant retinal tears using perfluoroperhydrophenanthrene. A multicenter case series Vitreon Collaborative Study Group. Ophthalmology. 1997 Jul;104(7):1159–65.
37. Shapiro MJ, Resnick KI. Identification, prevention, and treatment of silicone oil pupillary block after an inferior iridectomy. Am J Ophthalmol. 1991 Sep;112(3):357–358. PubMed PMID: 1882958.
38. Zivojnovic R. Silicone oil in vitreoretinal surgery. 1987. ISBN 0-89838-879-1.

30 Genetic Testing in Pediatric Retina

Hiroyuki Kondo

Abstract

Genetic testing is a powerful and helpful method to diagnose retinal disorders in pediatric patients. The expectation of mutation identification in these disorders depends on whether the appropriate genetic testing methods are used. Next-generation sequencing has recently become available, and the chance of identifying the genetic mutation would be increased. The general concerns about genetic testing include ethical issues and the patients' right to privacy on the results of the genetic testing should be carefully supported.

Keywords

Genetic testing · Mutation · Next-generation sequencing Exome sequencing · Target sequencing · Gene heterogeneity

30.1 Genetic Testing of Pediatric Retina

Genetic testing is a powerful and useful method to diagnose retinal diseases in pediatric patients accurately. The testing is useful when:

1. The clinical signs and symptoms are atypical or overlap those of other diseases, i.e., phenotypically mimicking disorders or spectrum disorders, and the ocular findings are usually ambiguous at the end stages (Figs. 30.1, 30.2, 30.3, 30.4 and 30.5).
2. A correct diagnosis offers optimal treatments decision (Fig. 30.6).
3. Determining the inheritance pattern is helpful for proper genetic counseling.

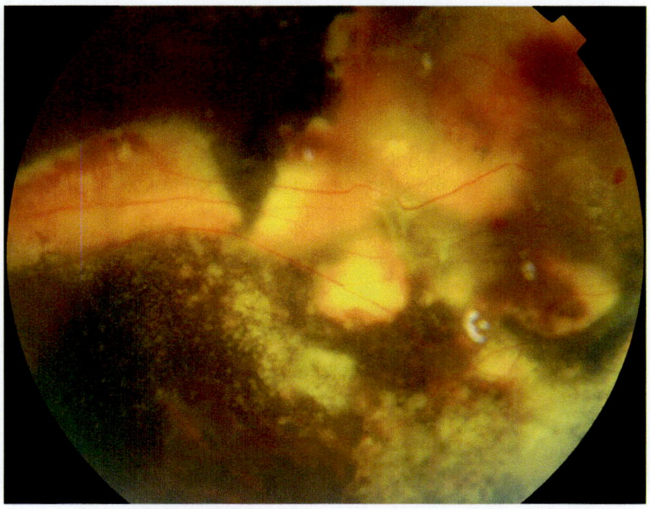

Fig. 30.1 Fundus photograph of the left eye of a patient with familial exudative vitreoretinopathy (FEVR) who was first suspected to have Coats disease. A 29-yearold female patient had an exudative retinal detachment and was blind in the right eye. At age of 29-years, an exudative retinal detachment developed in her left eye.Genetic testing revealed that she carried a mutation in the *FZD4* gene and a diagnosis of FEVR was made (Reprinted from [1])

Prior to genetic testing, it is mandatory to make a correct clinical diagnosis so that it can lead to the successful identification of the causative mutation(s). In addition to the retinal findings, the sex, age at onset, presence of systemic abnormalities, and inheritance pattern should be carefully assessed. Although sporadic cases may be due to non-genetic conditions, autosomal recessive, or X-linked recessive inheritance may underlie the clinical presentation. De novo mutations of autosomal dominant genes can also be found sporadically.

H. Kondo (✉)
Department of Ophthalmology, University of Occupational and Environmental Health, Kitakyushu, Japan
e-mail: kondohi@med.uoeh-u.ac.jp

W.-C. Wu, W.-C. Lam (eds.), *A Quick Guide to Pediatric Retina*, https://doi.org/10.1007/978-981-15-6552-6_30

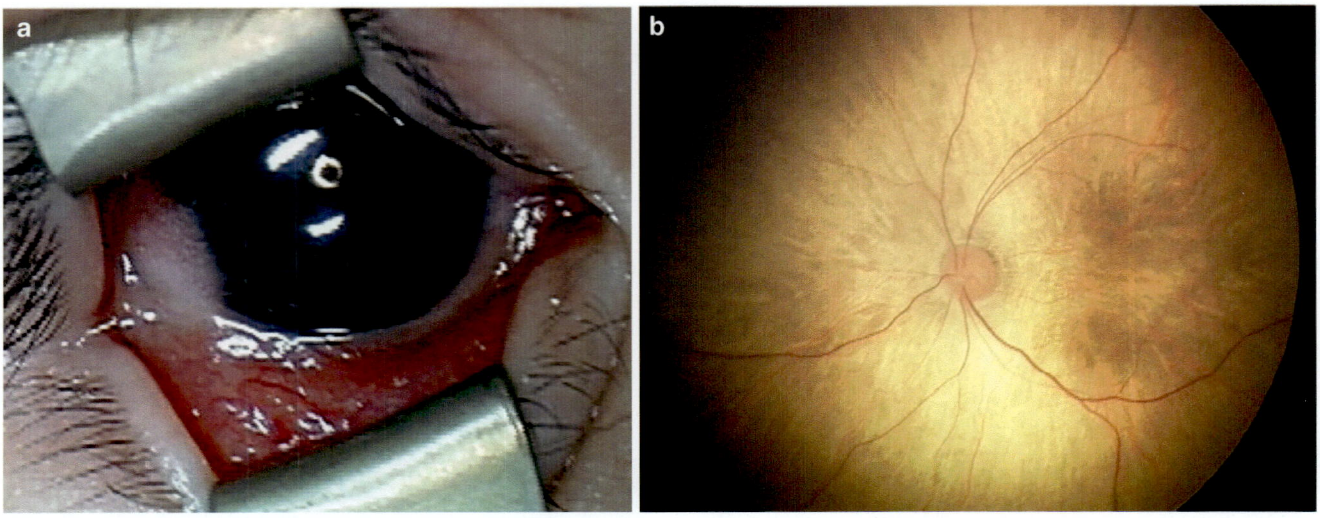

Fig. 30.2 Photographs of the exterior surface of the eye and fundus of a 3-month-old boy showing the findings of Goldenhar syndrome and ocular albinism. (**a**) Photograph of the exterior surface of the right eye showing a dermoid at the sclerocorneal margin. (**b**) Fundus photograph of the left eye showing depigmented retina suggestive of albinism. Genetic testing revealed a mutation in the *GPR143* gene and a diagnosis of ocular albinism was confirmed rather than syndromic albinism (Reprinted from [1])

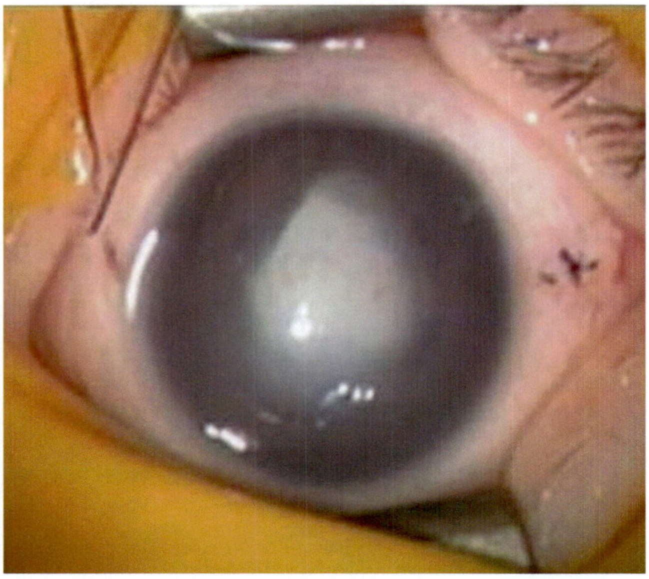

Fig. 30.3 Photograph of the external surface of the left eye of a three-month-old boy who was suspected to have Norrie disease. He had leukocoria with total retinal detachments in both eyes. A diagnosis of Norrie disease or familial exudative vitreoretinopathy was suspected. The final diagnosis was non-syndromic congenital retinal non-attachment due to the identification of a homozygous mutation in the *ATOH7* gene by genetic testing (Reprinted from [1])

30.2 Genes Causing Retinal Disorders in Children

There are several pediatric retinal disorders that are caused by mutations in a single gene (Table 30.1) while others result from mutations of different genes (Table 30.2). The clinical features of single-gene disorders tend to be uniform, and the causative mutation is more likely to be detected. Disorders associated with gene heterogeneity tend to have high clinical variations. The expectation of mutation identification in these disorders varies substantially even though a comprehensive screening can be performed (Table 30.2).

30.3 Strategies for Identifying Causative Mutations

DNA amplification by polymerase chain reaction (PCR) followed by DNA sequencing for targeted exons, the so-called Sanger sequencing, has been the standard practice for genetic testing [4]. However, all exons need to be examined individually and the efficiency is limited in terms of the cost and labor. If genes and exons have to be extensively screened for disorders of high gene heterogeneity, the role of Sanger sequencing in genetic testing is limited.

Recently, massive parallel DNA sequencing methodology, the so-called next-generation sequencing, has become commercialized [4]. In combination with microarray-based DNA capture methods that can target specific genomic regions, comprehensive screening has become possible for a set of genes (target sequencing) or for all protein-coding exons (exome sequencing). Computational results of next-generation sequencing will output a large number of variants most of which are non-pathogenic. The disease-causing variant(s) can be selected more accurately by filtering non-pathogenic variants with the help of web-based prediction programs and databases [5].

Mutations of a large-sized exon(s) deletion are missed by Sanger sequencing and exome sequencing. Alternatively, a long-range PCR can be applied if the deletion is already specified. A large gene deletion can be assessed theoretically by whole genome sequencing.

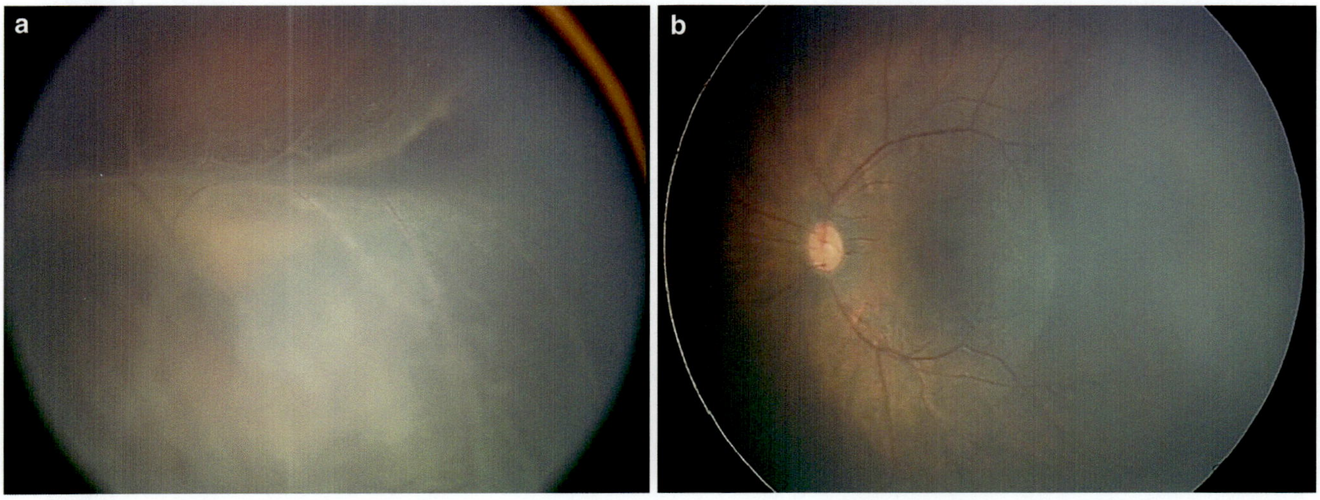

Fig. 30.4 Fundus photographs of both eyes of a 4-month-old boy. (**a**) Bullous retinal elevation suggestive of retinal detachment or retinoschisis can be seen in the right eye. (**b**) Left eye appears to be nearly normal. Genetic testing revealed that the patient carried a hemizygous mutation in the *RS1* gene, and the retinal appearance of the right eye was thought to be a retinoschisis. An immediate surgical management was postponed by the genetic testing (Reprinted from [1])

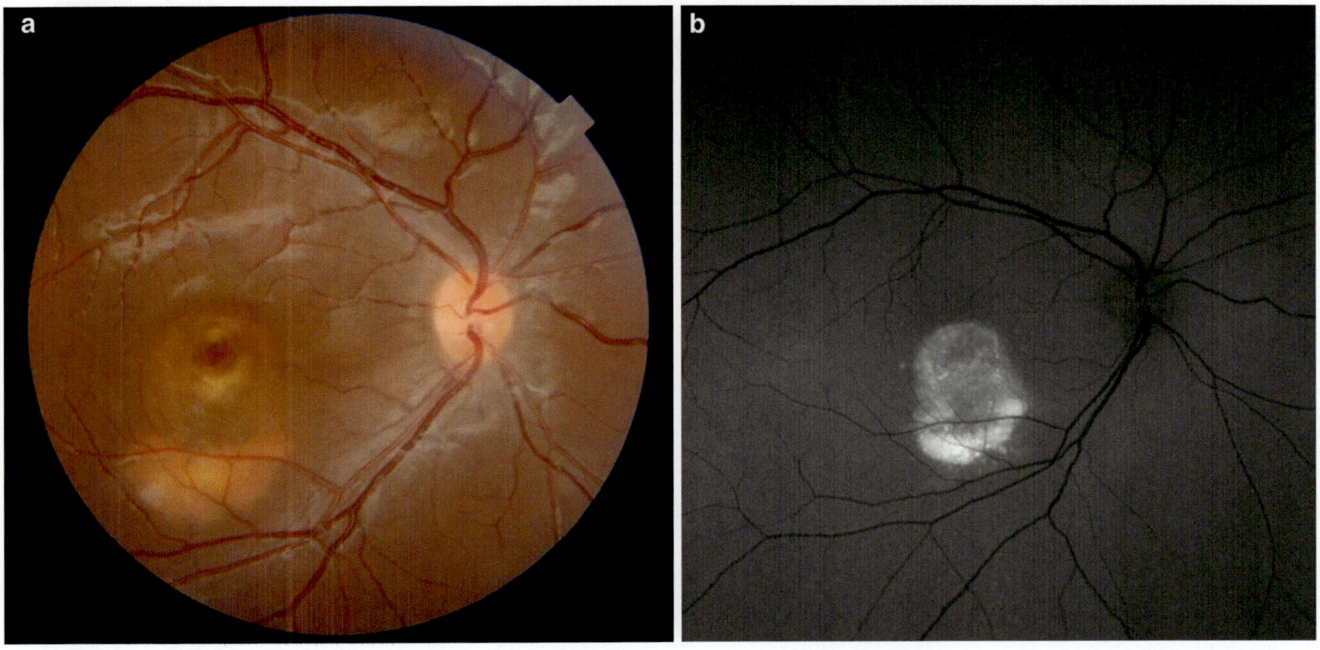

Fig. 30.5 Fundus photograph and autofluorescence of the right eye of an 11-year-old girl. Vitelliform macular dystrophy was suspected from the fundus photograph (**a**) and fundus autofluorescence (**b**). Bi-allelic mutations in the *BEST1* gene led to a diagnosis of autosomal recessive bestrophinopathy rather than autosomal dominant Best's vitelliform macular dystrophy. This information was used in genetic counseling (Reprinted from [1])

30.4 Issues to Be Considered

General concerns about genetic testing include ethical issues, e.g., possible discrimination and undesirable prospect of insurance and employment [6]. The patients right to privacy on the results of genetic testing should be carefully supported. Next-generation sequencing potentially provides off-target results of incidental findings of harmful genetic defects. The recommendations for the incidental findings are updated by a community of genetic analysis [7].

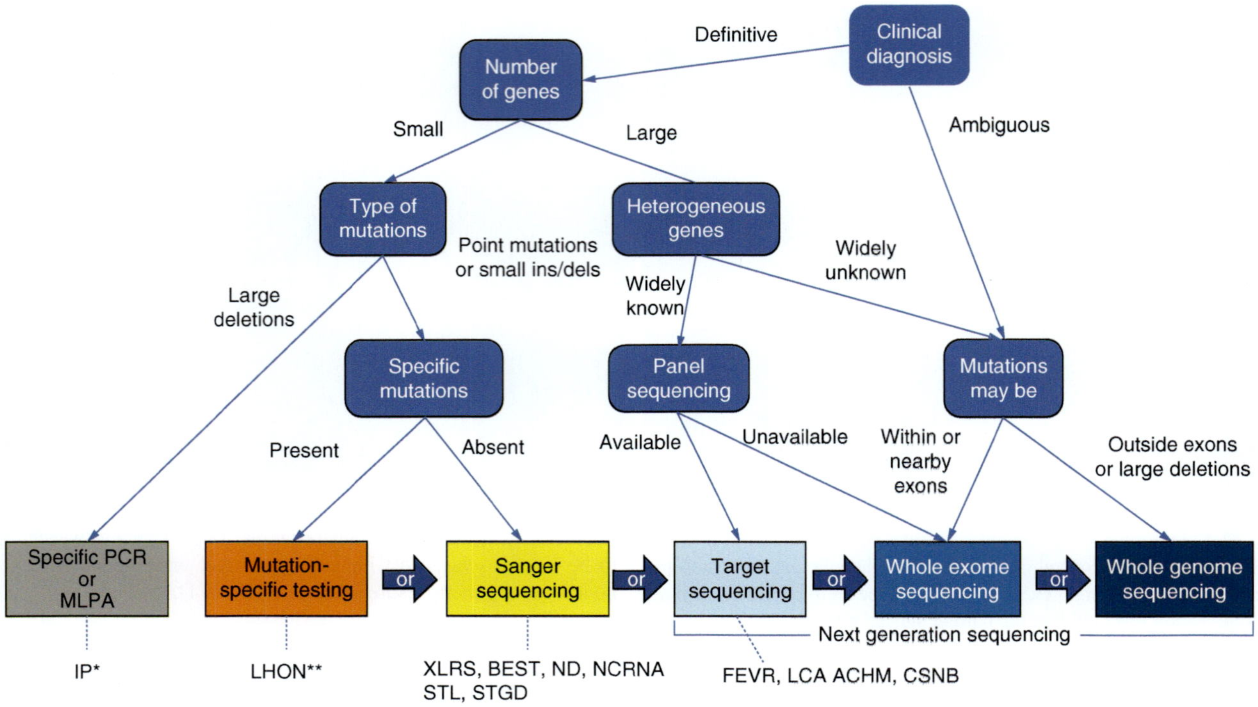

Fig. 30.6 Practical strategy for selecting methods of genetic testing in pediatric retinal disorders. Note that a set of genes in the target sequencing is usually custom made and the testing may be provided on a research basis and not always available. Instead, whole exome and genome sequencing have become more commercialized. *In IP, deletion encompassing exons 4–10 of the IKBKG gene account for 90% of known IP mutations [2] **Three specific mutations of the mitochondria gene account for >95% of LHON mutations [3]. *ACHM* achromatopsia, *BEST* Best's vitelliform macular dystrophy, *CSNB* congenital stationary night blindness, *FEVR* familial exudative vitreoretinopathy, *ins/dels* insertions and deletions, *IP* incontinentia pigmenti, *LCA* Leber's congenital amaurosis, *LHON* Leber's hereditary optic neuropathy, *MLPA* multiple ligation probe amplification (test for exon by exon copy number variation using multiplex PCR), *NCRNA* nonsyndromic congenital retinal nonattachment, *ND* Norrie disease, *STGD* Stargardt disease, *STL* Stickler syndrome, *XLRS* X-linked retinoschisis

Table 30.1 Single gene disease

Disease	Inheritance	Gene
BEST disease	AD	*BEST1*
Occult macular dystrophy	AD	*RP1L1*
Snowflake vitreoretinal degeneration	AD	*KCNJ13*
Wagner disease	AD	*VCAN*
Enhanced S-cone syndrome	AR	*NR2E3*
Gyrate chorioretinal atrophy	AR	*OAT*
Nonsyndromic congenital retinal nonattachment	AR	*ATOH7*
Stargardt disease	AR	*ABCA4*
Incontinentia pigmenti	XD	*IKBKG*
Blue cone monochromatopsia	XR	*OPN1LW/ OPN1MW*
Choroideremia	XR	CHM
Congenital retinoschisis	XR	*RS1*
Ocular albinism	XR	*GPR143*
Norrie disease	XR	*NDP*
Leber hereditary optic atrophy	MT	*mtDNA*

AD autosomal dominant, *AR* autosomal recessive, *MT* mitochondrial, *XD* X-linked dominant, *XR* X-linked recessive

Table 30.2 Disease of gene heterogeneity

Disease	Inheritance	Gene
Achromatopsia	AR	*CNGA3, CNGB3, GNAT2, PDE6H, PDE6C, ATF6*
Congenital stationary night blindness[a]	AD, AR, XR	*CABP4, CACNA1F, GNAT1, GNB3, GPR179, GRK1, GRM6, LRIT3, PDE6B, RDH5, RHO, RPGR, SAG, SLC24A1, TRPM1*
Familial exudative vitreoretinopathy	AD, AR, XR	*CTNNB1, FZD4, KIF11, LRP5, NDP, RCBTB1, TSPAN12, ZNF408*
Fundus albipunctatus	AR	*RDH5, RLBP1, RPE65*
Idiopathic foveal hypoplasia	AD, AR, XR	*GPR143, PAX6, SLC38A8*
Leber's congenital amaurosis	AR, (AD)	*AIPL1, CABP4, CCT2, CEP290, CLUAP1, CRB1, CRX, DTHD1, GDF6, GUCY2D, IFT140, IMPDH1, IQCB1, KCNJ13, LCA5, LRAT, NMNAT1, OTX2, PRPH2, RD3, RDH12, RPE65, RPGRIP1, SPATA7, TULP1*
Oculocutaneous albinism	AR, (AD)	*AP3B1, BLOC1S3, BLOC1S6, C10orf11, DTNBP1, HPS1, HPS3, HPS4, HPS5, HPS6, LYST, OCA2, SLC24A4, SLC45A2, TYR, TYRP1*
Stickler syndrome	AR, (AD)	*COL2A1, COL9A1, COL9A2, COL9A3, COL11A1, COL11A2*[b]

[a]Oguchi disease included, [b]No ocular symptoms shown

References

1. Kondo H. Genetic diagnosis for pediatric ocular disorders. J Eye [Japanese]. 2017;34(7):981–6.
2. Aradhya S, Courtois G, Rajkovic A, Lewis RA, Levy M, Israel A, et al. Atypical forms of incontinentia pigmenti in male individuals result from mutations of a cytosine tract in exon 10 of NEMO (IKK-gamma). Am J Hum Genet. 2001;68(3):765–71.
3. Hudson G, Carelli V, Spruijt L, Gerards M, Mowbray C, Achilli A, et al. Clinical expression of Leber hereditary optic neuropathy is affected by the mitochondrial DNA-haplogroup background. Am J Hum Genet. 2007;81(2):228–33.
4. Strachan T, Read A. Analyzing the structure and expression of genes and genomes. In: Human molecular genetics. 4th ed. New York: Garland Science; 2011. p. 213–54.
5. Richards S, Aziz N, Bale S, Bick D, Das S, Gastier-Foster J, et al. Standards and guidelines for the interpretation of sequence variants: a joint consensus recommendation of the American College of Medical Genetics and Genomics and the Association for Molecular Pathology. Genet Med. 2015;17(5):405–24.
6. Strachan T, Read A. Parmacogenetics, personalized medicine, and population screening. In: Human molecular genetics. 4th ed. New York: Garland Science; 2011. p. 603–38.
7. Green RC, Berg JS, Grody WW, Kalia SS, Korf BR, Martin CL, et al. ACMG recommendations for reporting of incidental findings in clinical exome and genome sequencing. Genet Med. 2013;15(7):565–74.

31 Pediatric Macular Hole

Mrinali P. Gupta and Philip J. Ferrone

Abstract

A macular hole is a full-thickness defect in the foveal neuroretinal tissue that can cause significant vision loss. While the majority of macular holes are "idiopathic" and age-related in nature, occurring as a result of a slow, degenerative process of progressive vitreoretinal traction, almost all macular holes encountered in the pediatric population are the result of direct ocular trauma. Owing to its disparate pathophysiology, the clinical course and prognosis of the pediatric traumatic macular hole is less predictable than that of idiopathic senile macular hole. Other traumatic ocular comorbidities may affect management and/or visual prognosis. Spontaneous closure may occur, and a period of observation is often undertaken, although considerations for deprivational amblyopia may prompt earlier intervention in younger patients. While surgical management is similar to that for idiopathic senile macular holes, the pediatric population poses unique surgical challenges including the adherent posterior hyaloid and limitations in the ability to position face-down postoperatively. This chapter provides an overview of pediatric traumatic macular holes, with attention to the key differences in epidemiology, anatomy, pathophysiology, diagnosis, and management in children, as compared to adults.

Keywords

Pediatric macular hole · Traumatic macular hole
Ocriplasmin · Plasmin · Transforming growth factor β
Autologous platelet-rich plasma

M. P. Gupta
Department of Ophthalmology, Weill Cornell Medical College, New York, NY, USA

P. J. Ferrone (✉)
Long Island Vitreo-Retinal Consultants, Great Neck, NY, USA

A macular hole is a full-thickness defect of the neuroretinal tissue involving the foveal center that can cause significant central vision loss. The first detailed ophthalmoscopic description of a macular hole presented by Noyes in 1871 involved a teenage girl whose eye had been struck by a cork from an ale bottle [1], and many early descriptions of macular holes similarly involved traumatic injuries. Since that time, it has become clear that the majority of macular holes are atraumatic "idiopathic" macular holes of the elderly. While multiple theories have been put forth regarding the pathogenesis of idiopathic macular holes, the predominant mechanism is felt to be anteroposterior traction from the vitreous, along with tangential tractional forces [2, 3]. In contrast, amongst pediatric patients, macular holes are generally traumatic in origin, although rarely other causes may be identified (Fig. 31.1). Accordingly, almost all of the literature on pediatric macular hole involves studies evaluating traumatic macular hole. This chapter will provide an overview of pediatric traumatic macular holes and their management.

Traumatic macular holes have been described in 1.4% of closed globe injuries and 0.15% of open globe injuries [4]. Blunt force is thought to create an axial deformation of the globe that causes both an anteroposterior reduction and equatorial expansion of the globe, resulting in horizontal forces to the posterior pole that cause a splitting of the foveal retinal layers. Vitreous traction may also be implicated to varying degrees [5–7]. The pathophysiology of the traumatic macular hole, therefore, is distinct from the slow, degenerative process of progressive vitreoretinal traction implicated in idiopathic senile macular holes. The progression and visual outcome of traumatic macular hole are likewise less predictable than that of idiopathic macular holes.

Clinically, slit-lamp biomicroscopy reveals a full-thickness defect in the central fovea. A Watzke test, performed by placing a narrow vertical slit beam through the fovea and asking the patient whether he/she detects a break in the line, is positive. Other traumatic injuries such as commotio retinae, retinal hemorrhage, vitreous hemorrhage, choroidal rupture, traumatic chorioretinal rupture, retinal

W.-C. Wu, W.-C. Lam (eds.), *A Quick Guide to Pediatric Retina*, https://doi.org/10.1007/978-981-15-6552-6_31

tears, retinal dialysis, and retinal detachment, may be noted. Optical coherence tomography (OCT) demonstrates the full-thickness retinal defect, as well as other features including the shape and size of the hole, status of the hyaloid, and associated macular changes. In comparison to adult idiopathic senile macular holes, posterior vitreous detachment (PVD) and operculum are typically absent in traumatic macular holes. Moreover, one study found that traumatic macular holes exhibited larger basal diameters and were more often eccentric and irregular or elliptical in shape [8].

Management of pediatric macular hole includes a period of observation followed by surgery, as the macular hole may close spontaneously within days or months. The rate of spontaneous closure for pediatric traumatic macular holes is higher than that for adult idiopathic macular holes as well as adult traumatic macular holes. In traumatic macular holes, studies have reported spontaneous closure rates ranging from 10 to 44% [5, 9] among traumatic macular holes in general, with higher rates in pediatric cases in particular [5, 10–12] (Figs. 31.2 and 31.3). One meta-analysis of traumatic macular holes found that 97% of patients with spontaneous closure were below age 30 years and that the median age among all patients with spontaneous closure was 15 years [12]. Other factors that may increase the likelihood of spontaneous closure include smaller diameter and absence of PVD, the latter of which is typical in traumatic macular holes [13]. Thus, a period of observation is generally recommended, especially in older patients (with less amblyopia risk) and in patients with small holes, good visual acuity, and/or posterior vitreous adhesion to the hole. There are at present no evidence-based guidelines prescribing the optimal duration of observation, although spontaneous closure typically occurs within 3 months and is rare after 6 months [12]. Younger patients may require earlier surgery due to deprivational amblyopia considerations.

The key surgical principles for macular hole repair are relief of anteroposterior traction forces from the vitreous and of tangential tractional forces from epiretinal membranes (if present) and internal limiting membrane (ILM), placement of a tamponade (air, gas, or oil), and postoperative prone positioning. This approach yields closure rates of over 90% for idiopathic macular holes [14]. Given the variable role of vitreous traction in traumatic macular hole, as compared to idiopathic macular hole, application of a similar surgical approach for traumatic macular holes yields more variable results, with success rates ranging from 45% to 100% (median 92.5%) in small studies including patient populations with a mean age ranging from 10 to 32 years [15]. Pars plana vitrectomy with separation of the posterior vitreous cortex from the retinal surface is essential for all macular hole surgery but is particularly challenging in the pediatric population, due to the well-formed vitreous humor and strong adhesion of the posterior hyaloid to the underlying retina. Intraoperative vitreoschisis, in which a layer of posterior vitreous cortex remains on the retinal surface after presumed induction of a PVD may also occur. Chromovitrectomy using triamcinolone acetonide injectable suspension (Triesence, Alcon, Ft. Worth, TX) may facilitate vitrectomy and confirmation of a complete hyaloidal separation without vitreoschisis. The vitreous cutter, a pick, a bent microvitreoretinal (MVR) blade, and/or forceps may be employed to engage or obtain an opening in the hyaloid from which the

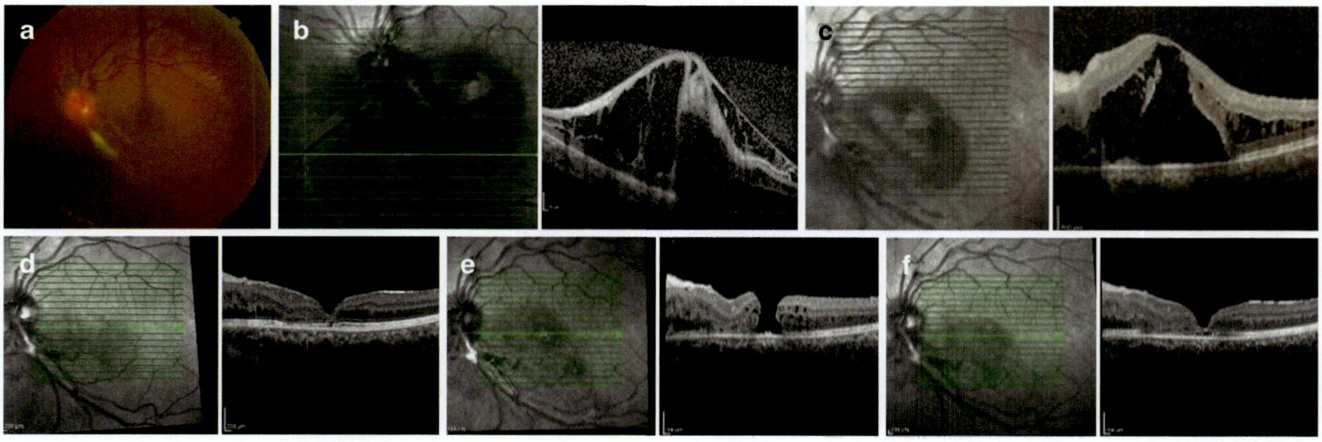

Fig. 31.1 Pediatric macular hole after pars plana vitrectomy for epiretinal membrane with cystoid edema associated with a combined hamartoma of the retina and retinal pigment epithelium (RPE). (**a**) Fundus photograph of a 3-year-old patient reveals a combined hamartoma of the retina and RPE in the left eye. (**b**) Optical coherence tomography (OCT) reveals a thick epiretinal membrane with underlying cystoid degeneration of the retina, schisis, and traction retinal detachment. (**c**) The patient underwent pars plana vitrectomy with membrane peeling. One month after surgery, OCT reveals interval removal of the epiretinal membrane and a large outer retinal defect with a thin inner retinal roof, adjacent cystoid and schisis changes, and localized retinal detachment. Visual acuity is 20/100. (**d**, **e**) Five months after surgery, OCT reveals a more compact retina with minimal cystic changes, but subsequent progression to a full-thickness macular hole occurred a short time later. Visual acuity is 20/80. The patient is observed, and OCT 1 year postoperatively reveals a spontaneously closed macular hole. Visual acuity is 20/60. (**f**) Four years postoperatively, OCT revealed the closed macular hole, and visual acuity is 20/20

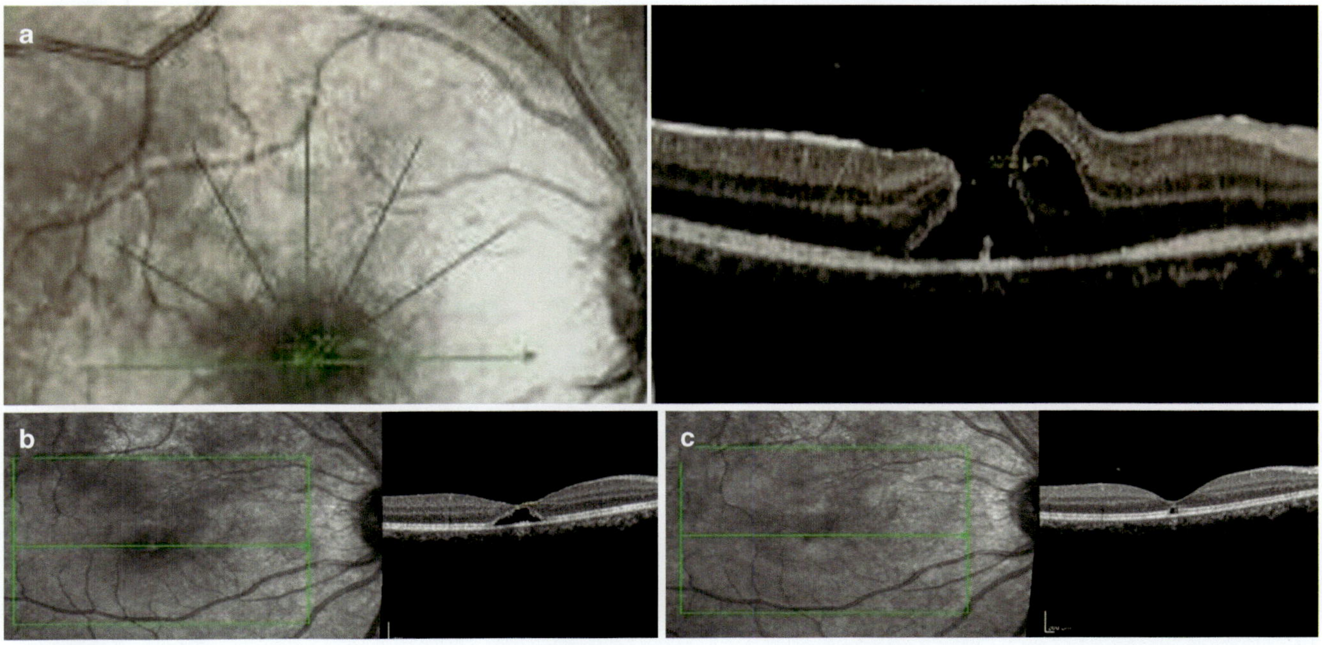

Fig. 31.2 Spontaneous closure of a pediatric traumatic macular hole. (**a**) Optical coherence tomography (OCT) of a 15-year-old female who sustained a soccer ball injury to the right eye reveals a full-thickness macular hole with slightly raised edges and cystic macular edema (CME). Visual acuity was 20/40. (**b**) After observation and treatment with topical nonsteroid anti-inflammatory drops, OCT reveals resolved CME and closed macular hole. Visual acuity was 20/25. (**c**) Eight months after the injury, OCT reveals a closed macular hole with a small residual defect in the ellipsoid zone. Visual acuity was 20/20

PVD can be induced. Iatrogenic retinal breaks are most likely to occur during induction of a PVD and are particularly problematic in the pediatric population, where they can incite intense proliferative vitreoretinopathy (PVR).

Peeling of the ILM has been shown to improve outcomes in idiopathic macular holes [16–18], potentially by reducing tangential traction, confirming complete removal of cortical vitreous and/or epiretinal membranes, and/or stimulating glial cell proliferation. Stains such as indocyanine green, triamcinolone acetonide, and brilliant blue may facilitate visualization and peeling of the ILM [19–21]. As with idiopathic macular holes, ILM peeling is also routinely employed for pediatric macular holes [22, 23]. Advanced techniques such as the inverted ILM flap technique have been described in larger pediatric traumatic macular holes [24]. The postoperative regime for a pediatric macular hole, like idiopathic macular holes, generally involves intraocular gas (air, SF6, or C3F8) tamponade in conjunction with prone (face-down) positioning for several days or more. The optimal tamponade agent (none, air, SF6, C3F8) and the duration of positioning remains controversial [17, 25–32]. Silicone oil tamponade may also be considered in pediatric macular hole cases, particularly in young patients incapable of positioning or in patients with large holes, recurrent holes, or holes that failed to close with an initial surgery.

Adjunctive agents including autologous plasmin or ocriplasmin (Jetrea, ThromboGenics, Iselin, NJ) and transforming growth factor β (TGF-β) or platelet concentrates (e.g., autologous platelet-rich plasma) [23, 33, 34] have also been employed in pediatric macular hole surgery. Intravitreal autologous plasmin and ocriplasmin have been administered perioperatively to facilitate separation of the hyaloid, albeit with limited data in the pediatric population. These agents act as proteases to cleave fibronectin and laminin, two key components of the vitreoretinal attachment [35]. Autologous plasmin-assisted pars plana vitrectomy for pediatric traumatic macular hole has been reported in small case series with successful closure and subjective improvement in ease of PVD induction [36–38]. Whereas autologous plasmin requires collection of the centrifugation of the patient's blood and collection of the plasmin-rich component, ocriplasmin is a commercially available recombinant truncated form of plasmin that has been FDA-approved for the treatment of adult patients with vitreoretinal traction and/or macular hole. Data regarding the use of ocriplasmin in the pediatric population is limited. A single, randomized, single-center, placebo-controlled, double-masked phase 2 study of ocriplasmin administered pre-operatively to pediatric patients included only one patient with pediatric traumatic macular hole. Overall, the study found no significant difference in rates of total macular PVD, vitreous liquefaction grade, or adverse effects in ocriplasmin versus placebo-treated eyes, but was limited by the heterogeneous diseases included and a small sample size [39]. Adverse effects reported in the adult ocri-

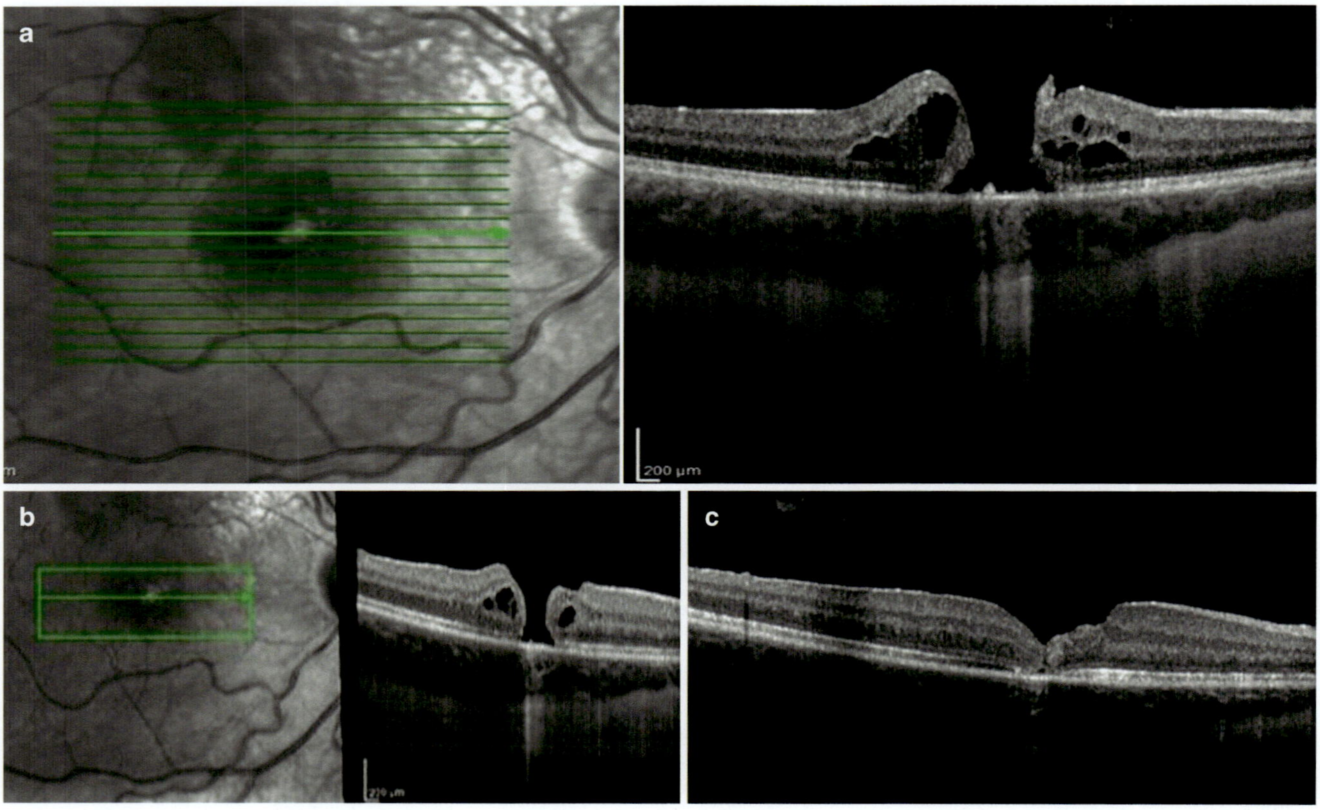

Fig. 31.3 Pediatric macular hole treated with vitrectomy using platelet-rich plasma. (**a**) Optical coherence tomography (OCT) of a 10-year-old boy who sustained a soccer ball injury 4 months previously to the right eye reveals a full-thickness macular hole with cystoid macular edema. Visual acuity is 20/100. (**b**) OCT 2 months after pars plana vitrectomy with internal membrane peel (ILM) and 20% SF6 gas tamponade with face-down positioning reveals a smaller but persistent full-thickness macular hole. Visual acuity is 20/60. (**c**) The patient undergoes a second pars plana vitrectomy with re-peeling of the ILM, platelet-rich plasma administration, and 10% C3F8 gas. OCT 2 months afterward reveals a closed macular hole with a focal area of retinal pigment epithelium atrophy. Visual acuity is 20/40

plasmin population after ocriplasmin use include retinal tear, retinal detachment, retinal vascular findings, electroretinogram abnormalities, and abnormalities in the ellipsoid zone, as well as lens subluxation [40], which was also found in one pediatric patient receiving ocriplasmin prior to vitrectomy [39]. Oncriplasmin is not approved by the FDA in the USA presently for use in the pediatric population.

Transforming growth factor β (TGF-β) and platelet concentrates (e.g., autologous platelet-rich plasma, obtained by collecting the platelet-rich supernatant after centrifuging the patient's blood) were used in early reports of surgery for pediatric traumatic macular holes to facilitate hole closure by stimulating fibroglial proliferation at the edge of the macular defect and/or providing support similar that that achieved by tamponade [23, 33, 34, 41, 42]. While there are no randomized controlled trials comparing outcomes for pediatric macular hole surgery with and without use of these adjuncts, such adjuncts may be considered for chronic or large holes, recurrent holes, holes that failed to close after a previous surgery (Fig. 31.3), or in patients such as young pediatric patients who are unable to position.

Acknowledgment MPG is supported by an unrestricted departmental grant from Research to Prevent Blindness.

References

1. Noyes HD. Detachment of retina with laceration at macula. Trans Am Ophthalmol Soc. 1871;1(8):128–9.
2. Gass JD. Idiopathic senile macular hole. Its early stages and pathogenesis. Arch Ophthalmol. 1988;106(5):629–39.
3. Johnson RN, Gass JD. Idiopathic macular holes. Observations, stages of formation, and implications for surgical intervention. Ophthalmology. 1988;95(7):917–24.
4. Kuhn F, Morris R, Witherspoon CD, Mann L. Epidemiology of blinding trauma in the United States Eye Injury Registry. Ophthalmic Epidemiol. 2006;13(3):209–16.

5. Yamashita T, Uemara A, Uchino E, Doi N, Ohba N. Spontaneous closure of traumatic macular hole. Am J Ophthalmol. 2002;133(2):230–5.
6. Hirata A, Tanihara H. Ruptured internal limiting membrane associated with blunt trauma revealed by indocyanine green staining. Graefes Arch Clin Exp Ophthalmol. 2004;242(6):527–30.
7. Johnson RN, McDonald HR, Lewis H, Grand MG, Murray TG, Mieler WF, et al. Traumatic macular hole: observations, pathogenesis, and results of vitrectomy surgery. Ophthalmology. 2001;108(5):853–7.
8. Huang J, Liu X, Wu Z, Sadda S. Comparison of full-thickness traumatic macular holes and idiopathic macular holes by optical coherence tomography. Graefes Arch Clin Exp Ophthalmol. 2010;248(8):1071–5.
9. Li XW, Lu N, Zhang L, Wang WW, Wang Y, Yan W, et al. Follow-up study of traumatic macular hole. Chin J Ophthalmol. 2008;44(9):786–9.
10. Miller JB, Yonekawa Y, Eliott D, Kim IK, Kim LA, Loewenstein JI, et al. Long-term follow-up and outcomes in traumatic macular holes. Am J Ophthalmol. 2015;160(6):1255–1258.e1251.
11. Mitamura Y, Saito W, Ishida M, Yamamoto S, Takeuchi S. Spontaneous closure of traumatic macular hole. Retina. 2001;21(4):385–9.
12. Gao M, Liu K, Lin Q, Liu H. Management modalities for traumatic macular hole: a systematic review and single-arm meta-analysis. Curr Eye Res. 2017;42(2):287–96.
13. Chen H, Chen W, Zheng K, Peng K, Xia H, Zhu L. Prediction of spontaneous closure of traumatic macular hole with spectral domain optical coherence tomography. Sci Rep. 2015;5:12343.
14. Williams GA. Macular holes: the latest in current management. Retina. 2006;26(6 Suppl):S9–12.
15. Liu W, Grzybowski A. Current management of traumatic macular holes. J Ophthalmol. 2017;2017:1748135.
16. Spiteri Cornish K, Lois N, Scott N, Burr J, Cook J, Boachie C, et al. Vitrectomy with internal limiting membrane (ILM) peeling versus vitrectomy with no peeling for idiopathic full-thickness macular hole (FTMH). Cochrane Database Syst Rev. 2013;(6):CD009306.
17. Park DW, Sipperley JO, Sneed SR, Dugel PU, Jacobsen J. Macular hole surgery with internal-limiting membrane peeling and intravitreous air. Ophthalmology. 1999;106(7):1392–7; discussion 1397-1398.
18. Spiteri Cornish K, Lois N, Scott NW, Burr J, Cook J, Boachie C, et al. Vitrectomy with internal limiting membrane peeling versus no peeling for idiopathic full-thickness macular hole. Ophthalmology. 2014;121(3):649–55.
19. Enaida H, Hisatomi T, Hata Y, Ueno A, Goto Y, Yamada T, et al. Brilliant blue G selectively stains the internal limiting membrane/brilliant blue G-assisted membrane peeling. Retina. 2006;26(6):631–6.
20. Kadonosono K, Itoh N, Uchio E, Nakamura S, Ohno S. Staining of internal limiting membrane in macular hole surgery. Arch Ophthalmol. 2000;118(8):1116–8.
21. Kimura H, Kuroda S, Nagata M. Triamcinolone acetonide-assisted peeling of the internal limiting membrane. Am J Ophthalmol. 2004;137(1):172–3.
22. Kuhn F, Morris R, Mester V, Witherspoon CD. Internal limiting membrane removal for traumatic macular holes. Ophthalmic Surg Lasers. 2001;32(4):308–15.
23. Wachtlin J, Jandeck C, Potthofer S, Kellner U, Foerster MH. Long-term results following pars plana vitrectomy with platelet concentrate in pediatric patients with traumatic macular hole. Am J Ophthalmol. 2003;136(1):197–9.
24. Abou Shousha MA. Inverted internal limiting membrane flap for large traumatic macular holes. Medicine. 2016;95(3):e2523.
25. Eckardt C, Eckert T, Eckardt U, Porkert U, Gesser C. Macular hole surgery with air tamponade and optical coherence tomography-based duration of face-down positioning. Retina. 2008;28(8):1087–96.
26. Essex RW, Kingston ZS, Moreno-Betancur M, Shadbolt B, Hunyor AP, Campbell WG, et al. The effect of postoperative face-down positioning and of long- versus short-acting gas in macular hole surgery: results of a registry-based study. Ophthalmology. 2016;123(5):1129–36.
27. Hikichi T, Kosaka S, Takami K, Ariga H, Ohtsuka H, Higuchi M, et al. 23- and 20-gauge vitrectomy with air tamponade with combined phacoemulsification for idiopathic macular hole: a single-surgeon study. Am J Ophthalmol. 2011;152(1):114–121.e111.
28. Hu Z, Xie P, Ding Y, Zheng X, Yuan D, Liu Q. Face-down or no face-down posturing following macular hole surgery: a meta-analysis. Acta Ophthalmol. 2016;94(4):326–33.
29. Kim SS, Smiddy WE, Feuer WJ, Shi W. Outcomes of sulfur hexafluoride (SF6) versus perfluoropropane (C3F8) gas tamponade for macular hole surgery. Retina. 2008;28(10):1408–15.
30. Modi A, Giridhar A, Gopalakrishnan M. Sulfurhexafluoride (SF6) versus perfluorfluoride (SF6) gas as tamponade in macular hole surgery. Retina. 2017;37(2):283–90.
31. Nadal J, Delas B, Pinero A. Vitrectomy without face-down posturing for idiopathic macular holes. Retina. 2012;32(5):918–21.
32. Wickens JC, Shah GK. Outcomes of macular hole surgery and shortened face down positioning. Retina. 2006;26(8):902–4.
33. Garcia-Arumi J, Corcostegui B, Cavero L, Sararols L. The role of vitreoretinal surgery in the treatment of posttraumatic macular hole. Retina. 1997;17(5):372–7.
34. Rubin JS, Glaser BM, Thompson JT, Sjaarda RN, Pappas SS, Murphy RP. Vitrectomy, fluid-gas exchange and transforming growth factor–beta-2 for the treatment of traumatic macular holes. Ophthalmology. 1995;102(12):1840–5.
35. Uemura A, Nakamura M, Kachi S, Nishizawa Y, Asami T, Miyake Y, et al. Effect of plasmin on laminin and fibronectin during plasmin-assisted vitrectomy. Arch Ophthalmol. 2005;123(2):209–13.
36. Margherio AR, Margherio RR, Hartzer M, Trese MT, Williams GA, Ferrone PJ. Plasmin enzyme-assisted vitrectomy in traumatic pediatric macular holes. Ophthalmology. 1998;105(9):1617–20.
37. Chow DR, Williams GA, Trese MT, Margherio RR, Ruby AJ, Ferrone PJ. Successful closure of traumatic macular holes. Retina. 1999;19(5):405–9.
38. Wu WC, Drenser KA, Trese MT, Williams GA, Capone A. Pediatric traumatic macular hole: results of autologous plasmin enzyme-assisted vitrectomy. Am J Ophthalmol. 2007;144(5):668–72.
39. Drenser K, Girach A, Capone A Jr. A randomized, placebo-controlled study of intravitreal ocriplasmin in pediatric patients scheduled for vitrectomy. Retina. 2016;36(3):565–75.
40. Hahn P, Chung MM, Flynn HW Jr, Huang SS, Kim JE, Mahmoud TH, et al. Safety profile of ocriplasmin for symptomatic vitreomacular adhesion: a comprehensive analysis of premarketing and postmarketing experiences. Retina. 2015;35(6):1128–34.
41. Finn AP, Chen X, Viehland C, Izatt JA, Toth CA, Vajzovic L. Combined internal limitin gmembrane flap and autologous plasma membrane concentrate to close a large traumatic macular hole in a pediatric patient. Retinal Cases Brief Rep. 2018. e-print ahead of publication.
42. Kapoor KG, Khan AN, Tieu BC, Khurshid GS. Revisiting autologous platelets as an adjuvant in macular hole repair: chronic macular holes without prone positioning. Ophthalmic Surg Lasers Imaging. 2012;43(4):291–5.

Non-accidental Trauma

32

Kimberly D. Tran, Ryan C. Young, Emmanuel Y. Chang, Lejla Vajzovic, Audina M. Berrocal, and C. Armitage Harper III

Abstract

Non-accidental trauma (NAT) is a leading cause of childhood traumatic injury in the United States. Retinal findings in NAT are common and well described, including extensive retinal hemorrhages in multiple layers, retinoschisis, perimacular retinal folds, vitreous and optic nerve hemorrhage. Management keystones include a multidisciplinary approach to the patient's multiple comorbidities, careful photographic and angiographic documentation of ophthalmic findings, amblyopia prevention and visual development, as well as interventions including photocoagulation and vitrectomy.

Keywords

Abusive head trauma · Non-accidental trauma Fluorescein angiography · Retinal hemorrhage · Pediatric retina

K. D. Tran · A. M. Berrocal
Department of Ophthalmology, Bascom Palmer Eye Institute, Miami, FL, USA

R. C. Young
Austin Retina Associates, Austin, TX, USA

E. Y. Chang
Retina and Vitreous of Texas and Baylor College of Medicine, Houston, TX, USA

L. Vajzovic
Department of Ophthalmology, Duke University Medical Center, Durham, NC, USA

C. Armitage Harper III (✉)
Austin Retina Associates, Austin, TX, USA

Department of Ophthalmology, University of Texas Health, San Antonio, TX, USA

Department of Ophthalmology, University of Texas, Austin, TX, USA
e-mail: caharper@austinretina.com

Abbreviations

FA	Fluorescein angiography
ILM	internal limiting membrane
NAT	non-accidental trauma
OCT	optical coherence tomography
RH	retinal hemorrhage

32.1 Introduction

Non-accidental trauma (NAT) is a leading cause of childhood traumatic injury in the United States [1, 2]. In 2016, an estimated 2.36 per 100,000 children died as a result of abuse and neglect. The ages most at risk are 0–3 years, and crying is the most common inciting event [3]. Shaking is thought to result in a shearing injury between the posterior vitreous face and the retina resulting in extensive retinal hemorrhages. The sensitivity and specificity of retinal hemorrhages (RH) in the diagnosis of child abuse have been reported at 75% and 93.2%, respectively [1]. In addition to shearing, the acceleration–deceleration forces involved with shaking are thought to cause retinal injury, similar to the mechanism responsible for the development of diffuse axonal brain injury in these infants. Additional findings include retinoschisis, perimacular retinal folds, vitreous and optic nerve hemorrhage [4–8] (Figs. 32.1, 32.2 and 32.3). Ischemia may lead to retinal neovascularization, vitreous hemorrhage, and tractional retinal detachment [9–12].

32.2 Evaluation

The evaluation of retinal hemorrhages in the setting of suspected NAT has important medical, social, and legal implications. The management of NAT requires a multidisciplinary team with careful documentation with Ret Cam photos, examination under anesthesia, as well as careful co-

W.-C. Wu, W.-C. Lam (eds.), *A Quick Guide to Pediatric Retina*, https://doi.org/10.1007/978-981-15-6552-6_32

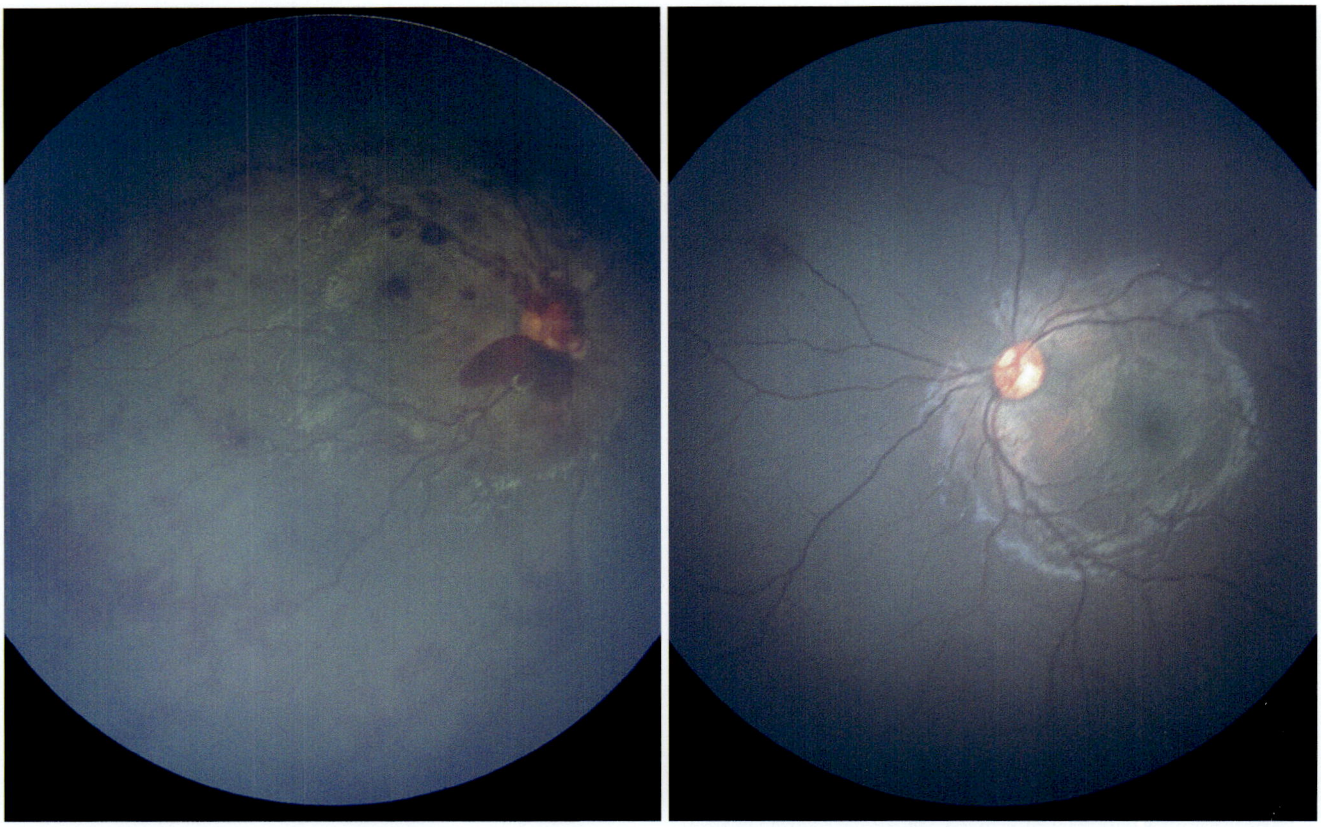

Fig. 32.1 This 10-month-old male was found at daycare with a decreasing level of consciousness and agonal breathing after NAT. He was diagnosed with subdural hemorrhage, hemispheric infarct, traumatic brain injury, cervical hemorrhage, rib fractures, and lung contusion. The color fundus photographs show sub-hyaloid hemorrhage, nerve head hemorrhage, and multiple bilateral intraretinal hemorrhages (Images courtesy of C. Armitage Harper III, MD)

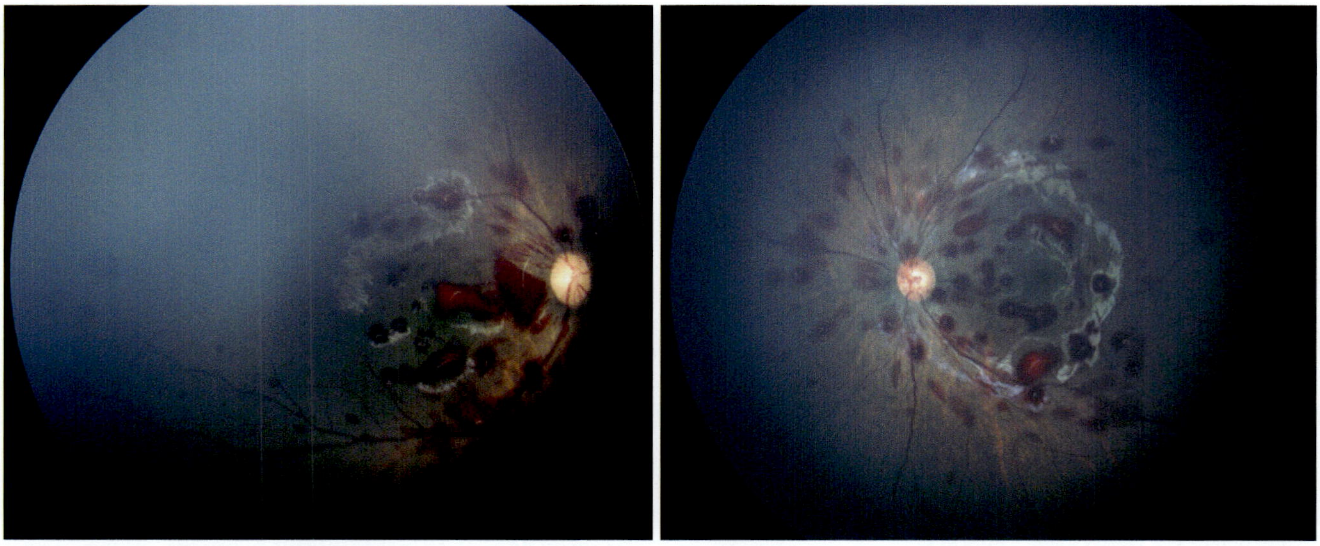

Fig. 32.2 This 6-month-old male was found non-responsive at home. He had been previously admitted for subdural hemorrhage after falling out of bed 2 months prior. He was diagnosed with anoxic brain injury and pronounced deceased on arrival to the hospital. The color fundus photographs show multiple bilateral preretinal, intraretinal, and subretinal hemorrhages (Images courtesy of C. Armitage Harper III, MD)

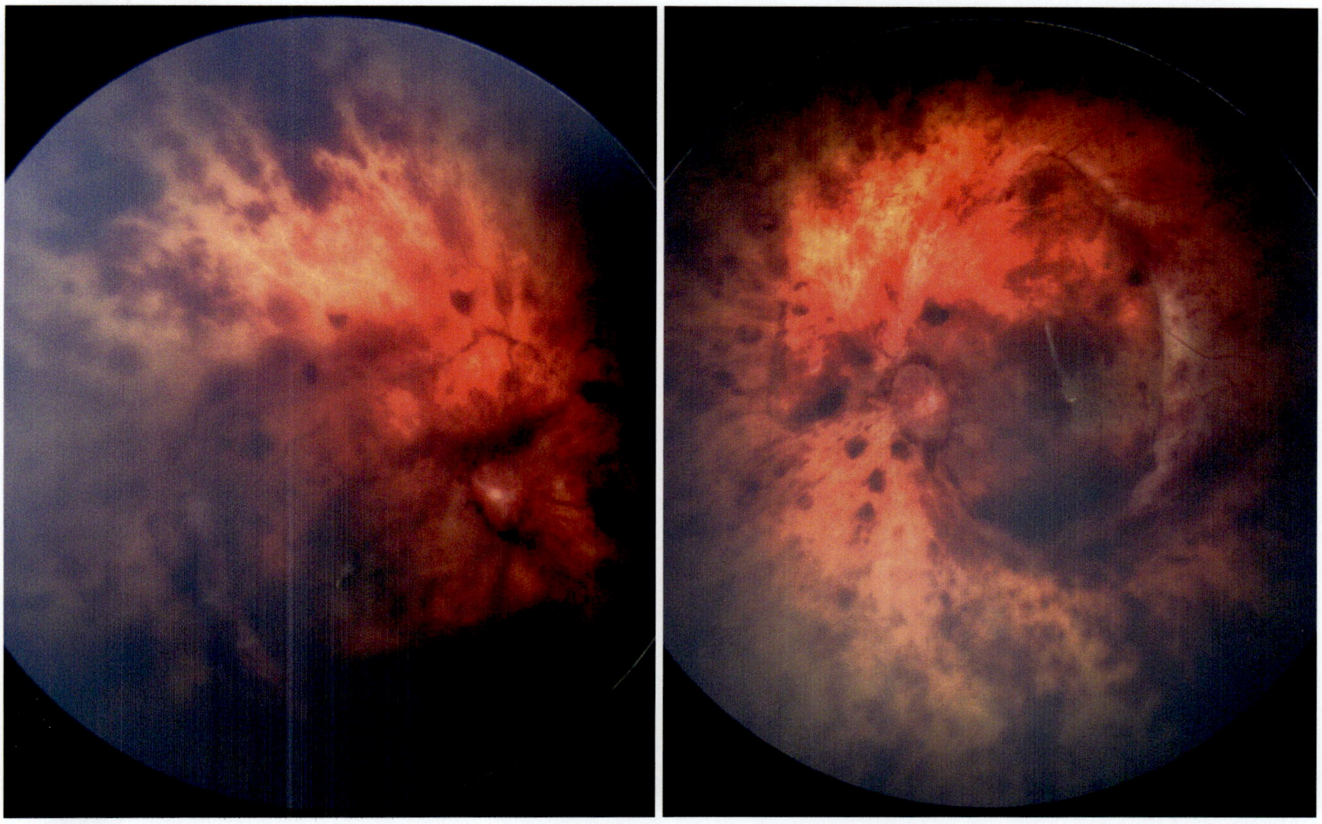

Fig. 32.3 This 12-month-old male with a history of benign macrocephaly and plagiocephaly was found non-responsive after falling from bed. He was diagnosed with severe anoxic encephalopathy, subdural hemorrhages and suffered cardiorespiratory arrest. The color fundus photographs show diffuse bilateral preretinal, intraretinal, and subretinal hemorrhages (Images courtesy of C. Armitage Harper III, MD)

management of the patient's comorbidities often including extensive neurologic, cardiopulmonary, and orthopedic injuries. Additional modalities for evaluation and documentation of ophthalmic findings include fluorescein angiography (FA) and optical coherence tomography (OCT). FA provides angiographic evidence of peripheral retinal nonperfusion in NAT [11–14]. These angiographic defects appear to persist even after other visible signs of trauma have resolved [12] (Figs. 32.4, 32.5, 32.6 and 32.7). OCT provides information about the density, thickness, and location of hemorrhage useful for management decisions and surgical repair. OCT can help assess whether the fovea is blocked by sub-hyaloid or sub-internal limiting membrane blood and assess whether there is a macular hole (Fig. 32.8).

32.3 Medical Management

Hemorrhage after NAT typically improves without further intervention, thus medical management centers on amblyopia prevention, and patients should be closely followed by pediatric ophthalmologists for visual development. Patient positioning sometimes is necessary in premacular hemorrhages to allow dependent clearance of vitreous hemorrhage from the visual axis if not surgically significant. However, in some cases, neovascularization may occur. The mechanism for neovascularization after NAT and how best to treat it is debated. Neovascularization can result from ischemia from retinoschisis (described also in juvenile retinoschisis [15–17] and senile retinoschisis [18]), as well as from ischemia from disruption of capillary networks [9]. Additionally, the tightly adherent posterior hyaloid face as well as preretinal hemorrhage may provide a scaffold for aberrant neovascularization and fibrous proliferation. In the setting of multiple reports of neovascularization after NAT [9, 10, 13, 19], Kiernan et al. suggested prophylactic photoablation to the nonperfused peripheral retina may be warranted, especially in children whose long-term follow-up cannot be certain. Laser photoablation, though effective, has well-documented adverse effects including the formation of cataract, vitreous hemorrhage, iris synechiae, constriction of visual field, strabismus, and high myopia. In some series, angiographic evidence of peripheral nonperfusion is documented without subsequent development of neovascularization [11, 12]. Thus, deciding who and when to treat will be an important area to elucidate.

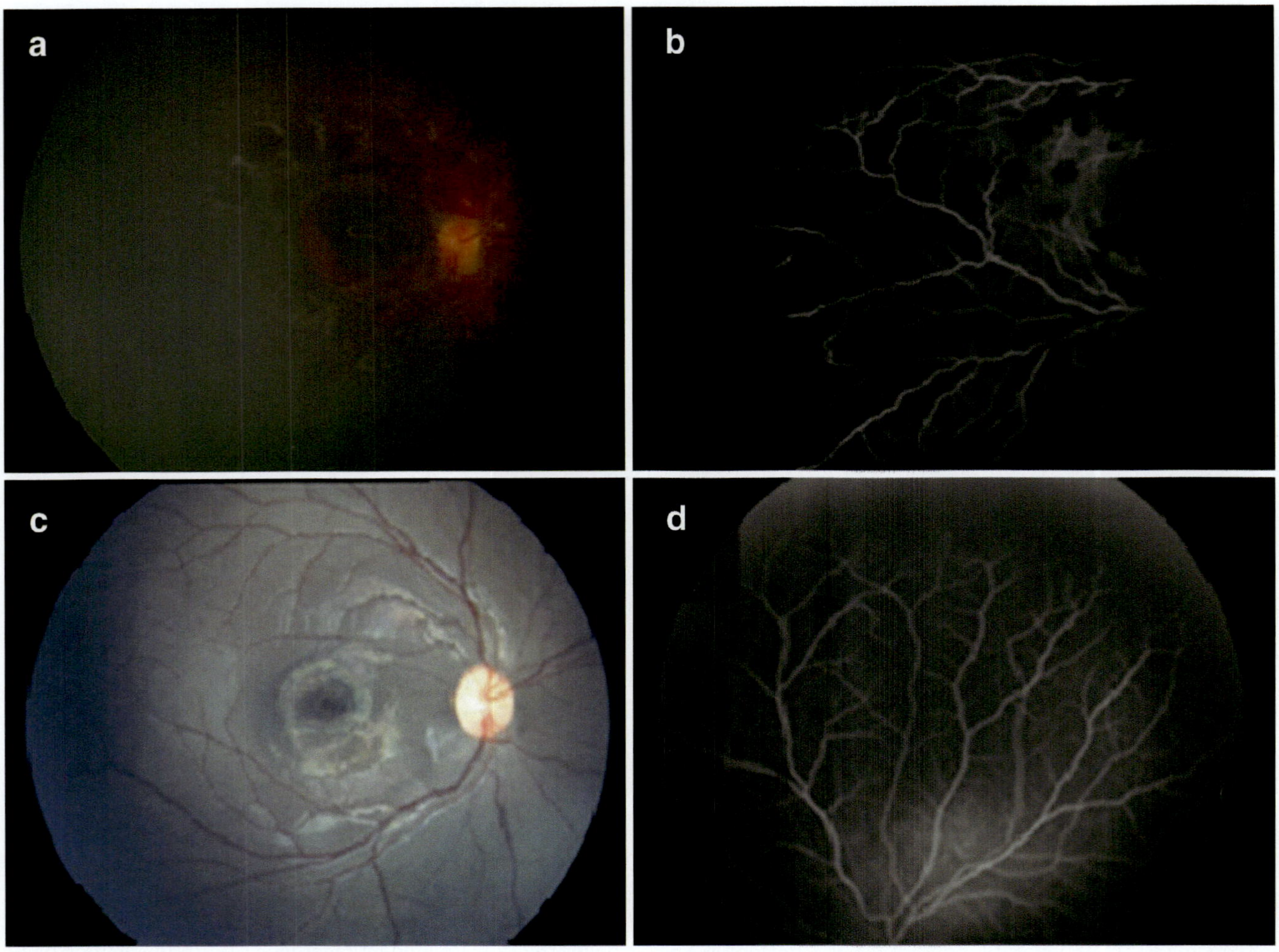

Fig. 32.4 This 5-month-old female was brought to the emergency room with a loss of consciousness and seizures after NAT. She was diagnosed with skull fractures and subdural hematoma. Four days after trauma, color photographs show showed diffuse retinal hemorrhages (**a**) and peripheral nonperfusion on FA (**b**). EUA 5 months later showed interval resolution of retinal hemorrhages (**c**), but persistent peripheral nonperfusion on FA (**d**). (Images courtesy of Audina M. Berrocal, MD. Reproduced from Tran K, Ko A, Read S, et al. The Use of Fluorescein Angiography to Evaluate Pediatric Abusive Head Trauma: An Observational Case Series. *Journal of Vitreoretinal Diseases*. 2017;1(5):321-327) [12]

32.4 Surgical Management

The use of vitrectomy in NAT is also widely debated. While RHs typically resolve within 4–6 weeks, preretinal hemorrhage may persist for weeks and vitreous hemorrhage for months. In the case of thick, non-clearing hemorrhage, surgical intervention may be warranted to reduce the risk of deprivation amblyopia and progressive tractional fibrotic changes [20–22] (Figs. 32.9, 32.10, 32.11 and 32.12). In smaller pediatric eyes, sclerotomies must be placed strategically to avoid iatrogenic damage to the crystalline lens and peripheral retina. The standard guidelines for port placement used for adults are not appropriate for pediatric patients, and Dr. Chang and colleagues have proposed a pediatric pars plana vitrectomy sclerotomy nomogram taking into account the pediatric patient's age and underlying diagnosis (Tables 32.1 and 32.2) [23]. Small gauge (i.e., 25 gauge) instrumentation is used to allow for optimal intraoperative maneuverability. During the vitrectomy, the hyaloid may be less adherent and a posterior vitreous detachment easier to induce due to prior trauma and the plasmin effects of the vitreous hemorrhage. If there is a large amount of sub-internal limiting membrane hemorrhage, one may consider peeling the internal limiting membrane. In some cases, immediate sequential bilateral vitreoretinal surgery (ISBVS), performed in both eyes sequentially during the same anesthesia session may be fea-

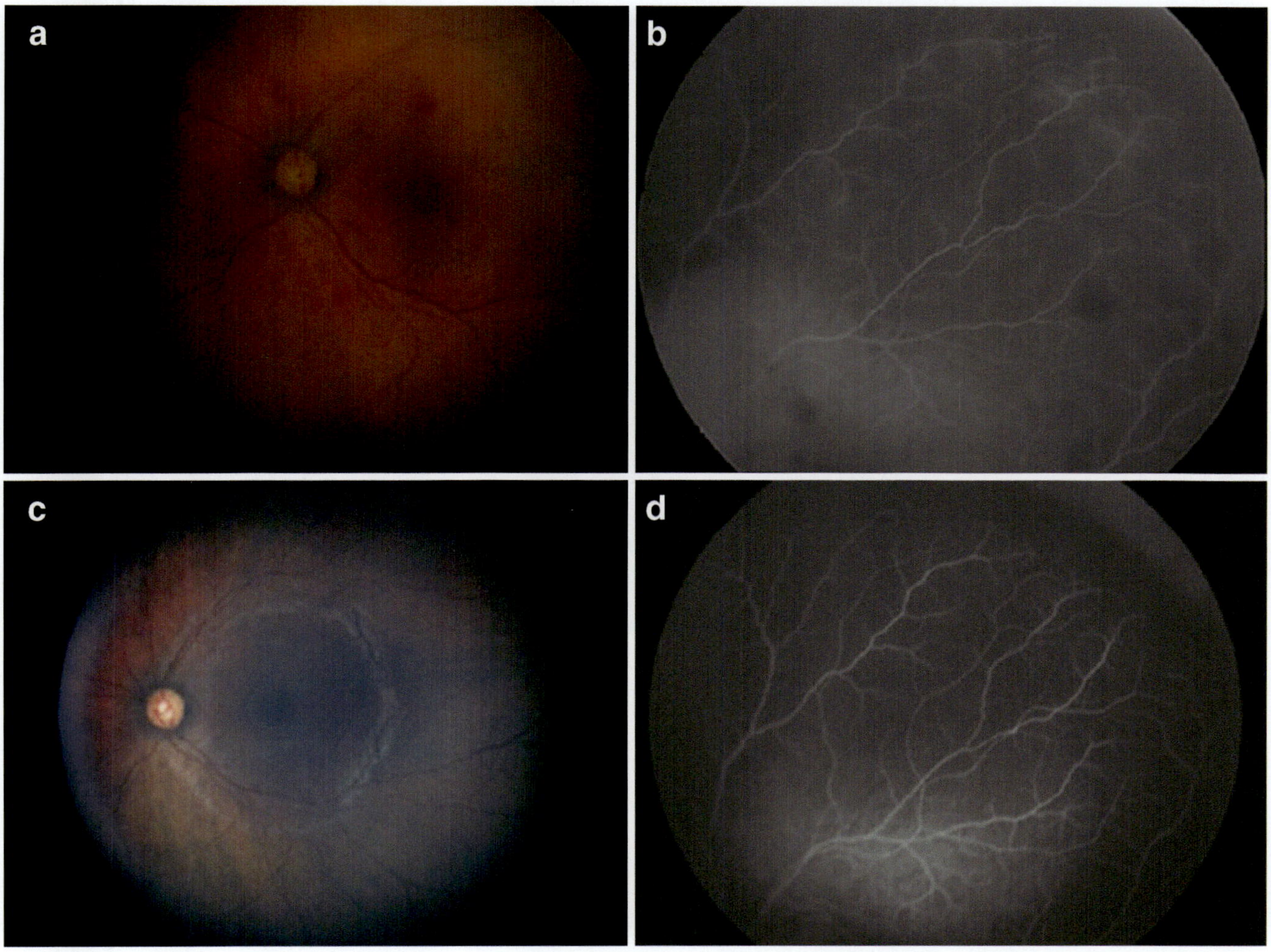

Fig. 32.5 This 6-week-old male was brought to the emergency department for new seizures after NAT. He was diagnosed with subdural and subarachnoid hemorrhages and fracture of the left radius. Two days after presentation, color photographs demonstrated retinal hemorrhages (**a**), peripheral nonperfusion, and late small vessel leakage on FA (**b**). Repeat EUA 3 months later showed interval resolution of retinal hemorrhages (**c**), but persistent peripheral nonperfusion on FA (**d**) (Images courtesy of Audina M. Berrocal, MD. Reproduced from Tran K, Ko A, Read S, et al. The Use of Fluorescein Angiography to Evaluate Pediatric Abusive Head Trauma: An Observational Case Series. *Journal of Vitreoretinal Diseases.* 2017;1(5):321-327) [12]

sible and safe for pediatric patients with bilateral vitreoretinal pathologic features when repeated general anesthesia is undesirable or impractical [24].

The potential benefit of vitrectomy must be weighed against the additional limitations to visual potential including cortical visual loss, optic atrophy, pigmentary changes in the macula, and retinal ischemia as well as potential complications of surgery including iatrogenic breaks and the patient's multiple systemic comorbidities associated with NAT. Additionally, vitrectomy plays an uncertain role in the prevention of neovascularization. A posterior vitreous detachment (PVD) is often difficult to attain, and thus the scaffold for neovascularization and fibrous proliferation may persist. However, removal of the formed vitreous may decrease the intraocular VEGF concentration and in this way decrease the risk of aberrant angiogenesis. Ocriplasmin is currently being studied as a surgical adjunct to vitrectomy in pediatric vitreoretinopathies to aid with the induction of PVD [25], and the use of intravitreal tissue plasminogen and SF6 have been described for pediatric sub-hyaloid hemorrhage associated with NAT [26].

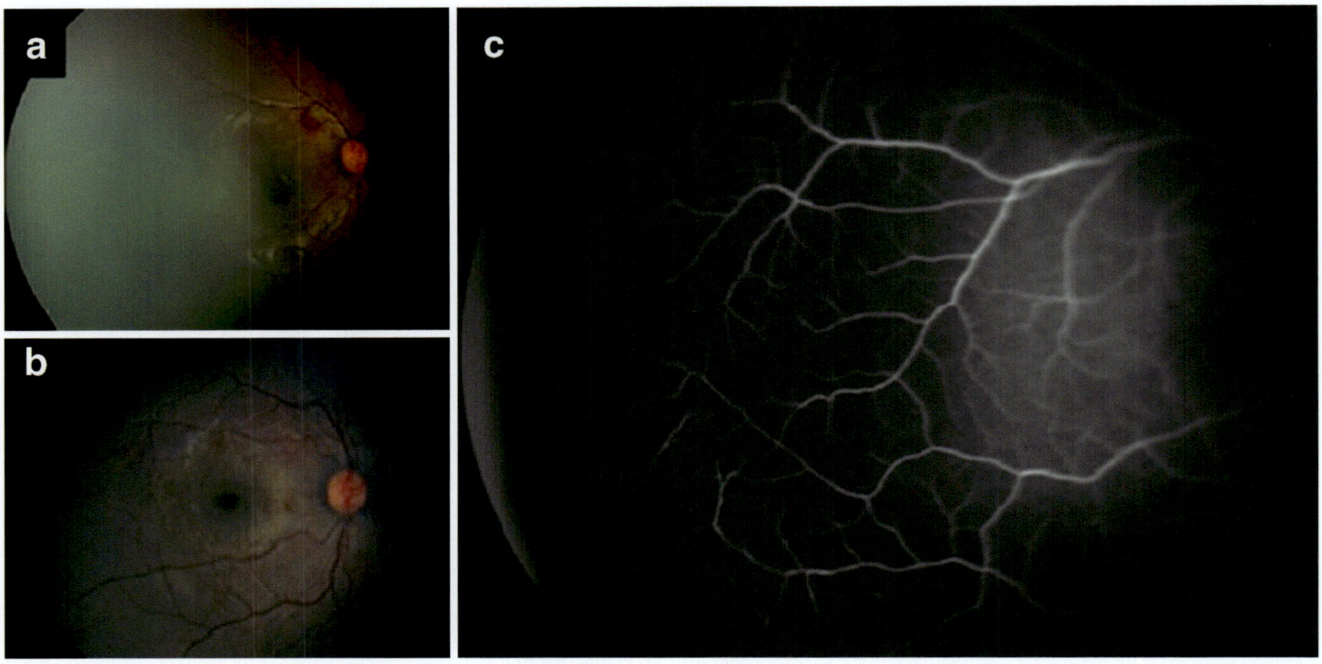

Fig. 32.6 This 4-month-old male was brought to the emergency department for shortness of breath and was diagnosed with multiple skull fractures, rib fractures, and pneumothorax after NAT. On presentation, retinal hemorrhages were noted (**a**). Follow-up EUA 3 months later showed interval resolution of retinal hemorrhages (**b**), but persistent peripheral nonperfusion on FA (**c**). (Images courtesy of Audina M. Berrocal, MD. Reproduced from Tran K, Ko A, Read S, et al. The Use of Fluorescein Angiography to Evaluate Pediatric Abusive Head Trauma: An Observational Case Series. *Journal of Vitreoretinal Diseases*. 2017;1(5):321-327) [12]

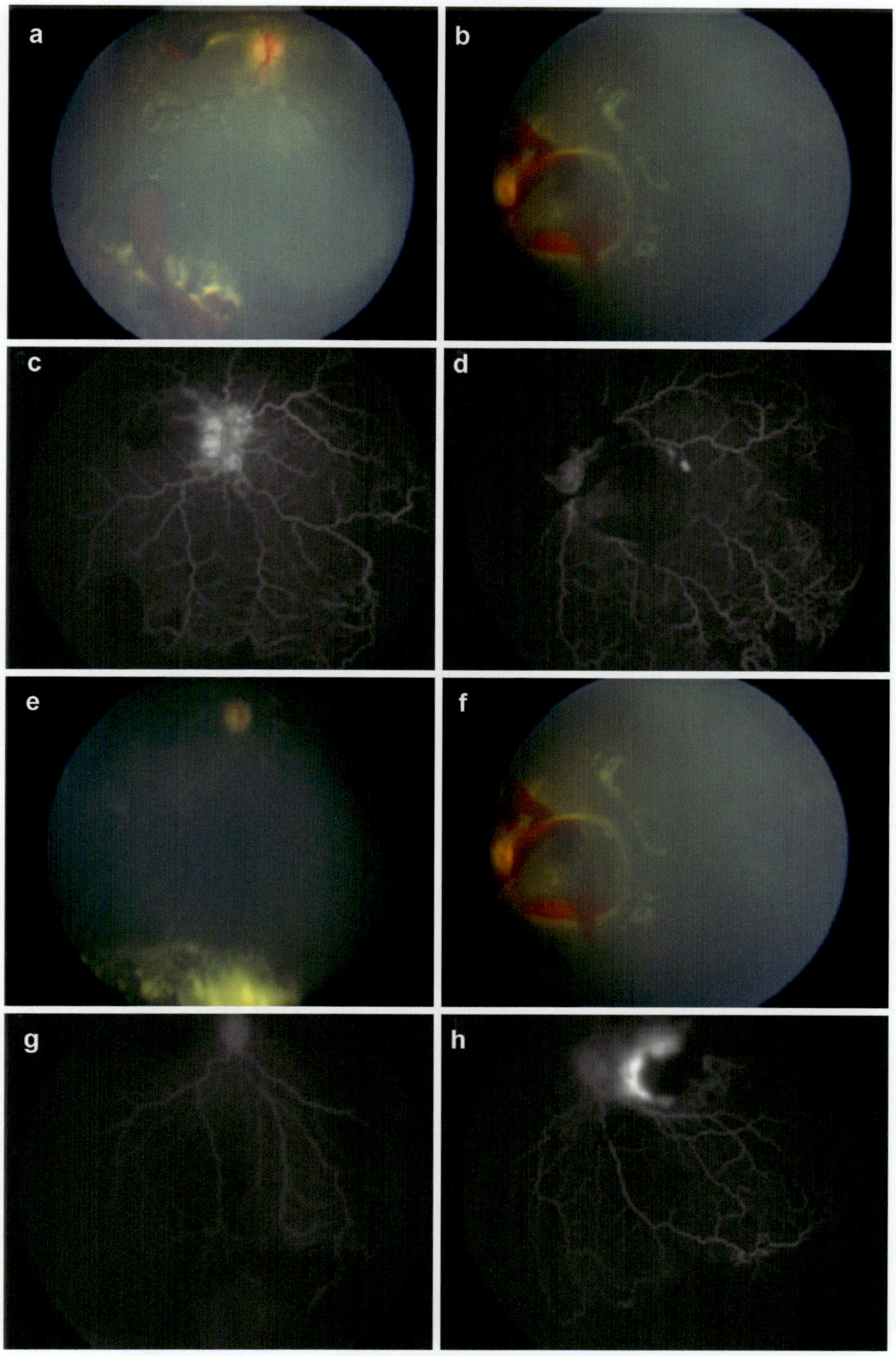

Fig. 32.7 This 2-year-old female was admitted to the intensive care unit with loss of consciousness after NAT. One month after trauma, color photographs showed diffuse preretinal, intraretinal, and subretinal hemorrhages within the macula and in all four quadrants (**a**, **b**). FA showed bilateral leakage from the optic nerve heads and peripheral nonperfusion 360 degrees extending 2DD posterior to the ora (**c**, **d**). On follow-up EUA 2 months later, the fundus exam showed fibrosis surrounding the optic nerves, subretinal fluid within the macula, interval improvement in peripheral retinal hemorrhages, but persistent areas of severe retinal ischemia with pinpoint areas of leakage and neovascularization in both eyes (**e**–**h**). (Images courtesy of Audina M. Berrocal, MD. Reproduced from Tran K, Ko A, Read S, et al. The Use of Fluorescein Angiography to Evaluate Pediatric Abusive Head Trauma: An Observational Case Series. *Journal of Vitreoretinal Diseases.* 2017;1(5):321-327) [12]

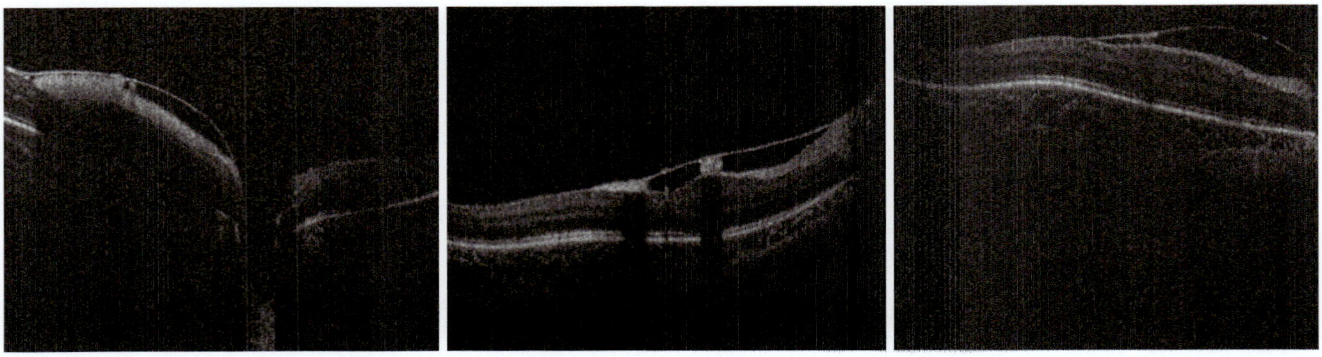

Fig. 32.8 This 4-month-old female presented 3 months after trauma with a history subdural hemorrhages and seizures after suspected non-accidental trauma. She was diagnosed with sub-hyaloid and intraretinal hemorrhages in both eyes. The original optical coherence tomography (OCT) from presentation was blocked by hemorrhage; however, the follow-up OCT shows sub-internal limiting membrane hemorrhage with shadowing obscuring foveal visualization. The patient was managed with observation and was closely followed by pediatric ophthalmology to evaluate for obstructive amblyopia. One month later, OCT shows the fovea is no longer blocked by hemorrhage, and there is no shadowing from sub-hyaloid hemorrhage. On last visit, OCT shows the fovea partially imaged but clearly without sub-hyaloid hemorrhage and with fair foveal contour (Images courtesy of Lejla Vajzovic, MD)

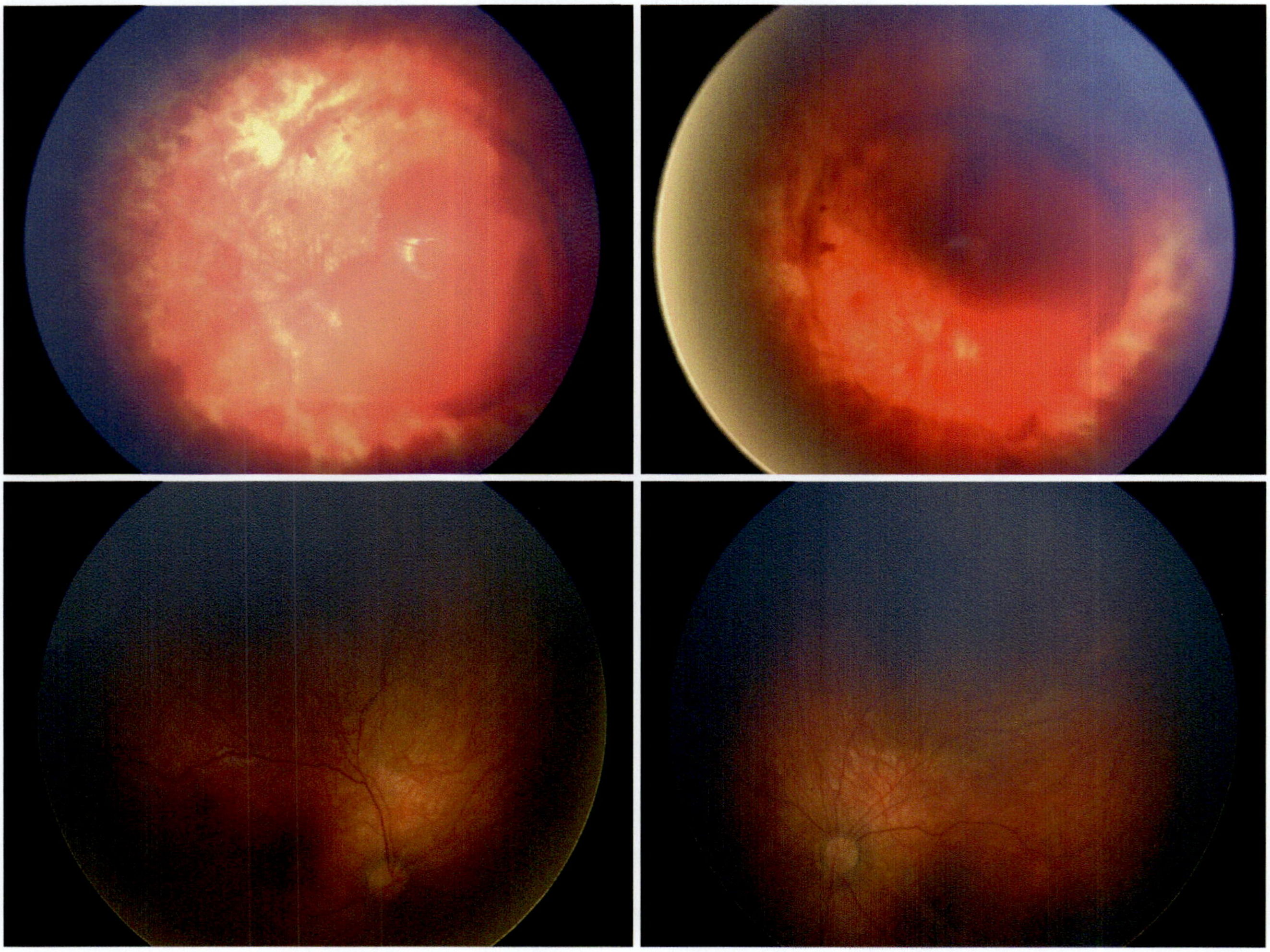

Fig. 32.9 This 4-month-old male was found to be non-responsive after NAT. He was diagnosed with subarachnoid and subdural hemorrhage, bilateral rib fractions, and left distal radius fracture. The color fundus photographs show vitreous hemorrhage, optic nerve hemorrhage, multiple intraretinal hemorrhages, and sub-internal limiting membrane hemorrhage. Four months after vitrectomy and membrane peel in both eyes, fundus photographs demonstrate resolution of previously noted hemorrhages, pale nerves, and attenuated vessels (Images courtesy of C. Armitage Harper III, MD)

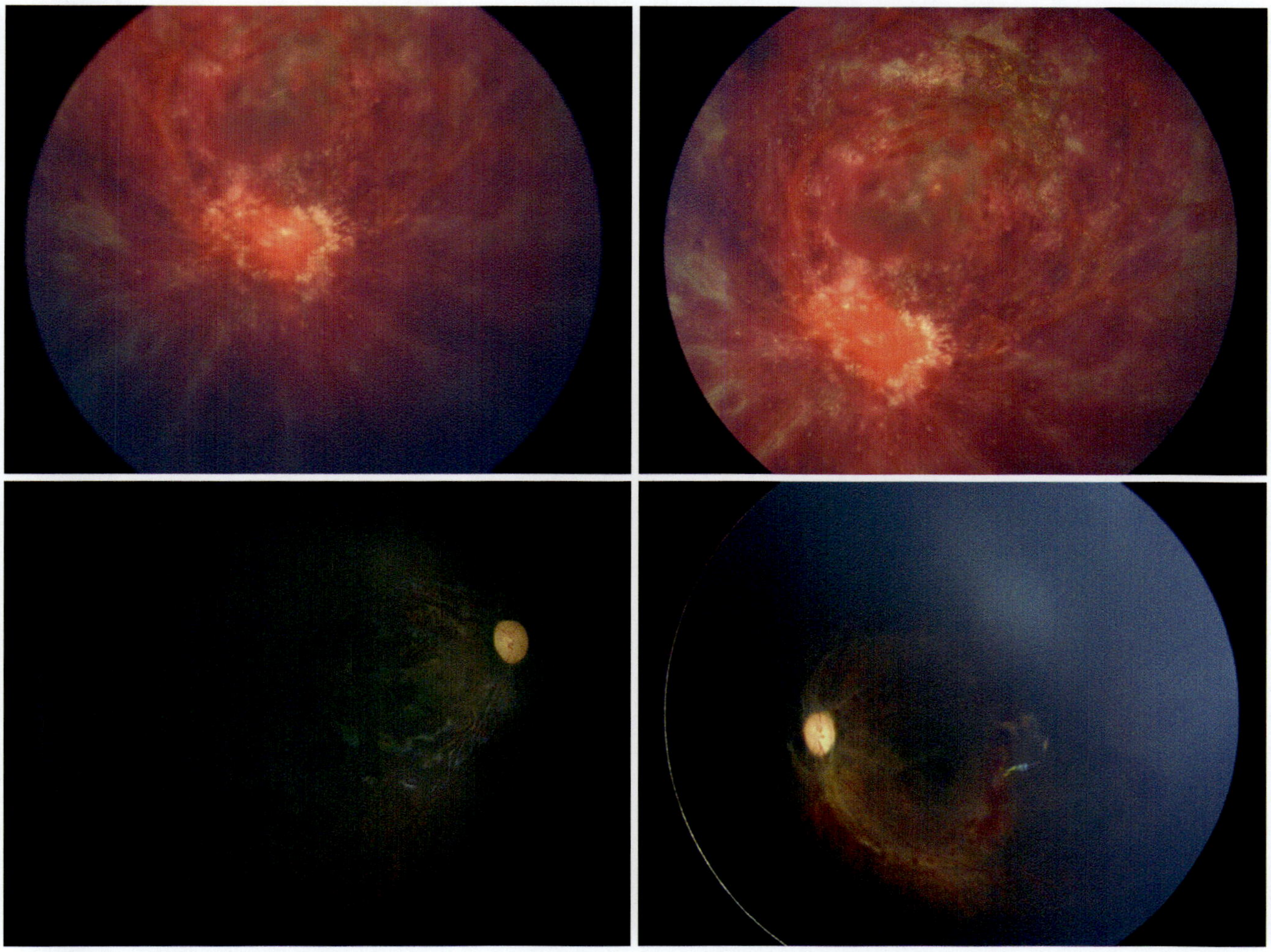

Fig. 32.10 This 3-month-old female was found to have spontaneous seizures after NAT. She was diagnosed with convulsive status epilepticus, subarachnoid and subdural hemorrhage, acute respiratory failure, anoxic brain injury. The color fundus photographs show vitreous hemorrhage, optic nerve hemorrhage, multiple intraretinal hemorrhages, and sub-internal limiting membrane hemorrhage. Four weeks after vitrectomy, color fundus photographs show interval improvement in the intraretinal hemorrhages, pale nerve, and attenuated vessels (Images courtesy of C. Armitage Harper III, MD)

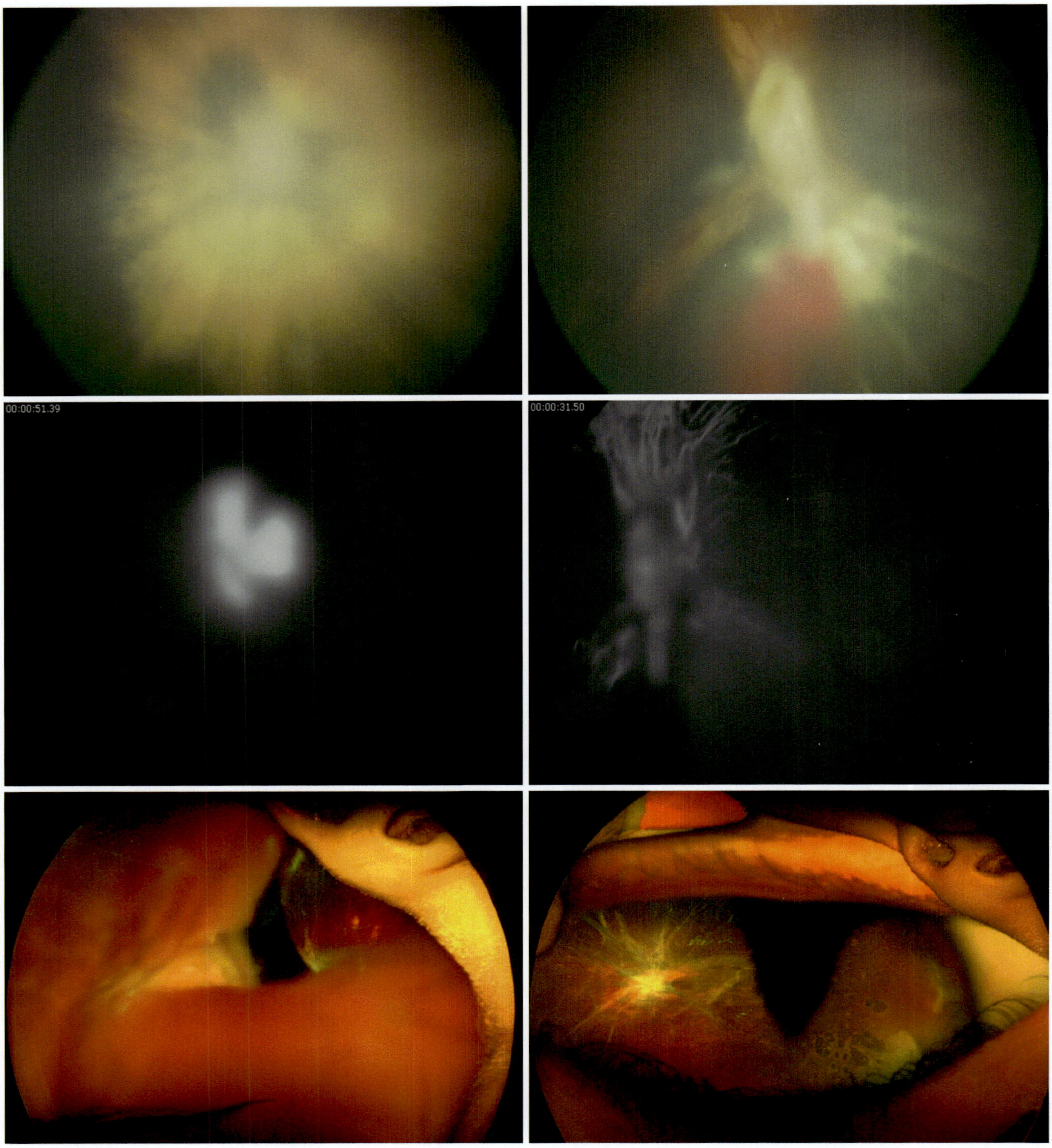

Fig. 32.11 This 4-month-old African-American female was found to have diffuse dense scattered intraretinal and mild preretinal hemorrhage after NAT. The patient was monitored, and the initial retinal hemorrhages improved significantly after several weeks. However, on follow-up at 2 months, the patient was diagnosed with vitreous hemorrhage and tractional retinal detachments resulting from ischemia and secondary re-neovascularization of the regressed hyaloidal artery. The color fundus photographs and fluorescein angiogram (FA) show bilateral persistent fetal vasculature syndrome (PFVS)-like tractional retinal detachments with leakage on FA. The patient underwent same-day bilateral vitrectomy, membrane peel, retinal cryopexy, and laser. Final postoperative color photographs at almost 3 years of age: right eye shows ischemic retina attached under fluid with optic atrophy. The left eye shows a settled re-attached trifold PFVS-like stalk configuration with ischemic retina under fluid (Images courtesy of Emmanuel Y. Chang, MD, PhD)

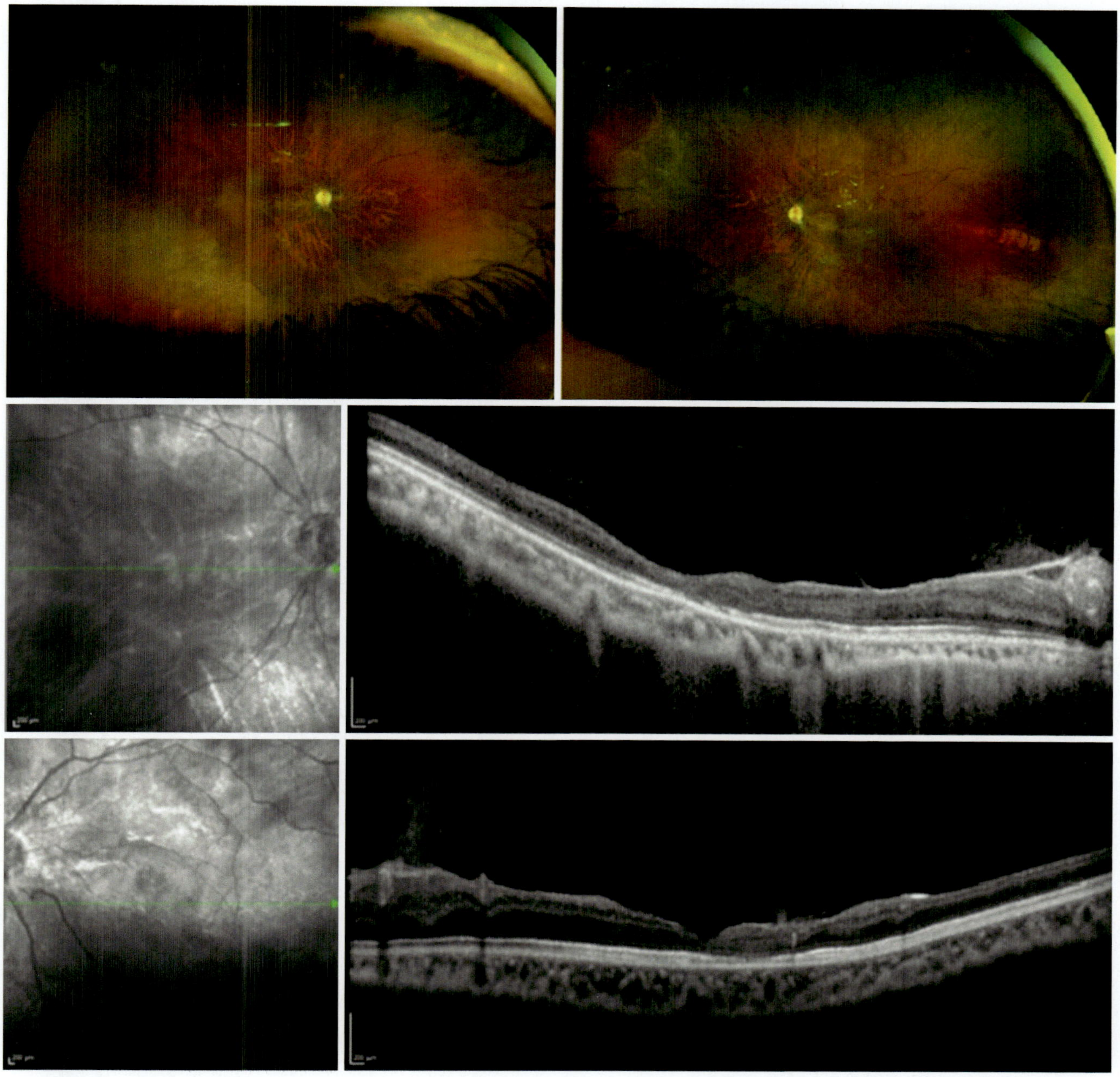

Fig. 32.12 This 8-year-old male was found down at 4 months old and diagnosed with large subdural hematomas and severe bilateral preretinal hemorrhages after NAT. He underwent bilateral vitrectomy 10 weeks after presentation due to the risk of amblyopia. At the last follow-up, the patient is 20/200 best-corrected visual acuity in both eyes with nystagmus. The color fundus photographs and optical coherence tomography (OCT) show bilateral disc pallor, foveal atrophy, and attenuated vessels (Images courtesy of C. Armitage Harper III, MD)

Table 32.1 Sclerotomy site placement for infants and children based on disease type and age (Images courtesy of Emmanuel Y. Chang, MD. Reproduced from Wright LM, Harper CA III, Chang EY. Management of Infantile and Childhood Retinopathies: Optimized Pars Plana Vitrectomy Sclerotomy Nomogram. *Ophthalmology Retina.* 2018; 2:1227-1234) [23]

	Distance posterior to the limbus,[a] mm				
Age	Control	FEVR[b]	PFV[b]	Coloboma[b]	Stidder syndrome/myoptia
1 month	0.75	0.75	0.75	0.5–0.75	1.5
2 months	1.0	0.75	1.0	0.5–0.75	2.0
3 months	1.0	0.75	1.0	0.5–0.75	2.0
4 months	1.5	1.0	1.0	0.5–0.75	2.0
5 months	1.5	1.0	1.0	0.5–0.75	2.5
6 months	1.5	1.0	1.0	0.5–0.75	2.5
7 months	1.5	1.5	1.5	0.5–0.75	2.5
8 months	2.0	1.5	1.5	0.5–0.75	2.5
9 months	2.0	1.5	1.5	1.0	2.5
10 months	2.0	1.5	1.5	1.0	2.5
11 months	2.0	2.0	1.5	1.0	2.5
12 months	2.0	2.0	1.5	1.0	2.5
18 months	2.5	2.0	1.5	1.5	3.0
2 years	2.5	2.5	2.0	2.0	3.0
3 years	3.0	2.5	2.0	2.0	3.5
4 years	3.0	3.0	2.0	2.5	3.5
5 years	3.0	3.0	2.0	2.5	3.5
6 years	3.5	3.5	2.5	3.0	3.5
7 years	3.5	3.5	2.5	3.0	4.0
8 years	3.5	3.5	2.5	3.0	4.0
9 years	3.5	3.5	2.5	3.5	4.0
10 years	3.5	3.5	2.5	3.5	4.0
11 years	3.5	3.5	2.5	3.5	4.0
12 years	3.5	4.0	2.5	3.5	4.0
13 years	4.0	4.0	2.5	3.5	4.0
14 years	4.0	4.0	2.5	4.0	4.0
15 years	4.0	4.0	2.5	4.0	4.0
16 years	4.0	4.0	3.0	4.0	4.0
17 years	4.0	4.0	3.0	4.0	4.0
18 years	4.0	4.0	3.0	4.0	4.0

FEVR familial exudative vitreoretin opathy, *PFV* persistent fetal vasculature, *ROP* retinopathy of prematurity

[a]Determination of ora-limbus distance is based on regression analyses of control and disease subjects, as measured from the limbus, permitting ≥1 mm from the ora serrate; we recommend nasal sclerotomies be placed 0.25–0.5 mm shorter than the recommended location

[b]We recommend variability in ora-limbus distance and possible anterior—posterior contraction among infants

Table 32.2 Sclerotomy or intravitreal injection site for retinopathy of prematurity (Images courtesy of Emmanuel Y. Chang, MD. Reproduced from Wright LM, Harper CA III, Chang EY. Management of Infantile and Childhood Retinopathies: Optimized Pars Plana Vitrectomy Sclerotomy Nomogram. *Ophthalmology Retina*. 2018; 2:1227-1234) [23]

PMA, weeks	Distance posterior to limbus,[a] mm
34	1.6–2.1
35	1.6–2.1
36	1.6–2.1
37	1.5–2.0
38	1.5–2.0
39	1.4–1.9
40	1.4–1.9
41	1.4–1.9
42	1.3–1.8
43	1.3–1.8
44	1.3–1.8
45	1.2–1.7
46	1.2–1.7
47	1.2–1.7
48	1.1–1.6

PMA postmenstrual age

[a]Determination of ora-limbus distance is based on regression analyses, as measured from the limbus, permitting ≥1 mm from the ora serata; we recommend nasal sclerotomies be 0.25–0.5 mm shorter than the recommended location. We recommend transillumination guided identification of the on serrata, given the variability in ora-limbus distance and possible anterior–posterior contraction among infants

References

1. Vinchon M, Defoort-Dhellemmes S, Desurmont M, Dhellemmes P. Accidental and nonaccidental head injuries in infants: a prospective study. J Neurosurg. 2005;102(4 Suppl):380–4.
2. Bishop NB. Traumatic brain injury: a primer for primary care physicians. Curr Probl Pediatr Adolesc Health Care. 2006;36(9):318–31.
3. Families USDoHHSAfCa, Administration on children Y, and families, bureau Cs. Child maltreatment 2016. 2016.
4. Adamsbaum C, Grabar S, Mejean N, Rey-Salmon C. Abusive head trauma: judicial admissions highlight violent and repetitive shaking. Pediatrics. 2010;126(3):546–55.
5. Vinchon M, de Foort-Dhellemmes S, Desurmont M, Delestret I. Confessed abuse versus witnessed accidents in infants: comparison of clinical, radiological, and ophthalmological data in corroborated cases. Childs Nerv Syst. 2010;26(5):637–45.
6. Maguire SA, Watts PO, Shaw AD, et al. Retinal haemorrhages and related findings in abusive and non-abusive head trauma: a systematic review. Eye (Lond). 2013;27(1):28–36.
7. Bhardwaj G, Chowdhury V, Jacobs MB, Moran KT, Martin FJ, Coroneo MT. A systematic review of the diagnostic accuracy of ocular signs in pediatric abusive head trauma. Ophthalmology. 2010;117(5):983–992.e917.
8. Emerson MV, Jakobs E, Green WR. Ocular autopsy and histopathologic features of child abuse. Ophthalmology. 2007;114(7):1384–94.
9. Brown SM, Shami M. Optic disc neovascularization following severe retinoschisis due to shaken baby syndrome. Arch Ophthalmol. 1999;117(6):838–9.
10. Caputo G, de Haller R, Metge F, Dureau P. Ischemic retinopathy and neovascular proliferation secondary to shaken baby syndrome. Retina. 2008;28(3 Suppl):S42–6.
11. Goldenberg DT, Wu D, Capone A, Drenser KA, Trese MT. Nonaccidental trauma and peripheral retinal nonperfusion. Ophthalmology. 2010;117(3):561–6.
12. Tran K, Ko A, Read S, et al. The use of fluorescein angiography to evaluate pediatric abusive head trauma: an observational case series. J Vitreoretinal Dis. 2017;1(5):321–7.
13. Kiernan DF, Blair MP, Shapiro MJ. Neovascularization after nonaccidental trauma. Ophthalmology. 2010;117(12):2443.e2441–2.
14. Bielory BP, Dubovy SR, Olmos LC, Hess DJ, Berrocal AM. Fluorescein angiographic and histopathologic findings of bilateral peripheral retinal nonperfusion in nonaccidental injury: a case series. Arch Ophthalmol. 2012;130(3):383–7.
15. Hung JY, Hilton GF. Neovascular glaucoma in a patient with X-linked juvenile retinoschisis. Ann Ophthalmol. 1980;12(9):1054–5.
16. Arkfeld DF, Brockhurst RJ. Vascularized vitreous membranes in congenital retinoschisis. Retina. 1987;7(1):20–3.
17. Pearson R, Jagger J. Sex linked juvenile retinoschisis with optic disc and peripheral retinal neovascularisation. Br J Ophthalmol. 1989;73(4):311–3.
18. Campo RV, Reeser FH, Flindall RJ. Vascular leakage, neovascularization, and vitreous hemorrhage in senile bullous retinoschisis. Am J Ophthalmol. 1983;95(6):826–32.
19. Hayden A, Tawansy K, Gonzalez J, Patel P, Chung M. Peripheral retinal non-perfusion in the shaken baby syndrome. Investigative Ophthalmol Visual Sci. 2004;45(13):271.
20. Maguire AM, Trese MT. Visual results of lens-sparing vitreoretinal surgery in infants. J Pediatr Ophthalmol Strabismus. 1993;30(1):28–32.
21. Capone A. Lens-sparing vitreous surgery for infantile amblyogenic vitreous hemorrhage. Retina. 2003;23(6):792–5.
22. Rahman W, Osbourne S, Bhan A, Orr GM, Gregson R. Vitrectomy in cases of nonaccidental injury. J Pediatr Ophthalmol Strabismus. 2010;47(3):163–7.
23. Wright L, Harper C III, Chang E. Management of infantile and childhood retinopathies: optimized pediatric pars plana vitrectomy sclerotomy nomogram. 2018;2:1227–34.
24. Yonekawa Y, Wu WC, Kusaka S, et al. Immediate sequential bilateral pediatric vitreoretinal surgery: an international multicenter study. Ophthalmology. 2016;123(8):1802–8.
25. Wong SC, Capone A. Microplasmin (ocriplasmin) in pediatric vitreoretinal surgery: update and review. Retina. 2013;33(2):339–48.
26. Conway MD, Peyman GA, Recasens M. Intravitreal tPA and SF6 promote clearing of premacular subhyaloid hemorrhages in shaken and battered baby syndrome. Ophthalmic Surg Lasers. 1999;30(6):435–41.

Rhegmatogenous Retinal Detachments in the Pediatric Population and Special Considerations for Pediatric Vitreoretinal Surgery

33

Nicola Y. Gan and Wai-Ching Lam

Abstract

In this chapter, the authors present a concise summary of the more commonly seen types of rhegmatogenous retinal detachments (RRD) one can encounter in pediatric patients. A spectrum of diseases and their management will be described, including Stickler syndrome, Marfan syndrome, choroidal coloboma, and atopic dermatitis associated RRD. As the pediatric eye is smaller than the adult eye, certain considerations must be borne in mind when performing pediatric vitreoretinal surgeries. A section on surgical management pearls is included at the end of this chapter.

Keywords

Pediatric · Retinal detachment · Vitreoretinal surgery Vitrectomy · Scleral buckling

33.1 Introduction

Retinal detachments in the pediatric population span a variety of congenital and acquired conditions with some not commonly seen in adults. In this chapter, we describe the more commonly encountered types of rhegmatogenous retinal detachments, and highlight important pearls in the diagnosis and management of each.

N. Y. Gan
Department of Ophthalmology, Tan Tock Seng Hospital, National Healthcare Group Eye Institute, Singapore, Singapore

W.-C. Lam (✉)
Department of Ophthalmology, The University of Hong Kong, Hong Kong, Hong Kong

Department of Ophthalmology and Vision Sciences, University of Toronto, Toronto, Canada

33.1.1 Epidemiology and Clinical Presentation

The causes of RRD can be divided into traumatic and non-traumatic. Non-traumatic causes include (1) myopia; (2) hereditary congenital anomalies (more common examples include Stickler syndrome, Marfan syndrome, and X-linked retinoschisis); (3) non-hereditary developmental anomalies, e.g., choroidal coloboma, cicatricial retinopathy of prematurity (ROP); and (4) previous intraocular surgery [1–6].

Delayed diagnosis is a significant feature of pediatric RRDs. Compared to adults, children with non-traumatic RRDs usually present at a later stage and with detachments of undetermined duration. At presentation, the macula is often involved or proliferative vitreoretinopathy (PVR) is present. The incidence of PVR has been reported in various studies to range from 40% to 45% [2, 6, 7]. Occasionally a child presents late with sensory strabismus as a result of an undiagnosed chronic retinal detachment. Bilateral involvement has also been reported to be more common in pediatric non-traumatic RRDs, with a range of 15–22% [2, 3].

Conversely, traumatic RRDs usually present acutely and with a known duration. In a large series of 127 eyes, Soheilian M et al. [2] reported a statistically significant higher male to female ratio in traumatic RRDs (9.8:1), but no significant difference in non-traumatic cases [2]. In a retrospective case series of 88 eyes in patients aged 0–16 years by Lee RWJ et al. [8], 53% of RRDs were related to trauma and 44% of these had retinal dialyses. Interestingly, in the idiopathic RRD group, 76% were found to have retinal dialysis. Previous series have reported similar findings [9, 10] suggesting that "spontaneous" dialyses are a separate clinical entity in the pediatric age group. It has been postulated that the temporal retina is the last area of the retina to vascularize; therefore, retinal dialyses may occur in children with a congenital predisposition [11]. If vitreous hemorrhage or cataract is absent, treatment of choice is usually a circumferential segmental scleral buckle [12]. It is recommended that the width of the buckle should extend from the ora serrata anteriorly to cover the entire width of the dialysis [13]. Anatomical

W.-C. Wu, W.-C. Lam (eds.), *A Quick Guide to Pediatric Retina*, https://doi.org/10.1007/978-981-15-6552-6_33

reattachment was reported in 67–88% of cases, with low rates of PVR [14, 15].

The reported overall anatomic success rate of surgical repair of pediatric RRDs ranges from 74.9% to 80% [2, 3]. Performing a pneumatic retinopexy (PR) may be considered in some older children with RRD. Warder D et al. [16] reported a retrospective, non-interventional comparative case series of PR done in 27 eyes, in 26 patients (9–18 years old) and found an overall anatomical success rate of 63% with a single procedure.

33.1.2 RRDs Associated with Congenital Developmental Anomalies

- *Epidemiology and Clinical Presentation*

The reported incidence of congenital developmental anomalies as a cause of pediatric RRD ranges from 12% to 56% [2, 3, 7, 17, 18]. In studies done in East Asian countries, e.g., Taiwan, the incidence reported is lower at 12–17% as there is a higher incidence of RRD associated with high myopia [3, 6].

In a retrospective case series of 127 eyes, Soheilian M et al. [2] reported that congenital-developmental anomalies comprise 52.5% of RRDs in children below the age of 10 years, with an overall incidence of 39.3%. Hereditary vitreoretinopathies comprise the majority with Stickler syndrome being the most common [2, 18].

33.1.2.1 Stickler Syndrome

Stickler et al. [19] described a pedigree combining ocular, facial, palatal, and skeletal changes in 1965. Prominent features of this disorder include generalized arthropathy, cleft palate, flat face, hearing loss, and spondylo-epiphyseal dysplasia. Abnormalities of the vitreous gel structure are pathognomonic of this disorder. The inheritance is usually in an autosomal dominant pattern, but it can also occur sporadically.

Type I Stickler syndrome has a membranous vitreous phenotype, is most common and is associated with gene mutations for synthesis of collagen type II (*COL2A1*) [20, 21]. The less common type II Stickler syndrome has a beaded vitreous phenotype (type 2 vitreous) and is associated with mutation in the *COL11A1* gene which codes for type XI collagen. Type III Stickler syndrome has no ocular findings.

Non-ocular features Facial features of patients with Stickler syndrome include abnormal nasal, maxillary, and mandibular bony development. Patients usually have an underdeveloped nasal bone with a saddle nose. Other skeletal abnormalities include epiphyseal dysplasia, lax joints, and early onset progressive arthritis [19, 20, 22, 23]. Neurosensory hearing loss also affects most patients over time [23, 24].

Ocular features In Stickler syndrome, early-onset cataract is common with a characteristic lamellar wedge-shaped lens opacity occurring symmetrically in both eyes reflecting the embryologic abnormality in this syndrome [23, 25]. Patients are usually highly myopic with peripheral retinal thinning and retinal breaks, including giant retinal tears. In type I Stickler syndrome, the vitreous gel is optically empty with the presence of a fibrillar retrolenticular membrane extending to the pars plana and the peripheral retina. In type II Stickler syndrome, vitreous changes present are beaded condensations in the retrolenticular space, with peripheral lattice degeneration and perivascular pigmentation.

RRD is the most serious ocular complication of Stickler syndrome and may occur early in life. Eight percent of affected children have RRD between the ages of 0 and 9 years and 26% between 10 and 19 years [23, 26]. The incidence of RRD varies between different reports and ranges between 10% and 73% [23, 25, 27–29]. There is a propensity for giant retinal tear formation (Fig. 33.1), but a spectrum of retinal breaks may be seen [18, 29, 30].

A detailed examination of both eyes is mandatory in patients with Stickler syndrome, with the need to consider prophylactic treatment of high-risk peripheral retinal pathology in the fellow eye. Bilateral RDs are common and range from 39% to 51% [18, 27, 29, 31].

Ang et al. 2008 [27] did a large retrospective study on 204 type I Stickler syndrome patients and concluded that prophylactic treatment (either unilateral or bilateral 360 degrees of cryotherapy applied to the post-oral retina) reduced the risk of developing a retinal detachment. They published a statisti-

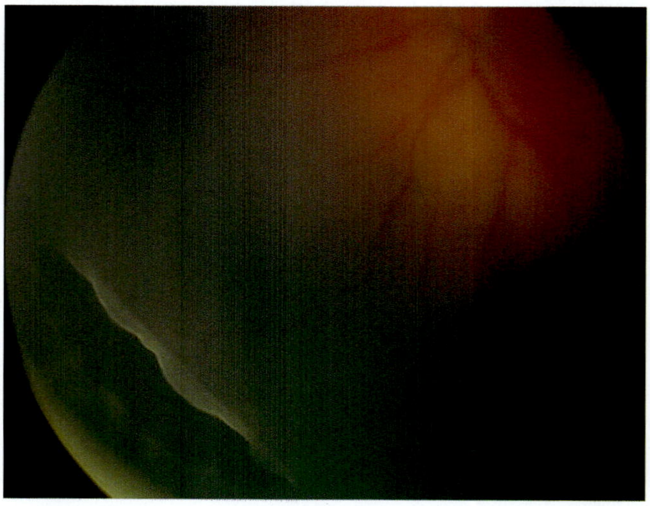

Fig. 33.1 Giant retinal tear with retinal detachment in a patient with Stickler syndrome

cally significant difference in the incidence of RD in patients with type I Stickler syndrome without prophylaxis (73%, 81 of 111) versus failure of prophylaxis in patients with bilateral cryotherapy (5 of 62 [8%]) and patients with unilateral cryotherapy (3 of 31 [10%]). However, this approach is unconventional and based on one study. We prefer to carry out prophylactic treatment only to high-risk lesions such as lattice degeneration.

Lastly, screening the family members of Stickler syndrome patients is also an important strategy to identify other affected members for prophylaxis or early treatment.

33.1.2.2 Marfan Syndrome

Marfan syndrome is an autosomal dominant disorder that involves the ocular, cardiovascular, and musculoskeletal systems. The genetic defect is found on the long arm of chromosome 15, known as fibrillin 1 gene (FBN1). The pathogenesis lies in a defect in the production of fibrillin, a glycoprotein that is an essential component of the microfibril assembly in the extracellular matrix. Microfibrils are essential in the deposition of elastin, which is present in the lens, zonules, and joint capsule [1, 32]. Fibrillin is also found in ocular structures such as the lamina cribrosa, sclera, choroid, and Bruch's membrane [33]. The revised Ghent nosology is most widely used to diagnose this syndrome [34].

Non-ocular features The cardiovascular manifestations include aortic dilatation and dissecting aneurysms. Mitral valve prolapse affects 60–70% of patients [35]. Musculoskeletal features include tall stature (>95th percentile by age/race/sex), joint laxity, hyper-extensible joints, arachnodactyly or long fingers, dolichostenomelia or long limbs, scoliosis, pectus deformities of the anterior chest wall, congenital contractures of the digits and elbows and generalized osteopenia [36].

Ocular features Non-traumatic ectopia lentis (Fig. 33.2) is the most common ocular presentation in Marfan syndrome and is seen in 50–80% of patients [37, 38]. Lens subluxation is usually towards the superotemporal meridian. Patients usually have poorly dilating pupils and iris transillumination defects. Axial myopia is common and Maumenee IH [37] found that 21% of eyes had myopia of 7 diopters or more.

Retinal detachment occurs in 5–11% of these patients and increases to 8–38% in those who have ectopia lentis or who have undergone cataract surgery [37–39]. Most develop RD at a young age [37]. In a large series, it has been reported that 70% of 160 patients with RD were below the age of 20 years. Bilateral RD is common and may reach 70% [40, 41].

Due to the high incidence of bilaterality, careful evaluation and monitoring of the fellow eye is recommended and prophylactic treatment may be justified [41]. Patients with

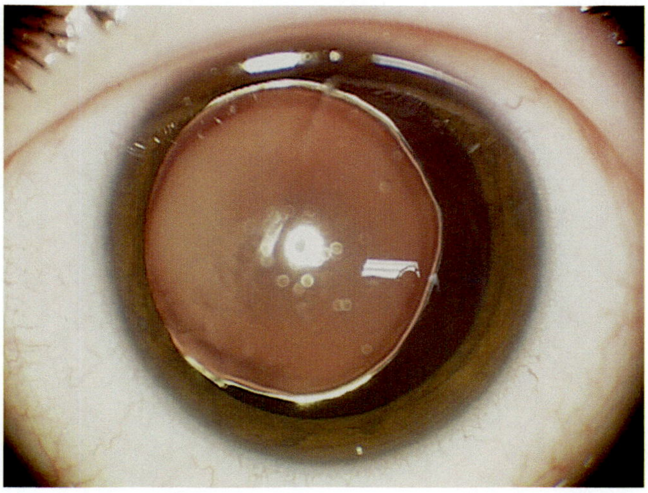

Fig. 33.2 Ectopia lentis in a patient with Marfan syndrome

Marfan syndrome tend to have more complex RRDs including giant retinal tears. The main difference between patients with Marfan syndrome versus Stickler syndrome is that the congenital vitreous anomaly seen in Stickler syndrome is absent. The pathogenesis of RD in Marfan is related to posterior vitreous detachment. The incidence of detachment is related to the level of myopia, and these patients have vitreous degenerative changes similar to that found in myopic eyes [37, 42]. Lens subluxation and lens extraction are also risk factors for developing retinal detachment [38].

Retinal detachments in Marfan syndrome can be a surgical challenge. Special considerations include a poorly dilating pupil and subluxed lens that can sometimes limit visualization of the retina. In eyes with minimal lens subluxation and well-dilated pupils, the RD can be successfully repaired using standard scleral buckling techniques. However, complex retinal detachments with severe lens subluxation are better managed with pars plana lensectomy, vitrectomy, and endotamponade using long-acting gas or silicone oil, with or without scleral buckling. With current advanced surgical techniques, anatomic success rates reported for repair of RDs in Marfan syndrome are comparable with non-Marfan eyes at 75–86% [40, 41].

33.1.2.3 Retino-choroidal Coloboma

Coloboma of the retina and choroid is a rare condition occurring in only 0.14% of the general population [43]. The prevalence of RRDs in this group of eyes has been reported to be 23–40% [44, 45].

A retino-choroidal coloboma is caused by incomplete closure of the embryonic fissure at the seventh week of gestation. It may also be associated with colobomas of the eyelid and iris. Histologically, the choroidal coloboma area is deficient in the normal choroid, retinal pigment epithelium (RPE), and retina (Fig. 33.3). The retina splits into two layers near the

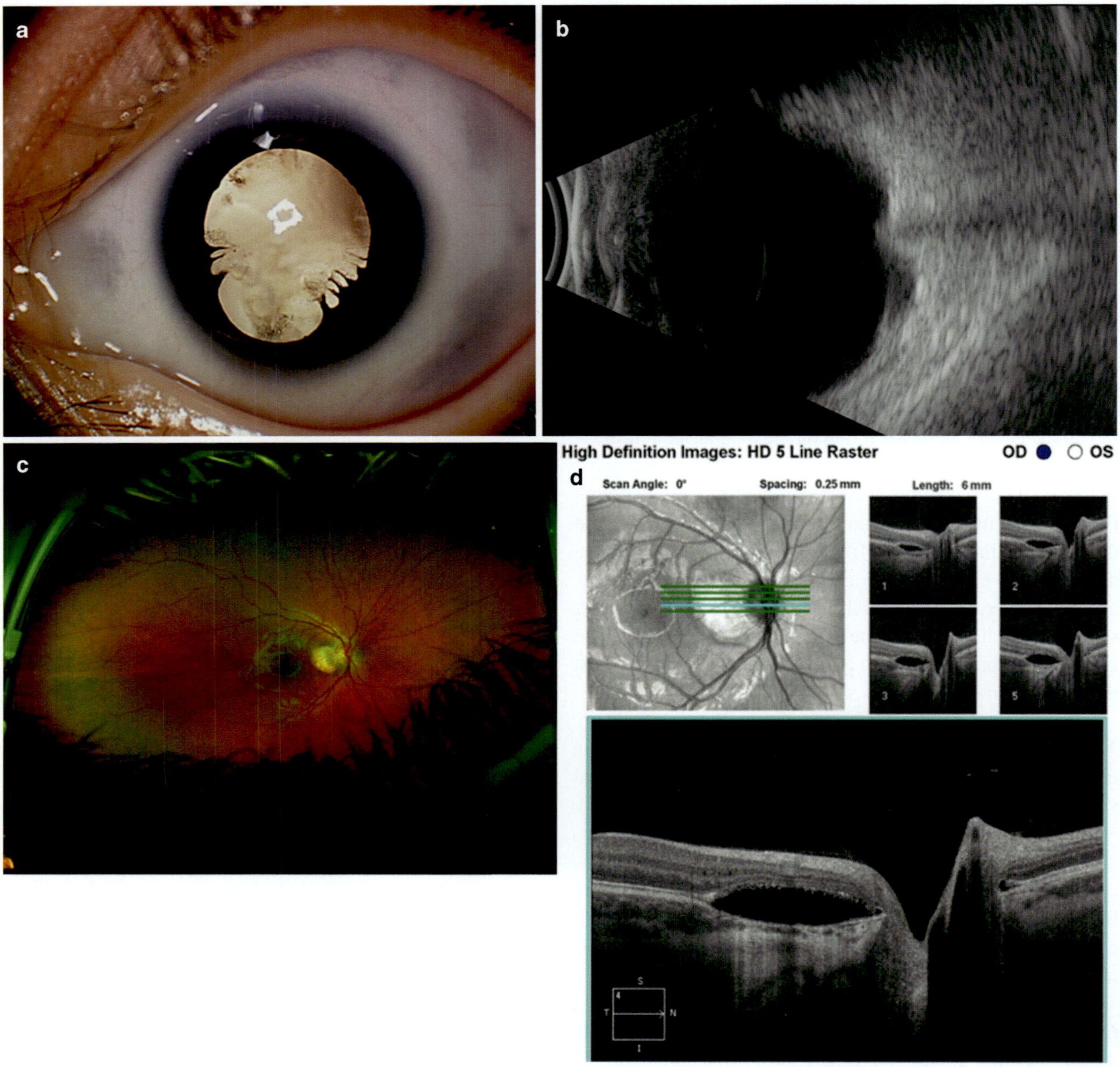

Fig. 33.3 (**a**) Iris coloboma with inferior key-hole defect, (**b**) Retino-choroidal coloboma adjacent to the optic disc seen as an excavation on B-scan ultrasound, (**c**) Peripapillary retino-choroidal coloboma, (**d**) OCT scan through the peripapillary retino-choroidal coloboma demonstrating a cavity due to a deficiency in the retina, retina pigment epithelium, and choroidal layers

margin of the coloboma; the inner neuroblastic layer shows the central continuation of the intercalary membrane (ICM) to the coloboma, whereas the outer neuroblastic layer turns back, becomes disorganized, and fuses with the RPE. The retina gradually thins into the ICM, with a high chance of breaks in the ICM developing along the edge of the coloboma, or towards the center [46, 47]. Retinal breaks within such abnormal tissue are hard to identify clinically due to the lack of contrast. A break in the ICM with communication between the sub-ICM space and the subretinal space can be demonstrated well on optical coherence tomography (OCT) [46–48].

Repair of coloboma-associated retinal detachment (Fig. 33.4) remains a surgical challenge to date, especially if the optic nerve is involved and if there are associated ocular anomalies such as microphthalmia, cataract, and lens coloboma [50]. For a retinal detachment occurring in a colobomatous eye that does not involve the area of the coloboma, surgical repair principles are the same.

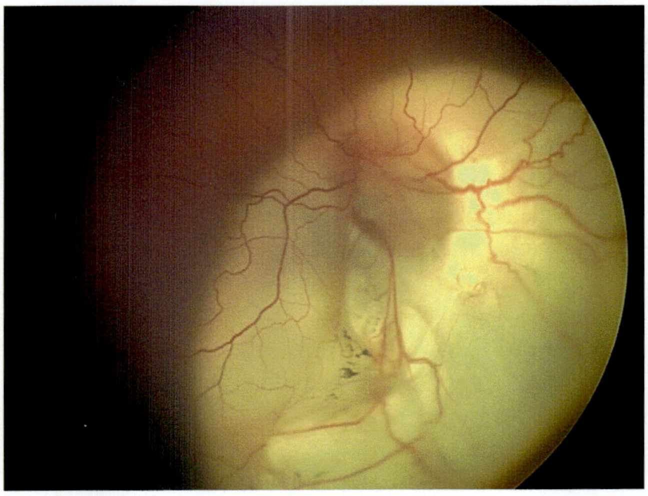

Fig. 33.4 Choroidal coloboma involving the optic disc with retinal detachment (Reproduced with permission from Gan et al. [49])

Previously, Wang K et al. [50] advised buckling the margin of the coloboma with two radial buckles. Patnaik et al. [51] reported success in a patient in which they buckled the entire coloboma. However, with the advent of small gauge pars plana vitrectomy, most coloboma-related retinal detachments are now repaired via the intraocular approach. The identification of breaks in the ICM is easier with intraocular visualization in a pars plana vitrectomy [52]. Direct closure of the breaks with cyanoacrylate glue has been described [53]. However, in most cases, direct closure is not possible. Glue is not effective in a split or atrophied ICM as only the inner layer of the schisis will be sealed and progressive atrophy may enlarge the hole as the ICM contracts. The best approach, therefore, would be to isolate the coloboma from the rest of the retina [48].

Meticulous removal of vitreous attachments and incision of the ICM to weaken it are important to relieve traction on the break within the ICM. Laser retinopexy can then be applied around the coloboma margin to create a border of chorioretinal adhesion. It is difficult to create chorioretinal adhesion directly around holes in the ICM as the choroid and RPE are absent. After creating a circumferential barrier of chorioretinal adhesion, endotamponade with gas [54] is preferred as silicone oil [52, 55] has the potential risk of getting into the subretinal space through the colobomatous defect.

In eyes where the coloboma involves the optic nerve, peripapillary endolaser photocoagulation through the papillomacular bundle may result in laser-induced retinal nerve fiber layer damage, leading to poor visual improvement even with retinal reattachment [56]. In these eyes, underlying amblyopia also limits functional recovery. McDonald et al. [56] suggested that postoperative laser treatment through the papillomacular bundle may be preferable. However, this is not easily performed in the clinic.

33.1.2.4 Atopic Dermatitis

Atopic dermatitis is associated with ocular complications including keratoconjunctivitis, blepharitis, keratoconus, uveitis, subcapsular cataracts, and retinal detachment. In patients with RD, causative retinal breaks are usually peripheral. Retinal dialysis or breaks in the ciliary epithelium of the pars plicata and pars plana [57–59] have been described. In addition, a high incidence of cataracts and proliferative vitreoretinopathy (PVR) may be found in these eyes [60].

Most patients with atopic dermatitis present with RD in adolescence or young adulthood. In a 12-year series of RDs in patients under 18 years old who attended a single center in Hong Kong, the average age of patients with atopic dermatitis related RRD was 14.67 ± 3.04 years [61]. The percentage of eyes with atopic dermatitis related RRD was 18.4% (9 of 49 eyes). In another case series of consecutive RDs in a single center in Japan from 1992 to 2011, the authors published the mean age of patients with atopic dermatitis related RRDs to be 22.9 years (range 12–57) at presentation [62].

Carmi et al. [63] found that the severity of atopic dermatitis [64], face involvement, and external ocular signs [for example periorbital darkening, infraorbital fold (Dennie–Morgan fold)] did not correlate to the incidence of ocular involvement.

Many theories have been published on the higher incidence of RD in patients with atopic dermatitis. Balyeat [65] attributed the cause to edema of the peripheral retina. A shock organ theory was proposed by Coles and Laval [66], which takes into account the common embryonic origin of the skin, lens, and vitreous. They postulate that the retina detaches as a result of diseased vitreous that does not hold the retina firmly in place. Takahashi et al. [64] believe that anterior vitreoretinal traction plays an important role in the pathogenesis of tractional retinal breaks in patients with atopic dermatitis and cataracts. They postulate that repeated rubbing of the eye causes chronic blunt trauma. This triggers an abnormal immune reaction and inflammation in the peripheral retina, causing chronic cyclitis. Cyclitis affects the anterior vitreous, which leads to contractions that produce retinal breaks [57, 64]. Direct slapping of the eye is also a cause of blunt trauma that can result in retinal dialyses in this group of patients [64].

In pediatric and adolescent eyes with no PVR, the authors' surgical procedure of choice is scleral buckling. It is important to note that the incidence of buckle-related infections has been reported to be higher in patients with atopic dermatitis. Oshima et al. [67] studied their scleral buckling procedures done from 1995 to 1997 and published an 18.8% (6 of 32) incidence of methicillin-resistant *staphylococcus aureus* (MRSA) infections in patients with atopic dermatitis, compared to 0.4% (1 of 261, $p < 0.001$) in patients without atopic dermatitis. The average interval from the scleral buckle surgery to the onset of infection was found to be 8.3 ± 9.1 days (range, 2–28 days) [67]. This can be attributed to the high incidence of staphylococcal or methicillin-resistant staphylococcal colonization of the skin in patients with atopic dermatitis. Previous studies have isolated *staphylococcus aureus* in 51–100% of patients with atopic dermatitis, compared to 2–25% in healthy subjects [68–70]. Moreover, in atopic dermatitis patients, the surgical drapes are usually hard to attach to the skin. The drapes often detach and expose the lid margins intraoperatively. This further increases the risk of contamination from pathogens on the skin, lids, and lashes [67].

Therefore, the authors advise that extra care should be taken to thoroughly clean the eyelashes and skin with povidone-iodine at the start of surgery. Buckle implants may be soaked in broad-spectrum antibiotics, for example, cefazolin and gentamicin, or vancomycin if MRSA has been isolated in previous skin swab cultures of the patient. In addition, the authors also give a dose of intravenous antibiotics peri-operatively (cefazolin or vancomycin) for prophylaxis. If buckle-related infection occurs, prompt removal of the buckle is recommended with repeat subconjunctival or intravitreal vancomycin injections. Early vitrectomy should be considered in selected cases [67].

33.2 Special Considerations for Pediatric Vitreoretinal Surgery

Pediatric vitreoretinal surgery has its unique set of challenges compared to surgery in the adult eye. Both vitrectomy and scleral buckling techniques may be used, but each has its advantages and disadvantages peculiar to the pediatric population. Endoscopic vitrectomy is another useful technique to have in a vitreoretinal surgeon's armamentarium, especially in complicated eyes with a poor view of the posterior segment. Enzymatic vitreolysis has been used as an adjunct to aid in complete vitreous separation and to reduce the risk of intraoperative retinal breaks. Finally, postoperative monitoring and visual rehabilitation are essential in maximizing functional outcomes.

33.2.1 Anatomical Considerations

Infants have smaller eyes with different surgical landmarks compared to adult eyes. These anatomical considerations must be taken into account when performing a vitrectomy in newborns or in infants. Surgical instrumentation for a vitrectomy can be approached via two ways, either anterior (trans-limbal) or posterior (trans pars plicata/pars plana).

The pars plana, through which vitreoretinal surgical instruments are usually safely introduced in adults, is not fully formed until approximately the age of 8–9 months [71]. As a rule of thumb, the sclerotomies are placed at 4 mm from the limbus only in children aged 4 years and older. The distance of the sclerotomies from the limbus is dependent on age and different practices may recommend different cutoffs (Table 33.1). Our practice is illustrated in the table below (Table 33.1) and can be easily remembered as adding 1 mm to the distance from the limbus with each year of age after the first year of life. Our sclerotomy approach is conservative and is applicable for a variety of eye sizes. For eyes with unusual anatomy such as microphthalmos in persistent fetal vasculature (PFV), or eyes with severe anterior segment abnormalities, trans-scleral illumination is another useful method to determine the location of the pars plana for safe sclerotomy entry [73] (Fig. 33.5).

As babies under 2 years of age have very thin sclera, trocar-cannula systems are utilized only at ≥2 years of age. Trocars are usually inserted perpendicular through the sclera as oblique placement of the trocars is associated with an increased risk of accidental trocar dislocation and lens trauma with the relatively thicker dimension of the children's lens. This is because the trocars have a shorter path through the pediatric sclera compared to that in the adult sclera [72]. Therefore, sutureless sclerotomies are not advisable in pediatric patients.

The posterior trans-pars plicata lens-sparing technique can only be considered if the surgeon can safely introduce the instruments without causing an iatrogenic retinal break.

Table 33.1 Recommendations for the distance of the sclerotomy from the limbus

	Distance of sclerotomy from limbus (millimeters)	
Age (months)	Meier and Weidemann [72]	Gan NY and Lam WC
<3	1.5	1.0
>3–6	2.0	1.0
>6–12	2.5	1.0
>12–24	3.0	2.0
>24	3.5	3.0

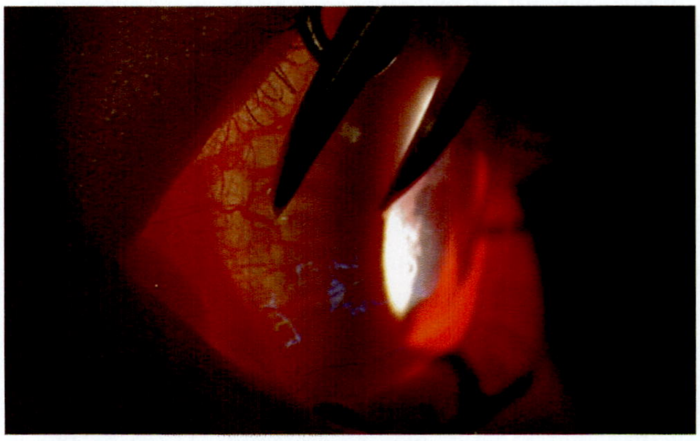

Fig. 33.5 Trans-scleral illumination to identify the pars plana (seen as the dark band) for safe sclerotomy entry

Creating an iatrogenic retinal break in pediatric cases is best avoided as a vigorous proliferative response often follows [74]. This trans-pars plicata approach may not be possible in patients with advanced retinal detachment (e.g., stage 5 retinopathy of prematurity (ROP) with extensive anterior traction, or severe anterior and posterior persistent fetal vasculature) or with a poor view posterior to the lens (e.g., in PFV with diffuse retrolental plaques). In these cases, the risk of instruments entering the subretinal space outweighs the benefits of performing lens-sparing surgery, and an anterior trans-limbal approach with lensectomy and vitrectomy is usually preferable.

In patients with advanced retinal detachment, lens removal necessitates a total capsulectomy. Residual capsule serves as a scaffold for pre-retinal membrane proliferation and secondary circumferential vitreoretinal contraction can result in ciliary body detachment and hypotony. Once formed, this contractile anterior ring is usually difficult to visualize and dissect safely. In cases with lenticulo-retinal apposition, the retina can generally be dissected away from the capsule without causing retinal breaks. Anterior dissection of pre-retinal proliferative membranes can then proceed [75].

33.2.2 Surgical Techniques

In pediatric eyes, the surgical method of choice should take into account the anatomical differences compared to adult eyes, in addition to increased vitreoretinal adhesion and increased propensity for membrane proliferation.

33.2.2.1 Vitrectomy

Babies and infants have lower systolic blood pressure compared to adults and surgeons must bear in mind that iatrogenic occlusion of the central retinal artery can be induced if the infusion pressure is too high or with prolonged scleral depression. Therefore, the optic nerve must be observed at all times to ensure patency of the central retinal artery [76]. In the anterior trans-limbal approach, the infusion is usually supplied via a self-retaining anterior chamber maintainer. A shelving corneal wound is made with a 20G MVR blade and the 20G anterior chamber maintainer anchored in the corneal wound via grooves on its side (Fig. 33.6). The infusion pressure should be optimized to reduce the risk of corneal clouding and retinal incarceration during the withdrawal of instruments.

The creation of a posterior vitreous detachment (PVD) is an important step in the successful management of a retinal detachment. This may be essential in managing RRD in older children. However, this is not recommended in eyes with ROP because of the very firmly adherent posterior vitreous. Forceful creation of a PVD when there is firmly adherent vitreous is not only challenging but also carries a high risk of inducing retinal tears [78].

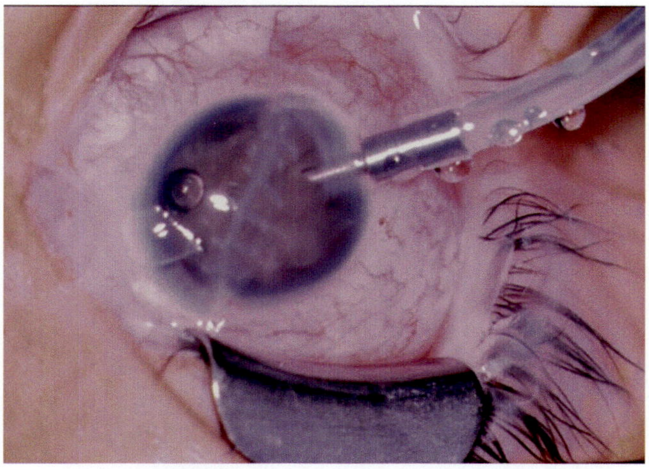

Fig. 33.6 Trans-limbal self-retaining anterior chamber maintainer in a patient with previous blunt trauma, corneal laceration, total RD, and 12 clock hours of anterior grade C PVR (Reproduced with permission from Gan et al. [77])

In eyes with proliferative vitreoretinopathy, it is preferable to perform segmentation instead of delamination when removing pre-retinal membranes due to the firm vitreoretinal attachments in children.

When using heavy liquids intraoperatively, perfluorodecalin ($C_{10}F_{18}$) is the preferred tool of choice in pediatric retinal detachments as it has the highest specific gravity of 1.93 g/cm^3 and is ideal for flattening the retina which is usually thicker in babies and children. Posterior drainage retinotomies are best avoided as extensive fibrous proliferation can occur postoperatively, leading to retinal redetachment. If a retinotomy is unavoidable, it is usually recommended to create one as close to the ora serrata as possible.

For vitreous tamponade, silicone oil should be avoided in cases of advanced retinal detachment such as stage 5 ROP or advanced posterior PFV with retinal detachment. The incomplete dissection of all the tractional components increases the risk of subretinal migration of silicone oil. Similarly, in the case of retinal detachment associated with coloboma, there is also an increased risk of subretinal migration of silicone oil through the colobomatous defect; therefore, the use of silicone oil should be avoided.

33.2.2.2 Scleral Buckling

A scleral buckle may be used as a primary cerclage or as an encircling band in combination with vitrectomy. When combined with a vitrectomy, the element of our choice for an encircling band in infants is a number 40 (2 mm) or 240 (2.5 mm) silicone band (Fig. 33.7), and the band is usually placed just anterior to the equator. If additional height is needed, number 20 segmental element can be added.

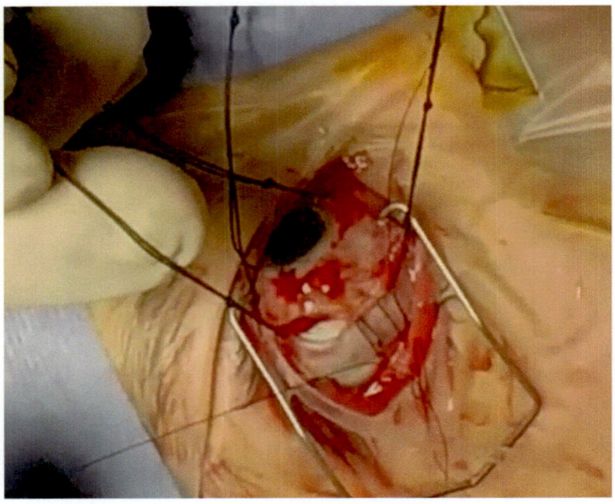

Fig. 33.7 Suturing an encircling scleral band in a child

In ROP-related detachments, the band is placed to support the ridge, akin to supporting a retinal tear, with the encircling element supporting the ridge along the anterior portion of the element. Sutures are imbricated to provide height [79]. Scleral belt loops are avoided in children as the sclera is thinner than in adults. In pediatric rhegmatogenous retinal detachments, we usually recommend a broad, low buckle with precise localization of the retinal break on the buckle. However, due to the more vigorous reproliferation in children, a slightly higher indent may be preferred by some, with care not to cause significant distortion of the globe and further opening of the retinal break [80].

Postoperative complications of scleral buckling in children include limitation of eye growth, development of amblyopia, and loss of vision from cycloplegic eyedrops. Some authors recommend dividing the encircling band approximately 3 months after the operation in children less than 2 years of age or in those whose eye growth is retarded. The band is preferably divided rather than removed as continued support may be provided by the encapsulated explant. In children with good visual potential in both eyes, atropine 1% eye drops should be avoided, instead a short-acting cycloplegic such as cyclopentolate 0.5–1% may be prescribed to reduce the risk of developing amblyopia [80]. Refractive errors are also treated aggressively in the postoperative period to maximize visual outcomes.

33.2.2.3 Endoscopic Vitrectomy

The conventional surgeon's perspective is to look down an operating microscope through the patient's anterior segment and into the vitreous cavity and retina using contact or non-contact viewing systems. The endoscope, however, allows direct visualization of the vitreous cavity by capturing images through its internal tip. This results in a side-on intraoperative view that is up to 90° off the conventional viewing axis of microscope-based systems.

Endoscopic vitrectomy is thus complementary to conventional top-down microscope-based viewing systems as it is able to bypass anterior segment opacities and provide undistorted and unobstructed views of the space between the vitreous base and the posterior iris [81]. The surgeon performs heads-up surgery and looks at a display screen to see the posterior segment and anterior structures including the vitreous base, pars plicata, pars plana, ciliary body, lens, posterior iris surface, and the anterior hyaloid face (Fig. 33.8). The on-screen image is, however, two-dimensional rather than three-dimensional, thus the surgeon needs to compensate by using non-stereoscopic clues such as shadows to judge distance [82].

Conventional top-down microscope viewing systems dissociate the surgeon's visual axis and source of illumination. Light is transmitted through the patient's clear vitreous, resulting in the vitreous appearing mostly transparent. In contrast, the illumination and surgeon's view of the reflected light that bounces off the retina/vitreous is co-axial in endoscopic vitrectomy. Vitreous and membranes appear more opaque because of the co-axial viewing and illumination, which is a bonus in pediatric detachments where removing adherent vitreous and membranes from the retinal surface is already challenging [81].

Endoscopy is particularly useful in advanced pediatric tractional retinal detachments in ROP or familial exudative vitreoretinopathy (FEVR), in which there is often a significant anteroposterior tractional component with the retinal detachment extending towards the anterior hyaloid and lens. The endoscope enables better visualization of the side profile of the retinal detachment, versus looking at the top edge of the retinal detachment with a conventional top-down view, thereby facilitating more direct and potentially more complete tissue dissection [83].

In ROP and PFV, extensive retrolental plaques may occur, blocking direct visualization of the underlying retina. Avoiding iatrogenic retinal breaks is critical in these cases. In PFV, the retina is also often drawn up along the hyaloidal stalk. Differentiating the limit of the retina along the stalk to allow safe transection is challenging with a bird's eye view in conventional microscope-based systems. With endoscopy, direct visualization enables the entire side profile of the hyaloidal stalk and its relationship to the retina to be seen with greater ease [84].

33.2.2.4 Enzymatic Vitreolysis

Pharmacologic vitreolysis has been attempted in pediatric eyes as an adjuvant to vitrectomy surgery. The hypothesis is that enzymatic vitreolysis can weaken the vitreoretinal junction, resulting in a more complete dissection of the hyaloid from the retina with less trauma to the retina and less iatro-

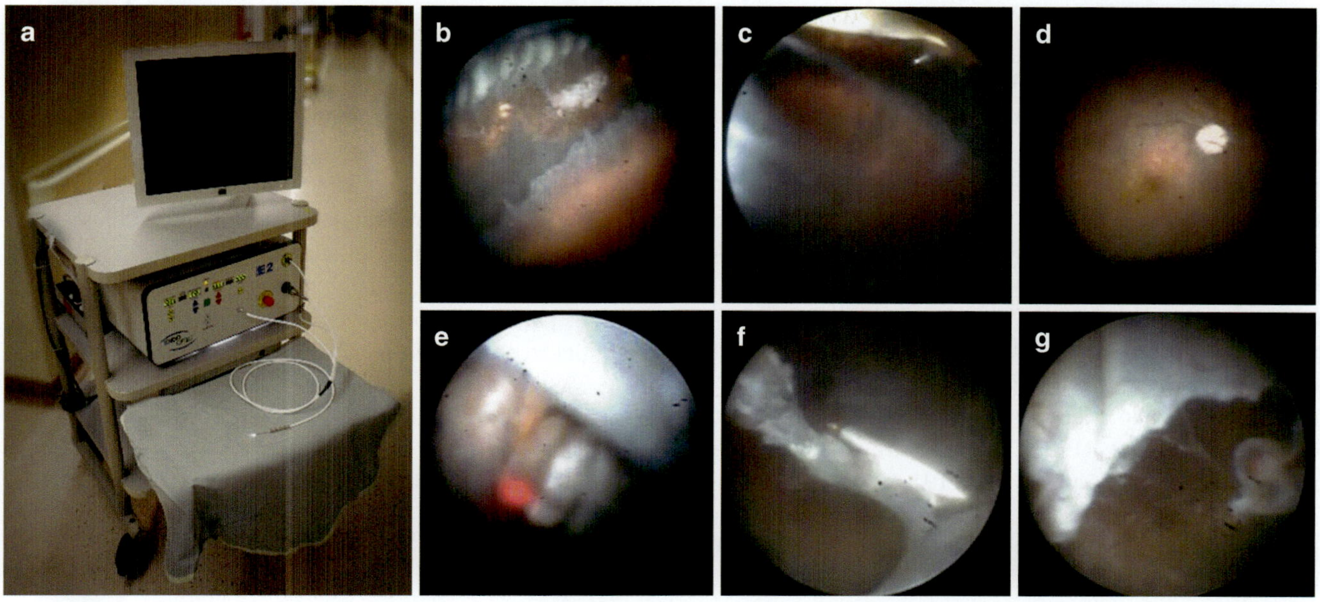

Fig. 33.8 (**a**) An endoscopy and laser unit used at the Hospital for Sick Children, Toronto, housing a Xenon light source, diode laser, video camera, and display screen, with the endoscope probe attached. (**b**) Endoscopic view of the ciliary body, pars plana, and ora serrata, (**c**) Wide angle view of a trans pars plana port and anterior retina, (**d**) Endoscopic view of the posterior pole, (**e**) Endoscopic cyclophotocoagulation with laser beam aiming at a ciliary process with the adjacent ciliary process appearing white post ablation, (**f**) Intraocular diathermy of vessels of anterior contracted retina with pre-equatorial band of PVR, (**g**) Relaxing retinectomy (Reproduced with permission from Gan et al. [77])

genic breaks. Plasmin-assisted vitrectomy has been described in patients with stage 5 ROP reducing iatrogenic breaks and improving anatomical outcomes in reoperations [85]; reducing the need for inner-wall retinectomies in congenital X-linked retinoschisis [86]; and improving the rates of complete posterior vitreous detachment with successful closure of pediatric traumatic macular holes [87, 88]. In these studies, autologous or maternal plasmin enzyme was used. Blood was drawn a few days prior to the surgery, centrifuged and purified followed by eluting of plasminogen and finally, conversion to plasmin with streptokinase.

Ocriplasmin is a recombinant protease enzyme that can lyse fibronectin and laminin, components of the vitreomacular interface. It is a stable, truncated form of plasmin and has several advantages over plasmin including its stability and smaller size, hence increased ability to penetrate tissues [89]. Its use as an intravitreal injection (125 μg) has been studied in two phase III randomized controlled trials for symptomatic vitreomacular adhesion (VMA) and vitreomacular traction (VMT) [90] and approved for use in more than 50 countries. The MIVI-TRUST study reported VMT release in 26.5% and closure of small full-thickness macular holes in 40.6% [90]. However, ellipsoid zone changes have been seen in some treated eyes, reportedly more common in those with resolution of VMT but mainly transient [91].

Drenser et al. [92] report a Phase 2 single-center, prospective, randomized, placebo-controlled, double-masked study with 22 pediatric patients randomized 2:1 to receive 175 μg of ocriplasmin injection or placebo 30–60 min before vitrectomy. They found that ocriplasmin was generally well tolerated. However, the primary efficacy endpoint of total macular PVD either before vitrectomy or after suction was seen in 50% (8 of 16) of ocriplasmin-treated eyes and 62.5% (5 of 8) of placebo-treated eyes. The study sample size was small in this study. Therefore, true efficacy of ocriplasmin as an adjunct cannot be adequately assessed.

As shown in the above small studies, enzymatic vitreolysis is a useful tool in complicated pediatric vitrectomies. However, large randomized controlled trials are still needed before pre-vitrectomy injection is an approved indication for ocriplasmin use.

33.2.3 Vitreous Tamponades

Heavy liquids are often used intraoperatively to unfold and stabilize the retina during surgery for retinal detachments. In pediatric retinal detachments where extensive proliferative vitreoretinopathy (PVR) may be present with intrinsic retinal thickening, F-decalin® ($C_{10}F_{18}$) is the author's preferred choice as it is the highest density heavy liquid (1.93 g/cm^3) and can stabilize the retina well. Another useful tool is visco-elastics. These may be used intraoperatively for retinal manipulation, to tease apart contracted retina and improve visualization for subsequent removal of PVR membranes.

In complex pediatric PVR-detachments, some advocate the use of heavy liquid perfluoro-n-octane as a short-term postoperative tamponade [93, 94]. In their series, Imaizumi et al. [94] described a staged surgery where perfluoro-n-octane (C_8F_{18}) was injected at primary surgery and removed after 1–4 postoperative weeks. During repeat surgery, gas tamponade was used depending on the surgeon's decision. The authors advocate this method as it allows patients to posture supine after surgery, and compared to silicone oil, reduces the pooling of inflammatory components over the inferior retina and the risk of postoperative inferior PVR. The lower rate of redetachment has also been attributed to extended apposition of the retina to the RPE, allowing more effective chorioretinal adhesion by retinopexy [95, 96]. However, the authors feel that this approach should be used bearing in mind that there is often increased inflammation in pediatric eyes.

33.2.4 Postoperative Care

In pediatric patients, postoperative care is an integral part of the treatment journey. Not only is compliance to the posturing and medication regimen important, visual rehabilitation also plays a large role in increasing functional success. In patients who have predisposing conditions that have caused deprivational amblyopia, the visual potential may be guarded. Postoperatively, all refractive errors must be corrected and amblyopia treated aggressively so that maximal visual potential may be achieved. In children with baseline good vision and who undergo vitrectomy with long-acting gas tamponade or silicone oil, deprivational amblyopia may set in while the gas or silicone oil is in the eye. Children may be refracted to give the best correct visual acuity with silicone oil. Once the gas resolves or silicone oil is removed, any amblyopia present should be treated together with pediatric ophthalmologists.

In children with poor visual prognosis despite undergoing all treatment and surgery, ophthalmologists should be aware of the community resources that are available for the parents to ease their child's integration into society. Useful resources include parent support groups, schools for children with special needs, national societies for the visually handicapped for access to visual aids, and learning of life-skills, for example, reading and writing braille.

For children with one good eye, parents must be taught the importance of avoiding contact sports, and to use polycarbonate lenses and sports goggles to avoid accidental trauma to the good eye.

33.3 Conclusion

The management of pediatric retinal detachments is often complicated, and sound surgical techniques combined with experience are keys to increased success. Compared to adults, surgical treatment usually entails a longer period of postoperative visual rehabilitation and requires close management with pediatric ophthalmologists in the treatment of associated amblyopia. Finally, managing the expectations of anxious parents and pediatric patients can be difficult, but is essential to ensure continued follow-up to enhance surgical outcomes.

Acknowledgments The authors would like to acknowledge our Medical Imaging Specialists, Cynthia VandenHoven, BAA, CRA and Leslie D. MacKeen BSc, CRA, from the Ophthalmic Imaging Unit at the Department of Ophthalmology and Vision Sciences, Hospital for Sick Children, Toronto for their contributions to the photographs in this chapter.

Declaration of any financial interest or conflict of interest The authors do not have any relevant financial interests to disclose and have no conflicts of interest. Reprint permission has been obtained from the Taiwan Journal of Ophthalmology for contents in this chapter.

References

1. Soliman MM, Macky TA. Pediatric rhegmatogenous retinal detachment. Int Ophth Clin. 2011;51(1):147–71.
2. Soheilian M, Ramezani A, Malihi M, et al. Clinical features and surgical outcomes in pediatric rhegmatogenous retinal detachment. Retina. 2009;29:545–51.
3. Chen SN, Jiunn-Feng H, Te-Cheng Y. Pediatric rhegmatogenous retinal detachment. Retina. 2006;26:410–4.
4. Chang PY, Yang CM, Yang CH, et al. Clinical characteristics and surgical outcomes of pediatric rhegmatogenous retinal detachment in Taiwan. Am J Ophthalmol. 2005;139:1067–72.
5. Gonzales CR, Singh S, Yu F, et al. Pediatric rhegmatogenous retinal detachment: clinical features and surgical outcomes. Retina. 2008;28:847–52.
6. Wang NK, Tsai CH, Chen YP, et al. Pediatric rhegmatogenous retinal detachment in East Asians. Ophthalmol. 2005;112:1890–5.
7. Fivgas GD, Capone A Jr. Pediatric rhegmatogenous retinal detachment. Retina. 2001;21:101–6.
8. Lee RWJ, Mayer EJ, Markham RH. The aetiology of paediatric rhegmatogenous retinal detachment: 15 years experience. Eye. 2008;22:636–40.
9. Daniel R, Kanski J, Glasspool M. Retinal detachment in children. Trans Ophthalmol Soc UK. 1974;94:325–34.
10. Winslow RL, Tasman W. Juvenile rhegmatogenous retinal detachment. Ophthalmol. 1978;85(6):607–18.
11. Cameron ME. Non-traumatic dialysis in the young. Br J Ophthalmol. 1960;44:540–6.

12. Meier P, Wiedemann P. Chapter 115. Surgery for pediatric vitreoretinal disorders. Injuries – indirect injury. In: Ryan SJ, editor. Part 1: Surgical retina, Section 3: Complicated forms of retinal detachment, vol. 3. 5th ed; 2012.
13. Chignell AH. Retinal dialysis. Br J Ophthalmol. 1973;57:572.
14. Haring G, Wiechens B. Long-term results after scleral buckling surgery in uncomplicated juvenile retinal detachment without proliferative vitreoretinopathy. Retina. 1998;18:501–5.
15. Wang NK, Chen YP, Yeung L, et al. Traumatic pediatric retinal detachment following open globe injury. Ophthalmologica. 2007;221:255–63.
16. Warder D, Muni R, Yong SO, Kertes PJ. Pneumatic retinopexy as a treatment for rhegmatogenous retinal detachment in paediatric patients. American Society of Retinal Specialists Annual Meeting 2015 poster.
17. Weinberg DV, Lyon AT, Greenwald MJ, et al. Rhegmatogenous retinal detachments in children: risk factors and surgical outcomes. Ophthalmology. 2003;115:164–8.
18. Soliman MM, Macky T. Pediatric rhegmatogenous retinal detachment: clinical features, management and visual outcome. EVRS Educ Electr J. 2005;2:5–12.
19. Stickler GB, Belau PG, Farrell FJ, et al. Hereditary progressive arthro-ophthalmopathy. Mayo Clin Proc. 1965;40:433–55.
20. Snead MP, Yates JR. Clinical and molecular features of Stickler syndrome. J Med Genet. 1999;36:353–9.
21. Richards AJ, Meredith S, Poulson A, et al. A novel mutation of COL2A1 resulting in dominantly inherited rhegmatogenous retinal detachment. Invest Ophthalmol Vis Sci. 2005;46:663–8.
22. Stickler GB, Pugh D. Hereditary progressive arthro-ophthalmopathy, II: Additional observations on vertebral abnormalities, a hearing defect, and a report of a similar case. Mayo Clin Proc. 1967;42:495–500.
23. Stickler GB, Hughes W, Houchin P. Clinical features of hereditary progressive arthro-ophthalmopathy (Stickler syndrome): a survey. Genet Med. 2001;3:192–6.
24. Liberfarb RM, Levy HP, Rose PS, et al. The Stickler syndrome: genotype/phenotype correlation in 10n families with Stickler syndrome resulting from seven mutations in the type II collagen gene locus COL2A1. Genet Med. 2003;5:21–7.
25. Parma ES, Korkko J, Hagler WS, et al. Radial perivascular retinal degeneration: a key to the clinical diagnosis of an ocular variant of Stickler syndrome with minimal or no systemic manifestations. Am J Ophthalmol. 2002;134:728–34.
26. Abeysiri P, Bunce C, da Cruz L. Outcomes of surgery for retinal detachment in patients with Stickler syndrome: a comparison of two sequential 20-year cohorts. Graefes Arch Clin Exp Ophthalmol. 2007;245:1633–8.
27. Ang A, Poulson AV, Goodburn SG, et al. Retinal detachment and prophylaxis in type I Stickler syndrome. Ophthalmol. 2008;115:164–8.
28. Donoso L, Edwards A, Frost A. Identification of a stop codon mutation in exon 2 of the collagen 2A1 gene in a large Stickler syndrome family. Am J Ophthalmol. 2002;134:720–7.
29. Scott JDS. Giant retinal tears of the retina. Trans Ophthalmol Soc UK. 1975;95:1142–4.
30. Billington BM, Leaver PK, McLeod D. Management of retinal detachment in the Wagner-Stickler syndrome. Trans Am Ophthalmol Soc UK. 1985;104:875–9.
31. Hirose T, Lee K, Schepens C. Wagner's hereditary vitreoretinal degeneration and retinal detachment. Arch Ophthalmol. 1973;89:176–85.
32. Remulla JF, Tolentino FI. Retinal detachment in Marfan's syndrome. Int Ophthalmol Clin. 2001;41:235–40.
33. Wheatley H, Traboulsy E, Flowers B. Immunohistochemical localization of fibrillin in human ocular tissue. Arch Ophthalmol. 1995;113:103–9.
34. Loeys BL, Dietz HC, Braverman AC, et al. The revised Ghent nosology for the Marfan syndrome. J Med Genet. 2010;47:476–85.
35. Pyeritz R, McKusick V. The Marfan syndrome: diagnosis and management. N Engl J Med. 1979;300:772–7.
36. Magid D, Pyeritz R, Fishman EK. Musculoskeletal manifestations of the Marfan syndrome: radiologic features. AJR Am J Roentgenol. 1990;155(1):99–104.
37. Maumanee IH. The eye in the Marfan syndrome. Trans Am Ophthalmol Soc. 1981;79:684–733.
38. Cross HE, Jensen AD. Ocular manifestations in the Marfan syndrome and homocystinuria. Am J Ophthalmol. 1973;75:405–20.
39. Jarret WH Jr. Dislocation of the lens: a study of 166 hospitalized cases. Arch Ophthalmol. 1967;78:289–96.
40. Sharma T, Gopal L, Shanmugam MP, et al. Retinal detachment in Marfan syndrome: clinical characteristics and surgical outcome. Retina. 2002;22:423–8.
41. Abboud EB. Retinal detachment surgery in Marfan syndrome. Retina. 1998;18:405–9.
42. Allen R, Straatsma B, Apt L, et al. Ocular manifestations of the Marfan syndrome. Trans Am Acad Ophthalmol Otolaryngol. 1967;71:18–38.
43. Yong W, Yu L, Chen F. Vitrectomy treatment of retinal detachments related to choroidal coloboma involving the disk. Retina. 2014;34:1091–5.
44. Jesberg DO, Schepens CL. Retinal detachment associated with coloboma of the choroid. Arch Ophthalmol. 1961;65:163–73.
45. Daufenbach DR, Rutum MS, Pulido JS, et al. Chorioretinal colobomas in a pediatric population. Ophthalmology. 1998;105:1455–8.
46. Gopal L, Khan B, Jain S, et al. A clinical and optical coherence tomography study of the margins of choroidal colobomas. Ophthalmology. 2007;114:571–80.
47. Gopal L. A clinical and optical coherence tomography study of choroidal colobomas. Curr Opin Ophthalmol. 2008;19:248–54.
48. Gopal L, Bardinath SS, Sharma T, et al. Surgical management of retinal detachments related to coloboma of the choroid. Ophthalmol. 1998;105:804–9.
49. Gan NY, Lam WC. Retinal detachments in the pediatric population. Taiwan J Ophthalmol. 2018;8(4):222–36.
50. Wang K, Hilton GF. Retinal detachment associated with coloboma of the choroid. Trans Am Ophthalmol Soc. 1985;83:49–62.
51. Patnaik B, Kalsi R. Retinal detachment with coloboma of the choroid. Indian J Ophthalmol. 1981;29:345–9.
52. Gopal L, Kini MM, Badrinath SS, Sharma T. Management of retinal detachment with choroidal coloboma. Ophthalmology. 1991;98:1622–7.
53. Hotta K, Hirakata A, Hida T. The management of retinal detachments associated with choroidal colobomas by vitrectomy with cyanoacrylate retinopexy. Jpn J Ophthalmol. 1998;42:323–6.
54. Jalall S, Das T. Selection of surgical technique for retinal detachment with coloboma of the choroid. Indian J Ophthalmol. 1994;42:27–30.
55. Gonvers M. Temporary use of silicone oil in the treatment of special cases of retinal detachment. Ophthalmologica. 1983;187:202–9.
56. McDonald HR, Lewis H, Brown G, et al. Vitreous surgery for retinal detachment associated with choroidal coloboma. Arch Ophthalmol. 1991;109:1399–402.
57. Katsura H, Hida T. Atopic dermatitis: retinal detachment associated with atopic dermatitis. Retina. 1984;4:148–51.
58. Matsuo T, Shiraga F, Matsuo N. Intraoperative observation of the vitreous base in patients with atopic dermatitis and retinal detachment. Retina. 1995;15(4):286–90.
59. Nakatsu A, Wada Y, Kondo T. Retinal detachment in patients with atopic dermatitis. 5-year retrospective survey. Ophthalmologica. 1995;209(3):160–4.
60. Hida T, Tano Y, Okinami S, Ogino N, Inoue M. Multicenter retrospective study of retinal detachment associated with atopic dermatitis. Jpn J Ophthalmol. 2000;44(4):407–18.

61. Fong AH, Yip PP, Kwok TY, Tsang CW. A 12-year review on the aetiology and surgical outcomes of paediatric rhegmatogenous retinal detachments in Hong Kong. Eye. 2016;30:355–61.
62. Sasoh M, Mizutani H, Matsubara H, Furuta M, Matsui Y, Yamanaka K, Kondo M. Clin Ophthalmol. 2015;9:1129–34.
63. Carmi E, Defossez-Tribout C, Ganry O, Cene S, Tramier B, Milazzo S, Lok C. Ocular complications of atopic dermatitis in children. Acta Derm Venereol. 2006;86:515–7.
64. Takahashi M, Suzuma K, Inaba I, Ogura Y, Yoneda K, Okamoto H. Retinal detachment associated with atopic dermatitis. Br J Ophthalmol. 1996;80:54–7.
65. Balyeat RM. Complete retinal detachment. Am J Ophthalmol. 1937;20:580–2.
66. Coles RS, Laval J. Retinal detachments occurring in cataract associated with neurodermatitis. Arch Ophthalmol. 1952;48:30–9.
67. Oshima Y, Ohji M, Inoue Y, Harada J, Motokura M, Saito Y, Emi K, Tano Y. Methicillin-resistant Staphylococcus aureus infections after scleral buckling procedures for retinal detachments associated with atopic dermatitis. Ophthalmology. 1999;106:142–7.
68. Leyden KK, Marples RR, Kligman AM. Staphylococcus aureus in the lesions of atopic dermatitis. Br J Dermatol. 1974;90:525–30.
69. Hanifin JM, Rogge JL. Staphylococcal infections in patients with atopic dermatitis. Arch Dermatol. 1977;113:1383–6.
70. Hoeger PH, Lenz E, Boutonnier A, Fournier JM. Staphylococcal skin colonization in children with atopic dermatitis: prevalence, persistence and transmission of toxigenic and nontoxigenic strains. J Infect Dis. 1992;165:1064–8.
71. Hairston RJ, Maguire AM, Vitale S, et al. Morphometric analysis of pars plana development in humans. Retina. 1997;17:135–8.
72. Meier P, Wiedemann P. Chapter 115. Surgery for pediatric vitreoretinal disorders. Surgical considerations and techniques – Posterior-segment surgical techniques. In: Ryan SJ, editor. Part 1: Surgical retina, Section 2: Retinal reattachment: general surgical principles and techniques, vol. 3. 5th ed; 2012.
73. Sharma A, Ali A, Henderson RH, Patel CK, VandenHoven C, Lam WC. Accuracy of scleral transillumination techniques to identify infant ciliary body for sclerostomy and intravitreal injections. Clin Exp Ophthalmol. 2019;47(4):478–83.
74. Trese MT, Capone A. Surgical approaches to infant and childhood retinal diseases: invasive methods. In: Hartnett ME, editor. Pediatric retina. Philadelphia, PA: Lippincott Williams & Wilkins; 2005..
75. Ranchod TM, Capone A. Tips and tricks in pediatric vitreoretinal surgery. Int Ophth Clinics. 2011;51(1):173–83.
76. Recchia FM, Scott IU, Brown GC, et al. Small-gauge pars plana vitrectomy: a report by the American Academy of Ophthalmology. Ophthalmol. 2010;117:1851–7.
77. Gan NY, Lam WC. Special considerations for pediatric vitreoretinal surgery. Taiwan J Ophthalmol. 2018;8(4):237–42.
78. Thompson JT. Advantages and limitations of small gauge vitrectomy. Surv Ophthalmol. 2011;56:162–72.
79. Trese MT, Capone A. Retinopathy of prematurity. Section II. Clinical assessment and management of retinal diseases requiring surgery in infants and children. In: Hartnett ME, editor. Pediatric Retina. Philadelphia, PA: Lippincott Williams & Wilkins; 2005.
80. Trese MT, Ferrone PJ. Pediatric vitreoretinal surgery. In: Duane's ophthalmology: Lippincott Williams & Wilkins; 2006.
81. Wong SC, Lee TC, Heier J, Ho AC. Endoscopic vitrectomy. Curr Opin Ophth. 2014;25:195–206.
82. Wong SC. Endoscopy in pediatric vitreoretinal surgery. Retina Today. 2015;Jul/Aug:40–2.
83. Wong SC, Lee TC. Chapter 13. Endoscopy and endoscopic-assisted vitreous surgery in infants and children. In: Hartnett ME, editor. Pediatric retina. Philadelphia, PA: Lippincott Williams & Wilkins; 2013.
84. Wong SC, Say E, Lee TC. Endoscopic vitrectomy. In: Ho AC, Garg S, editors. Expert techniques in ophthalmic surgery. 1st ed. Philadelphia, PA: JP Brothers Medical Publishers; 2014.
85. Wu WC, Drenser KA, Lai M, Capone A, Trese MT. Plasmin enzyme-assisted vitrectomy for primary and reoperated eyes with stage 5 retinopathy of prematurity. Retina. 2008;28(3 Suppl):S75–80.
86. Wu WC, Drenser KA, Capone A, Capone A, Williams GA, Trese MT. Plasmin enzyme-assisted vitreoretinal surgery in congenital X-linked retinoschisis. Surgical techniques based on a new classification system. Retina. 2007;27:1079–85.
87. Margherio AR, Margherio RR, Hartzer M, Trese MT, Williams GA, Ferrone PJ. Plasmin enzyme-assisted vitrectomy in traumatic pediatric macular holes. Ophthalmology. 1998;105:1617–20.
88. Wu WC, Drenser KA, Trese MT, Williams GA, Capone A. Pediatric traumatic macular hole: results of autologous plasmin enzyme-assisted vitrectomy. Am J Ophthalmol. 2007;144:668–72.
89. Stefanini FR, Maia M, Falabella P, Pfister M, Niemeyer M, Kashani AH, Humayun MS, Koss MJ. Profile of ocriplasmin and its potential in the treatment of vitreomacular adhesion. Clin Ophthalmol. 2014;8:847–56.
90. Stalmans P, Benz MS, Gandorfer A, Kampik A, Girach A, Pakola S, Haller JA, for the MIVI-TRUST Study Group. Enzymatic vitreolysis with ocriplasmin for vitreomacular traction and macular holes. N Engl J Med. 2012;367:606–15.
91. Sharma P, Juhn A, Houston SK, Fineman M, Chiang A, Ho A, Regillo C. Efficacy of intravitreal ocriplasmin on vitreomacular traction and full thickness macular holes. Am J Ophthalmol. 2015;159(5):861–7.
92. Drenser K, Girach A, Capone A. A randomized, placebo-controlled study of intravitreal ocriplasmin in pediatric patients scheduled for vitrectomy. Retina. 2016;36:565–75.
93. Sisk RA, Berrocal AM, Murray TG, Mavrofrides EC. Extended endo-tamponade with perfluoro-n-octane in pediatric retinal detachment. Ophthalmic Surg Lasers Imaging. 2010;3(9):1–3.
94. Imaizumi A, Kusaka S, Noguchi H, Shimomura Y, Sawaguchi S. Efficacy of short-term postoperative perfluoro-n-octane tamponade for pediatric complex retinal detachment. Am J Ophthalmol. 2014;157:384–9.
95. Chang S, Lincoff H, Zimmerman NJ, Fuchs W. Giant retinal tears: surgical techniques and results using perfluorocarbon liquid. Arch Ophthalmol. 1989;107(5):761–6.
96. Bottoni F, Bailo G, Arpa P, Prussiani A, Monticelli M, de Molfetta V. Management of giant retinal tears using perfluodecaline as a post-operative short-term vitreoretinal tamponade: a long-term follow-up study. Ophthalmic Surg. 1994;25(6):365–73.

Index

W.-C. Wu, W.-C. Lam (eds.), *A Quick Guide to Pediatric Retina*, https://doi.org/10.1007/978-981-15-6552-6

GPSR Compliance

The European Union's (EU) General Product Safety Regulation (GPSR) is a set of rules that requires consumer products to be safe and our obligations to ensure this.

If you have any concerns about our products, you can contact us on ProductSafety@springernature.com

In case Publisher is established outside the EU, the EU authorized representative is:

Springer Nature Customer Service Center GmbH
Europaplatz 3
69115 Heidelberg, Germany

Batch number: 10756367

Printed by Printforce, the Netherlands